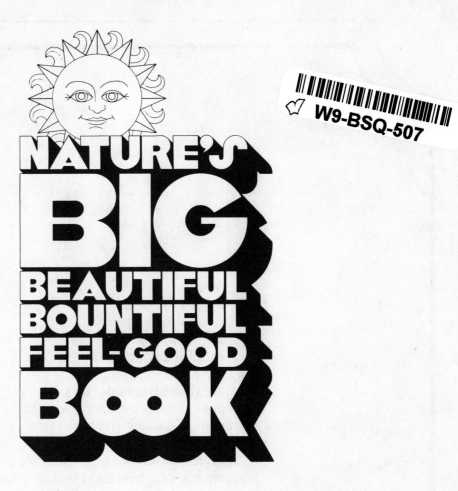

NATURE'S BIG BEAUTIFUL BOUNTIFUL FEEL-GOOD BOOK

W9-BSQ-507

By the editors of
    The Health Quarterly
    Nutritional Update
    Healthful Living Today
With the help of
    more than seventy doctors,
    biochemists, researchers, writers,
    nutritionists, reporters,
    herbalists, natural therapists,
    farmers, cooks, physical therapists,
    pioneers, prophets and consumer specialists
    who simply want you to feel good!

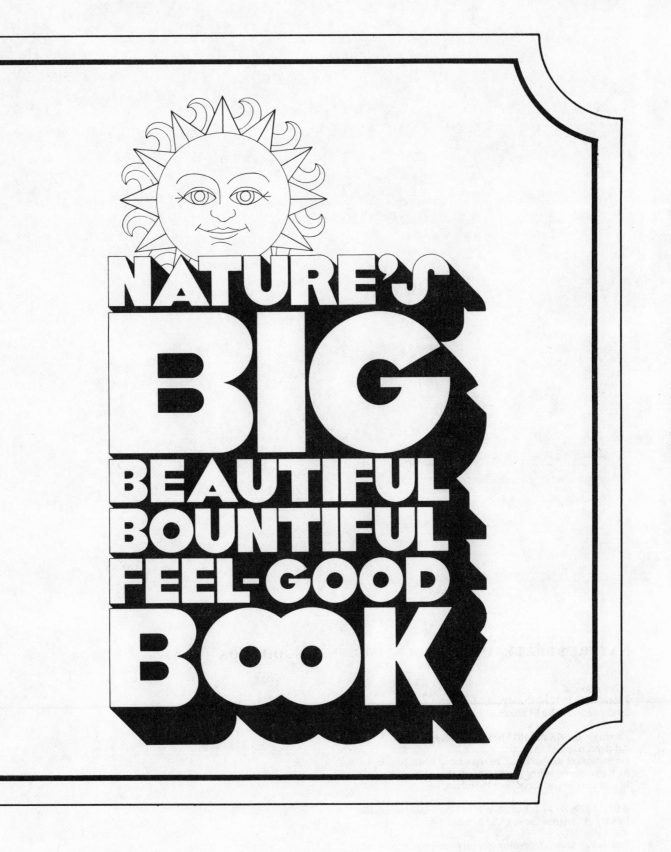

NATURE'S BIG BEAUTIFUL BOUNTIFUL FEEL-GOOD BOOK

Keats Publishing, Inc. ✻ New Canaan, Connecticut

NATURE'S BIG, BEAUTIFUL, BOUNTIFUL FEEL-GOOD BOOK

A Pivot Special
Published in 1977 by Keats Publishing, Inc.
36 Grove Street, New Canaan, Connecticut 06840

Copyright © 1976 and 1977 by Keats Publishing, Inc.
All rights reserved
No portions of this book may be reproduced in whole or in
part, by mimeograph or by any other means, without permission.
For information, address Keats Publishing, Inc.

ISBN: 0-87983-136-7 (hardcover); 0-87983-133-2 (paperback)
Library of Congress Catalog Card: 76-245-04

Permissions acknowledgements for previously published articles
and other materials may be found on page 322

Printed in the United States of America

Dedication

This book is dedicated to that Idea Whose
Time Has Come, to all of you whose powerful
conviction and example have formed the
groundswell, and to those teachers who light
the way.

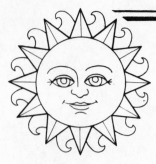

Table of Contents

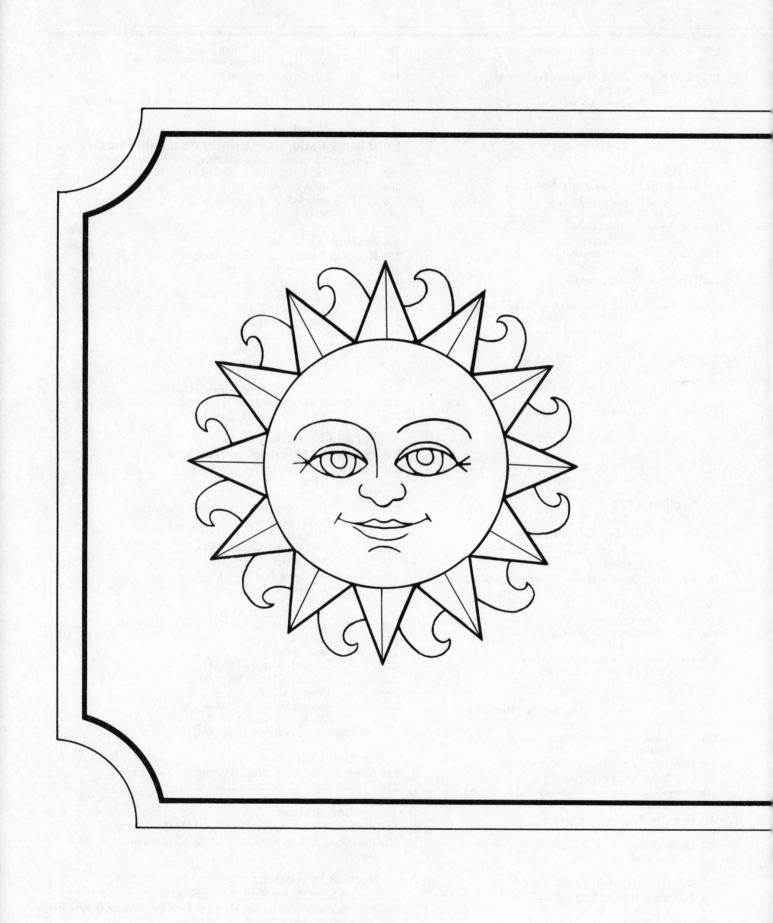

Publisher's Foreword

As is clear from the contents of this book, an idea of natural, healthful living must take root in a wide variety of fields. This concept draws its sustenance from ancient customs as well as from the most up-to-date laboratory research, and its disciplines range from biochemistry to herb gardening. This way of living is by nature holistic, a multidimensional picture.

It is a picture filled in by a loose core of doctors, scientists and researchers who are working behind the scenes to establish the physical principles of natural living, to document and draw scientifically acceptable conclusions. Say that this picture is of a tree. That core is the trunk of our tree of life, and its main stems and branches. Thousands of people throughout the world are devoted to writing and publishing this information as it becomes available. These are the green leaves budding on our tree. Merchants and agricultural and commercial suppliers concerned with offering us pure, nutritious, healthful products fertilize and nourish our tree.

The tree still grows. This book is a new leaf. Some of you may miss your favorite author or subject. But no one book occupied with healthful living could make a claim to completeness on such a broad and dynamic subject. Others may wonder at the inclusion of old classics whose discoveries have long been surpassed — but these are the foundation of our growth. Still others may resist the inclusion of new work which they condemn as faddism — but which may, in the future, bear fruit of another form.

What we have tried to accomplish is to give you a few footholds, and an outstretched hand. Come up into the tree and explore for yourselves. Find in this book some rope ladders to climb from branch to branch on; find a platform here and there to rest on for a while. Enjoy the view and fresh air up here, the fresh hope.

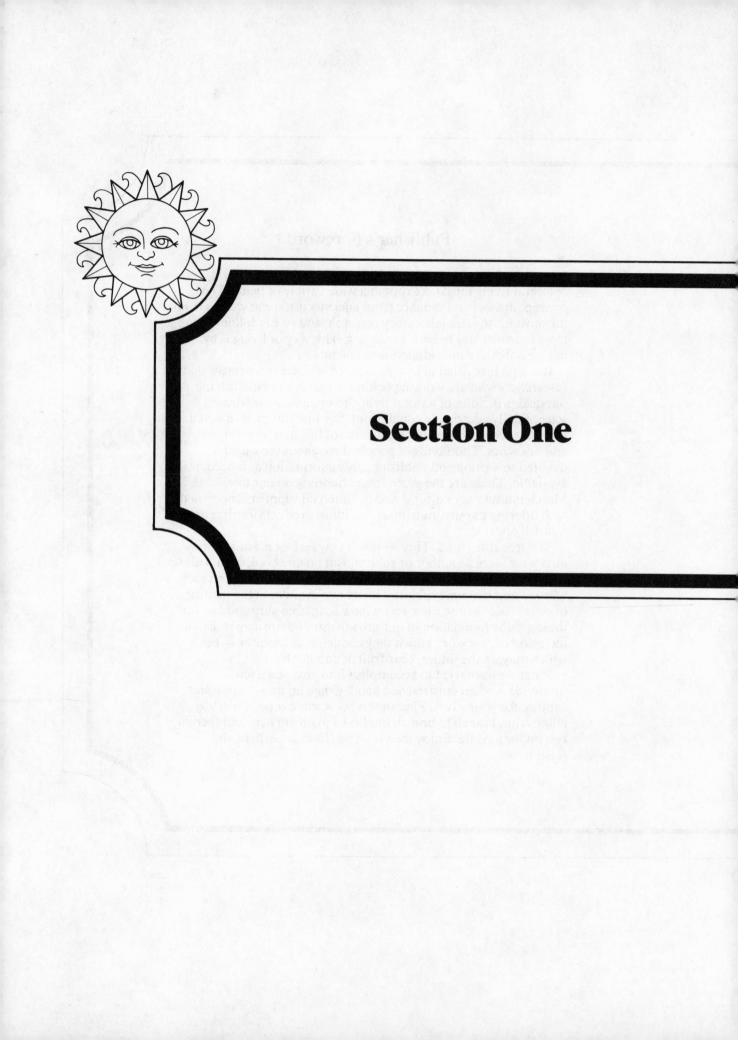

Section One

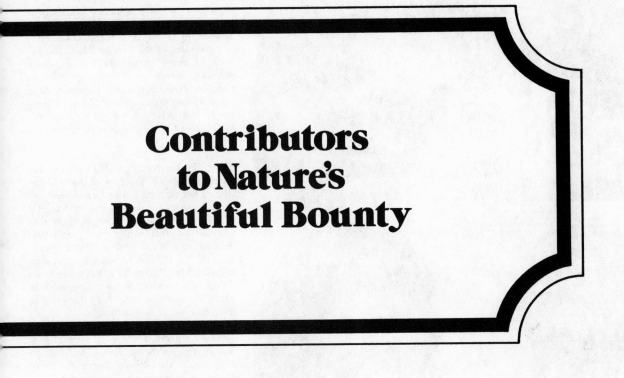

Contributors to Nature's Beautiful Bounty

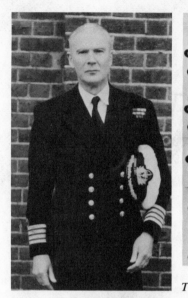

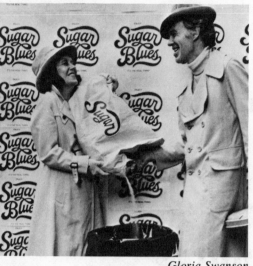

T.L. Cleave, M.D.

Gloria Swanson
and William Dufty

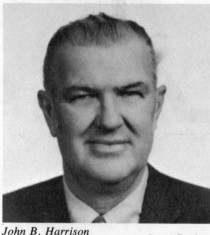

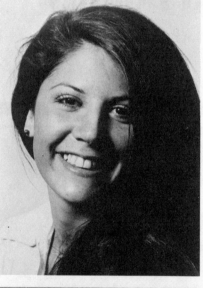

John B. Harrison

Janet Barkas

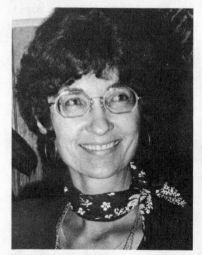

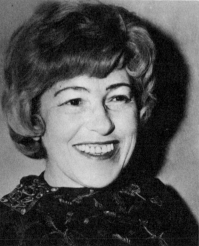

Sharon Cadwallader

Renée Taylor

Gayelord Hauser, at age eighty, continues to be a vital, marvelous example of the virtues of natural living and eating. He has been called one of the ''Makers of the Twentieth Century'' (by the *London Times*), and is equally well known in almost every country of the world. Many of us knew him for a long while as health advisor to Greta Garbo and other Hollywood stars of the thirties. He is the author of many bestsellers, among them *Mirror, Mirror On The Wall; Be Happier, Be Healthier; Look Younger, Live Longer;* and the *Gayelord Hauser Cookbook*. His newest book, just published, is *Gayelord Hauser's New Treasury of Secrets.*

Janet Barkas recently added a flavorful chapter to human history with the publication of her new book *The Vegetable Passion, A History of the Vegetarian State Of Mind,* which offers unique insights into vegetarian religious, philosophical, economic, ethical and aesthetic backgrounds. In addition to being a vegetarian herself, Ms. Barkas is a busy freelance writer whose articles have appeared in *McCall's* and *The New York Times.* She lives and works in Manhattan.

John B. Harrison wrote the popular gardening and soil book *Good Food Naturally* which the *Whole Earth Epilogue* describes in one word, ''wonderful!'' An Australian by birth, he emigrated to Canada, thirty-five years ago. Inspired by Louis Bromfield's *Pleasant Valley,* he determined to convert his British Columbia farm, Mylora, to organic methods. The measure of his success is the fact that this farm has been an organic showplace for twenty-five years. Mr. Harrison teaches at Vancouver City College and the Free University, and conducts organic farming classes for students who come to Mylora from all over the world, as well as managing the farm and a family of ten.

Dian Dincin Buchman, first learned about herbs from her Rumanian grandmother who was privy to Gypsy secrets, and from her doctor-father who practices drugless therapy. She is the author of *The Complete Herbal Guide to Health and Beauty* and the recently published paperback *Organic Makeup: The ABCs of Beauty.* She has written a health book for teen-agers *Feel Good/Look Great;* and is in the midst of a ''large health book'' called ''*The Stay Healthy Handbook.*''

Philippa Back belongs to English herbal societies, holds a Cordon Bleu certificate and a diploma in Food Hygiene. Putting her talents together, she has written *Choosing, Planting and Cultivating Herbs* and has co-authored *Herbs for Health and Cookery* and *The Complete Book of Herbs and Spices* with **Claire Loewenfeld,** who began herb researching in 1939. During wartime, and shortages of the usual vitamin C sources, Claire pioneered the use of rose hips. Later she treated children at the Great Ormond Street Hospital by using fruit and vegetable diets laced with herbs. The herbs that she and her husband grew at Chiltern Herb Farms were considered among the best in England.

William Dufty's career has been varied to say the least. He has danced in a Shubert chorus line, been a speechwriter, a labor organizer and an award-winning reporter for the *New York Post* for more than ten years. He has been writing books for at least twenty years, his most acclaimed being the Billie Holiday biography *Lady Sings the Blues.* Mr. Dufty's translation and introduction to the first U.S. publication of Sakurazawa-Ohsawa's book published in 1965 as *You Are Sanpaku,* has become a best-selling classic in the health field as well as on college campuses. The author's friendship with Gloria Swanson led him to write his latest book, *Sugar Blues.* We think you will agree that anyone who reads his book is unlikely to feel quite the same way again about sugar. Both Ms. Swanson's and Mr. Dufty's opinion of white sugar can be gathered from this photo we reprint in this section.

Sharon Cadwallader's books — *In Celebration of Small Things* and the *Whole Earth Cookbook* — are perhaps the best explanations of why simplicity is the only way to go, and "using well" (as she puts it), food, resources, space, etc. — the happiest and most effective way to live. Ms. Cadwallader, a mid-westerner by birth, went to college at San Jose State in California and lived for awhile in Central Mexico. She founded the Whole Earth Restaurant at the University of California in Santa Cruz and lives there now with her ten-year-old son.

Catharine Osgood Foster says that one day she woke up to the fact that she and her husband had been organic gardeners all along. On their Vermont farm, the compost piles, and stock which supplied manure were part of Yankee frugality and tradition. All of this experience is aptly passed on through articles and books such as *The Organic Gardener.*

Euell Gibbons relates that he originated his first wild food recipe at age five, and an intense thirst for knowledge about nature has always characterized him. After boyhood in New Mexico and college studies in botany on the West Coast and Hawaii, he pursued a teaching career in Pennsylvania. His study of wild life continued and finally led to his classic wild food guidebooks, *Stalking the Wild Asparagus* and *Stalking the Blue-Eyed Scallop.*

Max Warmbrand, N.D., was a successful nutritional doctor, lecturer, author and guest on radio and television. Aghast at the practice of polluting a sick person with drugs, he preferred to cleanse the body with a fruit and vegetable diet, tailor-made to each patient. His medical career was vigorous and lifelong, as was his writing career. Just being published at the time of his death was his latest book, *Overcoming Arthritis and Other Rheumatic Diseases.*

Renée Taylor's *Yoga . . . The Art of Living* has been re-issued in quality paperback. Miss Taylor is one of the few who has been privileged to visit the Hunzas as a guest of the royal family. Her lectures and books on the Hunza-yoga techniques for physical and mental exercise and relaxation have made her one of the best-known authorities on the subject. She has trained teachers and also taught yoga to large groups and has found time to write three books in addition to the new release mentioned above: *Hunza Health Secrets; How to Enjoy a Longer Life;* and *Hunza, the Himalayan Shangri-La.*

Ben Charles Harris, health enthusiast and author, is also one of America's most active herbalists, an interest he inherited from his grandfather. His other career is in pharmacy, and he has operated his own drug store in Worcester, Massachusetts for nearly forty years. Meanwhile, he wrote six books, served as Curator of Economic Botany at the Worcester Museum of Science, as President of the Boston Nutrition Society and the Natural Hygiene Sociey, conducted the activities of the Worcester Herb Club, and instigated or participated in several radio and TV programs concerning health and nature. He gives lectures and conducts nature field trips. Apparently

not quite busy enough, he says he is "now back as a student at Worcester State College."

Ken and Pat Kraft, a married couple, have gardened and written together for years all over the U.S.A. and Mexico. Their articles have appeared in the *New Yorker, Reader's Digest* and *American Heritage* as well as other major magazines. They have nine books to their credit. Since they have tried both chemical and organic gardening, they are able to base their advice on organic gardening on research and fact: they *know* it's the most successful way to grow your own food.

T.L. Cleave, a member of the Royal College of Physicians in England, has become famous throughout the world for being the first to discover the importance of dietary fiber. This original study led to his theory of a master disease related to other major diseases of our time, brought on by the consumption of refined carbohydrates. His book, *The Saccharine Disease,* is a medical landmark.

Jeanne Rose's education in herbal lore and use began when offhand comments by family members were passed along to her as a child. She was often skeptical. During recuperation from a serious automobile accident a friend gave her a little herb book to read. This was the turning point. Since then she has been using, smelling and writing about herbs in *Herbs & Things* and other books.

Roger J. Williams was the first man to identify, isolate and synthesize pantothenic acid, one of the most important B vitamins, and has also done important pioneer work on folic acid. He is a member of the National Academy of Sciences and former president of the American Chemical Society. He is the author of many books — among them *Nutrition In A Nutshell, Nutrition Against Disease* and *You Are Extraordinary.*

Linda Clark is so familiar to the public through her books and articles that we will just mention that her energy and concern — and daily writing — in the field of natural living and better nutrition have not waned. Author of sixteen books at this time, including *Know Your Nutrition,* one of the fastest selling books in the health field, and her newest book, *Natural Remedies for Common Ailments.*

Dr. Carl C. Pfeiffer, author of the recently released best-seller, *Mental and Elemental Nutrients,* is an eminent research scientist, clinician and writer for professional journals. He was at one time Chief of the Division of Neuropharmacology at the State of New Jersey's Bureau of Research in Neurology and Psychiatry, and was Deputy Director of that Bureau. Dr. Pfeiffer has been a leader in subdivid-

ing the schizophrenias into their biochemical parts, and the first to use the combination of zinc and vitamin B-6 in the effective treatment of mental disease. Dr. Pfeiffer is director of the Brain Bio Center today, where he devotes his time to a thriving clinical practice, public speaking engagements and writing on brain biochemistry and nutrition for laymen and his fellow professionals. With all this, he still finds

time to garden organically (or as he calls it, scientifically) and to build things.

Hilda Cherry Hills is an Argentinian by birth but has lived most of her life in England, and for a while in Africa. She has long been qualified as a physiotherapist, and a long series of hospital appointments and private practice encouraged her study of habits and living conditions which work against health and happiness. She is married to Lawrence Hills, a well-known gardening author and Director-Secretary of the Henry Doubleday Research Organization in England. Mr. Hills, who is a celiac (one who is allergic to protein in some grains) was the inspiration for her *Good*

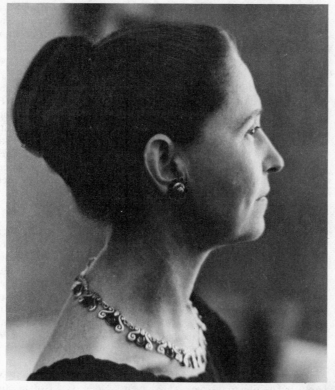

Beatrice
Trum Hunter

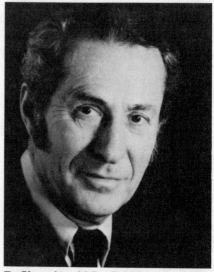

E. Cheraskin, M.D., D.M.D.

Jerome S. Mittelman, D.D.S.

Allan Cott, M.D.

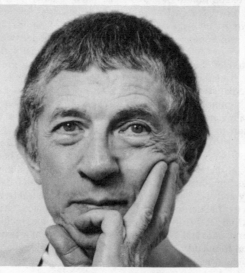

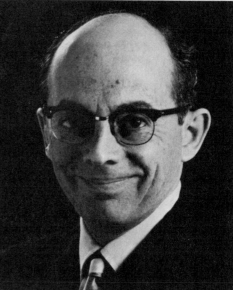

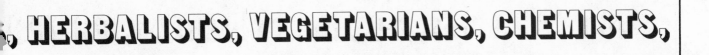
Food, Gluten Free, and the "testing ground" for the variety of special recipes and diets she has included.

Ed Flynn still works on "Madison Avenue," heading his own advertising agency in Teaneck, New Jersey, but he abandoned drinking, smoking and other facets of the Madison Avenue way of life several years ago. As a result, he has become an active spokesman for the health problems of the business man and for natural nutrition and a positve health regimen.

Dr. J. H. Tilden was born in 1851 and died in 1940, after having practiced

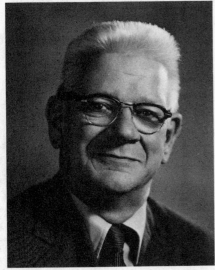

Carl C. Pfeiffer, M.D.

Irwin Stone

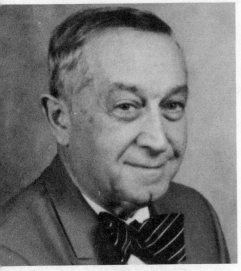

medicine for sixty-eight years. In many ways, he was super-modern. He knew that all diseases in man have a common source; he believed in the simplest of cures. He recognized the incipient dangers of refined foods and the overconsumption of food. He recommended diets high in vitamins not yet identified and isolated. Especially, he was aware of the necessity of the right combinations of food for the highest nutrition and the least digestive trouble. Altogether, a prophet before his time, indeed!

Nikki and David Goldbeck are a team in their professional as well as personal lives, writing and lecturing about food, nutrition and ecology. Nikki received her Cornell University degree in food and nutrition; David is a former elementary school teacher and still a practicing lawyer. They have written three books — *The Supermarket Handbook, The Dieter's Companion* and *The Good Breakfast Book.* Their traditional approach to the subjects they write about is so untraditional as to cause *The New York Times* to accuse them of trying to "re-invent the wheel."

Jerome S. Mittelman, D.D.S., is the first dental doctor to be president of The International Academy of Preventive Medicine, and is thus a familiar name to dentists and physicians alike. He helped to found the American Society for Preventive Dentistry, presently serving as Associate Editor of its journal.

Preventive dentistry has been taught and fought for by Jerome Mittelman for many years. He not only believes in it, but has a long-established practice of helping people to save their teeth and to have the healthiest mouths possible. His newsletter, *The Once Daily,* which he edits with his wife Beverly, is an inspiration to several thousand dentists, physicians and dental-surgeons, and is used by dental schools and as a study guide for various clubs and groups. His many published articles have also been dedicated to furthering a knowledge of the preventive concept of medicine.

Beatrice Trum Hunter has authored bestsellers in the consumer protection and nutrition fields, is one of the most-read experts on additives in our food. The scope of her knowledge is impressive and her wide expertise has given us *Consumer Beware! The Mirage of Safety* and *Gardening Without Poisons,* as well as *The Natural*

Foods Cookbook, the *Whole Grain Baking Sampler* and more. Through her research and wriiing she has become familiar with almost all the important aspects of natural, healthful living in the world today.

Irwin Stone preceded his famous book, *The Healing Factor,* with forty years of research on that ancient genetic mutation which left man unable to produce his own ascorbic acid (vitamin C) like the other animals do. Dr. Stone's massive documentation and sustained dedication to the subject helped make it possible for Linus Pauling's (Nobel Laureate) work, and elicited Albert Szent-Györgyi's (another Nobel Laureate) comment that mankind owes serious thanks to Irwin Stone.

E. Cheraskin, M.D., D.M.D. is professor and chairman of the department of oral medicine at the University of Alabama in Birmingham, and holds numerous scientific honors for his work in nutrition and preventive medicine. Included in the *World's Who's Who in Science* since 1966, he is a respected author as well. Some of his titles include: *Diet and Disease, Predictive Medicine, New Hope For Incurable Diseases and Psychodietetics.* **W.M. Ringsdorf Jr., D.M.D., M.S.** is associate professor of oral medicine at the University of Alabama in Birmingham, and has co-authored the majority of Dr. Cheraskin's previous books, as well as hundreds of articles appearing in professional journals.

Allan Cott, M.D. is one of the new generation of doctors who understands and applies orthomolecular treatment; in his case, specifically to learning disabilities. He has lectured on this subject, as well as on megavitamin treatment of childhood schizophrenia, and the use of controlled fasting in the Soviet Union. His work extends to include a private practice in New York City and a staff position at Gracie Square Hospital.

Barbara Farr has varied talents and the life she leads could be divided in two and still represent the work and interests of an average person. She is author of two cookbooks and a regular contributor to *Bestways Magazine,* all the while championing her hero the soybean (see her latest book titled *Super Soy!*). In her life and work she sets an admirable standard of "using her talents."

Richard Passwater appears frequently in *Prevention* magazine where his series of articles on the beneficial effects of Vitamin E first brought him praise from leading scientists such as Linus Pauling. Mr. Passwater's particular specialties lie in research on cancer, heart disease and retardation of aging. He has also been interested for a long time, in the problem of proper nutrition and athletics, and is now called in frequently to advise professional athletics on nutrition. You will find his newest book, *Supernutrition for Healthy Hearts* on sale at book stores and health stores everywhere.

Dr. Kurt Donsbach is totally dedicated to his work and philosophy which is that the only passport to good health is through preventive, organic medicine. A chiropractor and naturopath who received his degree from the Western States College, he has been involved for years in nutritional research, especially with the Lee Foundation in Milwaukee. Now practicing, lecturing and researching in Garden Grove, California, Dr. Donsbach is also writing prolifically to tell the world his story which can be summed up by his slogan: "Our Supplier is Nature, Over Two Billion Years of Quality Products."

Barbara Hegne is a newspaper woman and physicalculturist by profession(s), conducting classes regularly and writing for a Utah newspaper on fitness. She is presently on the home stretch of a new manuscript dealing with nutrition, diet and body improvement.

Lelord Kordel has written and lectured for more than thirty-five years on health, diet, psychosomatic medicine and nutriton. A world traveler, he has made a point of collecting health secrets from everywhere. He is the author of the widely-read *Eat and Grow Younger, Cook Right — Live Longer,* and *How to Keep Your Youthful Vitality After 40.* His newest book, *You're Younger Than You Think,* has just been published in hardcover.

Barbara Jurgensen and Murray Goodwin have yet to meet even though they have collaborated on what we feel is a most unusual book. Ms. Jurgensen is a Chicago housewife who had the idea of taking Robert Louis Stevenson's classic title, *A Child's Garden of Verses,* and using it as a take-off for a book of limericks and verses about pollution and other ecological prob-

lems. The result is *A Polluter's Garden of Verses.* Murray Goodwin did the general editing on the book and also contributed a sizeable number of verses of his own. Goodwin is an ex-Madison Avenue advertising creative director who saw the light — moved out of New York City and advertising, and "into" natural health. He now lives in Columbia, Maryland, where he works at free-lance writing, most of it not in advertising. Jerry McLaughlin, an artist whose work hangs in many major museums, did the illustrations for the book.

Ruth Stout — sister to Rex Stout the famous detective writer, has a bit of the Sherlock Holmes in her, too. She delights in "proving experts wrong and testing short cuts" when it comes to gardening. The mulching method is one of her more trumpeted triumphs. After years of gardening she has intimate knowledge of plants, knowing the personality and quirks of each, and sharing this knowledge in her best-selling book *How to Have a Green Thumb Without an Aching Back.* Ruth Stout has opened up mysteries of the soil for thousands of gardeners, expert and neophyte alike.

Dr. Irwin I. Lubowe practices medicine in the field of dermatology in New York City, and teaches at the New York Medical College. He is author of five books on skin, hair and cosmetics; his newest, *The Modern Guide to Skin Care and Beauty,* is already proving to be just the reference source everyone needs for skin problems.

Dr. Wilfrid E. Shute's work in treating more than 35,000 cardiac patients with Vitamin E is almost legendary at this point. Dr. Shute was a practicing physician for over forty years before his recent retirement and is the acknowledged authority on Vitamin E and its use in the treatment of burns, diabetes, skin ailments and circulatory diseases.

Martha H. Oliver is a nutritionist and biochemist and, according to the biography she furnished us, "comes from a long line of gardeners and good cooks." She is the author of *Add a Few Sprouts,* a new paperback that combines sprouting history and techniques with a host of recipes for inexpensive meals. Ms. Oliver lives with her husband and 2½-year-old daughter on a 140-acre organic farm in Fayette County, Pennsylvania, where she raises flowers and vegetables and gives

demonstrations of sprouting — that is, when she is not doing research for articles and her new book.

Charles Ewart — kept on top of what was happening in the world by spending seventeen years working for London newspapers, before becoming a free-lance writer. His interest in acupuncture found its object in Dr. Louis Moss (whose effectiveness Charles Ewart personnally experienced). Since then he has satisfied part of his original curiosity, in his book *The Healing Needles,* originally published in England and now available in paperback.

Dr. Melvin E. Page writes from a wealth of experience drawn from more than forty years of clinical observation, testing and

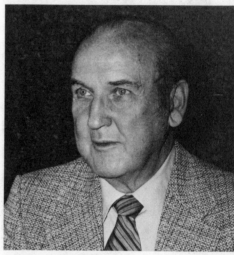

Wilfrid E. Shute M.D.

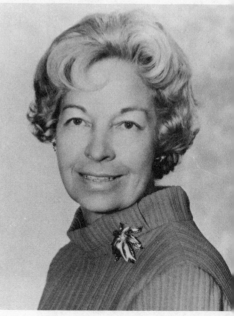

Gena Larson

treatment at the famed Page Clinic in St. Petersburg Beach, Florida. He believes that every human being has a built-in "blueprint" for good health and for resistance to disease, but that most of us spend our lives tearing up this blueprint with deadly living and eating patterns. He has spent his life, since graduating from the University of Michigan School of Dentistry, in an effort to correct that sitution via public-patient education, with books such as *Your Body Is Your Best Doctor* and *Degeneration-Regeneration*.

Gena Larson is one of the most knowledgeable lecturers and writers about a very special subject — nutrition for the young. Her pioneering work in the California grade school and high school system is known everywhere. As a result, she numbers thousands and thousands of young mothers and their children among her most devoted followers. She is the author of what is rapidly becoming a classic on the subject — *Better Food for Better Babies and Their Families*.

Doris Grant's contributions to better living and a healthier world include articles, books and the famous "Grant Loaf," the easy, no-knead whole grain bread that has given thousands of people a new understanding of what the "staff of life" should be like. She has been called England's Adelle Davis and is enormously respected in her own country and the world for her straightforward and authoritative research and writing in the field of consumerism.

Her book, *Your Daily Bread*, is a classic in England where it continues to be reprinted year after year.

Philip S. Chen, Ph.D., has taught organic chemistry at Madison and Atlantic Union Colleges and written nine books related to science and health. He has also written for many chemical journals and is the author of the widely used *Chemical Elements Wall Chart*. One of his greatest achievements is his intensive research into the food value of the soybean, and the results have had an important impact on agricultural and nutritional life in America. He is the author of *Soybeans for Health and A Longer Life*.

Malcolm Margolin is a writer on recreational and environmental subjects who formerly directed conservation projects for the East Bay Regional Park District in Oakland, California. Since graduating from Harvard College, he has worked at various jobs — carpenter, fruitpicker, small publisher, truck driver and tree planter. He is the author of the book, *The East Bay Out*, and has published articles in *Organic Gardening*, *Living Wilderness*, *The Nation* and *Science Digest*.

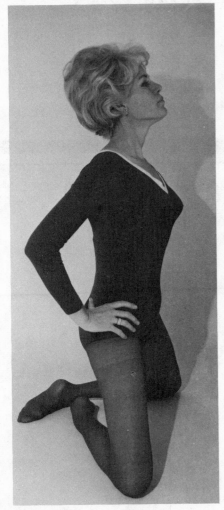

Barbara Hegne

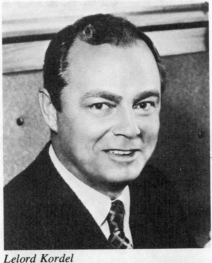

Lelord Kordel

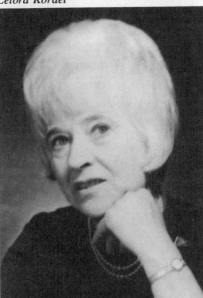

Doris Grant

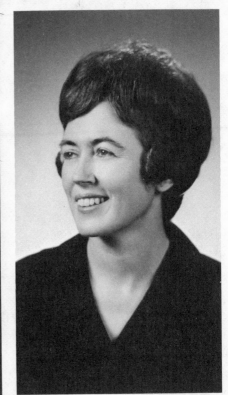

Barbara Jurgensen

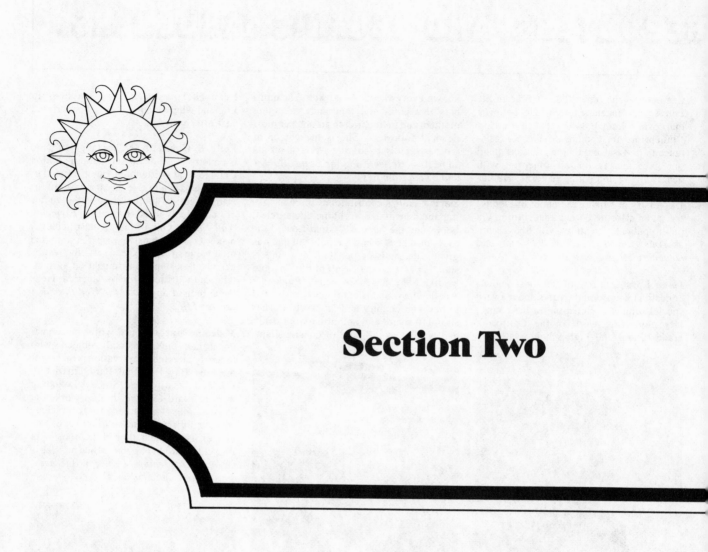

Section Two

Vitamins–Minerals–
Supplements–
In General and Particular

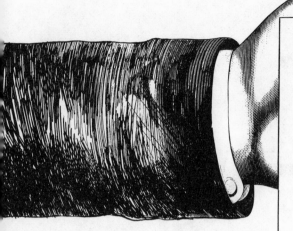

Nature's Helpers— A Handy Guide to the Familiar Vitamins, Minerals and Food Supplements

by Barbara Farr

I. THE VITAMINS

THE FAT-SOLUBLE VITAMINS: A, D, E & K

Fat-soluble vitamins are those which require the presence of both fat and bile salts in the body for proper assimilation. They can also be stored in fatty tissue, which makes it possible to ingest too much of vitamins A and D. Individual needs for these vitamins vary with individual metabolism and recommended allowances vary as well from 500 to 25,000 I.U. of vitamin A; 400 to 2,000 I.U. of vitamin D.

VITAMIN A is essential for healthy skin and hair and good eye-sight. "Night blindness" is one of the early symptoms of vitamin A deficiency. In addition, this vitamin is necessary for the proper development of bones and teeth, and for the health of the body's delicate mucous membranes. Thus, it decreases susceptibility to respiratory ailments. It is also essential for proper functioning of the genito-urinary and gastro-intestinal tracts.

Vitamin A requires the presence of dietary zinc, vitamins D and E, fats and bile salts for proper assimilation. A low-fat diet increases the need for vitamin A, and mineral oil ingestion causes excessive loss of all fat-soluble vitamins.

Vitamin A is found in fish liver oils, liver, egg yolks, butter and milk. It is also found in green and yellow vegetables, such as apricots, yams, carrots, tomatoes, chard and spinach. In fruits and vegetables, it is in the form of carotene, which the body converts to vitamin A. Foods containing carotene should be prepared carefully for maximum digestibility. Carrots, for instance, should be mature and well cooked in as little water as possible for optimum utilization of carotene.

VITAMIN D regulates absorption of calcium and phosphorus, which are important elements in the formation of healthy bones and teeth and the regulation of heart functions.

Vitamin D can be manufactured by the body in the presence of sunlight. Sunlight transforms ergosterol (a normal skin oil) into vitamin D, which is absorbed through the skin. Exposure to sunlight may be hindered, however, by air pollution, clothing, tinted glass, etc.

Vitamin D is found in fish liver oils, irradiated milk, bone meal, sardines, herring, salmon and other fatty fish. If one sunbathes to promote vitamin D, five or six hours should be allowed for the skin to absorb the vitamin before bathing.

VITAMIN E unites with oxygen to protect other chemicals from destruction or modification by oxygen. It is essential in preventing oxidation (rancidity) in unsaturated fats. While a diet high in poly-unsaturated fats would increase the need for vitamin E, the need is offset by the vitamin E naturally occurring in those fats. Vitamin E has been called the "vitamin in search of a disease." Although recognized as essential to human nutrition, its specific role is as yet unclear. It appears to be involved with enzyme actions in detoxifying drugs, and may be protective against air pollutants. In Canada, Drs. Shute, Shute and Vogelsgang have reported many benefits to cardiac patients through the use of vitamin E. They have also found vitamin E helpful in keeping circulation healthy, and in diabetes, hypertension, burns and the healing of scar tissue. Recent experiments have shown that vitamin E and vitamin C support each other, increasing their effect, particularly upon the heart, as they interact.

Vitamin E is found in oils from seeds and grains such as wheat germ oil. It is also present in green vegetables, milk and eggs. The strength of vitamin E is measured by the amount of alpha tocopherol present. Alpha tocopherol was the first component of vitamin E to be isolated, and other tocopherols have been discovered since then. There is no known toxic dose. Vitamin E spares, or reduces the requirement for Vitamin A.

VITAMIN K promotes normal blood coagulation. It is produced naturally in the intestine in the presence of fats, bile salts and friendly intestinal flora. Yogurt, kefir, and acidophilus milk all aid in the promotion of vitamin K production. It is found in alfalfa, green leafy plants and liver. A diet containing yogurt and polyunsaturated fats, and low in refined carbohydrates benefits vitamin K production. Oral antibiotics, frozen foods, aspirin and X rays destroy vitamin K.

THE B-VITAMIN COMPLEX

The B vitamins are complex indeed. To date, at least 22 separate units have been isolated. The function of these units is interrelated, however, so that the B vitamins should be taken together, preferably as they occur in nature. For almost all of the B vitamins, good sources are liver, brewer's yeast and whole grains.

The B vitamins are water soluble and excesses are excreted, so that toxic doses do not occur. In times of stress or trauma, however, there may be unusual excretion of B vitamins, so that the need for the complex increases. Also, their water-solubility makes them susceptible to destruction in cooking, especially if the cooking water is discarded.

VITAMIN B-1 (THIAMINE) is involved in the metabolism of carbohydrates, fats and protein. It is essential to the muscle tone of the digestive tract, normal growth, good appetite, and a healthy nervous system. A severe deficiency results in beri-beri. Milder deficiencies may result in fatigue, tingling and numbness, digestive problems, apathy, confusion, and irritability.

Sources of vitamin B-1 include liver, whole grains, brewer's yeast, meats, milk, egg yolks, wheat germ, and green leafy vegetables. B-1 is easily destroyed by alkalinity, and is extremely water-soluble. Be sure to use all cooking water and meat juices to conserve B-1.

VITAMIN B-2 (RIBOFLAVIN) is essential to proper enzyme formation, normal growth and tissue formation, and the metabolism of fats, carbohydrates and protein. Although it is less water-soluble than B-1, it is readily destroyed by alkalinity and sunlight. Deficiencies produce inflammation of the tongue and cornea, dermatitis, eye fatigue, oversensitivity to light and blurred vision.

Sources of B-2 include milk, organ meats, eggs, brewer's yeast, wheat germ, green leafy vegetables, legumes and nuts. Because sunlight is destructive to B-2, foods should be kept in dark, covered containers, which is why most milk is now in cardboard or amber glass containers.

VITAMIN B-3 (NIACIN) promotes good physical and mental health and aids in maintaining a healthy skin, tongue and digestive system. It can be produced in the body through conversion of the amino acid tryptophan, and is most effective in conjunction with the rest of the B complex. Niacin helps in oxidation of sugar and is essential to proper brain metabolism. It also helps regulate the blood sugar level in hypoglycemia. Niacin is used in treating arthritis, and has proved useful in maintaining low blood cholesterol. In conjunction with vitamin C, niacin is the basis for mega-vitamin therapy for various disorders, proving that individual requirements for this vitamin may vary enormously.

Severe niacin deficiency may result in pellagra. Deficiencies are characterized by weakness, diarrhea, dermatitis, and nervous and mental disorders.

Good sources of niacin are liver, rice bran, legumes, brewer's yeast and fish. In addition, tryptophan-containing foods such as eggs, meats, poultry and dairy products can aid in the body's manufacture of niacin. This important member of the B-complex family frequently produces a disconcerting effect after one takes it, causing a prickly flush that may last as long as fifteen minutes. The flush is harmless, and simply indicates stimulated circulation.

VITAMIN B-6 (PYRIDOXINE) is important to the metabolism of fats, carbohydrates, protein, and the formation of antibodies and red blood cells. It assists in the utilization of energy in brain and nerve tissues, and thus helps protect against stress and nervous disorders. It is necessary to adequate enzyme function, and may be related to cholesterol metabolism. Oral contraceptives and other drugs can increase the requirement for B-6. B-6 appears to function in relationship with zinc.

B-6 deficiencies may appear as weakness, dermatitis, nervousness, irritability, depression and a form of anemia.

B-6 is fairly stable to heat and acids, and a good supply of essential fatty acids can lessen the requirement for this vitamin. Good sources are brewer's yeast, whole grains, nuts, milk and meat.

VITAMIN B-12 (COBALAMIN) is the only vitamin containing the essential mineral, cobalt, which is essential for the function of all body cells, especially those in bone marrow, the gastro-intestinal tract, and nervous tissue. It is also necessary for tissue development and growth and the formation of red blood cells. It plays a role in the metabolism of fats, proteins and carbohydrates, as well as in the synthesis of choline and methionine. B-12 also increases tissue deposition of vitamin A. In order for assimilation of vitamin B-12 to occur, calcium must be present, and also a substance known as the "intrinsic factor" in the gastric juices. Lack of this intrinsic factor is responsible for non-absorption of the vitamin which can result in deficiency.

The most severe deficiency of B-12 results in pernicious anemia. Since its symptoms may be masked by folic acid, these B vitamins should always be taken in conjunction. Dietary pernicious anemia is rare except among those vegetarians who do not use any animal or dairy products. Lesser B-12 deficiencies may produce emotional disturbances, psychoses, neurological abnormalities and fatigue. Cases diagnosed as "senile dementia" often show startling response to B-12 therapy.

Sources of B-12 are liver, kidney, meats, fish, eggs, dairy products and brewer's yeast specially formulated to contain B-12.

FOLIC ACID is essential in red blood cell formation. It functions together with vitamin B-12 in protein metabolism, and is essential to the formation of nucleic acid. Some folic acid is manufactured in the intestinal tract. It is essential for proper brain function and appears to be crucial for mental and emotional stability. Stress, trauma, alcohol and contraceptive pills increase the need for folic acid. This vitamin should always be taken in conjunction with vitamin B-12.

Deficiency symptoms include irritability, forgetfulness, lesions at the corners of the mouth and mental dullness.

Sources of folic acid include liver, kidney, green leafy vegetables, legumes, whole grains, brewer's yeast and wheat germ. Folic acid is only slightly soluble

(continued on page 244)

Before

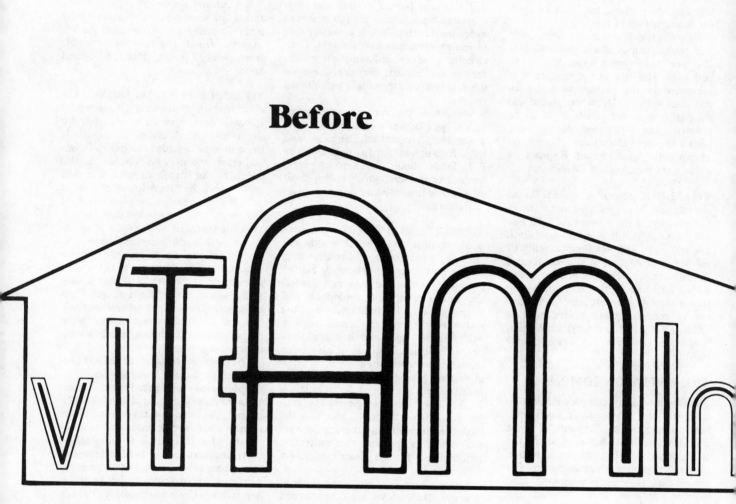

was a household word

by Melvin E. Page, D.D.S.
and H. Leon Abrams, Jr.

Among the many maladies which afflict mankind are the so-called "nutritional diseases" of which vitamin deficiencies are one class. These diseases can be prevented and cured merely by feeding the person enough fresh, wholesome, natural food products provided that his system can absorb them. . . . It is well known that a healthy body, though exposed to infectious diseases, is not likely to contract them. Disease germs can grow only in an unhealthy body. The process may be likened to a chain. When one link is broken, the strength of the whole chain is broken. A diet which results in a vitamin deficiency may be the link which breaks and thus brings on a nutritional disease which, if not corrected, will be fatal.

Hippocrates described scurvy in ancient times, and the disease seemed to especially plague armies in the field and cities that underwent siege for long periods of time. Later, following the discovery of America, when long sea voyages became com-

mon, scurvy became common among sailors. Little was known about what caused scurvy and less about its cure.

In 1553 Cartier made his second voyage to Newfoundland. Of his 103-man crew 100 developed agonizing scurvy and were in great anguish when the Iroquois Indians of Quebec came to their rescue with what was described as a "miraculous cure." The Iroquois Indians gave the sick sailors an infusion of bark and leaves of the pine tree. In 1553 Admiral Sir Richard Hawkins noted that during his career upon the high seas 10,000 seamen under his command had died of scurvy. He further recorded that in his experience sour oranges and lemons had been most effective in curing the disease. Yet these observations had no sweeping effect in bringing about an awareness of what could prevent scurvy, and the observations of this admiral went unheeded.

James Lind, a British naval surgeon, who later became the

chief physician of the Naval Hospital at Portsmouth, England, published in 1753 a book stating explicitly how scurvy could be eliminated simply be supplying sailors with lemon juice. He cited many case histories . . . . he proved that such things as mustard cress, tamarinds, oranges and lemons would prevent scurvy.

You might rightfully expect that Dr. Lind would have been highly honored and praised for his great contribution. The reverse was true. He was ridiculed and became frustrated. He remarked bitterly: "Some persons cannot be brought to believe that a disease so fatal and so dreadful can be cured or prevented by such easy means." They would have more faith in an elaborate composition dignified with the title of "an antiscorbutic golden elixir" or the like. The "some persons" to whom Dr. Lind referred were My Lords of the Admiralty and the other physicians. In fact, they ignored Dr. Lind's advice for forty years. One sea captain did take his advice—the now famous Captain James Cook, who stocked his ships with an ample supply of fresh fruits. The Royal Society honored Captain Cook in 1776 for his success, but the officials of the navy ignored the report. It was not until 1794, the year of Dr. Lind's death, that the first British navy squadron was supplied with lemon juice for a voyage of twenty-three weeks. On that voyage there was not one case of scurvy, yet another decade was to pass before regulations were enacted requiring the sailors to drink a daily ration of lemon juice to prevent scurvy. With this enactment, scurvy disappeared from the British Navy, and after the lapse of another sixty years, the same regulation was applied to the merchant marine fleet. A century after Captain Cook's great success in preventing scurvy on his ship, LeRoy de Mericourt praised Captain Cook's therapy before the French Academy of Medicine, but his words were received with great doubt and hostility. . . . It takes a long time for something new to become accepted. . . . The body chemistry approach to preventing degenerative disease is only gradually coming to be accepted and recognized — the day when it will be recognized is still in the future.

Scurvy was the first vitamin deficiency disease to be treated successfully before its exact cause was discovered, but there were others. The other major ones were beriberi and pellagra.

During the latter part of the last century beriberi became a prevalent disease in the Far East, especially in Indonesia. A Dutch doctor, Christian Eijkman, (1858-1930), was sent from Holland to investigate the ravages of beriberi. He felt certain that it was caused by a germ and he was determined to find the germ causing the disease. People suffering from beriberi develop nervous and paralytic symptoms and finally die an agonizing death. It was only by chance that Eijkman finally found out what caused beriberi. In his experiments, he was feeding chickens polished rice — rice left on the plates of patients — in an effort to find the germ that caused the disease

and they developed the disease. A new superintendent ordered this stopped as white rice was considered a superior food not to be wasted on chickens. Following this the chickens which had developed beriberi on the white rice, were fed brown or unpolished rice. To his amazement, the chickens fully recovered. He followed up this observation by checking prisoners who were fed the cheaper brown rice and only one case of beriberi was found. In another prison where polished rice was given the prisoners, only one had escaped beriberi. It was difficult for Eijkman to give up the germ theory for beriberi, and he did so only in 1906 but his observations proved that there was something in the brown covering of rice which prevented beriberi. . . . Yet Eijkman's discovery was not accepted at once — it took a long time. It was found that the "something" in brown rice which prevented beriberi was vitamin B. The word vitamin was coined by the Polish scientist, Casimur Funk, who was the first man to successfully isolate and extract the chemical factor in the rice polishings which prevents beriberi. . . .

Europe and the United States have not had to face the problem of beriberi, but they have been plagued with pellagra—a kindred disease to beriberi. Pellagra is characterized by dermatitis of the skin areas which are exposed to the air constantly—the hands, face, legs, and neck. Digestive troubles develop and are accompanied by dizziness. Eventually mental disturbances manifest themselves and are followed by insanity and death, often by suicide. At first it was definitely thought that the disease was caused by germs, that it was infectious in origin. Joseph Goldberger finally succeeded in proving that the disease was due exclusively to eating habits. It was prevalent in the deep South where the poorer people lived mainly on corn bread, salt pork and syrup. Of course, corn bread is a healthful food but life cannot be sustained on it alone. Salt pork loses much of its vitality in being cured, while syrup is merely liquid sugar. The diet did not supply something which was necessary for healthy living and whatever it lacked produced the deficiency disease of pellagra. It was found that if these people were fed large quantities of yeast, eggs and a well-rounded diet, they recovered rapidly. . . . In 1937 it was discovered that the element lacking from the diet of pellagra sufferers was nicotinic acid, often called PP — pellagra preventive — which is one of the B vitamins. Later a whole complex of B vitamins was found; this complexity is amply illustrated by the momentous discovery in recent years of vitamin B-12.

The discovery and isolation of vitamins falls within the Twentieth Century — in fact, new ones are still being discovered and some that have been discovered are little understood. The background leading to the discoveries was slow and tedious. It was due to the tenacity of purpose of a few conscientious scientists with the element of luck playing at hand. ☼

Vitamins

Should You Take Them and How Much?

by
Linda Clark

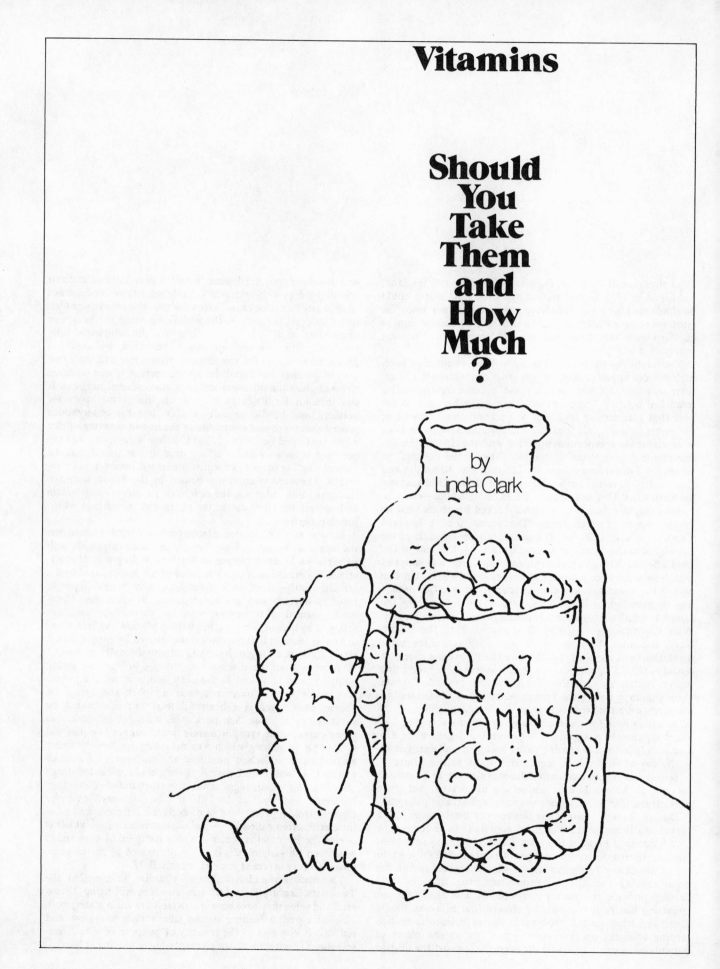

In this day and age, when food is so highly processed and so many natural elements are removed, it is my opinion, as well as that of nutritionists and nutritional doctors, that everyone needs vitamins, providing they are the right kind and taken in the right way.

To begin with, *natural* vitamins are not chemicals, but merely condensed food. For reducers, it saves eating many pounds of food. Someone asked Barbara Cartland, a nutrition columnist in England, "Is there danger of taking too many vitamins?"

Miss Cartland answered, "No! You can't take too many natural vitamins, which are food, not medicine. They are what should be on your plate, but owing to modern conditions: chemicals in the soil, the air, and the water, as well as vitamins being destroyed by processing, refrigerating and bad cooking, they are missing.

"You must supplement your diet. You eat every day, you therefore take your vitamins every day. It's not really a lot. Put all you eat in one day in a bucket, then put the vitamins you need in a small saucer. You will then see how few you have taken in proportion to all you consume."

Why don't more doctors advise you to take vitamins? The regrettable answer is that doctors are not taught nutrition in medical school and it is actually true that many patients, who are interested in and reading about vitamins in order to learn their values, know more about them than many doctors.

The need for vitamins today did not exist in the time of our ancestors. To begin with, our ancestors raised their own organic food with all the nutrients present and at that time there were no TV dinners, instant mixes, enriched bread or cereals. All food was *natural* and *whole*. Not so today. Our food has been tampered with so that our ancestors would never recognize it. It is torn apart, overheated, kept too long in cold storage, and subjected to removal of many of the most important nutrients.

It is then subjected to all sorts of camouflage: artificial coloring, artificial flavorings, preservatives, softeners, emulsifiers, alkalizers, acidifiers, hormones, dyes, antioxidants, hydrogenators (as in hydrogenated fats). All told there are some 3,000 additives allowed in our foods! Tests with animals show many of them are not safe, but the government refuses to ban them, sometimes for political, sometimes for financial reasons. Again, this may be why overweight is such a common problem. People are filling their stomachs with this junk, which is bulk only, instead of real, nourishing, wholesome food. If you don't believe it, read your labels on everything you buy. If it carries the name of a chemical you cannot pronounce, don't buy the product! No wonder we have hidden hunger, over-eat and need vitamins to supply the missing nutrients.

But there is still another reason why most people need vitamins these days. We are living in an era of stress; wars, the threat of the bomb, rising prices and taxes, crime, riots, hi-jackers — you name it, we have it. We worry, we hurry, we live constantly surrounded by stress of all kinds.

Roger J. Williams, Ph. D., found in animal studies at the University of Texas, that stresses and annoyances can increase our need to over-eat, over-drink, and also for added nutrients. The major protection necessary for our bodies is to supply these nutrients, *known and unknown*, to help maintain energy and prevent breakdown.

Many people pride themselves on the fact that they take one vitamin here, another one there. They may have occasional, or even regular injections of vitamin B12 and believe that they are doing all that is necessary. Well, they are only kidding themselves. Dr. Williams emphasizes that our bodies need, not single food elements, by themselves, but a complete assortment of them all! He says when he says *all*, he means *all*, that tests prove that if our diet lacks even one element, our bodies are not getting what they need. Vitamins (and minerals) work as a team. Nature grows them as a team. We should take them as a team. Otherwise, a one-sided diet will eventually exact its penalty from our body, struggling for health.

Only natural food contains all natural, known and unknown, vitamins and minerals. Synthetics do not contain them all. Synthetics have their place in temporary treatment for a disease state, but nutritional doctors feel that taken in high amounts too long, they can become the equivalent of whipping a tired horse. Natural vitamins are nothing more than concentrated food. If you must make a choice, choose whole food first, the supplements second. In food, variety is imperative. In order to get everything you need, one doctor has advised people to eat a different menu each day of the month. Too many people get into a rut and eat the same things every day. Buy yourself some paperback health-gourmet cookbooks at the health store and stretch your eating horizons. It's fun.

Which Vitamins Do What?

There are entire books written in an easy-to-understand manner, which are fascinating to read and tell what various vitamins have done for others. In general, here is a quickie outline:

Vitamin A: helps your skin, hair, vision and energy.

Vitamin D: is the sunshine vitamin and gives you strong bones and teeth and the well-being you feel after being outdoors.

Vitamin B: (There are many in this family.) In general, the B vitamins calm your nerves, help your digestion, and help you sleep, feel and look better. They also help thinning hair and a host of other ailments, including mental illness.

Vitamin E: is sold as the sex vitamin in Europe. It helps circulation, helps prevent heart attacks, cold feet, hot flushes during menopause and can prevent miscarriages.

Vitamin C: prevents infections and is now being considered in Europe as a rejuvenation vitamin.

Vitamin K: helps blood to clot and prevents hemorrhaging.

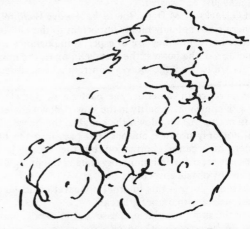

Are Any of These Vitamins Considered Dangerous?

In some cases, vitamins A and D in too-high doses have been found disturbing to *some* people. The effects vary with the individual.

Take vitamin A as an example. In 1932 Mead Johnson Co. offered $15,000 as an award to anyone who could find out how much vitamin A a person needs. There were no takers, and after 13 years the offer was withdrawn. One man in England was reported by Dr. Roger J. Williams as being healthy with no vitamin A at all; and a woman in

(continued on page 246)

Everyone talks about vitamins as the stars in the exciting drama of better health and nutrition. Now, we are coming to discover that minerals are almost as vital—if not more so—than vitamins. It it were not for minerals, the vitamins could hardly function in your body. Yet, many people have serious mineral deficiencies.

According to *U.S. Senate Document No. 264,* "It is bad news to learn from leading authorities that 99% of the American people are deficient in these minerals and that a marked deficiency in any one of the more important minerals actually results in disease! Any upset of the balance, any considerable lack of one or another element, however microscopic the body requirement may be, and we sicken, suffer, shorten our lives!"

Writing in *Modern Nutrition* Dr. J. F. Wischhusen says that minerals are needed to help protein to form; minerals enable the vagus nerve that controls stomach activity to function; minerals influence muscle contraction and nerve response; they control body liquids to permit nutrients to pass into the bloodstream; and they aid in blood coagulation.

Can Mineral Supplements Improve Your Health?

by Carlson Wade

Borden's Review of Nutrition Research (Vol. XVII, No. 4) tells us that minerals function as catalysts: that is, they are needed to change other nutrients in the body to utilized form. Without minerals, other vitamins, proteins, carbohydrates and fats, may just be "wasted."

Robert G. Jackson, M.D. in *How to Be Always Well,* tells us that "minerals are not only highly important to the well-being of the entire body, but they are of especial importance to the local structures of the bowels; the glands lining it, the muscles forming its walls, and the nerves controlling and directing these structures.

"In the absence of minerals, the bacteria of putrefaction multiply with enormous rapidity in the slowed-down current of food waste matter passing down the canal of the bowel. They [bacteria] not only produce poisons that pass into the blood and burden the organ of elimination, but they locally irritate and ultimately set up an inflammatory state in the lining of the bowel, called by physicians 'colitis.' "

Dr. Jackson feels that this internal upheaval could be controlled and healed with proper minerals.

Here are the more popular and essential minerals, and information on how they work to give you a strong, vigorous body and youthfully alert health.

CALCIUM

A constituent of bones and teeth, 99 percent of calcium is found in your bones and teeth. The remainder of a scant 1% circulates in the soft body tissues and the fluids. It is needed for normal bone and tooth development, for blood clotting, for enzymatic action, and for the regulation of fluid passage through walls of tissues and cells. Calcium in the blood is needed for the alternate contraction and relaxation of the heart muscles. *Note:* If you have a calcium deficiency, there may be a nervous symptomatic reaction.

Calcium is stored inside the ends of bones in long, needle-like crystals called trabeculae. When you are in a stress situation, your body draws calcium from these bones if you do not have enough from your daily diet. If you are deficient, your body will then draw calcium from your bones—usually first from the spine and pelvic area.

This causes a weakness that may lead to a vertebrae fracture. An early symptom is that of osteoporosis or brittle bones. Another calcium deficiency disease is osteomalacia—deformed bones, such as rickets in children, but also striking adults.

Calcium is a brother of phosphorus—in fact, it works so closely with this other mineral, that if there is an imbalance, *both* are impaired in function.

About half of all calcium taken into the body is excreted. So be sure to have enough calcium every day to meet your needs.

Note: Illnesses such as diarrhea may interfere with calcium absorption. Kidney trouble also interferes with the utilization of this mineral. Hormone imbalance, especially of the thyroid, parathyroid, and the adrenal cortical glands, also influences the storage and use of calcium. A valuable mineral, it is available in supplemental form by itself or in a multiple capsule.

PHOSPHORUS

Each body cell contains phosphorus. About 66 percent of phosphorus is found in your bones in the form of calcium phosphate while the balance occurs in soft tissues as organic and inorganic phosphate.

Organic phosphate compounds aid in converting oxidative energy into cellular work. As high energy phosphates, they also play an important role in the synthesis of protein, carbohydrate and fat, as well as in all forms of energy utilization; this includes contraction of muscles, secretions of glands, function of the kidneys, and generation of nerve impulses.

External and internal growth and repair are stimulated by this mineral; it also aids the bloodstream in neutralizing excess acidity to keep a healthy alkaline balance. Phosphorus seems to help lecithin (a fat-dissolving agent) in its formation, and also in the metabolization of fats and starches, thereby providing energy fuel for youthful vitality.

Phosphorus is an activator of enzymes which help in stomach digestive processes. Deficiency symptoms include loss of weight, poor mental stability, easy tiredness, low powers of virility and poor energy. Nervousness and insomnia may also occur.

IRON

Each of your billions of body tissues and muscle cells need iron to provide it with oxygen—the breath of life! Iron is a vital component of hemoglobin, the oxygen-carrying pigment of the red blood cell. Iron is also an essential component of respiratory enzymes which are needed for the production of energy in all cells.

Insufficient iron may lead to anemia, pale skin color, dim vision, and poor memory. (Remember, your brain also has cells and needs oxygen for proper function.)

Other iron deficiency symptoms are irregular heartbeat, bluish-white eyeballs, poor skin health. You have over 5 million red cells in just one cubic millimeter of blood—and iron is needed for each and every cell! Iron is stored, bound to protein, in the liver and intestines.

IODINE

This mineral is concentrated in the thyroid gland, and is present in the adrenal cortex, the ovaries, the lymph, and the cerebro-spinal fluid. Iodine is needed for normal gland func-

tion. A deficiency may cause goiter, sluggish metabolism, poor mentality. A serious deficiency may also interfere with proper fat utilization. Myoglobin (an iron substance resembling hemoglobin) combines with iodine to serve as a storage site for oxygen in muscular tissues. Iodine is also a constituent of chromatin (a portion of the cell nucleus) which is needed to maintain the youthful health of that cell.

SODIUM

Here is the valuable element that enters into the extracellular body fluids. It influences the osmotic pressure and fluid passage between tissues and blood, the acid-base body balance, and the heartbeat. Sodium is given off in wastes and perspiration, so you should also have an adequate replacement supply through approved mineral supplements containing this mineral.

Sodium combines with body chlorine to improve blood and lymph health; it also helps other blood minerals become more soluble and prevents them from clogging. Sodium enables your muscles to contract and also to respond to nerve impulses. Because sodium helps re-dissolve coagulated fibrin, it prevents a too-speedy blood coagulation. The fibrin is restored to a healthy liquid state by sodium. Signs of deficiency include poor blood color, nausea, edema, and poor healing of wounds.

POTASSIUM

This mineral works together with sodium in controlling body fluids and essential physiological and metabolic processes. Potassium also normalizes your heartbeat. It nourishes your muscles. *Note:* Both sodium and potassium must have a *balance*—sodium is mainly found in circulating liquids *outside* the cells—potassium is found mostly *inside* the cells. To prevent a "tug of war," you need to have enough of both minerals.

A unique function is that potassium helps your kidneys dispose of body waste substances.

MAGNESIUM

Writing in *Food, The Yearbook of Agriculture,* Dr. Ruth M. Leverton explains, "Magnesium is closely related to both calcium and phosphorus in its location and its functions in the body. About 70 percent of the magnesium in the body is in the bones. The rest is in the soft tissues and blood. Muscle tissue contains more magnesium than calcium. Magnesium acts as a starter for some of the chemical reactions within the body.

"It plays an important role as a coenzyme in the building of protein. There is some relation between magnesium and the hormone cortisone as they affect the amount of the phosphate in the blood. Animals on a diet deficient in magnesium become extremely nervous and give an exaggerated response to even small noises or disturbances. Such unnatural sensitiveness disappears when they are given enough magnesium.

"In extreme deficiencies, the blood vessels expand, the heart beats faster and causes such irritability that the animals die in convulsions."

Nature uses magnesium to calm your nervous system; it is a natural sedative during the hot, muggy "dog days." Your bones become firm with magnesium. Blood albumen forms with this valuable mineral—which acts as a catalyst in helping carbohydrates become properly assimilated instead of being stored as fat.

COPPER

This mineral is a nutritional partner of iron in helping to metabolize food into hemoglobin, the oxygen-carrying ingredient found in all red blood cells. It is found in the liver, bloodstream, and bile. The skin pigment, called melanin, is formed by iron and copper.

(continued on page 248)

The Almost Miraculous Qualities of Vitamin E Ointment

by Wilfrid E. Shute, M.D.

THAT EVERY CELL IN THE BODY must have Vitamin E is now firmly established. That the body needs many essential nutrients, amino acids, minerals and thirteen vitamins is now accepted by every biochemist. (The authority on this is Roger Williams, B.S., M.S., Ph.D., D.Sc. I recommend his book *Nutrition Against Disease* as a nutritional bible.)

That oxygen directly applied to damaged tissues can initiate and promote healing has also been well established. Hyperbaric oxygen applied locally can effectively shorten healing time in most chronic leg ulcers as well as in many decubitus ulcers. (Anyone who is interested in this form of treatment should consult the article by Dr. B.H. Fisher in *The Lancet* 2,405, 1969.)

Alpha tocopherol acts in a different manner to accomplish the same purpose, but has the advantage of acting not only locally as the pure oil or in an ointment base, but also systematically through the blood supply to the cell. It is not surprising, therefore, that by far the best treatment for burns is alpha tocopherol orally and by direct application.

The efficacy of alpha tocopherol is well illustrated by the experience of one of my nurses. This twenty-four-year-old very blonde nurse lay out in the sun on the beach on the first beautiful spring day. She was clad in a relatively scant bathing suit. She fell asleep and overstayed a reasonable time of exposure to the sun. The result was an intense sunburn over her face and neck and all the areas not covered by the bathing suit. She attempted to work the next morning but was nauseated and weak. She was brought to me by her co-worker in the electrocardiograph and laboratory division of the Shute Institute. She was running a fever, had a severe headache and was a very sick-looking girl.

Conventional treatment would probably have prescribed for her compresses of boric acid, doses of antihistamine, corticosteroid spray or cream and possibly painkiller medication. We put this nurse in one of the side rooms, covered all the burned areas liberally with Vitamin E ointment and covered her with a sheet. Within minutes she fell asleep. Within an hour her temperature was normal and her headache had vanished. She got up and went back to work.

Our nurse did not develop a single blister and she did not peel. This is all the more remarkable since it was about twenty hours after the burn that treatment was initiated.

Earlier I have related the unblind controlled experiment of a man familiar with the value of Vitamin E and Vitamin E ointment in treating burns. He applied the ointment to half the burn, and the difference between the two areas was obvious and striking. The owner of a company which wholesales Vitamin E products used the same technique on a severe barbecue burn on his thumb. The difference between the E-ointment-treated part of the burn and the other half was very obvious.

As I write this, my wife has suggested that I mention her ninety-one-year-old mother who, apart from some loss of hearing, is able to do all that the average sixty-year-old can do. She swims miles every day in the summer and is in the pool at least once a day when we are in Florida. She should be long since dead, for she had hypertension for years, developed a bundle branch block and then the dyspnea of congestive failure. Control of her hypertension with diuretics and 2,400 IU of alpha tocopherol a day, however, keep her well and vigorous.

Some six or seven years ago my mother-in-law accidentally upset a dish of boiling water on her foot which was in a sock and slipper. The whole dorsum was involved in a deep burn. Vitamin E ointment was applied within seconds, and today there is no visible trace of the burn.

Vitamin E has no equal for first- and second-degree burns and is a useful adjunctive therapy in third-degree burns. It has three unique characteristics. First, it lessens or takes away the associated pain a few minutes after application. Second, it keeps the burn from deepening, limiting the damage to the cells actually destroyed by the burning agent. Finally, it gives rapid epithelization and a scar that is not painful and does not contract. (Because it is antibacterial in vivo and in vitro, incidentally, it virtually removes the danger of infection.)

The majority of burn patients treated in this way do not need hospitalization. More important is the great reduction in the need for skin grafting. It is seldom necessary even in severe third-degree burns. Because the scars do not contract, there are no contraction deformities when the burns involve the axilla (armpit) or neck or groin. The color slides we show at medical conferences of the results of treating burns are unique and completely convincing.

The late Adelle Davis reported remarkable case histories emphasizing the value of tocopherol in the healing of burns without scars. Vitamin E, in fact, is such a useful product for domestic burns and sunburns that many who are familiar with it keep a tube in several rooms in the house, especially the kitchen, and never travel without it.

Vitamine E ointment has many uses in addition to its major role in the treatment of burns. It was first used in the treatment of ulcerations on the legs due to venous stasis (stagnation) or arterial insufficiency. These ulcers healed well with oral Vitamine E, but in most cases more rapidly with the addition of the local application of the ointment. However, the scars formed in these ulcer cases were surprising. They were the same size as the original ulcers, and they were soft, pliable and not tender.

When Vitamin E ointment is used on scars following abdominal surgery they will often virtually disappear. The ointment

(continued on page 249)

28

E

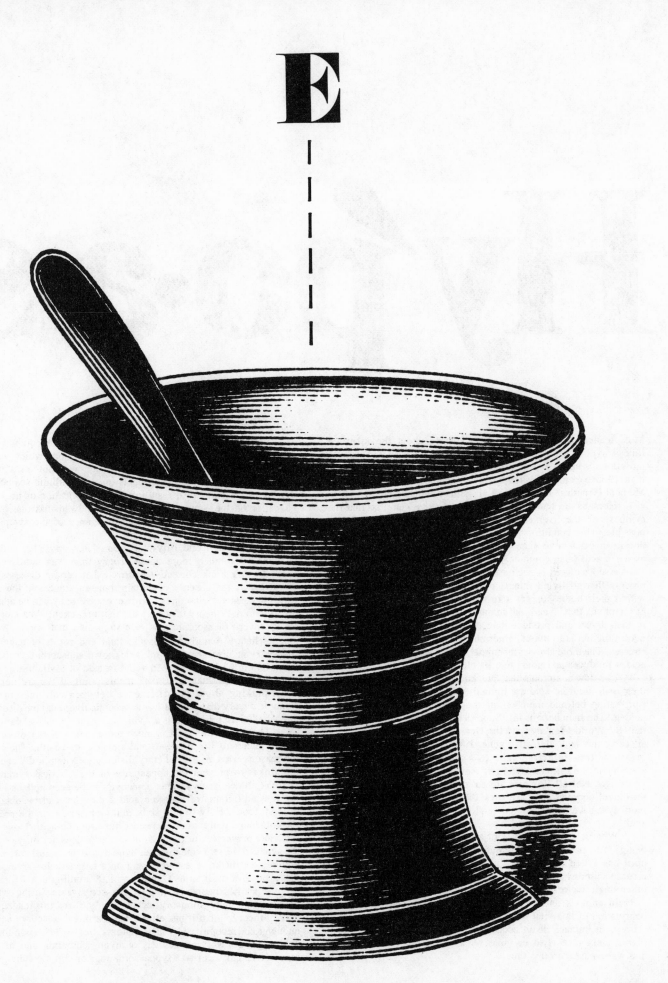

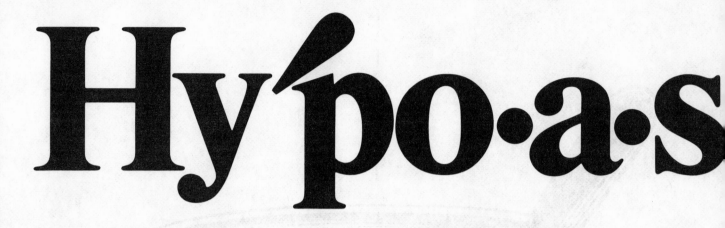

Hy'po·a·s

Most readers will not recall ever hearing about the inherited illness, hypoascorbemia; but don't feel too badly about that because most doctors have never heard of it either. Even though I described it in 1966 papers published by the Gregor Mendell Institute for Medical Genetics. Even though all human beings have it.

Humans are handicapped with a defective gene, so that the synthesis of the liver enzyme, L-gulunolactone oxidase, is not possible. This condition is known as hypoascorbemia, and it is due to this defective gene that we cannot manufacture our own ascorbic acid (also commonly known as vitamin C) in our liver.

Ascorbic acid is such a basic vital substance for the living process that all living things, plants and animals, must make it within their bodies or get it in their foods or they perish. It is as simple as that. Nearly all mammals manufacture ascorbic acid in their livers and produce it in rather large daily amounts. Its main function is to maintain normalcy in the face of biochemical stresses. The more stresses an animal undergoes, the more ascorbic acid it produces and pours into its bloodstream.

The few mammals that are known to be unable to make their own ascorbic acid are limited to the guinea pig, an Indian fruit-eating bat and members of the Primate Suborder, Anthropoidea. The members of this Suborder comprise Man, the Apes, the Old World Monkeys and the New World Monkeys, and they all carry the same defective gene. I have been able to trace the origin of this defective gene to a mutation occurring in an ancestor of the Primate Suborder, Anthropoidea about 60 million years ago. Not all Primates are so afflicted, as the members of the other Suborder of the Primates, the Prosimii, the very primitive monkeys, have the intact gene and can make their own ascorbic acid.

What is the significance of all this for our health and well-being? The presence of this defective gene in the human gene pool has killed more individuals, caused more misery and in recorded times has changed the course of history more than any other single factor.

In animals unable to make their own ascorbic acid, total deprivation of this vital material will cause a horrible death from scurvy. In humans death occurs in a few months but in guinea pigs it only takes two or three weeks. The body disintegrates and wastes away in this time.

For thousands of years witch doctors and folk medicine practitioners knew there was something in fresh foods which would prevent this daily plague. The knowledge was put on a more reasonable basis by the experiments on the scorbutic seamen of Dr. James Lind in 1740, resulting in the publication of his book "Treatise on the Scurvy" in 1753. He showed that one ounce of lemon juice would prevent the appearance of the symptoms of frank clinical scurvy.

One hundred and fifty-nine years later, in 1912, and not knowing very much more about scurvy than was published in 1753, Casmir Funk correctly theorized that certain diseases can be caused by the absence of certain trace substances in the diet, which he termed "vitamines". However he erred when he applied his "vitamine" theory to scurvy at this time, twenty years before the discovery of ascorbic acid. He suggested that scurvy was a simple dietary disturbance, is the fatal end result of a genetic liver-enzyme disease, and Funk's unknown antiscorbutic substances (vitamin C) is a liver metabolite instead of a vitamin.

The reader may well ask, at this point, if we are not just word-picking about the difference between calling scurvy a "simple dietary disturbance" or a "genetic liver-enzyme disease" and whether ascorbic acid is a "vitamin" or a "liver metabolite".

The answer is that it is much more than a matter of words; it is a matter of life or death and sickness or health. These are the reasons why: in the "dietary disturbance-vitamin C" theory, the aim is to prevent the appearance of the classical symptoms of frank clinical scurvy. This objective can be accomplished with the few milligrams of ascorbic acid a day that can be obtained in fresh foods. Fifty-five to sixty milligrams a day is the present recommended daily adult allowance for ascorbic acid. However, this mere prevention of frank clinical scurvy does not fully correct the genetic liver-enzyme disease, hypoascorbemia. Full correction requires the intake of ascorbic acid on a larger scale—grams per day instead of milligrams (1 gram = 1,000 milligrams).

What has happened in the past sixty years during which medicine has unquestionably accepted and utilized this inadequate dietary theory is that it has eliminated the threat of scurvy severe enough to be recognized by its symptoms, but has left a population suffering from varying degrees of hypoascorbemia and a false sense of health security. Hypoascorbemia, or chronic subclinical

World's Number 1 Disease!

or·be'mia

A New Slant On Vitamin C
by Irwin Stone

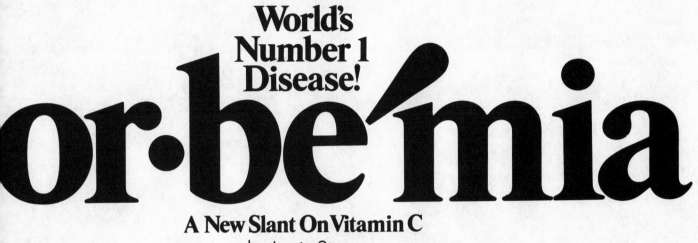

scurvy, is the more insidious because of a lack of obvious symptoms. Chronic subclinical scurvy is presently our most widespread disease and yet it is rarely spoken of and does not appear in recorded disease statistics. Chronic subclinical scurvy is the root of many of our most pressing medical problems. If chronic subclinical scurvy were eliminated by the simple proper use of ascorbic acid, it is believed that many of these medical problems would improve to an unimagined degree.

It is only in the last few years that the flaws in the vitamin theory have been recognized and the daily dosages have been challenged. The author was perhaps the first to put forth a definite challenge in his work on genetic diseases published in 1965-67. Recently Dr. Leon E. Rosenberg of Yale University Medical School working with the B vitamins and vitamin D distinguished between "vitamin deficiency" diseases (the true avitaminoses) and the "vitamin dependent" diseases. Successful treatment of the "vitamin dependent" diseases requires dosages ten to one thousand times more than is needed in the "vitamin deficiency" diseases. In the case of ascorbic acid, Dr. Linus Pauling's recent calculations indicate that humans should be getting 2.3 grams to 9.0 grams a day. The author's figures, based on the amount of ascorbic acid normally synthesized by the rat, suggests 3 to 5 grams per day, increasing to 15 grams or more a day under stress. For the past quarter century Dr. Frederick R. Klenner has been a pioneer in the use of large amounts of ascorbic acid to combat a variety of diseases. He has obtained fantastically successful clinical results using up to 100 grams or more of ascorbate a day both orally and intravenously. He recommends to his adult patients the continuous daily intake of 10 grams. For children he prescribes 1 gram of ascorbic acid a day for each year of age up to age 10 and then 10 grams daily thereafter. He reports unusual continuous good health and freedom from disease in his patients. He has published widely but the medical fraternity has chosen to ignore his work. As pointed out earlier, these amounts are greatly in excess of the daily 55 to 60 milligrams of ascorbic acid recommended as adequate by the vitamin C theorists.

Due to a lack of available space in this short article, coverage of the above topic has, by necessity, been brief. More detailed treatment of the history of ascorbic acid, the new genetic concepts of scurvy, facts about ascorbic acid and its use in the treatment of many diseases will be found by reference to the author's new book, *The Healing Factor "Vitamin C" Against Disease,* published by Grosset & Dunlap, New York City, 1972. Since these new genetic concepts provide the rationale for the use of massive daily doses of ascorbic acid (megascorbic therapy), completely new and unexplored fields of medicine and therapy are opened. The book contains many chapters devoted to megascorbic prophylaxis, megascorbic therapy and research protocols designed to obtain clinical data in many of our most serious medical problems. The discussions are fully documented by a large bibliography of citations from the medical literature of the past 40 years, since the discovery of ascorbic acid. Among the topics discussed and recommended for further clinical research are heart and vascular diseases, arthritis and rheumatism, the infectious diseases, diabetes and hypoglycemia, kidney diseases, cancer, mental illness, ulcers, allergies, smoking and others.

The versatile therapeutic properties of ascorbic acid have been long neglected by medical research because it has been considered a nutrient rather than a therapeutic metabolite. An organization such as the National Health Federation and its membership can do much to bring, by the power of public opinion, these neglected facts on ascorbic acid to the attention of Congress and the proper government agencies. Then medical research facilities can be used to explore the potential therapeutic properties of ascorbic acid and conduct the long neglected clinical research on the megascorbic therapy of a wide variety of diseases.

A Major Therapeutic Breakthrough

Another critical area that requires change is in the education of the doctors in the medical schools. The substitution of these new genetic concepts on frank clinical scurvy and chronic subclinical scurvy should be made in the present curriculum that now teaches the outdated "vitamin C-nutritional disease" theory. This would provide a new crop of doctors who could think more clearly in terms of medical genetics rather than nutrition and thus provide more enlightened care for their patients.

If properly conducted, the clinical research on megascorbic prophylaxis and megascorbic therapy could be the major therapeutic breakthrough of the latter quarter of the 20th Century.

Here are the latest discoveries about a vitamin that may help extend your prime of life.

Its name is *pyridoxine*. It is officially known as vitamin B[6]. It is a member of the B-complex family of vitamins. But that is just the start of its valuable function of being able to help reverse the aging process. Because this particular vitamin *slowly* vanishes, the aging process appears as a gradual symptom that could be reversed or delayed if adequate nourishment were available.

Vitamin B[6] acts as a sparkplug that enables your body to metabolize and process protein into usable amino acids so they can build and rebuild depleted tissues and cells. It also helps produce needed antibodies to help break down cholesterol so that it will not gather and cause arteriosclerosis.

As long ago as February 1971, the noted physician Paul Gyorgy, (he first identified vitamin B[6] and named it pyridoxine) said that "at present we are facing an almost explosive interest in the metabolic role of B[6] in man. There are large numbers of findings of various types accumulating, but a clear, overall picture of all connections and of their role is still missing."

Now more and more doctors are naming the value of B[6] as a youth-building substance. In particular, it has been related to the function of enzymes, those protein-substances that hold the key to youth.

When B[6] goes into the body, it is transformed into *pyridoxal phosphate*. This is a coenzyme. It activates the different enzymes throughout your body. Without B[6], most of the 1,000 enzymes in your body just could not function; or, if they did, they would do so very weakly. So B[6] is the key that unlocks the enzyme network into building body health.

Quoted in *The Enzymes*, a Soviet biochemist, A. E. Braunstein, says, "Pyridoxal phosphate (or transformed B[6]) holds an exceptional place among the coenzymes with regard to the unparalleled diversity of its catalytic function."

Now, this may be technical, but Dr. Braunstein helps clarify it by further saying that B[6] works by promoting the process of the metabolism of protein — which we all know is a building block of youth!

This is how it works. When you eat a protein food (meat, fish,

How Vitamin B6 May Help Delay The Aging Process

John Hildebrand

eggs, cheese, peas, beans, nuts, even some plant and seed foods), your body sends forth digestive secretions that break down the proteins and form them into amino acids. Next, these amino acids must be absorbed through the intestinal wall and then sent throughout the body to promote youth-building processes.

But for this absorption to take place, you must have a good supply of pyridoxal phosphate. Without this vitamin B^6 (which is what pyridoxal phosphate becomes in your system), protein cannot be absorbed through your system. Thus, the youth-building functions may be impeded and aging may follow at a more rapid rate.

Even if amino acids are absorbed, they need to be energized by vitamin B^6. Otherwise, they are too weak and cannot become the biological structures which you need to maintain, extend and prolong the prime of life. Furthermore, body enzymes need vitamin B^6 together with amino acids for their own nourishment. Enzymes are part of these nutrients. So you have a good supply of vitamin B^6 for overall body health.

Vitamin B^6 then works to send amino acids throughout your body, to nourish the endocrine and ductless glands, the viscera (internal organs), and the antibodies that help ward off illness. Vitamin B^6 strengthens cells and tissues, nourishes the blood vascular network, strengthens the skeletal structure and enters into the cellular integrity of muscle and skin tissue.

This biological process helps prevent or may even *reverse* the aging process — but in order for it to take place, vitamin B^6 is vital. Without vitamin B^6, the enzymes and other valuable substances would remain lifeless . . . as you would soon become.

Within your body, you have DNA and RNA, two valuable substances which are charged by Nature with carrying out the necessary growth, maintenance and regeneration of your body. These substances need vitamin B^6 for vigor. Without that vitamin, they might be unable to function. The result is that your body tissues would disintegrate. Such is the forerunner of illness and aging. Nature has given vitamin B^6 the power to feed DNA and RNA so that these processes can keep you youthfully alert. The more vitamin B^6 you have, the better these processes can function and the more chances you have for youthful vitality.

A vitamin B^6 dificiency, according to Drs. Arthur F. Wagner and Carl Folkers in *Vitamin and Coenzymes*, "reveals pathological alterations bearing a strong similarity to atherosclerosis."

But this is just one health risk. The doctors wrote that a vitamin B^6 deficiency causes serious health loss to the arteries. Arteriosclerosis "was detected microscopically in organs such as the heart, kidney, testes, ovaries, uterus, liver, adrenal and lung."

A more general array of health losses is described by Dr. Richard W. Vilter in *Modern Nutrition in Health and Disease*. The doctor notes that a vitamin B^6 deficiency may cause the development for forms of seborrheic dermatitis, muscular weakness, lowered resistance to infection, convulsive seizures, and faulty growth as well as abnormalities of the blood and urine.

Yes, these are extremes, but they do point out how valuable vitamin B^6 can be in helping to prevent such disorders.

Your body does have some vitamin B^6 but is reported by many doctors that there is a gradual leakage or loss as the person matures. For example, Dr. Ronald Searcy, director of diagnostic research at Hoffman-LaRoche, Inc., in *Diagnostic Biochemistry*, writes that as the person grows older, even in the middle 30s, the vitamin B^6 supply in the body has dropped.

This may suggest a serious relationship between aging and this vitamin. Namely, the less vitamin B^6 in the body, the more that body ages and falls vulnerable to ailments.

There are a wide variety of B-complex vitamins containing vitamin B^6 available. You might also choose such sources of B^6 as organ meats, liver (whole or desiccated), natural whole grains, natural brown rice, soybeans, barley, peanuts, walnuts, bananas, sunflower and other seeds, wheat germ and wheat bran.

A powerhouse of vitamin B^6 is found in brewer's yeast. Sprinkle it over cereals, use it in baking, mix it in a blender with almost any fruit or vegetable juice. Brewer's yeast is one of Nature's most effective youth foods with its rich treasure of vitamin B^6 as well as almost all other nutrients.

Nutritionist Dr. Roger J. Williams in *Nutrition Against Disease* hails vitamin B^6 or pyridoxine as being vital for the body's manufacture of lecithin, the substance that protects against age-causing cholesterol.

Dr. Williams says clearly, "From a consideration of the evidence we have reviewed, the surest guarantee against possible pernicious effects of various protein/fat-cholesterol combinations in whatever proportions, is the daily intake of a sufficient amount of pyridoxine."

Possibly, the most famous champion of vitamin B^6 is John N. Ellis, M.D., author of *The Doctor Who Looked At Hands*.

Dr. Ellis tells of a patient who was given 300 milligrams daily of vitamin B^6. She had suffered from edema of her hands, feet and legs. She had headaches, blurred vision, severe foot and leg cramps, also tingling and numbness of the hands.

Says Dr. Ellis, "For the next five weeks, the patient was given pyridoxine 300 milligrams daily with no other medication or supplement. Headaches subsided. Hands and feet became free of wrinkles, parethesia subsided in hands, muscle cramps subsided in feet and legs." Soon, she could wear a ring on her finger.

Dr. Ellis also says that vitamin B^6 is useful in relieving arthritis pain. "B^6 would relieve the edema, relieve the painful neuritis, improve hand function and reduce the size of joints of the fingers. It is of tremendous importance to note that symptomology associated with angina pectoris before the heart attack was relieved by B^6, and it is of equal importance to note that pain in the shoulders, arms and hands of patients was relieved by B^6 after the heart attack."

Your body needs a mineral such as magnesium for vitamin B^6 to work effectively. Dr. Ellis also points to potassium as a mineral intimately involved with vitamin B^6.

Your doctor can advise you how much B^6 you need. But an interesting potency was recommended by Dr. Gyorgy in the *American Journal of Clinical Nutrition* (10:71). Here is what he says,

"The levels of PLP (pyridoxal phosphate or the active coenzyme form of B^6) in the blood plasma showed *a gradual reduction in the aged*, accompanied by positive tryptophan load test (a biological defect traced to B^6 deficiency). But . . . large doses of pyridoxine restored all metabolic changes mentioned to normal."

How much for you? Dr. Gyorgy then declares emphatically:

"The present daily dietary allowance of B^6 should be changed from 2 to 2.5 milligrams to 25 milligrams per day as a precaution to prevent possible serious pathological conditions."

So there you have it — the need for vitamin B^6.

As stated above, you can get this needed vitamin in many foods. Be sure to get liver that is organic. Remember that unbleached soy products are good sources of vitamin B^6. Sprinkle wheat germ and sliced bananas with some peanuts (shelled) in a natural cereal such as granola and you've got a powerhouse of minerals, proteins, and the vital "youth vitamin" — vitamin B^6.

It's up to you!

☼

Does Your Diet Includ

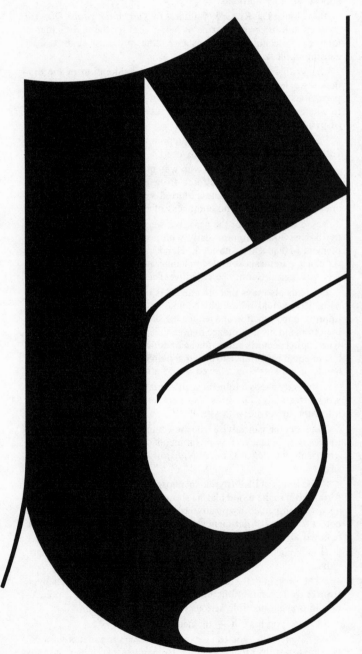

by Beatrice Trum Hunter

☐ Depending on the year of the pronouncement, the Food and Drug Administration has at various times stated that Vitamin E is worthless, nonessential, or adequately supplied in the average American diet. In earlier days, FDA repeated the ritualistic words that although vitamin E might be essential for animals, it had not been proven so for humans.

☐ By 1959, an impressive accretion of research data forced FDA to alter its position and to admit that, in the opinion of nutritional scientists, evidence showed that vitamin E was essential for humans. However, the agency hastened to add that "all practical diets in this country are amply supplied with this vitamin. There is no evidence that additional intake of vitamin E above that supplied by the daily diet is of any benefit." Anyone rash enough to write to FDA in that era, asking for information about vitamin E, automatically received a mailing piece on nutritional faddism along with the reply. The inference was clear that anyone interested in vitamin E, if not an outright faddist, was at least a potential victim for faddist propaganda.

☐ The glib reassurance, which FDA continues to give, that the average American diet supplies ample amounts of vitamin E, deserves analysis. The mere repetition of the reassurance doesn't make it so.

☐ Dr. Robert Harris, a respected authority on nutritional evaluation of food processing, stated in 1962 that "the literature relating to the effects of storage and processing on the retention of tocopherols [vitamin E] in foods is limited, controversial and inadequate. Most of the published data must be considered quantitative . . . since methods of analysis for total tocopherols only recently became precise."

☐ Dr. Harris said that vitamin E activity in food might be as much as 40 percent less than the total tocopherol content, and that data on true vitamin E activity of individual foods, both raw or processed, were essentially nonexistent. Later studies confirmed Dr. Harris' findings.

☐ FDA has stated that vitamin E deficiency is practically unknown in man. This statement needs to be challenged. Today's typical vitamin E consumption is reduced to only a fraction of what it was formerly, before the widespread practices of degermination, bleaching, processing, modification, and long-term storage of foods.

☐ Vitamin E is present in many foods, but the best sources are recognized in unrefined oils and grains. The average American does not use unrefined oils and grains, but, rather, refined ones. What happens to the vitamin E values in the refining and processing of oils and grains? One study measured the effect of heat treatment and storage of oils for tocopherol losses. After being heated for 30 minutes at 175°C., coconut oil lost 20 percent of its tocopherol; after storage for six months at 37°C., it lost 26 percent

nough Vitamin E?

of its tocopherol. Similar losses were noted in other oils after heat treatment and storage. Peanut oil lost 31 percent after heat treatment and 43 percent after storage; sesame oil, 36 percent and 42 percent.

☐ In another study, the oils from stored rice, corn and wheat flours were extracted and then measured for their vitamin E content. After eight days of storage, approximately half of the vitamin E content was lost.

☐ Grains, too, suffer severe tocopherol losses, both from processing and storage. Studies showed that wheat flour, bleached and aged with chlorine dioxide, lost 80 percent of its tocopherol. Dry breakfast cereals, produced with high heat for flaking, shredding and puffing, showed tocopherol losses up to 90 percent. How much vitamin E does the average American get from such sources?

☐ Another dietary source of vitamin E is from milk, but it is of lesser importance and unreliable. Studies of fluid cow's milk found its vitamin E content to vary, ranging from 1.06 mg. per quart in the middle of autumn to 0.21 mg. in early spring. In other forms of milk, vitamin E values are lower: 0.66 mg. in evaporated milk, and only 0.02 mg. in nonfat dry milk.

☐ Human milk has a higher tocopherol content than cow's milk, the average being 1.14 mg. of alpha tocopherol per quart. When mothers fail to breastfeed their infants, and depend on infant feeding formulas, they shortchange them nutritionally (and psychologically) in many respects. Vitamin E deficiency in infant feeding formulas has been a recognized problem, having been reported in the medical literature since the 1940s. Samples of infant feeding formulas (and infant cereals) were found to have very low levels of total and alpha tocopherols, believed to result from the severe losses inflicted from processing. The American Academy of Pediatrics and the Food and Nutrition Board of the National Academy of Sciences have both recommended that all infant feeding formulas should be supplemented with alpha tocopherol.

☐ What other foods in the typical American daily diet include some sources of vitamin E? Green vegetables contain this vitamin in limited amounts. But frozen foods, of all kinds, fried in vegetable oils showed severe losses of tocopherol during the time they were stored in freezers. One study, made at the request of the federal government, showed that frozen TV dinners were exceedingly deficient in vitamin E.

☐ The more food is processed, and the longer it is stored, the more severe are the losses for vitamin E. Note well the current trend: more and more processing of food, and longer shelf-life for food items. Currently, more than half of all food consumed by the average American is being used in the form of processed convenience foods. Even traditional fresh produce is declining in use. A prominent cook recently noted, "On a recent trip to California I learned that vegetables such as broccoli and fresh peas are slowly disappearing from the markets since most people only buy the frozen variety."

☐ Recent assays of vitamin E content of foods common on the American table indicate that the actual values may be far below the supposed ones. Researchers have found that the common practice of making calculations from food tables gives rise to gross errors in assessing adequate dietary intake.

☐ Using arbitrary figures of Recommended Daily Allowances (RDA) established by the Food and Nutrition Board of the National Research Council as a guideline up to 1973, borderline deficiencies of vitamin E were suspected in more than half the population of the United States. The average American diet was estimated as falling far short of those RDAs, which were 10 to 30 International Units (I.U.) daily for healthy people, with the higher figure recommended for males aged 18 to 75 or older, as well as for females during pregnancy or lactation periods. These estimates, revised and released in January 1974, drastically reduce the RDAs, with only 12 to 15 I.U. daily for males, pregnant and lactating women, and only 10 to 12 I.U. daily for other females. (The total vitamin E activity is estimated as 80 percent alpha tocopherol and 20 percent other tocopherols.) It should be noted that such recommended daily allowances are set by official boards and committees in various countries, and they are not always in agreement with one another; in fact, there is sometimes widespread disagreement.

☐ RDAs can be misleading. When such boards fail to set standards for certain nutrients, it is tacitly assumed that no human need exists. This is, of course, not necessarily true. It took the Food and Nutrition Board of the National Research Council some 30 to 40 years after the discoveries of vitamin B_6 and vitamin E before officially granting the need for these vitamins.

☐ Even detractors of the value of vitamin E concede that vitamin E supplementation is desirable in certain circumstances. Persons on diets that include high levels of polyunsaturated fats require a larger intake of vitamin E than other individuals. Premature infants suffering from hemolytic anemia (which destroys red blood cells) show very low levels of alpha tocopherol. This condition improves when such infants are supplied with vitamin E supplementation. Certain diseases and conditions are accompanied by low levels of vitamin E in the body, and are helped by vitamin E supplementation.

☐ Fats of abnormal types, indicative of a lack of vitamin E, were reported as having been detected in the blood plasma of 78 out of every 81 persons examined. These fats form as a result of the oxidation of polyunsaturated fats in the body. Of all subjects studied, 96 percent were found to be in a state of relative antioxidant deficiency. Is it possible that this condition is typical of the general population on the average American diet? ✿

VITAMIN

An identified nutrient found in raw seeds and nuts and cold-processed oils may hold the clue to natural "cholesterol washing" and longer life.

by Carlson Wade

Raw seeds and nuts and cold-processed oils are prime sources of a recently identified nutrient that goes by the name of vitamin F. While this is its unofficial identification, its functions have already been recognized as essential in helping to control cholesterol and preventing the buildup of the porridge-like sludge that contributes to the problem of atherosclerosis. Let's see how this works and how you can use foods containing vitamin F for youthful health and sparkling clean arteries.

Cholesterol is a tasteless, odorless, white fatty alcohol found in all animal fats and animal oils, in egg yolks, in milk and milk products. In pure form it is a white-like material. It does not dissolve in water.

Its word origin: *Chole,* Greek for "bile," and *sterol,* from the Greek for "solid." This is just what cholesterol is—a fat found first and abundantly in the digestive bile. (It is the stuff of which some gallstones are composed.)

If there is an increase of cholesterol, there is the risk of atherosclerosis. This is a condition in which cholesterol deposits on the arteries make them less elastic. There is a buildup of fatty material along with other "porridge" deposits in the smooth inner wall of the artery. This may cause the arteries to thicken and harden and the condition of atherosclerosis may set in.

Polyunsaturated oils made from plant sources (seeds, nuts, fruits, vegetables or grains) are prime sources of *essential fatty acids.* These are known, unofficially, as vitamin F. There are three basic vitamin F substances:

1. **Arachidonic Acid.** Useful in helping to control cholesterol and to melt down accumulated deposits from arterial walls throughout the body. This component of vitamin F is made up of the other two essential fatty acids.

2. **Linoleic Acid.** It has the beneficial effect of helping to lower cholesterol. It is also necessary for growth and reproduction, and protects against excessive dehydration or water-moisture loss. It also builds a better skin.

3. **Linolenic Acid.** Helps stimulate the manufacture of intestinal bacteria needed to produce B-complex vitamins for better skin and nerve health. It cooperates with the two listed preceding essential fatty acids to control cholesterol.

These three essential fatty acids that make up vitamin F enter into the metabolic process for your internal system's organs. They create the mechanism by which your body is able to help wash away excess cholesterol.

Where is vitamin F to be found? To begin with, this vitamin is highly sensitive to heat and processing. It is found solely in non-processed, natural and unadulterated seeds, nuts, fruits, vegetables and grains. It is highly abundant in the nonprocessed and cold-processed oils made from these foods. Such products are available in all health stores. These oils are prime sources of the precious cholesterol-washing vitamin F.

You should *substitute* plant oils for animal fats. The key here is to *substitute, not* to add. Doctors all agree that the effective lowering of cholesterol becomes possible when plant oils (rich in vitamin F) are used as fats in the diet.

Lecithin

Another good source of vitamin F is found in lecithin. This is a bland, water-soluble granular powder made from de-fatted soy beans. Lecithin is sold at all health stores. It contains phosphorus as well as other components that work in harmony with its supply of essential fatty acids to help create better body health and heart-saving cholesterol washing.

Writing in *Let's Eat Right To Keep Fit*, nutritionist-author Adelle Davis explains how vitamin F in lecithin can improve your health:

New Hope for Cholesterol Control

"Another cousin of the fat family, lecithin is supplied by all natural oils . . . Lecithin is an excellent source of the two B vitamins choline and inositol; if health is to be maintained, the more fat eaten, the larger must be the intake of these two vitamins. This substance can be made in the intestinal wall provided choline, inositol and essential fatty acids [or vitamin F] are supplied.

"Lecithin appears to be a homogenizing agent, capable of breaking fat and probably cholesterol into tiny particles which can pass readily into the tissues. There is evidence that coronary occlusion is associated with deficiencies of linoleic acid [one of the elements of vitamin F] and the two B vitamins, choline and inositol, and perhaps with a lack of lecithin itself.

"Huge particles of cholesterol get stuck in the walls of the arteries; they might be homogenized into tiny particles if sufficient nutrients were available for the normal production of lecithin. When oils are refined or hydrogenated, lecithin is discarded."

Here we see that lecithin as well as the essential fatty acids found in plant foods and plant oils are highly perishable. Therefore, to get your full bonus of vitamin F, the three essential fatty acids, you should use non-processed and unrefined oils. These are sold at all health stores.

The cold pressed method is favorable to the protection of vitamin F. By means of a hydraulic press, the nuts, grains, beans, seeds, olives, or vegetables are pressed so that their oils are extracted. A mechanical expeller press is used to squeeze the oils from the plant. Pressure is exerted on the oil seeds through a continuously revolving shaft against a fixed surface. Because this "expeller press" or "cold-pressed" method is used *without heat*, it produces oils that are as close to the natural state as possible. Such oils have the best color, odor, flavor and vitamin F content.

How To Use Oils

1. *Keep Temperature Low in Cooking.* Use lower heat when cooking with plant oils to preserve the valuable vitamin F content. Furthermore, high heat may cause the oil to splatter. (If this happens, add a few slices of onion or a fistful of parsley to the oil. They reduce splattering and add flavor at the same time.)

2. *Tenderizing.* Oil does help to tenderize meat. Tests have shown that meat marinated for an hour or longer with oil or a herb-seasoned mixture will remain more juicy and tender during roasting or barbecuing. Holes should first be punched in the meat, then the oil forced into the holes with a barbecue brush. This gives you some vitamin F. Remember that heating will cause evaporation to a large extent. But it is the natural way to tenderize meat.

3. *Salads.* When combined with apple cider vinegar or lemon juice and a bit of honey, oil becomes a vitamin F salad dressing that is good to your heart and arteries.

4. *Sauces.* Oil is especially good with tomato or tart bases, giving the sauce a silky-smooth texture. Use oil as a natural sauce for flavor and vitamin F, too.

Most health stores carry a wide variety of these plant oils that are non-processed and, therefore, good sources of cholesterol-washing vitamin F. Each oil has its own unique taste. You may even blend them together for exciting zest. Some vitamin F oils sold at health stores include: almond oil, apricot oil, corn oil, garlic 'n' oil, linseed oil, sesame seed oil, soy oil, sunflower oil, walnut oil, wheat germ oil.

Use these oils whenever a fat is called for. Use them raw, wherever possible.

It's the latest discovery of the natural way to help control cholesterol—*using vitamin F to wash arteries clean.*

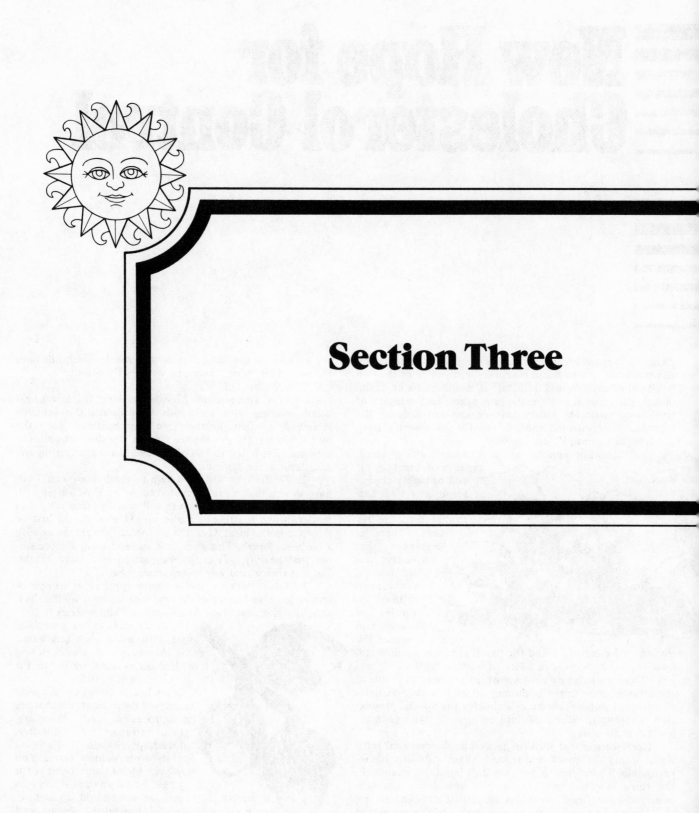

Section Three

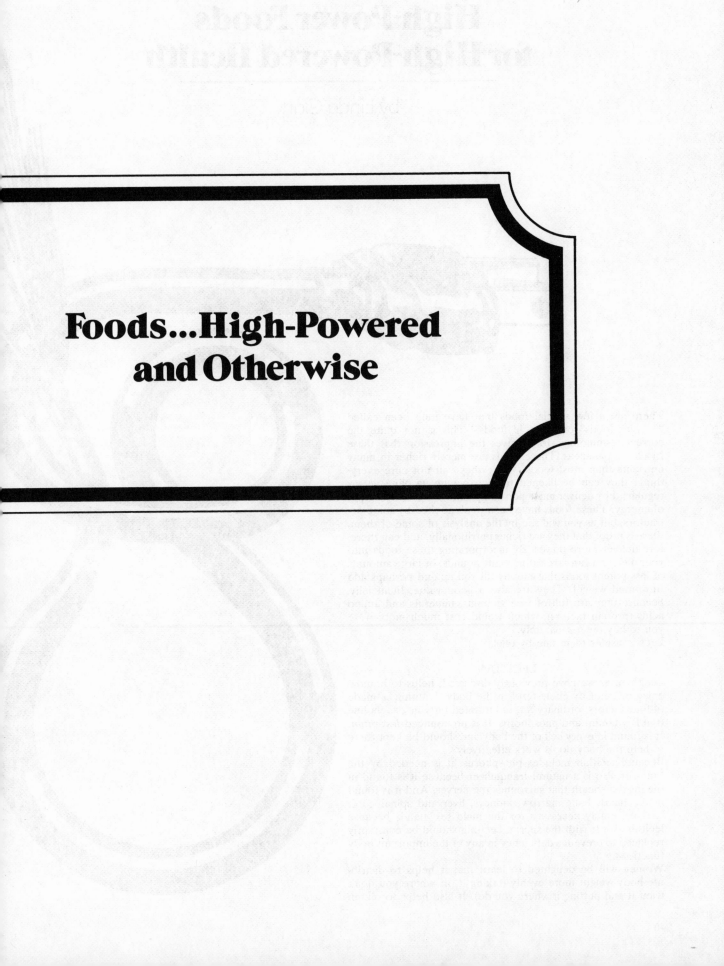

Foods...High-Powered
and Otherwise

High-Power Foods for High-Powered Health

by Linda Clark

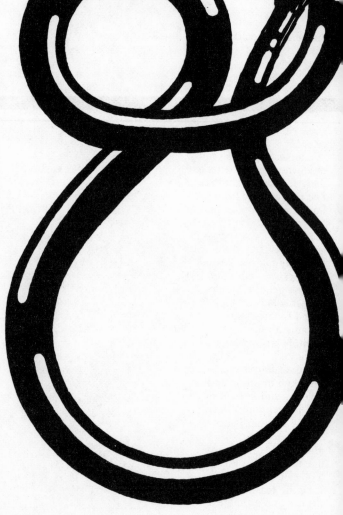

There are a few special foods that have long been called "wonder foods" or "miracle foods." This is not quite the correct terminology, for it gives the impression that these foods are panaceas. These foods are merely richer in many nutrients than most foods. While they will not cure everything, they can be likened to high octane gasoline versus regular: they deliver more pep and promote a greater output of energy. These foods have been pooh-poohed by some detractors, but as you will see by the analysis of some of them, there is proof that they are richer nutritionally, and can therefore deliver more power. By incorporating these foods into your diet, you can save eating many pounds, or large amounts of less potent foods that merely fill you up and perhaps add unwanted weight. They are also a good value, financially, because they are full of free vitamins, minerals and amino acids (protein factors), which would cost much more were you to buy them separately.

Let's consider them one by one.

LECITHIN

Lecithin, as we have previously discussed, helps to homogenize or emulsify cholesterol in the body. Lecithin is made of four factors: ordinary fat, unsaturated fatty acids, choline (the B vitamin) and phosphorus. It is pronounced *less-i-thin*. It is found in every cell of the body and should be kept there to help the body do its work effectively.

Because lecithin includes phosphorus, it is needed by the brain. It also is a natural tranquilizer because it is found in the myelin sheath that surrounds the nerves. And it is found in the heart, bone marrow, kidneys, liver and spinal cord. It is extremely necessary for the male sex glands because lecithin is lost with the sperm. Lecithin should be constantly replaced to prevent a deficiency in any of the important body functions.

Women will be delighted to learn that it helps to distribute body weight more evenly (taking it off where you don't want it and putting it where you do). It also helps to plump

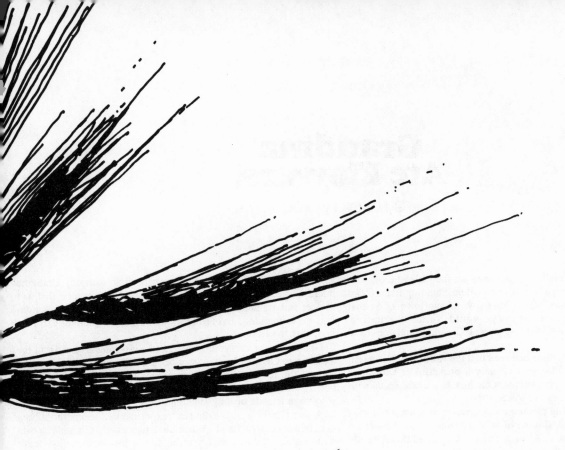

up the skin. Lecithin works slowly to accomplish its wonders, but it works exceedingly well. Cases of heart disturbance, high cholesterol, angina and myasthenia gravis have responded to lecithin. *Medical World News* has reported that it may be helpful in preventing gallstones.

Roger J. Williams, Ph.D., confirms what we have been saying about the effect of lecithin on cholesterol. He says not to shun cholesterol foods but to "consume more lecithin." He cites the work of Lester M. Morrison, M.D., who found that the cholesterol levels in the blood of twelve patients were lowered when the patients consumed about an ounce of lecithin daily for three months.

Lecithin is made from soybeans. It is available in three forms: liquid, powder and granules. The granules have been used for many years by Dr. Morrison and by Adelle Davis, who recommended three to six tablespoons daily to lower a high cholesterol level. She told of a ten-year-old girl with an abnormally high cholesterol level, as well as a heart condition. The girl was bedridden and had been given up by the doctors. Daily, several tablespoons of lecithin granules were sprinkled on her salads or added to juice, and she was given vitamins B and E and unsaturated oil. She recovered. Her cholesterol became normal and she was able to return to school.

Lecithin is tasteless in any form. Hans Wohlgemuth, a lecithin researcher, believes that liquid lecithin is effective in lesser amounts than the other forms. He believes that one teaspoonful taken morning and evening is enough to overcome a deficiency and keep it in the blood at all times for protection and prevention of lecithin-deficiency disturbances.

Liquid lecithin is not easy to take until you get used to it. It looks like honey and pours like honey, but there the similarity ends. It certainly does not taste like honey. (It tastes like nothing.) It also tends to stick to the roof of the mouth. You can try it in, or followed by, a tart fruit juice. If you take it by the teaspoonful, it will stick to the spoon. I usually tip the can and estimate a teaspoonful as it flows into my mouth. Then I follow with a tart fruit juice or hot drink. (When you

begin to follow the nutritional way of life, you cease to be fussy.) All types of lecithin are available at health stores.

HERE IS AN ANALYSIS OF LECITHIN:

	Content per 100 grams
Moisture (%)	1.33 gm
Protein (%)	4.53 gm
Ether extract (%)	99.95 gm
Crude fiber	Trace gm
Ash (%)	6.83 gm
Calcium (mgm/gm)	92 mg
Phosphorus (mgm/gm)	2140 mg
Copper (meg/gm)	100 meg
Total iron (meg/gm)	6.5 mg
Available iron (meg/gm)	0.360 mg
Manganese	0.00
Cobalt	0.00
Magnesium (mgm/gm)	164. mgm
Potassium (mgm/gm)	170. mgm
Iodine	0.00
U.S.P. units vitamin A (gm)	100. USP units
Thiamine (meg/gm)	11.5 meg
Riboflavin (meg/gm)	33. meg
Pantothenic acid (meg/gm)	5.59. meg
Niacin (meg/gm)	12. meg
Pyridoxine (meg/gm)	29. meg
Choline (mgm/gm)	2.931 mgm
Ascorbic acid	0.00
Vitamin K (gm)	589. units
Biotin (meg/gm)	0.00
Inositol (mgm/gm)	2.1 gm
Folic acid (meg/gm)	60. meg

(continued on page 250)

Grandma Ate Flowers!

by Lelord Kordel

Among my earliest childhood memories are the walks I took with my grandmother through her flower garden. Standing like golden giants against the fence was a long row of sunflowers. At that time, nobody in this country would think of eating sunflowers . . . nobody, that is, except Grandma and me—and the birds!

☐ For somewhere Grandma had read that the Russian and Turkish armies could march all day, with only a pocketful of sunflower seeds to sustain them. So she taught me how to hull the seeds with my teeth and fingers, as the soldiers did.

☐ One day, after lifting me numerous times to reach the tall sunflowers, Grandma picked some lilies of the valley and sat down on the grass to munch them. Always curious, I squatted down beside her and asked, "Are they good, Grandma?"

☐ "Good for a fast heart," she replied. "Is your heart fast?"

☐ "Only when I run. When is yours fast?"

☐ "Only when I lift a heavy boy sky-high a dozen times."

☐ Grandma laughed, tucking the rest of the flowers in her hair. "And tonight, for supper, we're having something even better to slow down a fast heart—asparagus!"

☐ That was my grandmother—a walking encyclopedia of the strangest information. Like the spring day she picked a bachelor's button, crushed it and rubbed it on my neck.

☐ "It's time I made an infusion of these," she said, "to keep mosquitoes away and to have on hand as a strengthening tonic."

☐ Infusion . . strengthening tonic . . . what odd-sounding words to a boy just learning to read. In the months and years that followed, I was also to discover the exotic names of plants that grew in Grandma's garden but rarely appeared in picture books—like comfrey and coltsfoot, horehound and hops, chamomile and mullein, filárée and nettle.

☐ But it was Grandma's vast storehouse of facts that never ceased to amaze me . . . and still does.

☐ Though I was only five years old, can I ever forget that day she sat on the back steps, her straight frame slumped a little, eating honeysuckle? When Grandma saw me peeking through the screen door, she patted the steps in an invitation to join her. With only a faint smile of welcome, she handed me some honeysuckle from the trellised vines around the porch. I was biting the ends off the flowers, sucking the drops of nectar and throwing the rest away, when I noticed that Grandma was eating the whole blossom.

☐ "Nothing like honeysuckle blooms," she said, "to lift the spirits when you're feeling spleenish and downcast." (Two more new words!)

☐ Grandma was always eager to convey her knowledge to others. "Spring crocus," she once told me, "was known as the 'bicarbonate of soda' of medieval times, before folks replaced it with more trustworthy flowers. I never did put much trust in a crocus."

☐ I never did get to ask what she meant by "more trustworthy" flowers, and why she didn't "trust" a crocus! For Grandma had boundless faith in the healing power of nature—a faith she imparted to all around her. But it wasn't faith alone that made her an "authority."

☐ When she and my grandfather were first married, Grandma made home remedies of the same natural substances that her mother and grandmother had used. Before long, she began searching, experimenting, trying out a new remedy or adding extra ingredients to old ones.

☐ Grandma read everything she could get her hands on, from the almanac to Grandpa's chemistry books, an assortment of herbals, and all the medical and scientific books and journals she could borrow from doctors, whom she had no faith in professionally, but who were friends of long standing.

☐ As her family grew, so did her "experiments." Sometimes both got a little out of hand. When that happened, Grandpa would remonstrate, "Why can't you be like other women and leave well-enough alone?"

☐ "Because well-enough isn't good enough," she would answer, "and I want to make it better!"

☐ How could Grandpa fight such "logic"? Secretly, I think, he loved those arguments.

☐ Like the day Grandma proudly invited us all to dinner, to savor her first flower recipes: unopened buds of day lilies dipped in beaten eggs and sautéed, green buds of sunflowers steamed and lightly buttered, a salad consisting of dandelion leaves and blossoms and the leaves and flowers of violets, nasturtiums, and borage.

☐ "How in blazes do you know that these conglomerations won't poison us?" Grandpa growled.

☐ "Because I've already tried them," Grandma said gaily.

☐ And she had. But make no mistake about it: before testing them herself, Grandma spent many months studying every scrap of information she could lay her hands on.

☐ "Don't you ever go popping flowers or anything else in your mouth unless you know what you're eating," she once warned me sternly. "Some flowers and weeds are good for you, and some can make you sick—even kill you. Until you learn the difference, you be sure to ask me."

☐ In addition to her vast knowledge, my grandmother had a great flair for the dramatic.

☐ "Ralphie Kurnick!" she once shouted at a friend who'd come to play with me. "You go straight home so your mamma can doctor that cold!"

☐ Sniffling sadly, Ralphie peered at me dejectedly through swollen, watery eyes, and started for the door.

☐ "Wait a minute," said Grandma, her face lighting up impishly. "What's Mother doing for that cold?"

☐ Ralphie rubbed his nose on his sleeve and mumbled, "Some pills and stuff."

☐ "Pills! Come back here, Ralphie! You can stay a while if you and Lee play in the garden."

☐ Soon Grandma joined us, carrying honey-sweetened lemonade, rose-hip-jelly sandwiches (on homemade bread) , and a basket of fresh violets.

☐ As we ate our sandwiches, Ralphie suddenly gawked and sput-

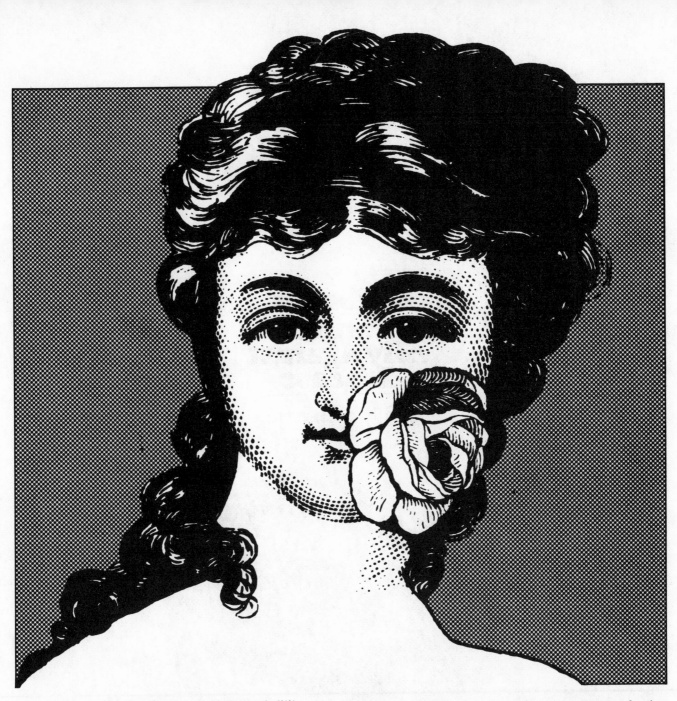

tered, "Your grandma's eating flowers, leaves and all!"

□ "Sure," I said matter-of-factly, "flowers taste good. May we have some, Grandma?"

□ Little did I realize that we'd played right into her hands. After giving us each a handful of violet blossoms and leaves, Grandma vanished into the kitchen.

□ As Ralphie downed his flower-snack—timidly at first, then with gusto—Grandma returned with a small bundle for him. How strange she must have sounded to the neighbors when she sent Ralphie home, shouting: "Now don't you forget, Ralphie! Tell your mother to give you the honey and horehound night and morning, and two garlic cloves, a spoonful of rose hips, and a fistful of violets every three hours!"

□ What a performance!

□ Needless to say, there were lots of people who scoffed at my grandmother, pitied her, laughed behind her back. Some of my friends, with an honesty that is the province of children and saints, even told me that their parents considered Grandma "tetched."

□ It never troubled me. They were all jealous, I concluded, because even at that early age, I realized that my grandmother was different.

□ She looked younger, prettier, healthier, and was more fun than other grandmothers. In an emergency or during an illness, she was always the one who knew what to do, promptly and decisively.

□ It was old, argumentative Grandpa who long ago advised, "Pay attention to your grandma and listen to what she tells you. Someday you'll realize that she's a woman far ahead of her time."

□ I recalled those words, one day, when a visitor asked Grandma, "Why do you trouble yourself with plants and home remedies when the drugstore carries plenty of patent medicine?"

□ "Patent fiddlesticks!" Grandma exploded.

□ I tugged at her apron and promised, "Don't worry about me, Grandma. I'll never take any patent fiddlesticks!"

□ A smile chased the indignation from her face, and she patted my head. "That's a good boy, Lee. You see that you don't."

□ More than sixty years have passed, and I still haven't broken that promise. Why should I? My grandmother remained hale and hearty until the day she died . . . at the age of one hundred and one!   ☼

Soybeans, Nature's Ally Against Disease

by Philip S. Chen, Ph.D.

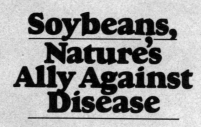

□ Not only is the soybean an excellent food from the standpoint of nutrition, but it also prevents or cures many of the common diseases which take a heavy toll of human lives each year and cause untold misery and suffering. Among these common diseases may be mentioned coronary disease, arteriosclerosis, diabetes, intestinal disturbances, and diseases due to food allergy.

□ Much research has revealed that one of the causes of both coronary disease and arteriosclerosis is the cholesterol which is found in all animal fats including meat, eggs and milk. On the other hand, soybeans, being of vegetable origin, contain phytosterol instead of cholesterol in the unsaponifiable portion of its oil. The use of soybeans in the human diet therefore does not contribute to coronary disease and arteriosclerosis.

□ Furthermore, credit is due the soybeans in that they contain a factor which aids in the cure of these diseases—phospholipids, which are used in the food industry under the name of lecithin.

□ The actual agent that is responsible for mobilizing cholesterol is not lecithin itself, however, but rather the choline molecule derived from it. Choline was claimed by Charles H. Best of the University of Toronto (*Chemical and Engineering News*, February 15, 1955), to be the missing factor responsible for liver damage in diabetic dogs and in rats on certain diets. Addition of choline prevented or cured the fatty livers. Further work, carried out in the United States, has shown that prolonged consumption of choline-poor diets eventually produces a shrunken, leathery liver, similar in many ways to cirrhosis of the liver in the chronic alcoholic.

□ In some species choline deficiency can produce kidney damage severe enough to cause uremia and death. Short periods of choline deficiency in a young animal may produce kidney damage resulting in development of high blood pressure.

□ Such a substance as choline, which is able to alter fat into another form or otherwise remove its accumulation in an organ, is known as a "lipotropic agent." In addition to choline, the soybean contains yet another lipotropic agent, namely, inositol. It is also a constituent of soy lecithin. Both of these lipotropic agents are members of the vitamin B complex, and are important factors for growth and lactation.

□ Choline and soybean lecithin are effective in preventing perosis or "slipped tendon" in poultry.

□ The soybean, by virtue of its high protein and very low starch content, has been extensively used in the dietary of diabetic patients. It was found that the soybean in some way causes a reduction in percentage and total quantity of sugar passed into the urine in diabetic persons on the usual dietary restrictions.

□ According to Dr. H. W. Dietrich of Texas, it is the lecithin in the soybean that is especially beneficial to diabetic patients. He found that soy lecithin and tocopherol given orally decrease insulin requirements and seem to have a favorable influence on diabetes.

□ Since lecithin has been found to counteract various substances, such as antibiotics and toxins, which interfere with phosphorylation (a chemical reaction by which blood sugar is utilized through its combination with phosphoric acid), he reasonably explains the action of lecithin as that of counteracting the effect of the diabetogenic hormone by partial restoration of the phosphorylating mechanism.

□ According to recent reports, both plant sterols and unsaturated fatty acids, of which the soybean is the best known food source, are found to lower the cholesterol content of the blood.

□ Much work has been done on the soybean's unique property of creating and maintaining a favorable intestinal flora. Dr. A. A. Horvath has summarized this work in "Some Recent Views about Soya Flour" from which we quote the following:

□ "As to the intestinal digestion it is of importance to mention that Von Noorden has demonstrated that the soybean is of very great service in changing the intestinal flora, helping materially in driving out the offensive germs which pollute our bodies and give rise to colitis and other acute and chronic infections besides headaches, skin troubles and a great variety of obstinate chronic maladies. This partly explains why Dr. Ruhrah obtained such good results from a soya diet in cases of summer diarrhea in children. Drs. Ribadeau-Dumas, Mathieu and Willemin of the Salpetriere Hospital in Paris made somewhat similar observations, and recently Prof. Mader recorded that on an exclusive diet of soya flour the intestinal flora is turning Gram-positive.

□ "In a recent personal letter to the writer, Dr. John Harvey Kellogg of the Battle Creek Sanitarium brings out the following interesting experience: 'We are making increasing use of the soy acidophilus with splendid results. I am sure it is very much superior to ordinary acidophilus milk as a means of changing the flora. It seems to stimulate greatly the growth of the acidophilus, whereas cow's milk is such an unfavorable medium that prolonged training is necessary to bring the organism up to a degree of activity sufficient to produce a good quality of buttermilk. The soy milk requires no such training. A slow-growing dying milk culture when placed in soy milk springs into rejuvenescence at once, producing a good quality of buttermilk in less than 24 hours. It seems evident that a medium which exercises such a stimulating effect upon the growth of acidophilus in vitro ought to be equally superior in the intestines. We find it of special value in old cases of toxemia in which the conditions are so unfavorable that the acidophilus has entirely disappeared. In such cases the soy acidophilus will reimplant the normal acidophilus flora within a week or two after other measures employed for months or even years have utterly failed.' "

□ According to E. C. Scott of Beltsville, Maryland, soybean oil is an ideal remedy for constipation. Below is his letter to the editor of *The Soybean Digest* (4(5):5, March 1944):

□ "I should like to recite my own personal experience in the use of soybean oil and offer it for possible consideration as one of the uses of soybeans after the war.

(continued on page 253)

KEFIR:
Yogurt Fanciers Are Finding That Marco Polo's Drink Makes You Feel Better!

by Beatrice Trum Hunter

Kefir is a rather well-known fermented milk drink long enjoyed throughout the Balkan countries. Moslems in the Caucasus thought that the ferment of kefir, or ''Grains of the Prophet Mohammed'' would lose its strength if people of other religions would use it. For this reason, the preparation of kefir remained a secret for a long time. It is thought that the word ''kefir'' came from keif, a Turkish word meaning ''good feeling,'' for the sense of well-being experienced after drinking this fermented milk product.

Outside of the Caucasus, kefir was scarcely known. Marco Polo mentioned kefir in his account of his Eastern travels. After that, for nearly five centuries, kefir was forgotten in the West. Renewed interest in kefir was displayed in the early nineteenth century when it was used therapeutically for tuberculosis at lung sanatoriums. Today, many of the qualities in kefir have become recognized as being similar to those in yogurt; however, kefir has some unique properties.

Kefir ''grains,'' the fermenting agent, are convoluted gelatinous particles obtained from fermented milk of a type commonly prepared in the countries of southwestern Asia. In appearance, they have been described as looking like cauliflower pieces, or coral-like. The kefir grains vary in size from the size of a grain of wheat to that of a hazelnut. They contain three kinds of lactic acid bacteria, and lactose-fermenting yeasts.

What are the unique properties of kefir? Kefir has a very low curd tension. This means that the curd breaks up very easily into extremely small particles. (The curd of yogurt holds together or breaks into lumps.) The small particle size of the kefir curd facilitates its digestion by presenting a large surface for the digestion agents to work on. This ease of digestion has led to many researchers recommending kefir as a food particularly beneficial to infants, convalescents, elderly persons, or persons with insufficient digestive activity.

It has been found that kefir stimulates the flow of saliva, probably due to its acid content and its slight amount of carbonation. Kefir increases the flow of digestive juices in the gastrointestinal tract, and stimulates peristalsis. Because of this latter virtue, kefir has been recommended as a post-operative food, since many abdominal operations cause the temporary cessation of peristalsis, accompanied by gas pains. A noted Danish dairy bacteriologist, Dr. Orla-Jenson, expressed the opinion that kefir has a *higher* nutritive value than yogurt due to the abundance of yeast cells digested and the beneficial effect on the intestinal flora.

In addition to the above virtues, kefir is different from yogurt in at least two other respects. Kefir is of a thin consistency, and generally is drunk, like buttermilk; yogurt is usually of a thicker consistency, and generally is eaten. In preparing milk for yogurt, it must be heated in order to destroy unfavorable microorganisms that would otherwise interfere with the fermentation. In preparing milk for kefir, the milk does *not* need to be heated. Hence, if one has access to Certified Raw Milk or a source of clean fresh raw milk, he has an ideal medium for culturing kefir.

In other respects, kefir has as many similar nutritional qualities and physiological effects as other cultured milk products. Kefir is laxative, and in Germany and in the Soviet Union it is used extensively with cases of chronic constipation. Kefir, like yogurt, is used for a wide variety of intestinal disorders. Kefir, like yogurt, also displays bactericidal powers against some virulent pathogenic organisms, and is also useful for reestablishing the ''friendly flora'' in the intestine after antibiotics have been administered.

Kefir grains are available in several forms. They are shipped commercially through the mail, suspended in milk. They are also sold in freeze-dried form. Although attempts have been made to process them in tablet, cake, and wafer forms, to date, such processed products appear to lose much of their value since the heat above 120° F. used in the processing, destroys lactic acid bacteria.

Homemade kefir: Obtain a supply of fresh kefir grains, suspended in milk. Culturing them is very simple. Add the kefir grains to whole or skim milk, stir, cover, and allow the mixture to remain at room temperature (65° to 76° F.) for two to three days. At the end of this time, the milk will have thickened. Pour it through a sieve. What drains through is the drinkable kefir. What remain in the seive are the active kefir grains, which can be used, over and over again, to culture future batches. Before transferring the grains to a new supply of milk, rinse them thoroughly in a sieve, using cool, running water. Drain off the excess water, and add the washed grains to the new batch of fresh milk you wish to culture. The proportion of grains to milk should be about one teacup of kefir grains to one quart of milk. As you continue to culture, the number of kefir grains will thrive and multiply. This increase takes place most rapidly when the kefir grains are cultured in skim or low-fat milk (less than 1 percent butterfat held at room temperature (68° to 70° F.).

If you wish to slow down the multiplication of kefir grains, hold the culturing milk at a lower temperature (55° to 60° F.). If you do this, you will only have to make batches of kefir weekly instead of every second or third day. Your choice may be determined by the amount of kefir you wish to consume.

When your grains multiply, and you find you have more than a teacupful for each quart of milk, you will have to come to a decision. You can allow the abundance of grains to remain, which will result in a thicker product. In time, the extra grains will have to

(continued on page 254)

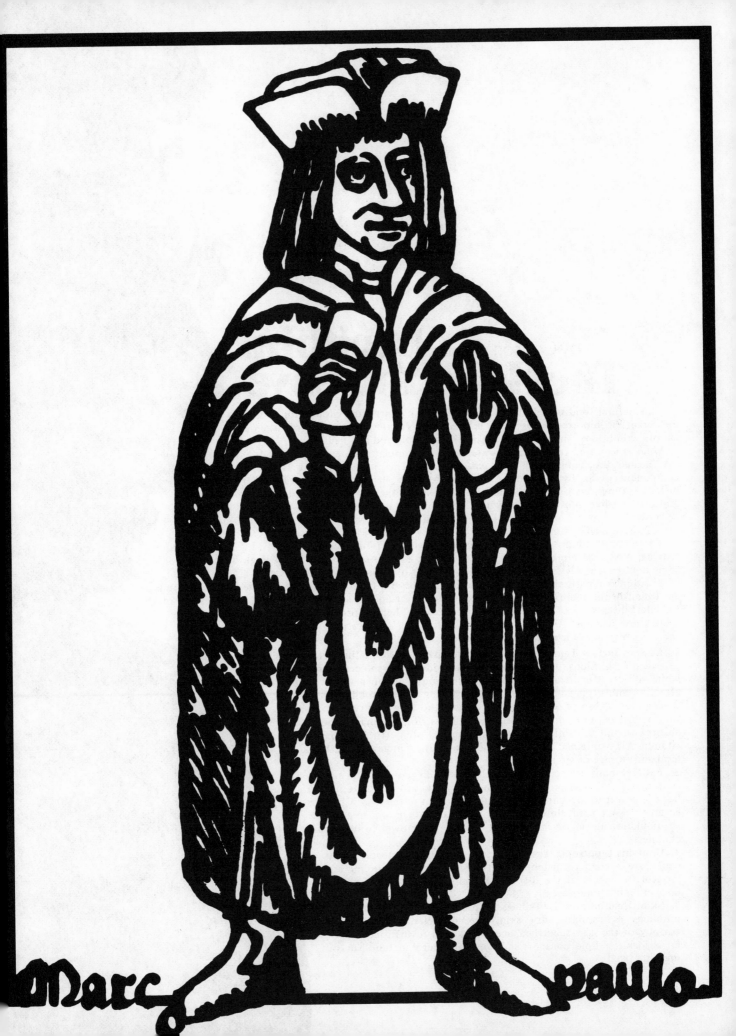

by Carlson Wade Lecithin: The Heart You Save

This natural food is considered to be helpful in controlling cholesterol. More important, it reportedly has been helpful in *preventing* the onset of atherosclerotic conditions. Many doctors regard this natural food as a heart saver.

What is lecithin? It is a bland, water-soluble, granular powder made from de-fatted soy beans. Biochemists call it a *phosphatide*. This means that it is an essential component of all living tissues and cells. As such, lecithin plays a valuable role in different functions of body chemistry. Lecithin is the most important member of a group of fat-like substances known as phosphatides or phospholipids. They are so called because they contain phosphorus (also nitrogen), together with the usual fat constituents of carbon, hydrogen and oxygen.

The name lecithin is taken from the Greek word *likithos* meaning "egg yolk." It is known that egg yolk has more than 6 percent lecithin. But, since egg yolk is also high in cholesterol, some doctors will advise against using it as a means of reducing body cholesterol.

Lecithin is a natural substance found in all cells and tissues. In the body, the largest amounts are found in the brain and nerve tissues, endocrine glands, kidneys and heart. Lecithin is one of the latest discoveries in the quest for substances that help to prolong the prime of life.

Research chemist, Dr. Philip S. Chen, author of *Heart Disease: Cause, Prevention and Recovery,* lauds lecithin for these reasons:

1. **Lowers Surface Tension.** Lecithin is effective in lowering the surface tension of aqueous solutions. The reason is that one side of the molecule prefers fat, while the other is attracted by water. This unique action makes lecithin an effective emulsifying agent, capable of dissolving cholesterol deposits.

2. **Improves Absorption.** Lecithin increases the digestibility and absorption of fats because of its emulsifying abilities. It also enhances both the absorption and utilization of vitamin A and carotene (the precursor of vitamin A as obtained from a meatless source). It increases the blood level and storage of vitamin A.

3. **Fat Metabolism.** Lecithin boosts the metabolism of fat. The enzyme, lecithinase, which is produced in the body, sets free choline, which has the power to prevent the accumulation of fat in the liver. Choline is able to alter fat into another form, or otherwise remove its accumulation in an organ. Lecithin contains the power to invigorate choline.

4. **Contains Lipotropic Agents.** Lecithin contains lipotropic agents which are needed to metabolize fat. It contains both choline and inositol (members of the B-complex family) which enter into the fat metabolization process.

5. **Skin Health.** Soy lecithin is helpful in treating such skin problems as psoriasis, dry skin, eczema, scleroderma, senile atrophy of the skin, seborrhea, acne and keloid formation, due to fat absorption, lipid transport and even cholesterol metabolism of the skin, itself.

May Be
Your Own

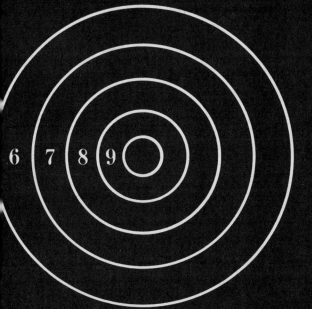

6. Diabetic Help. Lecithin reportedly may be able to decrease the needs of insulin requirements, by better absorption and metabolism of sugars and starches via the pancreas.

7. Lecithin improves the absorption of fat and lowers the susceptibility for problems of sprue (improper digestive absorption of fats and carbohydrates) and diarrhea.

8. Better Liver Function. Deranged fat metabolism often responds to soy lecithin and this helps improve problems of liver dysfunction.

9. Kidney Health. Lecithin helps correct a problem of deficiency in choline or other lipotropic agents which may cause hemorrhagic degeneration of the kidney.

10. Internal Cleansing. The lipotropic substances in soy lecithin often help clear up vitreous opacities (the forerunner of cholesterol deposits—a colorless thickening).

Dr. Chen quotes from *Phospholipids*, a publication of

(continued on page 255)

Piimä --
Remarkable Culture
from Nomad's Land

by Gena Larson

For centuries every successful dietary pattern has included lactic acid foods that were eaten regularly. Fermenting and culturing were among the earliest methods known to preserve foods beyond their natural season and help to add variety to meager diets. Nomadic peoples cultured their foods in order to transport them long distances without spoilage as they had no refrigeration or modern canning processes.

The health-giving properties of the lactic acid "buddy" bacteria were held in high esteem by the primitive peoples, and precious starters and fermenting formulas were handed down from mother to daughter or passed from friend to friend.

Yogurt, kefir, buttermilk and other raw cultured milk products have a fine curd which may permit them to be digested more quickly than plain milk.

These valuable cultured foods are particularly necessary after the use of antibiotics, to replenish the friendly bacteria in the bowel which have been destroyed by the medication.

Years ago a friend gave me a starter of a raw milk yogurt from Finland. This remarkable culture called piimä makes it possible to culture fresh raw milk at room temperature, thus preserving the valuable enzymes and other nutrients present in the unheated milk.

No special equipment is needed except an ordinary wide-mouth canning jar or a mayonnaise jar with a lid.

This precious culture has been used in our family continuously for the last twenty years and I have made starters for many friends both near and far.

Now I am so happy to tell you that a freeze-dried piimä yogurt starter is now (or soon will be) available in your health food store. If it isn't there yet, write me at this magazine for information about where it may be obtained. It comes in a handy little packet suitable for popping into an envelope and mailing to a friend. The starter can be stored for a long time in your refrigerator. To those who have lost their piimä starter by accident or from disuse this will be welcome news I know.

When you get your starter observe these precautions:

Use the freshest milk available. Milk warm from the cow is ideal but any cold fresh milk will become room temperature after a few hours. Do not heat it — ever. Do not use a yogurt maker. This would quickly kill the little organism.

Be sure there is no detergent residue left in your jars as this would prevent the milk from "setting up" or thickening. Also, if the milk contains an antibiotic it will not set.

It is quite a shock to the little organism to be freeze-dried. Treat it gently until it is revived.

To make your first bottle of piimä yogurt follow to the letter the directions on the package. If your kitchen is a cool 62° you may wish to reserve a high shelf in your kitchen cabinets for culturing where the temperature would be warmer — 72° to 78° is fine. In winter I sometimes bring my piimä in the living room, near a warm rock wall. In summer I culture on the kitchen counter, covering with a clean heavy towel to exclude the light which would destroy the riboflavin.

Piimä yogurt is a product that is compatible with and does not digest the other "friendly bacteria" (symbionts) of the small and large intestine.

Piimä will not set up in goat's milk, alas! Though I do have one friend who was able to make it successfully in half goat and half cow milk. You can make it from pasteurized milk although the flavor and nutrition do not compare with raw milk piimä. In an emergency, such as when traveling, if you cannot get raw milk use any milk you can get to preserve your starter. If possible make a new batch of piimä at least once or twice a week to keep your starter fresh and

working. If you have friends who own a cow, by all means give them a starter in case you need to borrow one back some day.

RECIPES

Piimä

To make the first bottle of piimä yogurt follow to the letter the directions on the package. After that proceed as follows:

Place 1/2 teaspoon prepared piimä in a pint, wide-mouth glass jar (or 1 teaspoon in a quart). Stir to make it smooth, then fill the jar with safe raw milk. Stir again to mix well, then cover and culture at room temperature for 16 to 20 hours, or until set like custard. Milk warm from the cow will culture faster but cold milk will culture in a few more hours. On a frosty winter morning I sometimes set my bottle of milk in a pan of lukewarm water for a few minutes before I start my culture, but under *no circumstances* warm the milk after it is mixed with your starter. Just be patient, it will get thick and firm at room temperature and all the valuable enzymes and nutrients will be preserved.

Piimä Cream

Each bottle of yogurt will have on the top about an inch of luscious cultured sour cream. This may be used to top a baked potato or fruit salad, as a salad ingredient or in any of your favorite sour cream dips, sauces, or dessert recipes.

If you require more cream than this just follow the directions for piimä yogurt, adding cream instead of milk to your starter. A very thick cream and a longer culturing time will make a product very like cream cheese, firm enough to be used as a spread for bread or to use in any recipe calling for cream cheese.

80 percent of the symbionts of the human bowel are lactobacillus bifidus. The other 20 percent are lactobacillus

(continued on page 256)

Garlic:
Don't "Put It Down," It's Good for You

by Lloyd J. Harris

Since World War I, extensive research has been carried out on garlic in many European and Asian countries. Part of this interest in garlic is a result of the successful use of garlic as an antiseptic in cases of gangrene and other serious infections. In the First War, garlic was applied to wounds to control suppuration (the formation and discharge of pus). In World War II, garlic was given credit for lowering the incidence of septic poisoning among wounded soldiers; not one case of gangrene or septic poisoning was reported among men receiving the garlic treatments.

The following information has been organized both according to areas of research (hypertension, cancer, the common cold, etc.), and within these areas, chronologically.

Gastro-Intestinal Disorders and Hypertension

During W.W.I, Marcovici, an army doctor on the Eastern front in 1915, carried out many experiments with garlic. For twenty-five years thereafter he used garlic therapy successfully in many gastro-intestinal disorders, and reported his findings in the *Medical Record* (January, 1941). In his experiments during the war with cases of dysentery, he administered one bulb of garlic per day, prepared in various forms. Rapid improvement followed both for subjective and objective symptoms. Evacuations decreased and appetite returned.

When garlic pills came on the market, Marcovici began to use them instead of fresh garlic. In 1925, Sandoz Company introduced Allisatin, a pill that contained the active principle of garlic, allicin, plus vegetable charcoal — the absorptive quality of this additive allowed the allicin to be released slowly enroute through the intestines, thus limiting the odor of the garlic. Marcovici used Allisatin successfully in dyspepsia, diarrhea, enterocolitis, fermentation, and as a treatment for symptoms of hypertension. His therapy consisted of two to four garlic tablets three times daily. Larger amounts were sometimes administered, but this increased the odor factor.

Later Marcovici was encouraged by clinical results with experiments undertaken at the Sero-therapeutic Institute of Vienna. These experiments were conducted with rabbits.

THE EXPERIMENT: Rabbits were fed dried garlic powder for several days. Dysentery toxins were then administered intravenously. Results: 2.5 grams daily of powdered garlic for three days prior to injections protected animals against a ten-fold dose of dysentery toxin. The garlic cured rabbits when it was given concomitantly with toxin (but not before injections). Many of these rabbits became ill, but none died. All of the control group given toxin but no garlic, died.

Marcovici also found garlic effective against hypertension. One of the symptoms of hypertension is high blood pressure. The exact causes of high blood pressure are complex, and many of those who studied garlic's power to reduce blood pressure could not agree on how it did the job. Marcovici said that the effects of garlic were not due to any specific vasodilatory effect of garlic, as claimed by Loeper and Debray who in 1921, experimented successfully with a garlic tincture in cases of high blood pressure. Marcovici claimed that the lowering of blood pressure was the result of garlic's power to control and purify intestinal putrefaction. Marcovici worked with aged hypertensive patients who suffered high blood pressure, chronic constipation, chronic appendicitis and fecal stasis. As a result of these intestinal problems, the incompletely digested food undergoes pathological putrefaction, and toxins are absorbed and carried into the bloodstream; this causes symptoms of headache, dizziness, fatigue, capillary spasms, etc. By controlling this putrefaction, garlic was, for Marcovici and others, a valuable treatment for all the symptoms associated with hypertension.

Marcovici's findings were confirmed by other researchers. In 1929, Ortner in Germany used garlic to lower blood pressure in eighty cases of hypertension. Other researchers

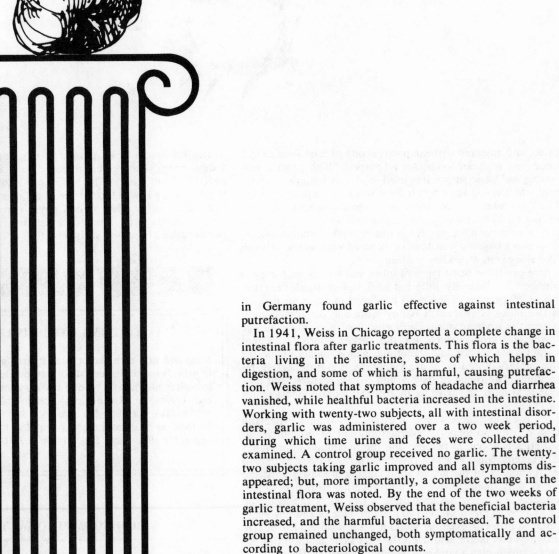

in Germany found garlic effective against intestinal putrefaction.

In 1941, Weiss in Chicago reported a complete change in intestinal flora after garlic treatments. This flora is the bacteria living in the intestine, some of which helps in digestion, and some of which is harmful, causing putrefaction. Weiss noted that symptoms of headache and diarrhea vanished, while healthful bacteria increased in the intestine. Working with twenty-two subjects, all with intestinal disorders, garlic was administered over a two week period, during which time urine and feces were collected and examined. A control group received no garlic. The twenty-two subjects taking garlic improved and all symptoms disappeared; but, more importantly, a complete change in the intestinal flora was noted. By the end of the two weeks of garlic treatment, Weiss observed that the beneficial bacteria increased, and the harmful bacteria decreased. The control group remained unchanged, both symptomatically and according to bacteriological counts.

In 1941, Damsau also worked with garlic to lower blood pressure. Experiments with cats having high blood pressure showed that intraperitoneal injections of garlic concentrate gave an immediate reduction in blood pressure. Control animals remained high. Damsau also made the link between garlic's ability to control putrefaction and the lowering of blood pressure.

Some researchers, such as G. Piotrowsky, have claimed however, that garlic actually dilates the blood vessels, thus reducing pressure. This would be very important in the treatment of fatty deposits in arteriosclerosis. In the journal, *Praxis* (July, 1948), Piotrowsky, working at the University of Geneva, claimed success in lowering blood pressure with garlic in experiments with 100 patients. His treatments began with large doses of garlic, decreasing over a two week period. Symptoms of dizziness, angina-like pains, head and backache were gone in three to five days.

(continued on page 257)

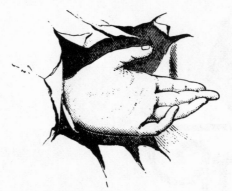

Miso, or fermented soybean paste, is one of East Asia's most important soybean foods. An all-purpose, high protein seasoning and basic staple, it is used in almost unlimited versatility; like bouillon or a rich meat stock in soups and stews; like Worcestershire, soy sauce or ketchup in sauces, dips and dressings; like cheese in casseroles and spreads; like chutney or relish as a topping for grains or fresh vegetable slices; as a gravy base with sautéed or steamed vegetables; or even like vinegar as a pickling medium.

There are three basic types of miso, and within each type a number of distinctly different and widely used varieties. About 80 percent of the miso produced in Japan at present is rice miso, 11 percent is barley miso, and the remaining 9 percent is soybean miso. Each miso has its own distinctive flavor and aroma which, for the darker, more traditional varieties are savory, and sometimes almost meaty, while for the lighter-colored types are subtly sweet and delicately refreshing. The range of flavors and colors, textures and aromas is at least as varied as that of the world's finest wines or cheeses.

Miso is a remarkable source of essential nutrients, especially high quality protein; the average amount of protein in all varieties is about 13 percent and the maximum approaches 20 percent. Miso is also a favorable protein booster due to its abundance of the amino acids lacking in most grains; the use of only small amounts of miso together with rice, bread, noodles or other grain preparations can boost the available protein by as much as 30 to 40 percent. One of the few vegetarian sources of essential vitamin B-12, miso is also rich in enzymes and lactic acid bacteria—the same as found in yogurt—which play a vital role in aiding digestion. Easy to use, it can be stored almost indefinitely at room temperature without refrigeration.

All miso is prepared in basically the same way, using a two-part fermentation process. A grain, such as rice, is soaked overnight, steamed until tender and mixed with spores of a special variety of mold; spread in shallow trays in a warm, humid room for about 45 hours, the inoculated grain, or koji, is crumbled and combined with an approximately equal volume of cooked soybeans, salt and water, some of the soybean cooking liquid and a small amount of mature miso which speeds the fermentation process. The ingredients are mashed together (formerly underfoot like grapes in large wooden tubs), packed into 6-foot deep cedar vats and allowed to ferment, traditionally for one to three years.

Red miso is made with a small proportion of rice koji and a large proportion of salt, and is fermented for a long time. Sweet white miso, by comparison, contains a large amount of rice koji and a small amount of salt, and is fermented for a short time. Miso can be prepared quite easily at home, especially if you use ready-made koji, now available in the West at many health food stores and Japanese food markets. For red or barley miso, a good flavor can be attained if the miso ferments through one entire summer, although the flavor generally improves with time.

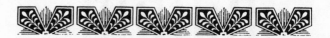

COOKING WITH MISO

Miso can add rich flavor plus hearty aroma to many of your favorite dishes. Miso may be easily substituted for salt in almost any type of cookery; use 1 tablespoon red, barley, or Hatcho miso (or 2 tablespoons sweet white miso) for each ½ teaspoon salt. Miso may also be used as is, uncooked, as a topping for grains, fresh vegetable slices, and (regular or deep-fried) tofu.

MUSHROOM MISO SAUTÉ

2 tablespoons oil
10 mushrooms, thinly sliced
1 tablespoon red, barley, or Hatcho miso
1½ to 2 teaspoons honey or natural sugar

Heat a skillet or wok and coat with the oil. Add mushrooms and sauté over medium heat for 1 minute, or until tender. Reduce heat to low, add miso and sweetening, and cook, stirring constantly for about 1 minute more, or until mushrooms are evenly coated with miso. Allow to cool to room temperature. Serve as a topping for brown rice, tofu, or fresh vegetable slices.

Any of the following vegetables may be substituted for the mushrooms: onions, lotus root, burdock root, squash or (kobocha) pumpkin, or sweet potatoes. Makes ½ cup.

Remarkable Miso and How to Use It

by William Shurtleff and Akiko Aoyagi

MISO-SESAME-AVOCADO SPREAD

2 teaspoons red, barley, or Hatcho miso
6 tablespoons sesame butter
½ avocado
¼ tomato, minced
1 tablespoon minced onion
1 teaspoon lemon juice
½ clove of garlic, crushed
1 tablespoon minced parsley or ¼ cup alfalfa sprouts

Combine the first seven ingredients; mash together until smooth. Serve topped with a sprinkling of the parsley or sprouts. Makes ¾ cup.

FLOATING CLOUD MISO DRESSING

6 tablespoons oil
2 tablespoons (rice) vinegar or lemon juice
2 tablespoons red, barley, or Hatcho miso
¼ teaspoon sesame oil
½ clove of garlic, crushed
Dash of powdered ginger
Dash of dry mustard

Combine all ingredients; whisk or shake well. Good on all tossed green salads, especially those with Chinese cabbage. Tomatoes and (deep-fried) tofu make excellent accompaniments. Or try marinating hot green beans overnight in this dressing, then serving drained and chilled on lettuce. Makes about ½ cup.

THICK FRENCH ONION SOUP with MISO

2 tablespoons oil
6 onions, thinly sliced
3 tablespoons red, barley, or Hatcho miso, dissolved in 2 cups warm water
1 tablespoon butter
2 ounces cheese, grated or minced

Heat a large casserole or heavy pot and coat with the oil. Add onions, cover, and simmer over very low heat for 3½ hours, stirring every 20 or 30 minutes. Mix in dissolved miso and butter, return just to the boil, and remove from heat. Allow to cool, then refrigerate overnight. Stir in the cheese, bring to a boil and simmer, stirring constantly, for about 1 minute, or until cheese melts. Serve hot or, for a richer, sweeter flavor allow to cool to room temperature before serving.

For variety, add 9 ounces diced deep-fried or regular tofu and, if desired, 2 lightly beaten eggs 15 minutes before adding miso. Increase miso to 4 tablespoons. Serves 4.

RICH NOODLE CASSEROLE with MISO-SOUR CREAM and CHIVES

1 cup sour cream
3 tablespoons red, barley, or Hatcho miso
2 eggs, lightly beaten
6 tablespoons minced chives
1½ cups cottage cheese
4¼ ounces (*soba* buckwheat) noodles, cooked, drained, and cooled
2 to 3 tablespoons butter

Preheat oven to 350°. Combine the first five ingredients, mixing well, then gently stir into the cooked noodles. Place into a buttered casserole and top with dabs of remaining butter. Bake covered for 20 minutes, then uncover and bake for about 15 minutes more or until nicely browned. Serves 5 to 6.

BAKED APPLES FILLED with SESAME-RAISIN MISO

5 large apples
Sesame-Raisin Miso:
    1½ tablespoons sesame butter
    ¼ cup raisins
    1 tablespoon red, barley, or Hatcho miso
    1 tablespoon butter
    3 tablespoons natural sugar
    2 tablespoons water
    1 tablespoon sake or white wine (optional)
    ¼ teaspoon cinnamon (optional)

Preheat oven to 350°. Core apples to about seven-eighths of their depth. Mix the ingredients for sesame-raisin miso, then pack the mixture firmly into the hollow center of each apple. Wrap apples in aluminum foil, place on a cookie tin and bake for about 20 minutes. Serve hot or chilled. Serves 5.

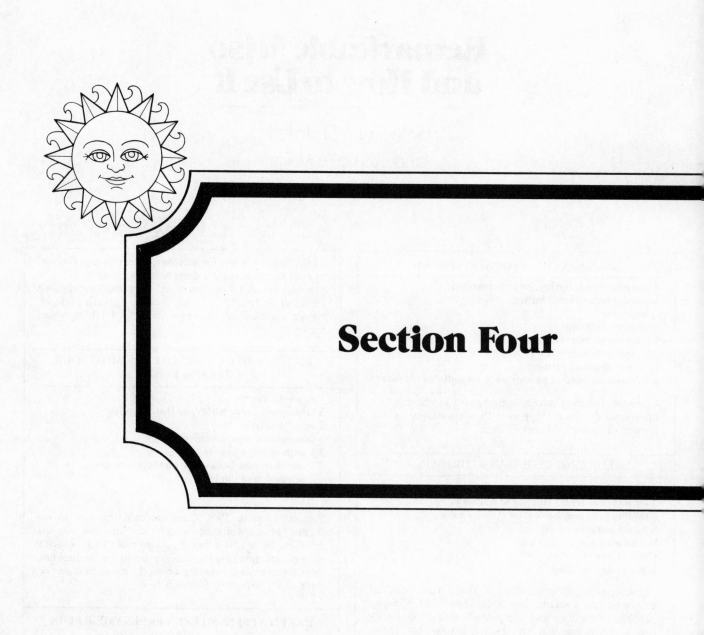

Section Four

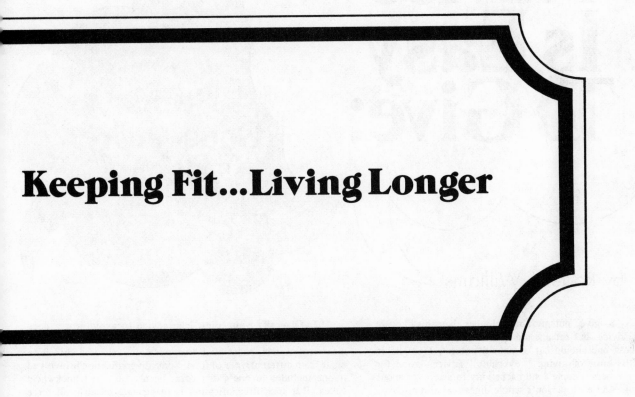

Keeping Fit...Living Longer

Advice Is Easy To Give;

Giving Good Advice Is Harder!

by Roger J. Williams

Advice is easy to give, but my aim is higher than this. I want to give *good* advice. If I become too specific about *exactly* what, when, and how one should eat or should not eat, I am liable to fall into the error of giving "reversible" advice—good for some, bad for others. People's stomachs vary in size over about a six-fold range and each person's whole digestive, assimilative, and metabolic apparatus is sufficiently different so that such advice as, "Eat more roughage" or "Eat less frequently" or "Eat a heavy breakfast" may be of the reversible kind. A faddist usually thinks everyone should eat just as he eats. I am not a faddist.

Although each of us is a distinctive individual with distinctive needs, there is some advice which is applicable to all. For people in general, I will list these pieces of advice under five main headings.

1. Don't be a hypochondriac or a worry wart. Maybe if you are reasonably well and youthful enough for your age you ought to eat about as you do already and thank God for your good health. Worry and concern (about anything, including your health) can help unhinge what good health you have and can make a good nutritional situation deteriorate into a bad one. Worry is able to alter the working of our body chemistry so that the demands for specific nutrients may become augmented. Experimental animals put under stress need, for example, an increased supply of pantothenate to keep their bodily machinery working properly.

There is probably no such thing as nutrition which is perfect in every respect, and undue striving for absolute perfection may have an unfortunate effect. Physicians are too often run ragged by people who should worry less about their own health and should be more concerned about what to do with the relatively good health they already possess.

2. Diversify your diet. The advice to avoid worry does not preclude the use of intelligent care. Diversification of diet means, of course, substantial diversification; selection should be made from different *types* of food. Some diversification is involved if one includes in one's diet corn, beans, rice, and buckwheat cakes. But such diversification is inadequate because all these are seed products and thus belong in the same general category. A much wider diversification is possible when one considers the following types of foodstuffs: (1) milk and dairy products; (2) seed (including nut) products; (3) meats (not exclusively muscle) from mammals and fowls; (4) fish and marine products; (5) leafy (green) vegetables; (6) root and tuber vegetables, including carrots and potatoes (yellowness is associated with a source of vitamin A); (7) fruits of all kinds, including melons and tomatoes; (8) fungi—yeast, mushrooms, truffles; (9) eggs.

No one should feel under obligation to sample all these foods every day or every month; they are listed merely to indicate that a wide range exists from which to choose. Some people's idea of an excellent meal (to be repeated as often as feasible) is a selection of steak or prime rib roast, baked or French fried potatoes, a dab of salad (mostly for looks), and topped with coffee and, to avoid extra calories, perhaps a little sherbert rather than a heavier dessert like ice cream. Such people need to have their eyes opened to the facts of diversity and to the listings given above.

It is possible that individual adults who appear to eat unwisely (from the standpoint of accepted nutritional standards) and yet live to advanced age in good health, have been unusually well nourished during youth, and that this foundation of good health is sufficiently strong to withstand considerable abuse in later life. Many of our biologically distant relatives, the insects, exhibit this characteristic in their nutritional history; in the larval stage their nutrition may require every mineral, amino acid, and vitamin in the book, but after they become adult, they can live on pure sugar alone!

The fact (and it does appear to be one) that some individuals can thrive on relatively monotonous and one-sided diets, tends to make it difficult for the general public to accept at their face value the preachments of nutritionists. The idea that what one individual can do, others should be able to do equally well, is subject to such a multitude of exceptions, however, that we should not be surprised by one more.

3. Use and cultivate your body wisdom. It is probable that appetite-controlling mechanisms are *exceedingly important* in helping us get what we individually need in our food. If they were all abolished, our lives would probably soon be snuffed out one way or another. In the case of individuals who have lived to advanced age without ever having given nutrition any study or followed any rules of good nutrition, their superior body wisdoms have probably turned the trick. That people do differ in their body wisdoms is apparent from the fact that some people tend to eat and drink unwisely to their own ruination while others have no difficulty whatever avoiding these excesses.

Part of what is suggested by the phrase "use your body wisdom" involves showing a certain amount of independence and choice in the selection of food. When one knows and feels that one has had enough, and yet continues to eat just to be sociable or to please the hostess, one is not using his body wisdom. If the general public (including hostesses) were educated to the point that everyone could eat, without embarrassment or social pressure, exactly what their body wisdom told them to eat, everyone's nutrition would probably be substantially improved. This would not work for those whose appetite mechanisms are already seriously deranged, nor would I imply that body wisdom should be expected to supersede common sense.

The question: how to *cultivate* one's body wisdom (particularly with respect to eating), is one about which we have relatively little direct knowledge. We do know, however, that *good nutrition builds body wisdom,* so one way to cultivate better body wisdom is to follow more closely the accepted rules of good nutrition.

Consistent moderate exercise, especially of a recreational nature is an *important way* of improving one's body wisdom. Exercise stimulates the circulation of the blood, and thus causes the blood to bring better nourishment (and oxygen supply) to all the tissues, including those that are concerned in regulating appetite. Mental relaxation does things to us chemically, and improves our bodily functioning.

Dean Roscoe Pound, Harvard nonagenarian, who wrote a five-volume work on American jurisprudence between the ages of 86 and 89, is said to have walked thousands of miles all over Scotland, Ireland, and France. In his earlier years he participated in many extensive bicycle trips.

Thomas Parr in England, one of the longest-lived men in recorded medical history (1483-1635), was accustomed to thresh grain at the age of 130 and continued to be active until his death at 152. He lived under nine British kings and a monument to his memory is in Westminster Abbey. In view of the known relationships between exercise, obesity, and longevity, the fact seems to be inescapable that sedentarianism is crippling many lives today. It may be very humorous when Robert Hutchins says that he overcomes the urge to exercise by taking a nap, but it is not funny when millions of Americans follow his example, and thereby lose their health, vigor, and part of their body wisdom.

4. Avoid too much refined food. In view of such advice the question arises: "How much is too much?" Students of nutrition would not all agree on the same answer though they would agree that for children the restrictions on refined foods should be relatively severe. When a child (or even an adult) substitutes a soft drink (which is mostly sugar-water) for milk as a mealtime beverage, this is a serious breach of good nutritional sense.

When we consume essentially refined fuel—sugar, alcohol, refined foods—we crowd out of our diets the vital lubricants: amino acids, vitamins, and minerals.

The use of large amounts of processed foods is not recommended for those who have reason to be seriously concerned about their nutrition. Prepared foods are often toasted which tends to destroy at least one of the potentially important vitamins. Processed foods are often claimed to have various specified percentages of those nutrients which the Food and Drug Administration has recognized as established needs, but no attention is paid to other nutrients which informed experts know are also necessary. If we could gather our oranges, apples, carrots, wheat, lettuce, oysters, eggs, fish, pork, and beef, etc., in our own backyards, process them ourselves when necessary and eat them in the fresh state, this might be ideal. Not everything we like grows in the same locality in the same season, but fortunately the use of frozen foods and modern transportation makes it possible for us to get great variety.

Canning is also an invaluable expedient, and modern canning preserves a large part of the food value of everything that is canned. There is, however some sense to the maxim "Eat some raw food every day," because there may be "unknowns" that are altered or destroyed by cooking. Cooking with plenty of water and then discarding the water is a bad practice since substantial amounts of minerals and vitamins are lost.

5. Use nutritional supplements when, on the basis of informed opinion, it seems desirable. There are two reasons for using nutritional supplements: first, to combat ailments including illnesses associated with aging. Parts of our working machinery tend to wear unequally as we age, and the use of supplements may cancel or diminish the difficulties which result. The treatment of disease or illness should be in the hands of a physician.

The second reason for using nutritional supplements involves *insurance* against all ills which may have a nutritional basis. While one may be well and give promise of remaining so, a prudent person provides for the "ifs" of life. No one can be sure, especially if refined foods are used, that he will never be affected adversely by deficient nutrition.

Inexpensive Health Insurance

It is for this reason that many reasonably healthy people use nutritional supplements regularly. There is room here for individual preference and judgement. Whether we like it or not, trivial matters such as aversion or liking for "pills," enter into people's decisions. Their financial circumstances and their thrift with respect to such expenditures also play a part. People are notoriously inconsistent in their expenditures. Some would not hesitate a moment to spend several dollars for a good steak or a bottle of liquor, but would shrink from the expenditure of a similar amount for several months' supply of a nutritional supplement—even though it might constitute cheap health insurance.☼

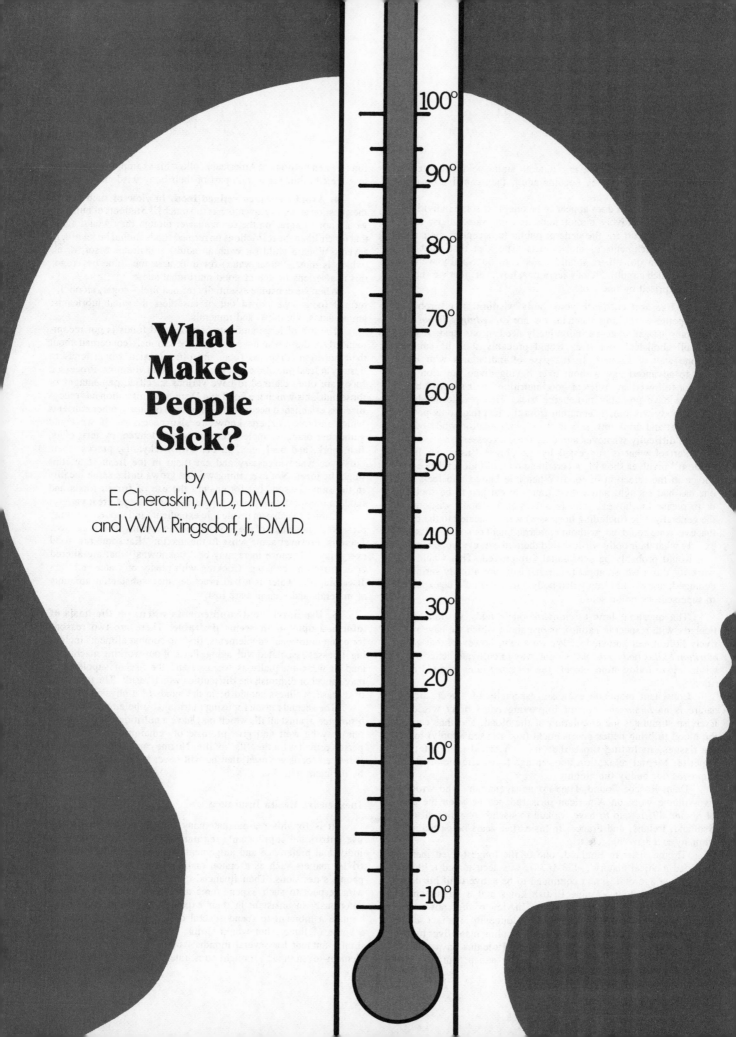

What Makes People Sick?

by
E. Cheraskin, M.D., D.M.D.
and W.M. Ringsdorf, Jr., D.M.D.

We have been told that many adult Americans are afflicted by chronic disease. The singular statistic seldom cited is that, in the final analysis, one out of one eventually dies! This is not of concern here. What is frustrating is that most adult Americans living today in the United States are agonized with one or another infirmity which, according to the best medical scholars, is incurable!

Just sheer common sense would dictate that, for every *effect*, there must be a *cause*. Hence, it follows that incurable disease, as an *effect*, must have a *cause!*

Thus, it is imperative that we grapple with the question, "What *causes* disease?" There are many avenues of approach to an answer. Perhaps the best source is the man in the street, for two reasons. First, he reflects modern medical opinion. Second, as a non-expert, he does not suffer with the near-sightedness which commonly besets those of us professionally involved with medicine.

And so we confront the layman with the question, "What makes disease?" The answer, with surprising regularity, is that man's ills stem from the external world. Take, for example, such oft-heard clichés as "I caught a cold," or "Flu is going around in the neighborhood," or "He contracted tuberculosis." It is not mere whimsy that man's ills are blamed on the world about him; his successes and accomplishments he attributes to his own deeds. Where and why did man inherit such a philosophy? There are two very good reasons. First, castigating the external world for his misery relieves him of responsibility. Thus, disease is no longer man's inherent weakness. Second, there is historic medical precedence for such thinking.

Before the Germ Theory

In the beginning, health and disease were acknowledged to be God-given. When man sinned, he was cursed with disease. When he behaved, he remained unscathed. Life and death were intimately tied to religious beliefs.

However, with the advent of scientific medicine, the explanation slowly changed. Increasingly more attention was directed *within* the body as the root of disease. In other words, the body was viewed as the "soil" in which disease occurs. While most of the ancient theories have now been discredited, the denominator which has persisted (even to this day) is that the *internal* world of man is intimately associated with his disorders.

The Germ Theory

For approximately twenty-five hundred years, medicine has been probing for the roots of disease. Until the advent of bacteriology, disease was ascribed to a turbulence in man's *internal* environment. Then came Pasteur and his colleagues and the birth of the germ theory. This neat and simple concept suggested that germs are seeds which beget disease. The proposition had its problems gaining acceptance, but it won out finally because it was simple, effective and comfortable. Now man could blame the cosmos and so regard his infirmities as part of destiny.

Beyond the Germ Theory

There is no question that germs are involved in many illnesses. However, the mere microbial involvement does not willy-nilly argue that the germ is the mainspring. Moreover, the germ theory does not resolve the many contradictions found in nature. Why, for example, can two seeming similar souls breathe the very same germs at precisely the same time and only one "catches a cold"? There are paradoxes in the field of microbial diseases where it is clear that microorganisms play a role. But, more importantly, how does one explain the rising problems of chronic disease where bacteriology plays less of a role?

What is the cause of arteriosclerosis (hardening of the arteries) and rheumatoid arthritis (rheumatism)?

These and many other enigmas now lead us to a theory of disease beyond the germ hypothesis. As a matter of fact, the modern interpretation of disease is a union of the before-the-germ-theory and the germ-theory. It recognizes that disease, gauged by symptoms and signs, is the end result of an environmental challenge. The peripheral threat may be microbial but it may also be physical, chemical or psychic. In this connection, the new philosophy concedes the importance of the world about man but enlarges the scope of challenges. Hence, the present concept of disease incorporates the germ theory. At the same time, the modern theory of illness appreciates the fact that the capacity of the person to withstand the external bombardment of disease is an equally vital ingredient. This latter factor is cloaked in such terms as host resistance, host susceptibility, tissue tolerance, constitution, or predisposition. In other words, the testimony is now clear that disease is of a multifactorial nature. This means that more than one element operates in the genesis of sickness. It follows, therefore, that disease may be aborted by eliminating any one or a combination of the contributing variables.

There is sound historic support for a multicausal explanation for illness. In the case of diphtheria, for example, there are two possible solutions. If it were feasible to rid the world of the diphtheritic organism, there would obviously be no diphtheria. One could wipe out the disease completely and forever. Unfortunately, as history has demonstrated, this is impossible. The alternative is to heighten host resistance, or minimize susceptibility, in such a manner that the very same microbe no longer creates the disease. This is precisely the basis for vaccination. That vaccination has worked is evidenced by the almost total abolition of diphtheria.

Vaccination is a workable solution for the acute infectious diseases like diphtheria, whooping cough, measles, smallpox, yellow fever, cholera, and infantile paralysis. However, the chronic disease problems such as cancer, heart disease, arthritis, and others, are more complex. Surely, the environmental factors are not as sharply defined in this group as with the communicable diseases (acute infectious disorders). It follows that greater attention must be given to the individual's constitution in such killing and crippling areas as cancer, heart disease, arthritis, and blindness.

Resistance and Susceptibility

In one sense, resistance and susceptibility are nothing more than opposites. It really matters little, *descriptively*, whether one succumbs because resistance is lowered or susceptibility is increased. But, viewed *analytically*, there is a big difference. An agent, which when added, increased protection against disease and, when eliminated, diminishes protection, is called a *resistance* factor. For example, vitamin C safeguards against scurvy; its absence invites scurvy. Hence, vitamin C is a resistance factor. Conversely, an agent which when added reduces protection against disease and when avoided increases protection is a *susceptibility* factor. Dietary sugar is not good for the diabetic patient. Abstinence is helpful. Hence, according to the above definition, sugar may be viewed as a susceptibility factor.

There are, to be sure, many obvious and very likely not-so-obvious factors which constitute the basis for host resistance and susceptibility. Surely, genetics plays a cardinal role. Certainly, hormones are intimately involved in man's constitution. Host state can be radically altered by physical activity and pollution. One area which is receiving increasing attention by scientists and is spilling over into lay thinking is diet and its contribution to health and disease.

(continued on page 258)

Toxemia,
the One Disease Everyone Has

by J.H.Tilden, M.D.

The medical world has built an infinite literature without any (except erroneous and vacillating) idea of cause. Medicine is rich in science, but now, as well as in the past time, it suffers from a dearth of practical ideas. The average doctor is often educated out of all the common-sense he was born with. This, however, is not his fault. It is the fault of the system. He is an educated automaton. He has facts — scientific facts galore — without ideas. Ford had mechanical facts — not more, perhaps, than thousands of other mechanics, but he joined them in an idea that made him a multimillionaire. Millions have facts, but no ideas. Thousands of doctors have all the scientific data needed, but they have not harnessed their science to common-sense and philosophy.

Without a clear conception of cause, cure must remain the riddle that it is.

The late Sir James Mackenzie — while living, the greatest clinician in the world — declared: "In medical research the object is mainly the prevention and cure of disease." If cause is not known, how is prevention or cure possible — as, for example, by producing a mild form of smallpox or other so-called disease by poisoning a healthy person by introducing into his body the pathological products of said disease? Certainly only pathological thinking can arrive at such conclusions. Vaccines and autogenous remedies are made from the products of disease, and the idea that disease can be made to cure itself is an end-product of pathological thinking. This statement is not so incongruous after we consider the fact that all search and research work by medical scientists to find cause, has been made in dead and dying people. As ridiculous as it may appear, medical science has gone, and is still going, to the dead and dying to find cause.

If prevention and cure mean producing disease, surely prevention and cure are not desirable. If prevention can be accomplished, then cures will not be needed.

At the time of his death, Mackenzie was laboring to discover prevention. A more worthy work cannot be imagined. But the tragedy of his life was that he died from a preventable disease; and he could have cured this disease that killed him if his conception of cause had been in line with the Truth of Toxemia — the primary cause of all disease.

In spite of Mackenzie's ambition to put the profession in possession of truth concerning prevention and cure, he died without a correct idea of even in what direction to look for this desirable knowledge, as evidenced by such statements as: "Our problems being the prevention of disease, we require a complete knowledge of disease in all its aspects before we can take steps to prevent its occurrence." There is the crux of the whole subject. It is not disease; it is cause "in all its aspects" that we need to know before we can take steps to prevent "disease." Mackenzie stated the following concerning diagnosis:

But it appears to be unlikely that in the present state of medicine there would be any great dissimilarity in the proportions of diagnosed and undiagnosed cases in many series of investigations such as we have made. The proportion depends, not on the skill or training of individual practitioners, but on the unsatisfactory state of all medical knowledge. The similarity of the statistical records from the institute and from private practice goes far to support this view. In spite of the additional time given at the institute to the examination of cases which are undiagnosable in general practice, and the assistance given by the special departments — clinical groups — in their investigation, they remain profoundly obscure, although we know that it is from among them that there will gradually emerge the cases of advanced organic disease and the end-results which form so large a proportion of the inmates of hospital wards. And the tragedy is that many of them suffer from no serious disabilities, and might, but for our ignorance, be checked on their downward course.

Isn't that about as sharp a criticism of medical inefficiency as Tilden has ever made?

This brings vividly to mind the statement, made only a short time ago, by Dr. Cabot, of Boston, that he himself was mistaken in his diagnoses about fifty per cent of the time — that he had proved it by post-mortems. Such a statement as this, coming from a man of his standing, means much. To me it means that diagnosis is a meaningless term; for, as used, it means discovering what pathological effects — what changes — have been brought about by an undiscovered cause. Diagnosis means, in a few words, discovering effects which, when found, throw no light whatever on cause.

Again I quote Mackenzie: "The knowledge of disease is so incomplete that we do not yet even know what steps should be taken to advance our knowledge." This being true, there is little excuse for laws to shut out or prevent

(continued on page 259)

TOXEMIA
Essentially Catarrhal:
Stomach / Bowels / Liver / Lungs
Infections / Fevers / Cancer
Skin Diseases • Metabolic • Rheumatism
Diabetes • Blood Dyscrasias
Deficiencies • Gland Overfunction
Cardiorenal: Kidney
Heart / Arteriosclerosis • Tuberculosis
Neuropathic diseases:
Organic / Functional

NUTRITIONAL: OVEREATING / WRONG FOOD / WRONG
COMBINATIONS / MINERAL DEFICIENCIES / VITAMIN DEFICIENCIES
COFFEE, TEA, ALCOHOL • TOBACCO AND DRUGS
BACTERIAL ACTIVITY • TAPROOT ENERVATION • UNCONGENIAL
ENVIRONMENT • KILLING EMOTIONS: FEAR / RAGE
JEALOUSY / WORRY • PHYSICAL EXCESSES • SENSUAL EXCESSES
PHYSICAL DEFECTS • POSTURAL TENSION • INJURIES
THE UNPOISED STATE

THE TREE OF TOXEMIA
IN THE SOIL OF HUMAN HABITS AND BEHAVIOR

Nutrition And Your Baby's First Years

by Gena Larson

Nursing Your Baby

The one best food is mother's milk. Mother's milk is more easily digested and always available at the proper temperature. Night feedings are easier for the new mother—no waiting to heat a cold bottle while the baby cries with hunger. Travel is safer for the breast-fed baby—no danger of a change in formula.

Nursing is certainly the most economical way to feed your baby. You might like to add up, sometime, the cost of feeding a prepared baby formula and baby food for six months. Enough to pay for household help for the new mother, or to take the whole family on a three-weeks' vacation? Yes, indeed!

Another advantage in nursing your baby is time saved each day. No sterilizing of bottles. No preparing and warming formulas. Just your own high quality milk, formulated especially for your own little one. Always ready. Always the correct temperature. This is a real blessing in the first few weeks after the two of you return home from the hospital. You will need time to regain your strength and to get acquainted with your precious child.

Once you have decided upon nursing your baby, tell your doctor upon the *first* visit. If you find he is not the least bit enthusiastic about your decision, find out why. There will still be time to shop around for another doctor who will support your efforts in this vital function. If your doctor is encouraging but not too knowledgeable about nursing, continue with your plans to nurse and educate *him* as you study and learn about it.

Sometimes well-meaning friends or relatives will try to discourage a young mother from nursing her child. This is a time when the husband can lend moral support and encouragement and say to all: "We have decided that our child is going to be nursed!"

For the mother, breast-feeding may help prevent cancer. Statistics show that women who nurse their babies are far less likely to get breast cancer.

Another result of nursing your baby can be seen for at least thirty years. One can examine the stool of any person, up to the age of thirty years, and tell by the presence or absence of certain essential bacteria whether or not that person was nursed as a child.

Before birth the placenta provides antibodies against a variety of infectious conditions. Breast-feeding promotes this process and should be continued for at least six months, after which the infant starts to manufacture his own antibodies. The well-nourished mother will have milk that is entirely adequate to sustain a high degree of health in the child.

One month before the birth of your baby, begin bathing the breasts, particularly the nipples, with a mild solution of sea salt and water. (¼ teaspoon to one cup water.) This will strengthen them for nursing.

The *ONLY* time it may not be wise to nurse is when a child is born with a serious illness, such as leukemia, heart or brain malfunction. Then it may be better not to nurse as the defective gene (or diet) that produced the defective child may hamper milk quality and production.

If the baby cannot be nursed, find a safe source of certified raw goat's milk or cow's milk. Dilute with bottled water in the amount specified by your doctor and add blackstrap molasses in a proper amount to regulate the baby's bowels. A tiny bit of brewers' yeast may be added for extra nutrients.

When safe raw milks are not available or the baby cannot tolerate them, for various reasons, some other way to nourish the baby must be found. Some infants thrive on the raw seed or nut milks, mixed with safe water, molasses and brewers' yeast. Other babies do well on a lightly cooked vegetable broth made from zucchini, carrots and parsley. This is strained into fresh raw carrot juice and diluted with water. Mashed avocado, diluted with mineral-rich water has also been used successfully by some mothers.

(continued on page 260)

Cholesterol and the Frequently Maligned Egg

by Carl C. Pfeiffer, Ph.D., M.D.

A strong case has been made against the consumption of eggs in an effort to reduce cholesterol intake. Doctors, voluntary health-oriented associations and even some nutritionists have convinced the public that eating eggs, with their appreciable cholesterol, will increase serum cholesterol and increase the risk of coronary heart disease. Probably as a consequence of this advice, the average American consumption of eggs per person in 1973 was estimated at 292, a 5 percent drop from the previous year. As recently as 1945, the average American was eating 403 eggs a year. We recommend 2 eggs per day or 700 per year!

Inspite of all this publicity concerning the bad effect of eggs on blood cholesterol, let's look at the accurate assay of the effects of eggs (or egg yolks) on the cholesterol levels of normal people. (All 275 mg of cholesterol in the egg is contained in the yolk.)

Svacha et al. at Auburn, Alabama fed three eggs per day to fourteen normal men, several of whom smoked tobacco habitually. Only the smokers had a significant total rise of 27 mg percent in serum cholesterol (9 mg per egg). Nonsmokers had a nonsignificant rise of only 2 mg percent (0.7 mg per egg). It should also be noted that smokers inhale poisonous cadmium, which antagonizes zinc, one of the useful trace metals contained in egg yolk.

In yet another study, Takeuchi and Yamamura of Osaka, Japan compared the responses of thirty-one young men with ten middle-aged men when each group was given nine egg yolks per person per day. The young men had an average rise in cholesterol of 17 mg percent (2 mg per egg) while the middle-aged men had a rise of 35 mg percent (4 mg per egg). The mean cholesterol levels at the start were 185 mg percent for the young and 195 mg percent for the middle-aged men.

These scientific studies in man contrast with the statement of Dr. Castelli, director of the laboratory in the Framingham study: "I have lowered my cholesterol from 250 to 200 mg percent partly by eliminating eggs and other measures, such as diet and exercise." Trager, in *The Bellybook,* says, without presenting a scientific basis for the statement: "If a man eliminates 2 eggs per day he can lower his cholesterol by something like 25 mg percent," and "Every 100 mg of cholesterol a man eats per day raises his serum cholesterol by 5 mg percent." If this last statement were true, then the men eating three eggs in Auburn, Alabama, should have had a rise in their cholesterol of 275 X 3 eggs X 5 mg%÷100 mg percent or a 41 mg percent rise! Actually the result was 2 mg percent for nonsmokers and 27 mg percent for smokers! What a difference!

The Japanese men cited above as eating nine yolks a day should have had a rise of 275 X 9 yolks X 5 mg%÷100=124 mg%. Actually, the rise was only 17 mg percent for young men and 35 mg percent for the middle-aged men. An easy answer lies in the fact that the egg yolk is a balanced nutritional delight which contains not only cholesterol but lecithin, zinc, iron, sulfur and other trace elements which provide the biochemical cement to build the native cholesterol into steroid hormones and other useful body bastions against disease.

The egg is an ideal natural food supplied in a hard (calcium and magnesium) disposable (for your compost pile) shell. If the shell were made of tough protein (as is the turtle's) the present-day consumer would get only frozen yolks and whites, and the shell would be snatched away by processors for use as animal food. At present, feeding the hens limestone (which is cheaper than egg shell) supplies the needed calcium. The brittle egg shell has almost completely prevented commercial adulteration of the egg. Only healthy hens will lay eggs, so the egg farmer goes to great pains to see that his hens are healthy. The only trace of adulteration is that American hens are fed additional B carotene and vitamin A in order to produce an egg with a deep orange yolk. Of some interest is the fact that the bones of the baby chick get their calcium, phosphorus, magnesium, sulfur, selenium, fluoride and iron from the yolk of the egg.

At six months of age the human infant's first dose of iron and sulfur ordinarily comes from the feeding of cooked egg yolk. This is needed since milk is deficient in iron. The egg also has a built-in warning device in that, when old or stored in heat, the sulfur compounds start to decompose, become noticeable, and the smell of "rotten eggs" warns the consumer. Believe it or not, this smell of rotten eggs is one of the reasons that we recommend two eggs per person daily. The odor means that sulfur is present. Man needs sulfur and its natural contaminant, selenium for skin, hair, fingernails and toenails, to build the amino acid taurine in the cells and brain and to make sulfonated compounds for the joints. The essential amino acids containing sulfur (cysteine and methionine) are not enough. Grandma, when she gave sulfur and molasses each springtime, was correct in believing that the body needs sulfur.

A whole chicken develops from one egg

Chicken eggs provide excellent food, since the protein balance is of the best biological value possible. The egg has the amino acid pattern in the proportion closest to the needs of your body. The egg is low in fat, rich in protein and vitamin A, low in calories and economical (much cheaper and higher quality protein than meat). It is, furthermore, a good source of vitamin B-12 if you are a vegetarian. (B-12 is found only in animal products.) It also contains (some in larger amounts than others) choline, tryptophan (precursor of niacin), pyridoxine (B-6), biotin, folic acid (a B vitamin), riboflavin (B-2), thiamin (B-1) pantothenic acid (a B vitamin), selenium, zinc, phosphorous, calcium and sulfur.

The yolk of an egg is almost the only food that will blacken a silver spoon because of its high sulfur content. (One other is hot red pepper.) So if you need sulfur for your skin and fingernails, you have little choice but to eat two eggs a day. As

(continued on page 263)

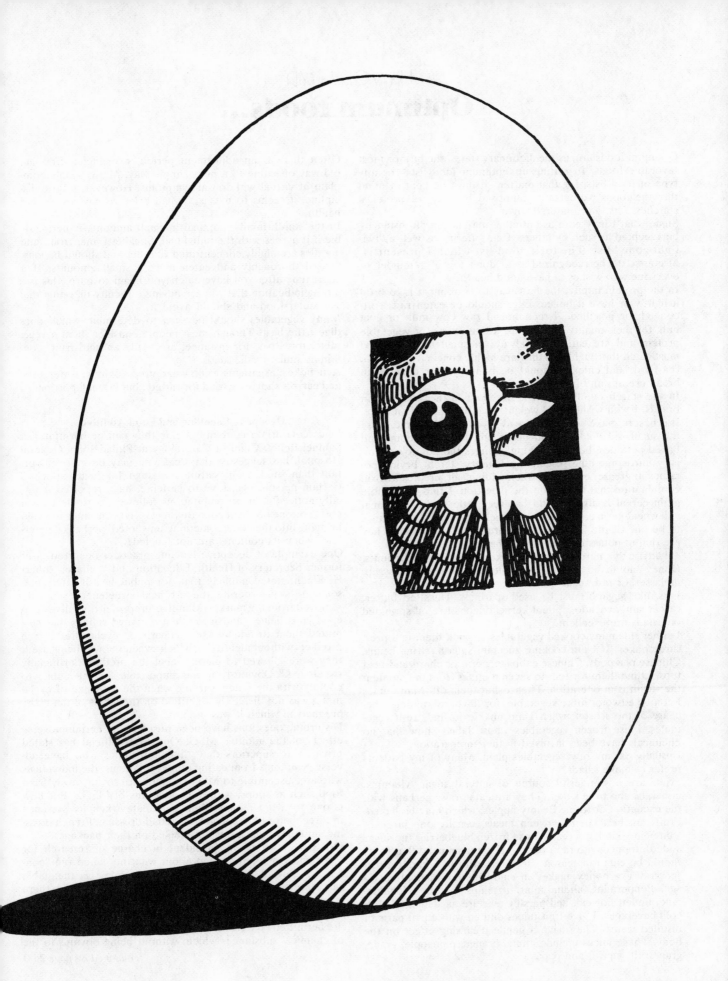

Henry G. Bieler, M.D.

Optimum Foods...

Optimum foods are, as the dictionary states, the best or most favorable foods. In setting up optimum food lists—or any type of food lists, for that matter—it must be kept in mind that the foods we eat are comprised basically of proteins, starches, fats, and (natural) sugar.

Since what I may note as optimum may not in all instances be accepted as such by others, I am offering as well a "twilight-zone" list. The toxic food list which I present is, of course, to be recognized as a "don't touch" reminder to everyone who wishes to have good health.

In the protein family, the best way to cook meat is to broil it lightly or have it boiled. Eggs should be eaten raw, soft-cooked, or poached. I recommend raw cow milk or goat milk for their quality. Pecans are a fine source of vegetable protein and are eaten raw, always in small amounts, and masticated thoroughly, as they are highly concentrated. Fish, sea food, and chicken should be boiled, never covered in bread crumbs and fried in grease.

In the starch family, wheat is excellent in the whole grain breads, if you wish to add weight. Rye bread builds muscle. It is best to make your own bread if you can find time. I use the small red potatoes and boil them. I never recommend baked potatoes, because baking changes the potato's chemistry into something resembling laundry starch. Frying potatoes in grease, especially when adding salt, creates a toxic combination that is hard on the digestion. I find that whole grain cereal is alkaline and has very little starch. Oatmeal and wheat-germ cereals are also excellent. I consider bananas to be one of the finest natural starch foods available. They are rich in potassium and should be eaten ripe.

I advise that natural sugars be taken only in small amounts. Honey should be raw and not filtered. Pure maple syrup, molasses, or raw sugar is allowed.

Fats, like sugars, must be used sparingly. Unsalted butter, raw cream, avocado, apricot kernel oil, or olive oil sprinkled on salads are excellent.

I either steam my cooked vegetables or cook them in a pressure cooker. If I am cooking zucchini squash, string beans, Chinese pea pods, Chinese cabbage, corn, or chard and beet tops, I time them for four to seven minutes from the moment the steam is in operation. Then I shut them off. Many times I combine two or more vegetables for flavor. Sometimes, because of the season, when I am unable to find fresh vegetables, I use frozen vegetables whose labels show that no chemicals have been involved in their preparation.

I usually eat my raw vegetables plain. Many of my patients prefer to make salads.

Fruits are a wonderful source of natural sugar, vitamins, minerals, and pure water. They are eaten raw, perhaps with the exception of Rome Beauty apples, which may be baked. Fruits are best eaten between meals, usually one piece of fruit of any kind at a time—I use frozen blueberries (no sugar added), topped with raw cream. I also recommend that fruits should be eaten in season. Herb tea, with or without a teaspoon of raw honey, makes an enjoyable hot or cold beverage. Peppermint, alfalfa mint, rosehips, comfrey, chamomile, linden flowers, and parsley teas are all delightful. For cold beverages, I give fruit juices diluted with equal parts of distilled water. They have a gentle cleansing effect on the body. These juices include apple, orange, pineapple, grape, grapefruit, guava, and papaya.

Often there is an adjustment period in changing from an old way of eating to a new, simple way. Many people complain of virtual withdrawal symptoms. However, a little discipline, it seems to me, is a small price to pay for vibrant health.

In the starch family, oatmeal in small amounts is permissible if it agrees with the individual. Spaghetti, macaroni, and noodles are highly concentrated starches and should be masticated thoroughly and eaten in very small amounts. If a short time after you have eaten you begin to burp, this is a strong indication that you are having difficulty digesting that particular food and should avoid it.

Many vegetables should be *tried* to determine which ones digest the best. Though most people consider them a vegetable, tomatoes, for instance, are really an acid fruit, containing much oxalic acid.

Artichokes, asparagus, yellow and green onions, watercress, and carrots should be tried for variety, but in small portions.

Deceptive Labelling and Food Additives

Since cola drinks contain caffeine they can be harmful. Dr. Samuel Bellet, Chief of Cardiology at Philadelphia General Hospital, has suggested that "caffeine may be more important than smoking in setting the stage for heart attacks." Certain persons, sensitive to caffeine, have reported markedly noticeable heart palpitations following a single cup of coffee or one bottle of cola. But how is the consumer to avoid bringing into the home something unwanted, perhaps deleterious, when its contents are not labeled?

One example of deceptive labeling practices occurred after former Secretary of Health, Education and Welfare, Robert H. Finch, stated publicly that, for public-health safety reasons, he was ordering the artificial sweetener cyclamate removed from the market. Manufacturers of artificially sweetened jams, jellies, and fruits then obtained rulings that permitted them to add *either* saccharin or cyclamates to the products without identifying which sweetener was being used; they were allowed to merely label the product "artificially sweetened." Obviously it was impossible for the public to comply with the Finch warning when the presence of cyclamates was not distinctly identified on the labels of the many products in which it was used.

Disturbing questions have been raised about certain adverse effects of the additive MSG. One FDA official has stated privately to superiors that "like individuals who have adverse symptoms from eating other food items, the individuals who are susceptible to MSG should learn to stay away from food such as soups, with large amounts of MSG." But how is one to avoid monosodium glutamate when its presence in three major food categories—salad dressing, French dressing, and mayonnaise—is not labeled on their packages?

Dr. Roy Newton, vice-president in charge of research for Swift and Company, talked about what he called the "confusers." One of the "confusers" he cited "...is that table salt is poisonous under some conditions." To my mind, there is no doubt about large amounts of salt being injurious to the human system. Many others agree with me that food products are permitted on our store shelves that contain small amounts of chemical substances which, without being obvious to the

(continued on page 263)

For Optimum Health

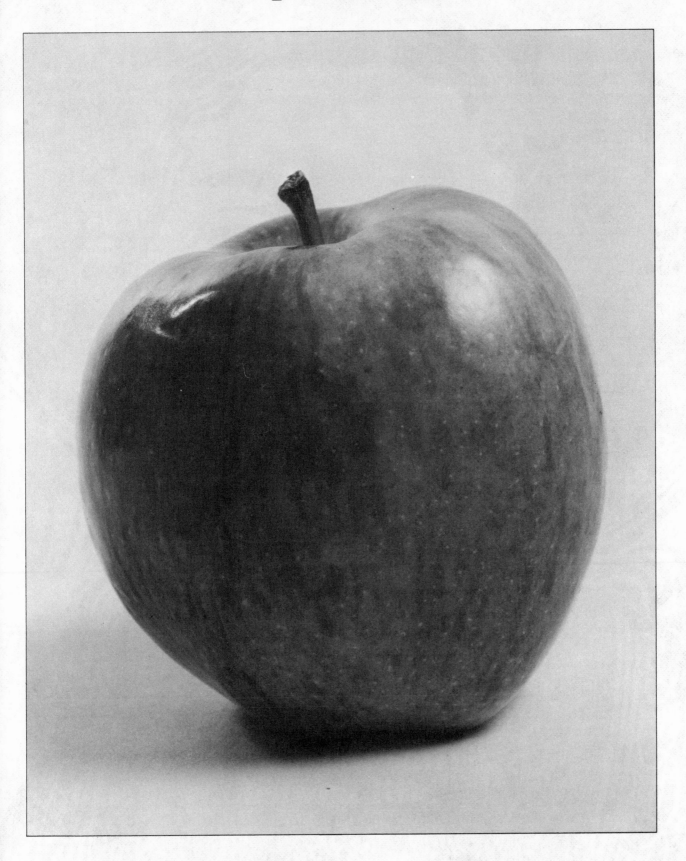

Grandma's Natural Remedies: Time-Tested and Still Trusted

by Kurt W. Donsbach, D.C., N.D.

Many years ago, I was privileged to know and observe the wisdom of an old Indian medicine man practicing his profession in a primitive area of Idaho. This accomplished and successful Indian herbalist used only herbs found in nature, which he carefully gathered and prepared himself. Almost every time I went to see him he would have a huge stainless steel container simmering on the stove. The aroma of herbs permeated the room and the gallon jugs into which he poured the finished product lined the wall.

I was forced to use much finesse in trying to inveigle him into revealing his secrets, as he was quite suspicious and cantankerous by nature. In fact, the first time I met him I spent the first half hour convincing him that I was not an agent of the FDA. It was only after a mutual friend, Dory Detton, solemnly vouched for my character, that the old man finally consented to accept me as a kindred soul.

To get back to the major lesson I learned from this Indian herbalist—he said that to cure most of the ills of the modern white man, all that was really necessary was to give him a good laxative. How simple, and yet how indicative of one of the most prevalent ills of our time. It is difficult for any serious ailment to attack the human system when the bowels are open. The other favorite remedy of this herbalist was a liver-cleansing regimen, which has been of assistance to me ever since.

Now for some common ailments and the old, time-honored remedies which are still practical.

BOILS—These usually are indicative of toxic wastes in the body, but also are a signal of thyroid deficiency. Calcium and magnesium are always indicated, and I often use a complex product consisting of kelp, dulse, hydrolyzed fish proteins and other factors to supply synergistic material for the normal functioning of the thyroid. Potato poultices are also excellent as an immediate relief and a means of bringing the boil to a head. The potato, peeling and all, should be finely grated and a small pack applied directly on the boil. Cover with gauze and hold in place with tape. Change twice a day.

MOTION SICKNESS and **SEASICKNESS**—Abstinence from a heavy meal, particularly heavy meats, just before taking the trip, and a preparatory period of three days using a vitamin C complex containing 250 milligrams of vitamin C eight times a day can usually control even serious cases. I have personally seen this work several times.

ULCERS—It is beyond me where the research work demonstrating the efficacy of cabbage juice in treating ulcers is buried. If the ulcer sufferer will drink the juice of a raw head of cabbage every day, relief will be quick and sure in not more than ten days, although longer use is advised for long-lasting results. Another time-honored remedy is fenugreek and comfrey tea. Our source tells us this should be used at the rate of at least three cups per day. Fifteen drops of pure extract of aloe vera taken three times a day has provided relief for many in these gastric irritations. It is, of course, understood by all that such measures alone, without refraining from smoking and consumption of alcohol and without eating a proper diet, would be inadequate at best.

HEMORRHOIDS—A disorder which is often miraculously relieved by cleansing the liver. Many herbs are particularly recommended for this: mandrake, chicory, black cohosh, red sage, quassia, golden seal. Collinsonia is also recommended for hemorrhoids. A more common name for collinsonia is "stone root." This appears to be helpful in strengthening the tone of the blood vessels.

PARASITES OR WORMS—Garlic taken by mouth and also used in a high enema is effective. Raw pumpkin seeds are also helpful. Quassia and red sage are worthy of consideration and have proven their worth in practice.

DIARRHEA—Two tablespoons of pure carob in heated milk or added to a custard is a practical and safe approach to this disturbance. Fifteen drops of essence of peppermint in 4 ounces of hot water, repeated every two hours until relief is obtained, may also be used.

NATURAL LAXATIVE FOR BABIES—Equal parts of butter and honey blended together, or equal parts of safflower oil and honey. Dosage is ½ to 1 teaspoonful, repeated as needed. This causes no griping, contains no harsh irritants and most of all, it tastes good. (Note: Kleiner's *Physiology* states that even a relatively small amount of mineral oil will remove all carotene present in the food eaten and cause a deficiency of vitamin A. Mineral oil should never be used in any way by humans.)

ARTHRITIS—Several rules apply here, but the following are basically good, and also simple: (1) Eat a raw potato every day. (2) Use 1 tablespoon of raw wheat germ oil three times a day. (3) Take 2 teaspoons of concentrated sea water every day (available at health stores. To avoid pollution, do not collect your own). (4) Eliminate citrus foods and pasteurized milk from the diet.

COLDS—Mix 10 drops of spirits of camphor in one pint hot water. Sip within twenty minutes. This helps open the pores of the skin allowing the toxins to be eliminated. Always use copious quantities of vitamin C complex—500 to 1000 milligrams per hour.

COUGH SYRUP—Mix 2 ounces apple cider vinegar, 2 ounces of honey and 2 ounces of safflower oil. This is both soothing and healthful. Some add cayenne pepper or the herb lobelia to this concoction.

GALLSTONES—Allow me to warn you that the following formula is capable of dislodging a gallstone and it may be too large to pass down the duct. Such an occurrence leaves the patient in acute distress which may be intolerable. (1) No food of solid nature for three days. (2) For two days drink 1 pint of organic apple juice every two hours for six doses and use a mild herbal laxative each evening. (3) First thing in the morning on the third day, drink 2 glasses of apple juice and follow with 4 ounces of olive oil. (4) If there are no results by four p.m., repeat the morning procedure. This may also be repeated next morning. Success is noted when small greenish pebbles are found in the stool.

A Woman's World

The foregoing is but a brief glimpse into the natural world of home remedies. In almost every household the world over can be found time-tested and trusted recipes of relief often reverently referred to as "Grandma's remedies"; one more solid affirmation that it is truly "a woman's world." ☼

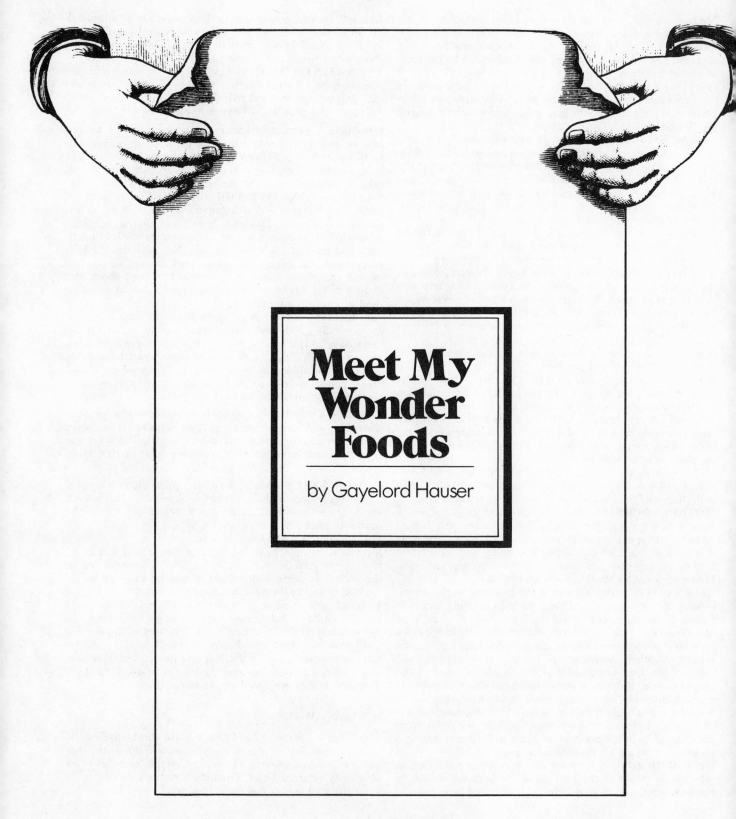

Meet My Wonder Foods

by Gayelord Hauser

There are certain foods I call "wonder foods" because they are so full of concentrated goodness, so inexpensive, so readily available, that they are indeed wonderful. They provide excellent quantities of many of the hard-to-get B vitamins; or they are rich in easily digested protein—and ease of digestion is of great importance, especially in the second half of life. They also provide generous quantities of calcium and iron, two minerals that become more and more difficult to obtain from ordinary foods. These wonder foods can also easily be eaten every day without becoming tiresome, and they can be mixed with other foods to add valuable nutritive factors. I talk a great deal about them, for I am convinced that if they are used generously, they will so improve the nutritive quality of the diet that your health is bound to be benefited. Wonder foods can also help you to look younger and live longer.

Brewer's Yeast
This wonder food has been found to contain 17 different vitamins, including all of the B family; 16 amino acids; and 14 minerals, including the "trace" minerals, held to be essential. It also contains 36 percent protein (sirloin steak, not counting the bone, may contain as little as 23 percent protein). Brewer's yeast contains only 1 percent fat, whereas sirloin steak contains 22 percent!

The calorie requirement of the average woman is about 2,000 per day. One tablespoon of brewer's yeast adds up to only one-hundredth of this calorie requirement, but it provides over one third of my generous daily allowance of vitamin B1 (thiamine) and very nearly one fifth each of the vitamin B2 (riboflavin) and niacin allowances.

Remember, the amount of brewer's yeast we are talking about is just *one tablespoonful*—8 grams, only 22 calories! Think how easy it is to add to your B vitamins and iron. To be sure that you get a true abundance, simply stir a tablespoonful of brewer's yeast into a glass of tomato juice, fruit juice, or buttermilk, or sprinkle it over your salad or your whole-grain cereal.

The figures given here are derived from ordinary brewer's yeast. Specially cultured strains, sometimes referred to as food yeast, are even richer in B vitamins. When you purchase brewer's yeast, examine the label carefully. It should always give you in 8 grams (a little over one-fourth ounce) not less than 0.78 milligram of vitamin B1, 0.44 milligram of vitamin B2, and 2.9 milligrams of niacin. Do not be confused if the label states the quantity in micrograms. There are 1,000 micrograms in one milligram; therefore, 0.78 milligram would be 780 micrograms. If you encounter micrograms and want to transpose them into milligrams, just move the decimal point three places to the left. The food yeasts, which are richer in vitamins than ordinary brewer's yeast, cost only a little more and are cheaper in the long run because they give you more vitamins. Moreover, they are more convenient to store, since you need a smaller quantity. If you do not care for the flavor of ordinary brewer's yeast, you can obtain it in a pleasantly flavored form.

I use the terms *brewer's yeast* and *food yeast* because these indicate a palatable form of yeast. Many kinds of yeast are produced, primarily for baking, that have an unpleasant, bitter taste. If you have trouble finding brewer's yeast, any diet or health-food shop will have it on hand. *Under no circumstances should you ever eat fresh yeast, which is intended for baking.*

If you have never supplemented your diet with brewer's yeast or food yeast, start slowly. Many poorly nourished people lack the enzymes necessary to digest yeast, and may be troubled with indigestion and bloating. If you are a beginner, start slowly with a very small amount, a half teaspoon or less,

Powdered Skim Milk
Powdered skim milk has many properties that cause me to classify it as a wonder food. First and foremost, it gives you protein of high biologic quality, practically free from fat, and in combination with rich quantities of calcium and riboflavin (vitamin B2). Moreover, its vital nutritive factors are in a form readily available to the body and easily digested. Of secondary importance is its convenient physical form; being a dry powder, it can be kept on hand at all times. It is well to store it in an airtight container, preferably a metal one with a screw-on closure provided with a rubber liner. This will exclude the moisture of the air and light, prevent the product from "staling" or becoming lumpy, and also preserve its riboflavin content.

Add powdered skim milk (also called nonfat dry milk) to fresh milk, sauces, soups, custards, waffles, muffins, and all breads; no change of recipe is necessary. It is also delicious whipped into potatoes.

A nourishing beverage for everyone—youngsters and oldsters alike—can be made by mixing one-half cup of powdered skim milk into a quart of whole or skimmed fluid milk. If whole milk is used, the calories are increased by only about 20 percent, whereas the vital food factors are increased by the following percentages: protein, 62.3; calcium, 62.5; iron, 50; vitamin B1, 60; vitamin B2, 100; niacin, 63.

Yogurt
Yogurt is an important wonder food because it is an excellent source of easily assimilated, high-quality protein and contributes significant quantities of calcium and riboflavin to the diet. Yogurt fills a need that has long existed—for that between-meal or bedtime snack when so many people eat what I call "foodless foods"—devil's food cakes, or cinnamon toast made with white bread lavishly sprinkled with white sugar. A taste for yogurt is acquired quickly; you will become fonder and fonder of it as time goes on. It is a good hunger satisfier and, most important of all, contributes much-needed vital food factors with every mouthful. A cup of yogurt fortified with powdered skim milk provides only about 7 percent of the calories for a 2,000-calorie-a-day diet; at the same time it provides, in terms of my generous daily allowances: protein, 17.5 percent; calcium, 50 percent; and vitamin B2,

(continued on page 265)

Human need for iodine has long been recognized. When iodine is undersupplied or absent, the body fails to manufacture thyroid hormone, and a goiter condition results. Certain geographic areas, the so-called "goiter belts" have soils that are seriously deficient in iodine. Crops consumed on such soils, when eaten by animals and humans, may induce thyroid problems that result from iodine deficiency.

However, too much iodine also creates problems. There is a fairly narrow range between too little and too much. A safe daily intake of iodine for humans is estimated to be somewhere between a minimum of 50 micrograms and a maximum of 1000 micrograms. An intake from 100 to 300 micrograms daily is generally regarded as desirable.

In order to overcome the problems created by iodine deficiency, potassium iodide was added to table salt. This step bears a striking similarity to the program of iron fortification of flours and baked goods. In both cases, oversimplified solutions were offered to complex problems. The programs were well-intentioned, but launched before adequate information was available regarding the need, effectiveness and safety of the programs. Both programs have been vigorously espoused by governmental officials and health-interest groups, although opposed by some who have attempted to demonstrate the shortcomings and dangers of the programs. Both the iodization of salt and the fortification of flour represent "gunshot approaches" which aim at a target group. In the case of the former, it is goiter-prone individuals; in the case of the latter, anemia-prone individuals. Both programs medicate the entire population, whether or not people need such supplementation. Such programs might be more wisely controlled by physicians than by grocers. Both programs succeed in placing certain individuals at special risk, if the elements of iodine or iron are oversupplied. And, upon close scrutiny, excesses can result from a combination of current agricultural practices, food processing, inadvertent contamination, and current dietary choices by American consumers.

How Did the Program for Iodized Salt Develop?

Actually, the idea of using iodized salt to combat goiter is not a new one. As early as 1831, J. B. Boussingault, a French physician, suggested its use to combat endemic goiter in South America. Several decades later, iodized salt was introduced in some European countries, notably in Austria, France and Italy. However, these early efforts were abandoned. Perhaps the programs had been poorly controlled, and possibly too much iodine had been used.

A long period followed when no iodine supplementation in salt was used. Then, the idea was reactivated. The U. S. Public Health Service reviewed health data which had been gathered by draft boards during World War I. In 1922, the USPHS issued a report which, among other health problems, described a high incidence of goiter in various geographical regions of America. Goiter was prevalent in 43 states. In some areas, more than 80 percent of the school children examined showed enlarged thyroids.

Also, shortly after World War I, two physicians, O. P. Kimball and David Marine, demonstrated experimentally that goiter could be induced in tadpoles on an iodine-free diet. Their findings were reinforced by studies they made of Ohio school children, and with office patients they examined. As

Iodine in Our Diets
...Too Little or Too Much?

by Beatrice Trum Hunter

a result, Kimball and Marine enthusiastically campaigned for the use of iodized salt, which they felt would eliminate the scourge of goiter. Elsewhere, health officials took up the cudgels, and a vigorous campaign was begun to encourage the use of iodized salt. The plan succeeded. By 1941, iodized salt was used in more than 75 percent of American households.

Pitfalls of the Program

Not all goiter is caused by an iodine deficiency. The appearance of goiter may only be the highly visible and dramatic expression of a general disturbance of the organism. Many patients who suffer from goiter frequently suffer simultaneously from imbalances of the pituitary and adrenal glands, and of the hypothalmus, and from liver malfunction. (H. Haubold, *Landwirtschaftliche Forschung*, 5 Sonderheft, 1954)

The problem is oversimplified with the popular notion that lack of iodine in the diet is the sole cause of goiter. Goiter is a reaction on the part of the thyroid to a disturbance in the metabolism of iodine. Lack of iodine in food or water may be one factor. However, for various reasons, even when an organism receives adequate amounts of iodine, the individual may be incapable of utilizing a supply normally.

Goiter may be related to vitamin A deficiency. The thyroid influences the metabolism of vitamin A, as well as its precursor, carotene. Vitamin A can inhibit the action exercised by thyroxine, the iodine substance extracted from the thyroid gland.

Modern agricultural practices may be involved. When the metabolic rate of an animal's body is slowed down, more fat can be produced and deposited. A thyroid-blocking drug has been developed which, when fed to a steer in the feedlot, gives the animal a "push" for the market by putting on more weight with less food. (*Journal of Clinical Physiology*, Spring 1962)

Another agricultural practice may be involved. Certain plants, for example, which may be particularly rich in iodine, may *cause* goiter in animals feeding on them. Selected white clovers, on the average, were found to contain *14 times more iodine* than ordinary white clover. According to classical chemical analysis, such an iodine-containing crop would be thought to be very favorable for proper thyroid functioning of animals grazing on such forage. However, biological tests of the animals showed that just the opposite was true. These selected white clovers were found to produce thiocyanate in the blood of the animals, which *prevented utilization of the iodine by the thyroid gland*. Other forage crops are also known to have such a goiter-producing factor. This can exert a profound effect on the animals, and their milk or meat products consumed by humans. (André Voisin, *Soil, Grass and Cancer*, Philosophical Library, 1959)

Despite the use of iodized salt, hyperthyroidism (Basedow's Disease, excessive functional activity of the thyroid gland) sometimes occurs in goiter patients *after treatment with iodine salts*.

Some people think that goiter occurs only in areas far from

(continued on page 266)

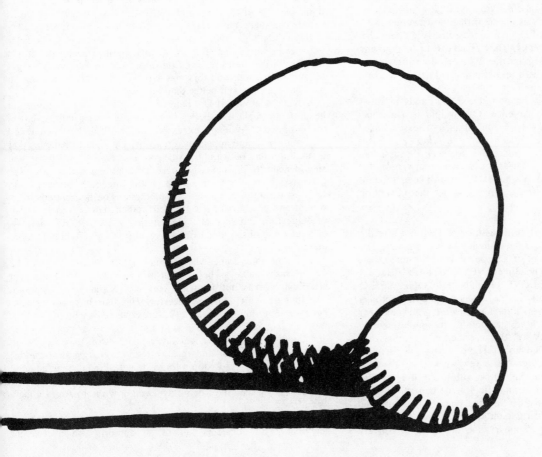

The Real Reason Why You Are

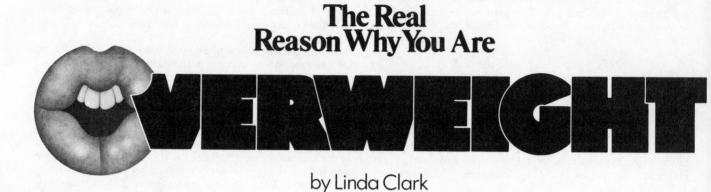

OVERWEIGHT

by Linda Clark

The guests at the party looked like peas in a pod. Most of the men were slightly pasty-faced, with thinning hair and a paunch. They were gulping down their cocktails and reaching out for more hors d'oeuvres. There was a startling similarity among the women present; their hair had been faultlessly set at a beauty salon; their nails perfectly manicured. They were fashionably dressed, slim as reeds, and heavily made up. At first glance, they appeared to be "well preserved" until you looked closer. Behind the facade, something alarming became apparent.

Almost every women had dry skin and straw-like, lustreless hair, even though the beauty operator had tried to hide this with conditioner and sprays. Even worse, on closer inspection, they looked discontented, nervous and trying to appear frantically gay for the benefit of their audience. Each sipped her drink daintily and looked hungrily at the hors d'oeuvre tray, fighting the temptation to eat the whole lot. It was apparent that these women were dieting. They looked sylph-like, but it was clearly evident that underneath they felt like wrecks. They pretended to be enjoying themselves, but once they were outside the host's door, they probably gave vent to their long pent-up ill humor and irritation, common by-products of a reducing diet.

This picture as you know, is reproduced thousands of times in every hamlet and city in America. Overweight is a national — even an international — epidemic. It is a disease caused by a condition *which is preventable and controllable,* and this unique approach, to my knowledge, has not been discussed in any book prior to this one. When you see the real reason for overweight, you will say, "How simple! Why hadn't I ever thought of that before?" There is a simple explanation for the prevention and control of overweight.

Another and Another — Let me assure you I am not offering you one more palliative. There have already been too many. The other day I picked up a copy of a popular women's magazine. On the cover were large red headlines: NEW DIET BY A DOCTOR HELPS YOU LOSE ELEVEN POUNDS IN ONE WEEK! Women were lining up to buy the magazine, hoping that perhaps *this* diet, *this* time, would work. Such articles are gold mines for magazine publishers, but they are just another disappointment to the poor would-be reducer. Why? Because the real cause has not even been guessed or touched upon. There are thousands upon thousands of reducing diets, but after a few weeks, and the loss of a few pounds, the reducer can't stick with it any longer. She becomes ravenous *and* nervous until finally she can stand it no longer, the minute her family has left the house, she shuts the front door and opens the refrigerator door. She starts stuffing herself until she is no longer hungry and no longer a convert

to *that* diet. As the pounds pile up again, within a few weeks she is trying another. But, meanwhile the interludes are blissful for her, and her family, who have been scapegoats for the case of nerves they have been forced to endure from a miserable, irritable, unhappy dieter. Is it really worth it?

Being thin these days is an image all women seem to try to attain. And some of them don't even need to reduce; they just want to keep up with their friends. Reducing becomes an obsession. Many women try to look like the too-thin models in the chic fashion magazine. Unlike those people who are compulsive eaters, others are obsessed by compulsive reducing, the opposite extreme. These unfortunates weigh daily, and if they gain a pound or less (weight can fluctuate temporarily in either direction without being serious), these women panic. I know three of them. They can think of little else. They feel guilt-ridden when they eat. Such people can make themselves and their families miserable.

If you can't get into a dress you wore 20 years ago because you have changed an inch or so in your measurements, forget it! Childbirth, even improved nutrition, can make some changes in your dimensions and this may be a sign you are either normal for your age, or even better than you were 20 years ago.

Salvator Cutolo, M.D., believes that many people should not be thin. He feels it is better to be a little overweight, even up to 10 pounds. Although excessive weight is to be discouraged for both health and appearance reasons, Dr. Cutolo believes that a small surplus of weight gives you a reserve of energy if you should need it. Women who are emaciated or too thin are more nervous and harder to live with. I am sure both husbands and families would prefer wives and mothers to be five pounds overweight and be cheerful and relaxed, rather than to make a fetish of being thin and snap at their families or feel irritable because of a reducing obsession. Life is too short. Decide which is more important.

The time may come when being slightly overweight will be just as fashionable as being over-thin is today. Why? Look at a woman who is not scrawny. Her skin is plump and smooth, like that of a girl. She is cheerful. Her hair has more sheen, her eyes more shine, and her nerves are covered by a bit of padding; they are not raw. Any man will tell you she is more lovable and cuddlesome. As she is more relaxed, so is her family. In short, she *feels* better and thus with more energy and sparkle, she *looks* better. And, don't forget that following the reducing cult can also cause premature aging.

One woman who likes being overweight wrote to Ann Landers as follows:

"Dear Ann Landers: I'm burning over that letter from the screwball who considers herself an authority on overweight women. That nitwit should not be suggesting psychiatric help for fat ladies, she should go to a psychiatrist herself and find out why she is so hostile.

"A person can't pick up a magazine or a newspaper anymore without being hit in the eyes with an article on why women overeat. These articles give the impression that overweight people are mentally ill or they feel rejected and unloved and food is their source of comfort and solace.

"God gave us taste buds because He wanted us to enjoy food. I am overweight because I love to cook and I can eat a meal just 'tasting'. I refuse to apologize for my size and I don't hide in the house. My husband loves me the way I am and he has never suggested that I go on a diet. I would rather be 20 pounds overweight than ruin my health with pills and end up looking like a broomstick with hair."

WHY DO PEOPLE OVEREAT? It is undeniably true that many people overeat as an escape from a disagreeable life situation. It is also true that they may feel unloved.

—Children sometimes overeat to satisfy a nagging or over-indulgent mother.

—Adults may overeat because of loneliness or lack of interest in life. Senior citizens, if they live alone, may not eat enough; on the other hand they may eat too much. I know an elderly woman, who upon awakening, begins deciding what she is going to eat for the day merely because she has no other interest. She *lives to eat*. An interest in others, or a new hobby, or some volunteer work would quickly cure this food-fixation.

—Some people dislike their work and overeat for consolation.

—Others, and this is common, are stress-ridden and overeat for compensation.

—Rewarding yourself with food or drink for bad luck, rejection or lack of love, appreciation, or attention from others, or other emotional disturbances is one of the easiest ways to gain weight. One woman, a successful wife and mother, really enjoyed her role. She was a former model, beautiful, with a perfect figure. She was admired by all, including her husband. Due to circumstances beyond her control, her husband left her. She lost interest in her appearance, ate constantly to forget her grief and now looks like a stuffed pin cushion. Her interest in her children also waned. Had she not given in to psychologically negative influences, she could have had her choice of suitors. But she has lost all interest in life except eating for consolation.

Again, finding a new interest in life, perhaps helping others to replace self-pity, would solve the problem for those living in an emotional vacuum.

—There are also other simple reasons for over-eating. Some people cannot bear to see food wasted and they gobble up everything in sight whether they are hungry or not. Probably these people were always urged, as children, to clean up their plates.

—Some people consider food as a sign of prosperity. One woman I know is grossly overweight. Although she tries every diet which comes along, she doesn't stick with it long. She and her husband own a restaurant and she supervises the food daily. Her will power holds out only so long and then she can't resist the food around her. But there is a reason. This woman was rejected by her mother when she was a small girl and placed in an orphanage. She had little to eat in the institution which was run on a tight budget. So she admits that the cause of her overweight is a double problem: an old grievance of feeling unwanted by her mother, and the fact that she was often hungry simply because there was a scarcity of food. My guess is that after her marriage, she was the deciding factor in choosing a restaurant as a family business. She loves food; she loves to cook and the restaurant is a big success. She is fat, but beautiful. And perhaps it is better for her to stay that way, who knows?

WHAT ABOUT HYPNOSIS? Does hypnosis work for reducers? Sometimes, sometimes not. If a person does not wish to overcome an emotional block to success, hypnosis, which aims at reconditioning the subconscious mind, may prove useless. The woman I have just mentioned submitted to hypnosis by a successful doctor because it had helped others lose weight. She, however, did not lose one ounce.

DO REDUCING DRUGS HELP? What about reducing pills for people who have no will power? Wouldn't they solve the problem? If you take reducing drugs, either with your doctor's permission or without it, watch it! Reports indicate that reducing drugs, including appetite depressants, may increase the pulse rate and cause shakiness in some people. Henry Brill, M.D., states: "Over-use can result in excessive beating of the heart, high blood pressure, nervousness, emotional tension, even hallucinations."

James B. Landis, of a well-known drug company, warns that even pep pills can affect the appetite center of the brain and may cause a psychosis similar to schizophrenia.

The American Medical Association warns that diet pills, including thyroid, hormones, digitalis and diuretics, may not work and can be dangerous. At least 60 deaths have resulted from taking diet pills.

IS OVERWEIGHT INHERITED? Some of you may blame your tendency to be overweight on your inheritance. It could be. Genes are a factor. Dr. Jean Mayer, of Harvard University, states that certain animals have a tendency to put on more weight than others, even though the diet is identical with animals which are not overweight. If your parents and grandparents tended toward fat, it may be a genetic inheritance; or it may be due to the fact that the love for fat-producing food runs in the family. The German diet, for example produces more corpulence, usually, than the Scandinavian diet. And because of national inheritances, some foods agree better with some people.

The Scandinavians have thrived on sea foods for generations. The Italians, living in their warm, sunny climate, thrive on fruits and vegetables. Orientals have subsisted on refined rice for centuries with no noticeable bad effects, whereas others find it a nutritionally inadequate food. (Orientals do fortify their diet with other foods.)

Your body type is another consideration. Some types just naturally gain weight more easily than others. If you are one, your eating must, of course, differ from those who can eat anything they wish without gaining.

WHAT ABOUT YOUR FRAME? Don't jump to conclusions that you are overweight because the height-weight chart says you should weigh so-and-so. The age-height-weight tables are not absolute. Some take into account the size of your frame; others do not. If you have a larger frame and heavier bones, obviously your weight, as judged by the weight of your frame and bones, will be influenced. You may be overweight, according to the chart, but not fat. A reducing diet is not for you.

How About Your Metabolism? You have heard again and again the advice, "Consult your doctor before going on a reducing diet." There are good reasons for this. One reason is, though it usually occurs in the minority, that there are physical disturbances which can cause overweight. This is often the cause in the extremely fat person. It may be due to glandular imbalance, dysfunction of the brain center regulating food intake, or a metabolic disturbance. In the latter case, the fat person may not digest or assimilate his food properly.

(continued on page 267)

Supernutrition and Staying Young Longer

by Richard Passwater

Sufficient knowledge is available today to increase the number of years that we exist, and more importantly, to guarantee an increase in the number of years that we *live*. The single greatest inhibitor of enjoyment to most people is *premature* old age. Some people at fifty years of age look like seventy and feel like eighty; this need not be so. Why is it that some people seem ageless? Science has learned what causes the signs of old age and has also learned to retard their advance.

Dr. Alex Comfort, England's leading gerontologist, in 1964 wrote in his famous treatise *Aging: The Biology of Senescence,* "If we kept throughout life the same resistance to stress, injury, and disease that we had at the age of ten, about one-half of us here today might expect to survive in seven hundred years time."

Contrary to popular belief, neither the maximum life span nor the average age of death for people living past the age of twenty has increased significantly since 1800. The average age at death increased steadily until 1950, but this was due to an improved childhood mortality rate.

For people born in 1950 the estimated mean life span is 68.2 years; for those born in 1955, it is 69.6; for 1960, it is 69.7; for 1965, it is 70.2; and for 1970, it is 70.9.

Can the people who reach seventy years today expect to live longer than people reaching that same age in previous decades? If you examine the percentage of people living to eighty-five years after they have reached seventy years, you will note little increase in the last twenty-five years. Based on the number of survivors reaching a given age out of each 100,000 live births, we find that the percentage of seventy-year-olds reaching eighty-five was 23 in 1950, 24 in 1960, and 24 in 1968 (the latest official figures available).

In terms of estimated years of life remaining for an individual reaching fifty-five years, there is only a difference of two years between the figures for 1900 and those for 1968. For someone reaching sixty years of age, there is only a one-year difference in life expectancy between the eighteenth century and today.

Age Is Not an Accurate Index of Health

Although growth proceeds at predictable rates, aging does not. Some people are old at forty; others are young at sixty. Measuring one's age chronologically has its limitations. It does not describe a person's appearance, vigor, or life expectancy accurately. Dr. Robert E. Rothenberg, author of the book, *Health in the Later Years,* (1965), points out that it would be more logical to determine the present health of a person carefully and estimate the number of years left to him. If this were the practice, then the person of sixty with twenty years of life left could be said to be ten years younger than the forty-year-old with only ten years remaining.

Studies conducted at the University of Maryland indicate people with high blood pressure may be twenty years older physiologically than people of the same age with normal blood pressure, according to Dr. Nathan Shock of the Gerontology Research Center of NIH. Hardening of the arteries (arteriosclerosis) was at one time believed to be associated with aging. This is often true, but arteriosclerosis actually results from a chemical imbalance and not because of chronological aging. Many very old people, including octogenarians and nonagenarians, are free from arteriosclerosis and have normal blood pressures. These people are also "young" in spirit and vitality. Studies similar to those conducted at the University of Maryland have revealed that much of the human deterioration once believed to be the result of time is due to disease. Older people are more prone to most diseases; but as knowledge from gerontological studies is applied to larger and larger segments of the population, it is expected that many currently prevalent diseases will disappear completely. Then, nearly perfect health until a natural disease-free death occurs at the end of the maximum life span will be a reality—many diseases will have been avoided, not by specific treatment, but by improving the body's own defense mechanisms.

Why Slow the Aging Process?

Long life does not interest most of us unless we can be reasonably sure we are going to continue to be vital. The potential cumulative effect and benefit of having the population increase its percentage of able and mature people, still active in the pursuit of a better world is, however, immense. By slowing down the aging process, we can succeed in preserving the quality of life. Crippling diseases due to neglect and undernutrition can be decreased, postponed, or eliminated by slowing the aging process. Arthritis, once thought to be age related, is related more to deficiencies of vitamins B-6, C, and pantothenic acid. It is not a matter of answering the question, "Why do you want to live longer?" It is a question of "Why should you want to die sooner?"

Critical Stages in the Aging Process

From birth to about fifteen or sixteen years of age, human growth is quite rapid. At the age of approximately twenty-five, the human body reaches its maximum strength and physical skill. Normally, this strength and physical skill diminish slowly until about forty-five years of age, the critical point in aging. From this point on, the aging process begins to accelerate. At fifty-five, the aging rate again increases its momentum significantly until age seventy or so, when the aging rate levels off.

During youth, cells that are spent or "die" are replaced by an equal number of new cells. In early youth, there is actually an excess of new cells which causes growth. HGH, the human growth hormone, controls the rate of production of new cells. Although growth proceeds at predictable rates, aging does not. Aging reduces the number of healthy cells in the body and leads to a loss of reserve in body functions, meaning that the body is less able to withstand a challenge or shock. As a person ages, his blood sugar level may remain fairly constant, but his ability to handle the challenge of a large amount of sugar, as measured by the glucose tolerance test, diminishes. Other values (blood volume, red-cell content, and osmotic pressure) that seem to be constant throughout life

(continued on page 268)

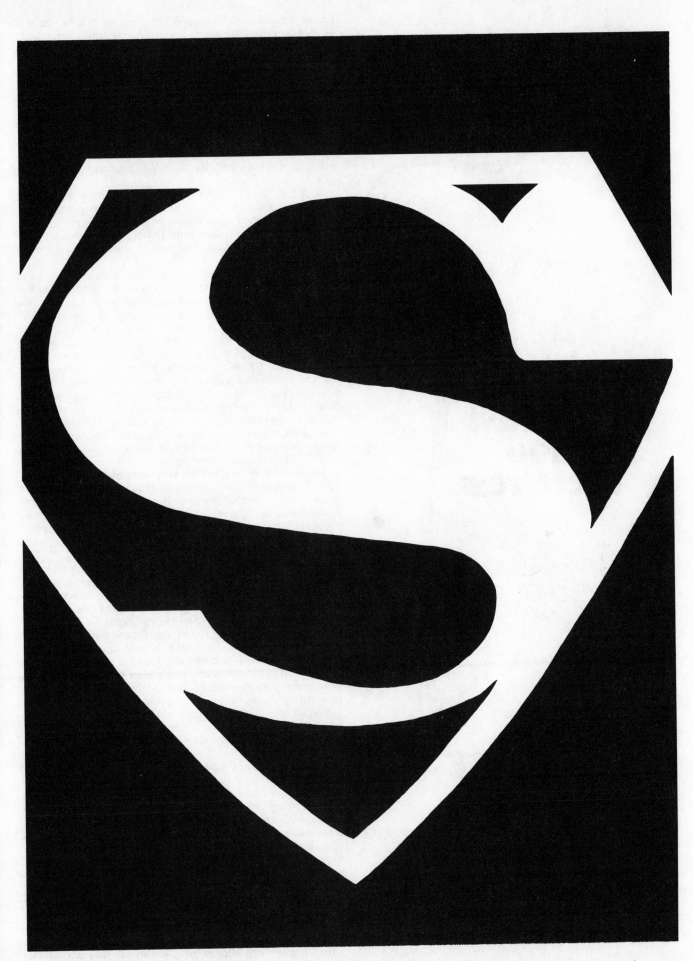

When You Fast You Feel Great

by
Allan Cott, M.D.
with Jerome Agel
and Eugene Boe

I have been blessed with good health all my life, but after a fast [of only drinking water, preferably mineral] I am acutely aware of a sense of well-being.

My own experience is like that of so many others who observe that after even a few days of going without food they feel better physically, mentally and spiritually.

And now we are discovering what the animal kingdom has always known—fasting can be therapeutic.

Unless humans intervene, animals use nature's way to heal themselves. They find a quiet place to rest and they stop eating when they are ill. Even domesticated dogs and cats will resist strenuous efforts of worried masters to force them to eat.

So-called "dumb" cows are smart enough to quit eating when they are sick; sometimes they will keep their jaws clamped shut when cattle raisers or veterinarians try to force-feed them. Hunters have reported seeing a wounded elephant lean against a tree and watch his companions eat without joining them.

Man is the only "animal" who persists in eating when he is sick, even though he may have no appetite and food makes him nauseous. Though our ailing bodies reject food, we are still urged by everyone around us to "keep up your strength" or "build resistance"—keep eating, in other words.

The medical orthodoxy continues to take a jaundiced view of fasting, particularly as a therapeutic tool. This perplexed the late Alice Chase, who wrote on fasting for health: "The medical profession, ruling over the health of mankind, appears willing to subject the sick to the trial of all sorts of drugs, surgery, electric shock, and other forms of treatment that are experimental, even heroic—and sometimes useless. They are unwilling to open their minds and eyes to the more kindly procedures such as *rest of the body, mind and emotions"*—which fasting provides.

The orthodoxy opposes the treatment of the sick by non-medical practitioners. It has used its muscle to put many of these "healers" out of business. But under the supervision of naturopaths and hygienists many sick people have fasted and recovered from really serious ailments after their doctors had all but given up on them. Fasting and new eating habits were just what the doctor *hadn't* ordered.

But even when something appears to work, the profession is still not impressed. The "cure" has to be proved according to orthodox guidelines. Empirical data are not acceptable and scientific journals will not publish papers based on such data; the material is dismissed as "anecdotal."

To me it is even more regrettable that so many of my colleagues are not even interested in investigating something new that has been found to yield desirable results. But when the medical profession shifts gears from treating sickness to preventing sickness—and *it must!*—I have every confidence that fasting will be increasingly prescribed.

People who have chronically abused their bodies with too much food and the wrong kinds of food say that after their first fast they felt really well for the first time that they could remember.

Here again we can take a lesson from the animals. Many species—hedgehogs, bears, woodchucks, female polar bears —hibernate for months without a morsel of food. Birds and beasts of prey get along nicely without food for two weeks or longer. Dogs have fasted for 60 days. Fishes, turtles, and salamanders can go without food for even longer periods of time. But the record may be held by some species of reptiles; they can survive for a whole year without eating. (Tadpoles and caterpillars fast before they become frogs and butterflies.)

The incredibly energetic salmon takes no nourishment as it fights its way upstream to spawn. The journey may last for months and take it through 3000 miles of rapids and waterfalls.

In common with salmon, people discover they have amazing resources of energy during—*and after*—fasting. When we lose a lot of weight, we are naturally going to feel more energetic because our strength isn't being sapped carrying around all that "waste" poundage.

While fasting, Dick Gregory ran in the Boston Marathon. In England a man named Park Barner ran in the 52½-mile "double marathon," from London to Brighton, on a stomach that had been completely empty for 24 hours. "Not only did he finish without having his energy run dry," the magazine *Runner's World* reported, "he ran almost a half hour faster than his previous best for 50 miles. Two weeks later, in a 36-miler, he used the same fasting technique. He passed the marathon mark within minutes of his best time at that distance, and went on another ten miles at the same pace." In the days when the University of Chicago had a football team, Anton Carlson, the distinguished professor of physiology, discovered that a fast of three or four days before a game usually increased the energy and endurance of the players.

Dick Gregory has proposed a provocative idea for the rehabilitation of prisoners, many of whom suffer from malnutrition. "Prisoners who engage in purifying fasts," he advocates, "could be credited with good-behavior time. The penal system that initiates these suggestions just might find it is on top of a tremendous breakthrough in the area of rehabilitation. It just might find that difficulties in rehabilitation stem more from the jailhouse kitchen than from any other source."

Fasting is a calming experience. It is restful. It relieves anxiety and tension. It is rarely depressing and it is often downright exhilarating. A colleague at Mount Sinai Hospital, in New York, tells us that fasting relaxes his muscle spasms, enabling him to reach a plateau in yoga exercises that would otherwise have been a long time in coming.

We have long ago discarded the myth of fat people being jolly people. We know they didn't become fat through just the joy of eating. Anxieties usually lead to overeating, and it is the aftermath of overeating that brings on fresh anxieties focused on health. Quick weight loss from fasting can dissipate these anxieties.

I don't know just how it happens, but many fears seem to disappear or diminish after fasting. I have heard reports of people who lost their fears of flying and crowds and darkness and heights.

One of my patients, who was a recent Harvard graduate, had been a stutterer since he was three years old; on the fifth day of my prescribed fast, his stuttering stopped—and it has not recurred.

Nearly half the population (a staggering 100 million of us) complain of sleeping problems. They sometimes or always have trouble getting to and/or staying asleep. During and after a fast many insomniacs discover they are sleeping better than they have for years. This should not be surprising. Fasting, which has been described as "nature's tranquilizer," relaxes the nervous system and eases the anxieties that account for much sleeplessness. The internal organs are at rest, and this rest is conducive to sleep. Much insomnia can be traced to the consequences of overeating or eating the wrong food: heartburn, bloating, acid indigestion. Because the body operates more efficiently during and after a fast, many people find they do not *require* as much sleep as they used to.

Fasting can be a cheap "high"—the cheapest "high." A state of ketosis, difficult to distinguish from intoxication, can be reached. "Groovy" people refer to it as "a trip," a drugless road to euphoria; they seek "good vibes" and ecstatic visions. They also find that longer fasts can bring on the desired state of susceptibility to spiritual renewal. They flush out their systems and break dope and junk-food "habits." (Their mentor, Herman Hesse's Siddhartha, fasted.)

We are the most antiseptic people on Earth—externally. Others find excessive our germ-consciousness and preoccupation with cleanliness. I wish we all were as concerned with internal cleanliness. In a fast of a week or so we can get rid of toxins that accumulate from food we eat and the very air we breathe. It is a detoxifying strategy that gives the system "a clean bill of health."

Cutting down on weight is one sure way to lower blood pressure and cholesterol levels. A brief period of fasting can bring down these levels dramatically. A 28-year-old man, as one example, lowered his cholesterol level from 232 to 165 milligrams in the three weeks it took him to shed 35 of his 209 pounds. Follow-up fasts help to maintain the lowered levels.

Fasting may be effective in treating many more varieties of sickness than orthodox medical circles are ever likely to concede. I am dismayed by the number of my colleagues who brand all naturopaths and chiropractors and hygienists as "charlatans." On the other hand, I am also turned off by the extreme "naturalists," who claim the expertise of orthodox medicine is totally misguided. Both groups have something to contribute; they could be learning from each other.

All kinds of skin disorders are said to benefit from fasting. It isn't that fasting by itself cures acne or eczema or psoriasis. But the abstention from eating leads the way to a refeeding diet that can discover which foods or combinations of foods are causing the trouble. Skin irritations are often caused by habitual overeating, particularly of starches and sugars, or by some specific food or foods to which the person is sensitized. Many clear up after a cleansing fast and a new diet.

When I was in Moscow, I learned about the use of fasting in the treatment of venereal and dermatological diseases in the clinic of Lumumba University. At University Hospital in Lund, Sweden, researchers saw bald patients—both men and women—start to grow hair again after fasts of only ten days.

Sufferers from such assorted ailments as constipation, hay fever, asthma, peptic ulcers, arthritis, and colitis avow that their symptoms either disappeared or were greatly alleviated after a fast. I have read in the literature that "the value of the fast for the sufferer with hay fever and asthma is so fully established that we can only wonder why it is not more generally resorted to."

Interestingly, *Christian Century* magazine advised its readers to fast out of enlightened self-interest and not "the pieties of traditional Christianity." The objective was not to observe Lenten sacrifices but to lose weight, improve health, and make the body more vibrant and beautiful. "Fast because it is good for you," the magazine urged; it can be an "exercise to get the body in shape to be alive to itself. This process frees the self to be more sensitive to the Creation, to ourselves, and to our histories."

Fasting: The Ultimate Diet

Roland Crahay, professor of psychology and sociology at Warocque-Mons Institute, in Belgium, has studied the psychology of fasting, and often quotes the credo of the famous Buchinger Clinics, in Germany and Spain:

> We must restore fasting to the place it occupied in an ancient hierarchy of values "above medicine." We must rediscover it and restore it to honor because it is a necessity. A beneficial fast of several weeks, as practiced in the earliest days of the Church, was to give strength, life, and health to the body and soul of all Christians who had the courage to practice it.

(The giant Chicago-based pharmaceutical firm Abbott Laboratories published the Buchinger credo in its house organ.)

In *The Great Escape,* "a source book of delights and pleasures for the mind and body," fasting is celebrated as "the ultimate diet . . . the only one that really works, not only for losing weight but for achieving a beautiful high and for getting a look into your cosmic consciousness. Try fasting."

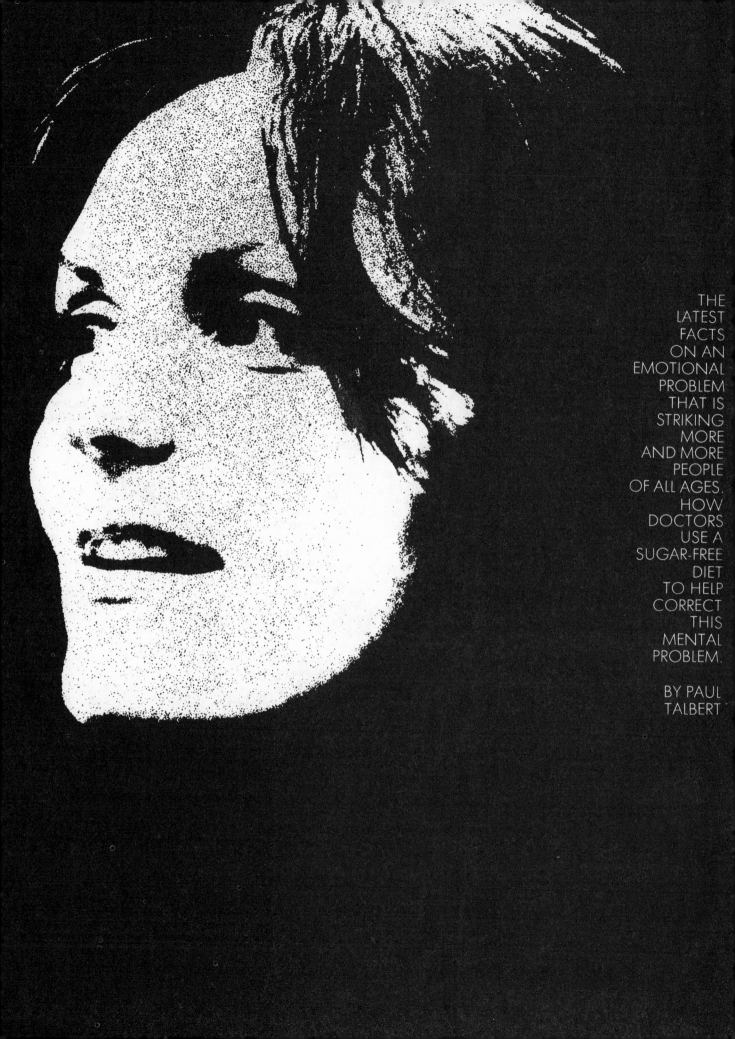

THE
LATEST
FACTS
ON AN
EMOTIONAL
PROBLEM
THAT IS
STRIKING
MORE
AND MORE
PEOPLE
OF ALL AGES.
HOW
DOCTORS
USE A
SUGAR-FREE
DIET
TO HELP
CORRECT
THIS
MENTAL
PROBLEM.

BY PAUL
TALBERT

"There is probably no illness today which causes such widespread suffering, so much inefficiency and loss of time, so many accidents, so many family break-ups and so many suicides as that of hypoglycemia."

These words were spoken by Stephen P. Gyland, M.D., when he addressed an American Medical Association meeting in New York. Dr. Gyland says that while hypoglycemia, or *low blood sugar*, has been recognized since early 1920, "it has remained the stepchild of medicine and is too often not even recognized or then properly treated."

Dr. Gyland was alerting the public to this disguised source of emotional disorders. Hypoglycemia has often been linked to such other emotionally-related problems as alcoholism, drug addiction, juvenile delinquency, mental illness, phobias, chronic fatigue, asthma and allergies, to name just a few. In the light of recent medical research, the list is growing.

The word hypoglycemia actually means "below normal blood sugar." *Hypo*—below or lower than normal. *Glycemia*—sugar in the bloodstream. It is the reverse of diabetes in which there is an excess of sugar in the bloodstream.

While the symptoms are varied, some of the more pronounced difficulties include the following, either singly or in overlapping reactions:

*Fatigue *Inability to concentrate *Excessive hunger *Anxiety *Overweight *Depression *Muscular tension *Restlessness *Poor coordination *Underachievement *Difficulty in speaking *Physical convulsions *Emotional disturbances.

Anyone with such problems should immediately consult a doctor. The earlier the treatment, the greater are hopes for healing.

Hypoglycemia is a symptom of an imbalance of the endocrine glands, specifically the pancreas (the

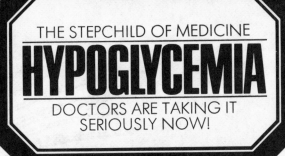

gland located behind the lower part of the stomach). The pancreas has become over-sensitive or over-active and produces an excess amount of insulin, the hormone involved with sugar metabolism. This problem causes the sugar in the body (or *glucose*, as it is called, and which is made from ingested food) to be burned up too rapidly. The preceding listed emotional-physical symptoms occur in varying degrees of severity.

The brain cells depend wholly upon blood sugar or glucose for nourishment. When there is a deprivation of sugar, the brain is usually the first to suffer and emotional disorders occur.

The special 5-hour glucose tolerance test. Many physicians are giving this special test to help chart the amount of sugar in the blood. The doctor who interprets your chart can tell from it how your body handles sugar and whether the levels are abnormal. Many physicians give such tests. You should also enquire at a local hospital to recommend an endocrinologist who could help you. Many physicians can perform the tests right in their own offices. It may well save your emotional health!

The hormonal imbalance of hypoglycemia is often the trigger that sets off a mental illness.

Severe Mental Disturbances. The noted E.M. Abrahamson, M.D., in his classic *Body, Mind And Sugar* (sold at health stores), says that low blood sugar affects the nerve tissue and leads to such neurotic and psychic complaints as:

1. *Psychasthenia*—a neurotic condition characterized by obsessions, phobias or irrational compulsions.

2. *Neurasthenia*—a neurotic condition, feeling of inferiority.

3. *Narcolepsy*—stupor, attacks of deep sleep, migraine headaches, epilepsy, seizure of fits, loss of consciousness.

4. *Psychosis*—mental disease and any serious mental derangement or disturbance.

Harry H. Salzer, M.D., writing in the *Ohio State Medical Technical Bulletin,* points out three major divisions of symptoms that can be traced to hypoglycemia:

1. *Psychiatric Symptoms*: Depression, insomnia, anxiety, irritability, lack of concentration, lack of self-control, crying spells, phobias, forgetfulness, confusion, anti-social behavior and even suicidal tendencies.

2. *Neurological Symptoms*: Headaches, dizziness, trembling, numbness, blurred vision, staggering, fainting or blackouts, muscular twitching.

3. *Intensive Somatic Symptoms*: These include exhaustion, bloating, abdominal spasms, muscle and joint pains, backaches, muscle cramps, colitis and convulsions.

Dr. Salzer says that hypoglycemia can duplicate many neuro-psychiatric disorders. He says that some were incorrectly diagnosed as having such illnesses as schizophrenia, manic depression, psychosis and psychopathic personality. When placed on a high-protein and low-sugar, low-carbohydrate food program, they recovered from emotional and physical disorders.

What is responsible for low blood sugar in the first place? Basically, it is the breakdown of the pancreas brought on by over-stimulating the islands of langerhans (cells in the pancreas) by excessive intake of sweets, processed starches, coffee, tobacco, alcohol and soft drinks. It also is traced to the use of processed foods which are saturated with sugar and starch.

The Abrahamson Diet for Improving Blood Sugar and Emotional Health

Dr. Abrahamson presents a special diet that he used for his patients in order to ease problems of emotional upset caused by low blood sugar. Here is the Abrahamson Diet:

On arising—Medium orange, half grapefruit or 4 ounces of fruit juice.

Breakfast—Fruit or 4 ounces of juice, 1 egg with or without 2 slices of ham or bacon; only 1 slice of bread or toast with plenty of butter; beverage.

Two hours after breakfast—4 ounces of juice.

Lunch—Meat, fish, cheese or eggs; salad (large serving of lettuce, tomato or Waldorf salad with mayonnaise or French dressing); vegetables if desired; only 1 slice of bread or toast with plenty of butter; dessert; beverage.

3 hours after lunch—8 ounces of milk.

1 hour before dinner—4 ounces of juice.

Dinner—Soup, if desired (not thickened with flour); vegetables; liberal portion of meat, fish or poultry; only 1 slice of bread if desired; dessert; beverage.

2-3 hours after dinner—8 ounces of milk.

(continued on page 270)

□ Community water utilities realize that they are in a new world of mounting pollution as the problems of supplying safe, clean water grow in quality and quantity.

□ About 75 percent of our water, for domestic and agricultural use, comes from the earth's surface — from lakes, rivers or reservoirs. This water is pumped up from underground and then stored in the form of wells. It is known as ground water, and it is subject to pollution as a result of what is known as "overdrafts." These occur when coastal fresh water levels are low, and therefore polluted sea water seeps into the storage wells. This leads to forms of municipal sewage in these well waters.

□ Another major source of pollution in our domestic wells can be traced to the dumping of untreated or insufficiently treated sewage into our waterways. We all know that in many communities, everything — all waste — goes down the same drain — domestic wastes, industrial waste, storm sewer drainage from run-off, and so on. Such wastes may or may not go through a sewage treatment plant, which means that this polluted disposal, untreated, seeps into our stored well water, thus affecting the water you take from your tap for drinking, bathing and other home purposes.

□ Pollution of our waterways therefore becomes a matter of growing concern as a variety of new chemicals and trace elements find their way into our raw water sources; and keeping water safe in the midst of this increasing pollution, urbanization and rapidly growing population has become a task beset with what appears to be overwhelming problems.

□ The major number of the nation's water treatments are obsolete. They were engineered to cope with the water problems of a half-century and more ago. Their primary objectives at the time of installation were to cope with the dangers of bacteria and suspended solids. They are incapable of solving the problems arising from dangerous chemicals, viruses and metals now present in available source waters.

□ Water treatment experts are in agreement that the pollution problem has and is mounting with such intensity that municipal facilities and their piping facilities, now and in the foreseeable future, cannot deliver water acceptable for domestic use, and that this job will have to be done in the home. The solution proposes three types of water: **1.** Raw water to be used for outside irrigation and cleaning; **2.** Conditioned water for laundry and other inside cleaning; **3.** Pure water for drinking and cooking. It is agreed that the only certain, feasible, economic solution to your conditioned and pure water needs is to provide for them in the house or apartment.

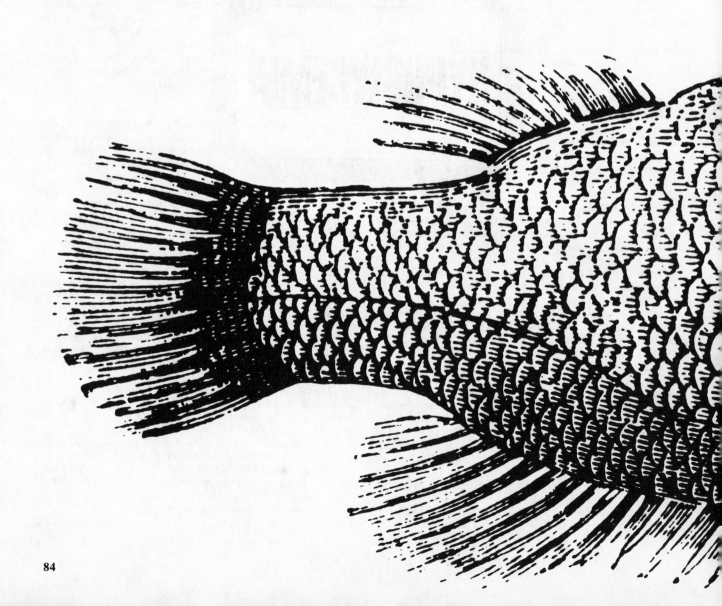

□ One of the principal obstacles in municipal water problems, obviously, is that of proper, constant supervision which unfortunately costs money. It is because of the lack of proper funding that many state health departments no longer have the personnel or equipment to make the necessary checks for appropriate pollution control or to make them on any kind of frequency basis.

□ Politics in many instances is a controlling factor, stemming largely from the fact that almost 80 percent of our water utilities are municipally owned, which means that they are subject to political controls which relate rate structures to votes rather than costs, and that tie water revenues to supporting the municipality and its political structure rather than dedicating such revenues to improved water service for the benefit of those who actually pay for it. When you get right down to it, a water department is a water utility. It can take care of itself if left to do so. Unfortunately, too often it is not.

□ **How Safe Is Your Drinking Water?** For truly good health, you should have at your disposal safe, pure drinking water. You may think you are getting this every time you open your taps at home, but this is in most instances not the case. Here are some reports culled from papers issued by the *U.S. Environmental Protection Agency:*

□ • In March, 1973, two severe community problems traceable to unsafe drinking water occurred in Florida. In one, 97 cases of typhoid were reported at a migrant work camp some 25 miles south of Miami. The other case was the discovery of high bacterial counts in Miami Beach drinking water, with the resulting warning to drink only boiled water.

□ • Throughout the 1960s, there were 128 reported outbreaks of disease or poisoning traceable to drinking water. Twenty people died. About 374 became ill. It is reasonable to assume that many other illnesses went unreported.

□ • A recent U.S. Public Health Service study revealed that 56 percent (over one-half) of 969 public waterworks surveyed had physical deficiencies; more than half (51 percent) failed to disinfect their water. One-sixth (18 percent) exceeded one or more mandatory limits in federal drinking water standards.

□ • The same USPHS study exposed the fact that most polluted waterways were found in smaller areas which suffered from insufficient staff, equipment and funds for improvement. There are about 40,000 American waterworks. Of these, only 1,300 are large systems to serve 106 million people. The rest supply some 54

(continued on page 271)

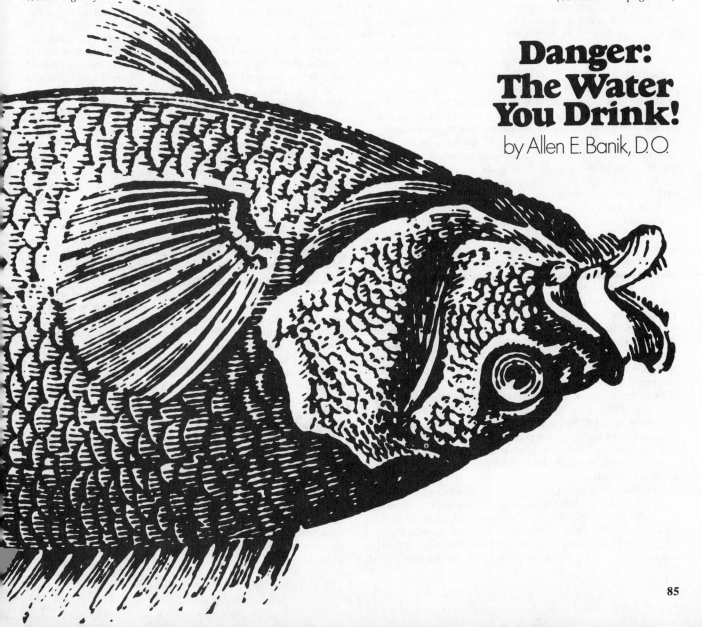

Danger: The Water You Drink!
by Allen E. Banik, D.O.

Total Rebuilding Essential

When we tell an arthritis patient that it takes time to get well, that painkilling drugs must be discontinued, and that a certain amount of pain cannot be avoided, the answer we most often get is, "What difference does it make? I am full of pain anyway. I'll do anything as long as it will get me well."

This is the only sensible way to look at it. If you are suffering from this most debilitating and often deforming disease, what more could you wish than to get well? Many of those who find their way to our care come only after their joints have been greatly damaged; then they realize that their only hope is to buckle down and do what is needed.

How is our program started? First, *all drugs must be discontinued.* This is an important step toward correction. It is essential that we realize from the very start that any drug or remedy that suppresses symptoms of disease such as pain, fever, etc., undermines the recuperative powers of the body, impairing its ability to rebuild itself.

Patients in search of well-being must realize that the pains or other symptoms are nature's attempts to rectify an unhealthy condition, and that they are only hurting themselves when they resort to measures that suppress these efforts of the organism. The aim of patients must be *not merely to obtain relief from pain or gain temporary comfort, but to rebuild the health of the body.*

All Drugs Hazardous

At this point it is essential to emphasize that not only the drugs specifically used in the treatment of arthritis or its associated diseases, but all potent drugs (those that influence or modify disease symptoms), are inherently toxic and must be avoided. People seldom realize that drugs taken in the past, for no matter what ailment, often contribute to the development of this, and other, chronic diseases. Dr. David P. Barr, in a lecture presented to the annual meeting of the American Medical Association, June 8, 1955, discussing the hazards inherent in the use of potent drugs, made this amply clear when he stated that "past use of drugs may be responsible for the late appearance of symptoms or for the development of a chronic disease such as lupus erythematosus or periarteritis."

Dr. Barr continued: "It seems inevitable that with the increasing potency of drugs and the multitude of different reactions caused by single agents that there could be production of syndromes strikingly like those of previously known diseases." He then emphasized that "adverse actions of drugs might be implicated in the pathogenesis (causes) of collagen diseases."

Dr. Jacob M. Leavitt, noted New York gastroenterologist, in some of his unpublished communications, explains that the concept of the collagen diseases (diseases of the bones and connective tissues) deals with many of our chronic and degenerative ailments such as arthritis, lumbago, myositis, neuritis, rheumatic fever, hardening of the arteries, heart trouble, as well as with profound nutritional changes. He stresses the fact that there is a definite interrelationship between these disorders, and emphasizes that a common denominator or an impaired or vitiated metabolism is usually operating in all of them.

In some cases, especially where drugs have been used over an extensive period of time and the patient has become dependent upon them, withdrawal may at first be more difficult and will have to be instituted gradually. Complete withdrawal, however, is imperative if lasting benefits are to be obtained.

Health and Body-Building Food

There was a time when the average doctor replying to the question, "Has food anything to do with arthritis?" would answer most emphatically, "No!" There are many doctors who continue to insist that food has nothing to do with arthritis, but there are others who believe that the wrong kind of food may contribute to the onset of this disease, while a change to the right kind of food can make all the difference between recovery or failure to get well.

A Well-Regulated Nutritional Program

The first step is to change to wholesome natural foods. The diet should at all times include the use of an abundance of fresh vegetables and fruits, and these should, whenever possible, be eaten raw. When used in their uncooked, natural state, they supply not only highly valuable protein and easily digestible starches, but also the essential minerals, vitamins and enzymes. These foods plus small quantities of the more concentrated protein foods (such as lean fish, fowl or any lean meat, lentils, chick-peas or the bland, unprocessed cheeses) and wholesome natural carbohydrate foods, such as potatoes, natural brown rice or any of the whole grain cereals, provide a well-rounded, healthful diet. All processed and refined substances such as the denatured cereals, cakes, pastries, spaghetti, sweets, ice cream; all kinds of white flour products, polished white rice and white sugar concoctions, must be excluded. The rich, highly concentrated foods, such as butter, cream, eggs, various fatty cheeses, as well as the fatty meats and fish, should be omitted or used only to a very limited degree.

Planning a Heathful Diet, Sensible Eating Habits

In planning meals for arthritis patients, various factors must be considered. Weight, habits of eating, hunger, physical activities; work, as well as the general health of the person, play a part in determining diet. This is why it is important for those who can possibly do so, to place themselves under the care of a doctor or practitioner who is fully conversant with sound hygienic principles of health. With experienced guidance these patients will be able to make much more rapid progress.

Those who cannot avail themselves of this help must still

New, and Natural, Hope for the Arthritic

by Max Warmbrand, D.O.

realize that only when they adhere to a diet providing all the essential nutrients in their natural and easily-digestible form, will they succeed in obtaining lasting results.

To make sure that an arthritis sufferer derives all the good from his or her food, sensible eating habits must be established. The arthritis sufferer must learn to eat slowly, chew his food thoroughly, eat only when hungry, and make sure not to overeat. The foods eaten should be properly combined — the fewer combinations at a given meal, the better.

Skipping Meals Beneficial

New patients should, if possible, start by abstaining completely from all solid foods for at least one, two or even several days, and should revert periodically to a liquid diet. Restricting food intake to fresh fruit juices, fresh vegetable juices, or the pleasant aromatic herb teas — gently sweetened with honey and flavored with a dash of lemon — rests the digestive system, promotes the elimination of toxins, and prepares the body for more rapid and effective rebuilding.

Some patients ask whether the body on a restricted diet is deprived of essential nutrients. All we can say is that what matters is not how little we eat, but the kinds of food we eat. If we eat only the best of foods, and receive adequate liquid nourishment, a little goes a long way. Remember that a tree grows for thousands of years on one spot, receiving the nutrients it needs during all its life from the soil where it stands. Of course, it also gets nutrients from the atmosphere, but so do we. The tree absorbs the carbon dioxide while we benefit from the oxygen we breathe.

Once in a while we suggest that patients restrict themselves to water, only for a day or two, or even for several days. When this is too difficult, a fruit juice diet, using the juices of freshly-squeezed fruits such as orange, grapefruit, apple, grape or any other wholesome fresh fruit, will do. Sometimes fresh fruits may be used in place of juices, taking one kind of fruit about every two to three hours for one, two or even several days. After this preliminary start, a diet that meets the needs of the individual case should be planned. Those who are overweight or who are not too hungry, may begin by taking one kind of fresh fruit whenever hungry or about every two to three hours during the day. Only one kind of fruit should be eaten at a time. Make a raw vegetable salad the major part of your meal. Then, add to it a moderate portion of protein or one of the easily digestible starches, plus one or two steamed vegetables. This provides a fine meal and supplies all the nutrients needed.

No butter, salt, or any of the other conventional seasonings should be added to the vegetables. We have no objection to the addition of small amounts of soybean oil, sunflower oil, wheat germ oil or freshly squeezed lemon juice

(continued on page 273)

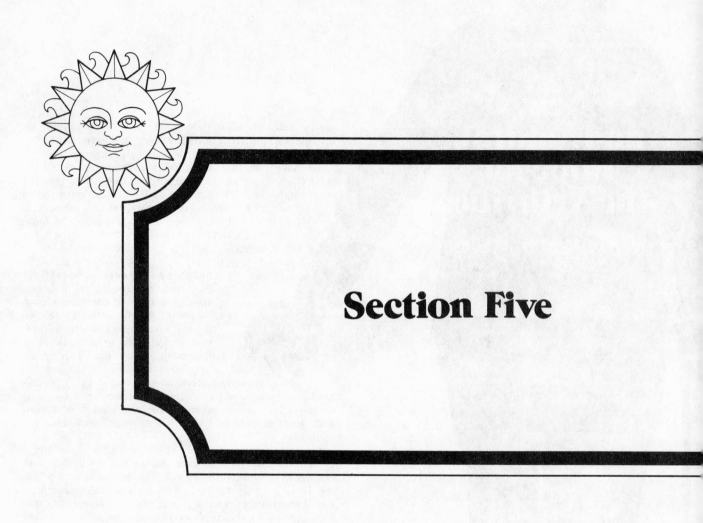

Section Five

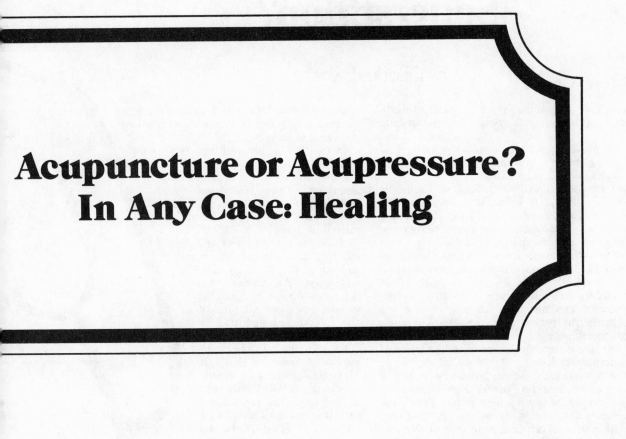

Acupuncture or Acupressure?
In Any Case: Healing

Acupuncture: Science or Superstition?

by Charles Ewart

What is acupuncture? A genuine system of curative medicine, or a mass of hocus-pocus rooted in folklore and superstition?

Dr. Moss has proved that it is a valuable method of relieving and curing many complaints, and has staked his professional standing on this conviction.

Acupuncture has been practised throughout China, its country of origin, for 5,000 years. It is taught in the medical faculties of the Republic's universities, is included in the Chinese medical curriculum, and is practised by more than half a million doctors. When Chairman Mao won power, one of his first measures was to proclaim that acupuncture should predominate in China, in association with western medicine.

In 1971 considerable publicity was given to a complicated lung operation in China in which acupuncture was used to anaesthetize the patient, who remained conscious throughout the operation.

Oddly enough, it was through the agony and suffering of war that acupuncture was discovered by the Chinese.

Five thousand years ago, when Britain was still a primitive society of small warring tribes, the Chinese had a civilization and culture of a very high order. They were peace-loving people, but even so, from time to time they had to fight, either to repel invaders, or to recover territory that had been occupied. The weapons used were normally spears and bows and arrows, which inflicted ugly wounds.

The High Priests, like those in biblical times in the Middle East, were also the physicians, and they observed among the wounded that injured men often said that since being wounded, an illness, from which they might have suffered for years, had disappeared.

For example, a wound in a specific part of the foot would reduce blood pressure or relieve a headache or toothache, or an injury on the outside of the knee joint would cure migraine.

Over the years the High Priests made more and more observations of the phenomena of a wound in one part of the body curing a long standing complaint at another point.

But it was not, they discovered, the size of the wound that mattered, but the precise position. Only a pin-prick in the right place was enough to effect relief. Thus acupuncture was discovered.

At first the surgeon-priests used fish bones and sharpened splinters of bamboo to effect the pricks. Later came finely honed needles. The war lords and nobility were treated with needles forged from gold and silver.

With the perfection of the science of acupuncture it was discovered that the needles need only be inserted in a point of skin measuring about one-tenth of an inch.

Altogether nearly 800 points of acupuncture have been discovered by the Chinese, and each one is named after its discoverer. When stimulated by the insertion of a needle each of these points has a beneficial effect on various illnesses.

Like most techniques and discoveries, acupuncture has waxed and waned in popularity, but by and large the Chinese have stuck faithfully to the five-thousand-year-old dictum of the Yellow Emperor: "I desire that all remedies apart from acupuncture be suppressed. I command that this method and knowledge should be recorded and transmitted to future generations and that its laws should be recorded so that it will be easy to practise it and difficult to forget it."

The laws and method have remained, although they have now been linked to western medical techniques.

Slowly the practice has spread throughout the rest of the world. In France there are four medical societies of acupuncture whose membership exceeds 1,000, and it is possible to get acupuncture treatment on the health service. It is taught in at least four Russian universities, and only recently it received official blessing in Japan. In Switzerland and Germany it has been used for many years, and there is growing interest in it in America.

But in Britain practitioners have to rely on their own faith, and frequently have to face up to the scorn and disbelief of the medical profession.

The major problem with acupuncture

(continued on page 275)

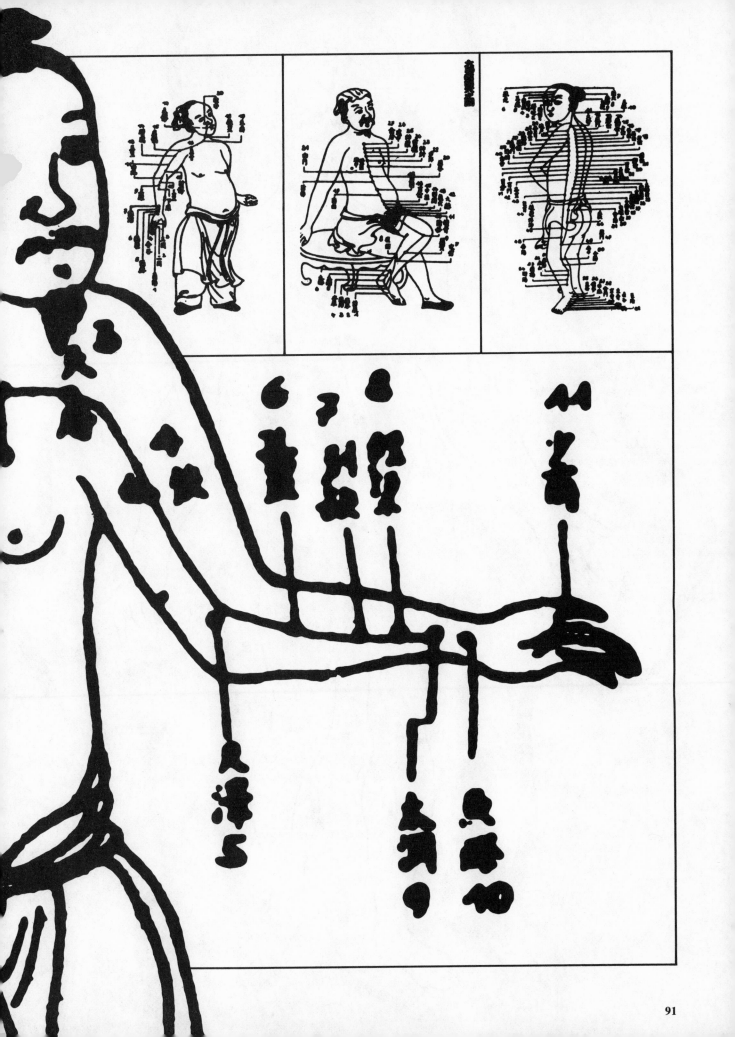

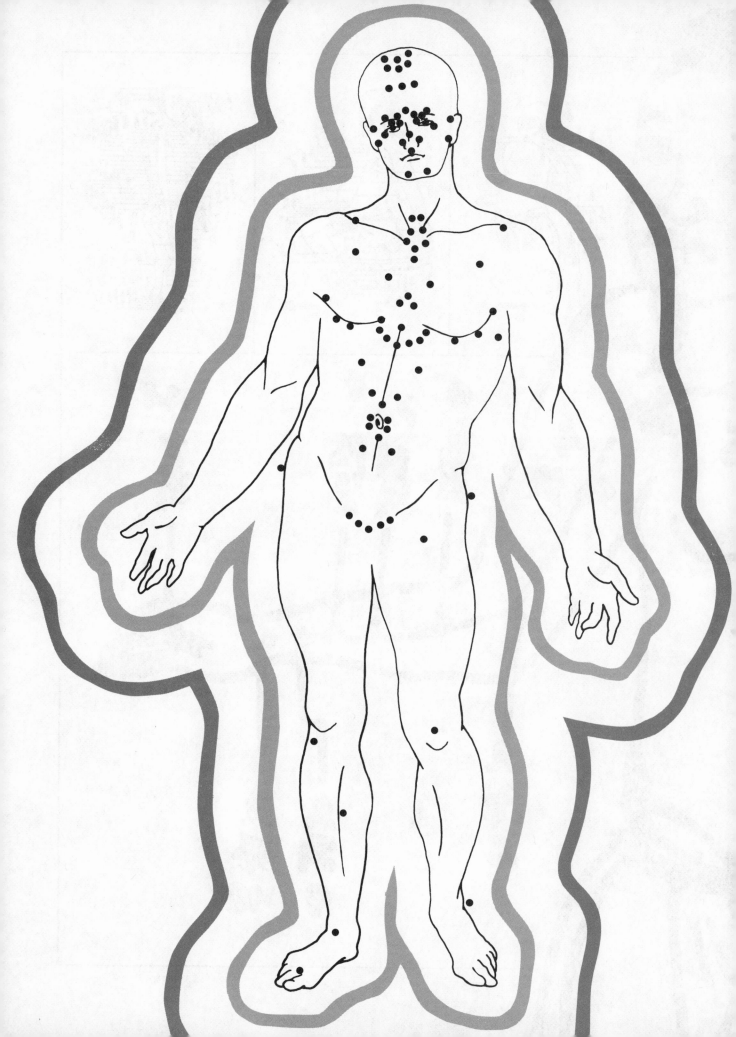

As we learn more about caring for our bodies in natural ways to acquire and maintain good health, the possibility of helping ourselves out of an ache, pain or ailment becomes more and more important. Doctors are busier than ever and house calls are out of style. Each family should have health information for emergency purposes if a doctor is not available or until he is available. For the last twenty years, acupressure, or acupuncture without needles, has spread to many countries, and many testify to the fact that it is helpful therapy and that nearly anyone can use it with benefit.

Acupressure is a method of contacting the electrical centers in the body. Balance and order must be established before health becomes established. Acupuncture is a proven system used for centuries by the Orientals to create a smooth flow of vibratory energy throughout the body by contacting various points on the pathways which relate to various organs, glands and cells. The acupuncturist, of course, uses steel needles which are inserted at certain points identified with the various body areas and their disturbances. By changing their distorted vibrational nature, balance is restored and the body can repair itself.

Contact healing, or acupressure, also treats the various points of the body which relate to various areas, glands and organs. However, instead of using needles, this method is a do-it-yourself technique of pressing your fingertip on these contact points. If the organ, area or gland the point represents is in trouble, that point will be sore, indicating an energy leak at that exit.

Once you have located a painful spot, just put your fingertip on it, press firmly and hold it there. Do not move it, or you will move off of the zone which needs help. This pressure closes an energy leak. As soon as you close the leak, the polarity is reversed and the energy flows back into the part of the body which was losing it. You should feel a warmth build up in the organ you are treating, indicating that regeneration and repair are beginning to take place. When there is no longer any tenderness at the contact point you can feel assured that the regeneration is complete.

Acupuncture may, or may not, require more than one treatment. Acupressure usually does need even more time. The reversal of symptoms seldom takes place in one treatment. But the more you treat and the longer you treat, the sooner the job is done to help you feel fit again. At the very least, the system is safe and simple and free. You have nothing to lose and much to gain if you will be consistent and faithful until you witness a restored feeling of well-being.

There are several ways of using the fingers: the tip of your index finger, your third finger, or for even more strength, reinforce your index finger by placing the third finger on top of the index finger or use the two fingertips side by side. At some points it is much easier to use the tip of your thumb.

Always use only the amount of pressure you can tolerate. Pressure on contacts should be firm but not hard enough to be acutely painful. Remember, you cannot overtreat. The longer and the more often, the better. In all severe, acute or chronic conditions, treat daily for the first week; then two or three times weekly; finally once weekly. This is determined by your own needs. Sometimes much time is necessary; other times a condition will respond so fast as to be unbelievable. When the tenderness is gone, the congestion has been relieved.

There are 102 pressure points on the body. The diagrams and legends of a few have been chosen here from *The Healing Benefits of Acupressure* for interest and experiment. Since each individual is differently built, your contact points may be slightly different in location than those on the diagrams. Tenderness indicates the spot that needs to be corrected. ☼

The Healing Art of Acupressure

by F.M. Houston, D.C.

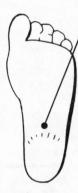

40 energy, inflammation

Located in the center of the bottom of each foot just in front of the heel prominence. These contacts connect energy from the earth to man and can travel clear to the brain. They are very important in all inflammatory conditions, such as colitis, cystitis, peritonitis and phlebitis.

13M duodenal ulcer, pneumonia

On top and center of the nose where the bone ends and the cartilage begins (single contact). This treats the occipital lobe of the brain where pneumonia has its origin before descending into the lungs. This contact also goes to the first twelve inches of the small intestine called the duodenum. 13M is for either pneumonia or duodenal ulcer. For ulcers press once daily until improved.

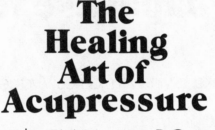

34 brain, energy, food poisoning

Treats the eyes, the frontal lobe of the brain and affects the consciousness and intestines. These two contacts are located directly above the center of the eyebrows against the frontal bone of the forehead. Also for food poisoning. If you become sleepy while driving, press #34's for a few minutes.

16M anti-sneeze, paralysis

A single contact located under the center of the nose. It is the point for the anterior pituitary and works on certain types of paralysis. It is also the anti-sneeze center.

50 Systemic diabetes, tension

Ask a friend or family member to stand behind you and place his thumbs at the base of your neck on each side simultaneously. Press inward and down at approximately a 45-degree angle, directing the contact toward #21. This contact is painful in everyone because everyone today suffers from tension. To release congestion in neck and brain and for mental fatigue. Also used to sober up an alcoholic and for insomnia and diabetes.

79 energy, tension

Located midway between the base of the neck and shoulders. Treat for tension in shoulders and arms, and also body warmth and energy.

Shiatzu: An Introduction to the Japanese Version

by Yukiko Irwin with James Wagenvoord

Since its beginnings, Oriental medicine has been closely related to the philosophy of Oneness and the idea of yin and yang forces of the environment and the body. The belief was that diminished health occurred only when the equilibrium between yin and yang was broken. The approach to healing was preventive, to keep the body in harmony. If, however, the harmony was lost, it had to be restored. This attitude of prevention has been carried down through the years to shiatzu, for it is first and foremost a method to maintain health and keep the body in harmony.

The ancient Chinese healers and philosophers made intensive studies of human ailments. The system which grew out of these studies was quite different from that developed by modern Western medicine thousands of years later. The Oriental approach is empirical: practices are based on experience and observation. The Chinese sages observed that certain ailments affected certain points on the surface of the body: various points became hot, cold, numb, hard, painful, oily, dry, discolored or stained. They located 657 such points on the body and observed that some of these points appeared to be related to one another. Acting like medical map makers, they charted the lines between these related points and determined that there are twelve pathways or meridians con-

necting the points on each half of the body. In addition to these twelve pairs of body meridians, they traced out two coordinating meridians which bisect the body. One, known as the meridian of conception, runs up from the base of the trunk, up the center of the abdomen, the center of the chest, and ends at a point in the front center of the lower jaw. The second, the governor meridian, begins in the center of the upper gum, traces up and over the center of the skull, down the spine, and ends at the base of the tailbone. The meridian of conception was so named because the sexual organs are located along this line. It acts mainly on yin energy. The governor meridian received its name because of the extreme significance of the spine as the main pillar of the body. It acts mainly on yang energy. These two bisecting meridians control the energy which flows constantly through the twelve pairs of body meridians. Interconnected, the twelve pairs of body meridians or pathways form the single energy system which maintains the health of the body.

The accuracy of the sages' observation is attested to by the fact that their idea of the functions of these meridians corresponds in many cases to the functions of the various networks discovered so many centuries later by Western medicine, i.e., the circulatory and nervous systems, the endocrine system, the reproductive system, etc.

The early sages believed that the meridians were pathways through which the energy of the universe circulated throughout the body organs and kept the universe and the body in harmony. They conceived that illness or pain occurred when the pathways became blocked, disrupting the energy flow and breaking the body's harmony. By inserting extremely fine needles into the body at the affected points on the pathways and into related points, they believed that the pathways' blockage was broken and the flow of energy was restored. They also believed that periodic treatment of a healthy person helped to preserve the flow of energy and to prevent illness. This grew into the science of acupuncture.

Over the years acupuncture has become a sophisticated medical discipline still based upon its early concept—that it is necessary to maintain balance between all areas of the body within itself as well as within the external environment.

Chinese acupuncture was introduced to Japan 1,300 years ago. Shiatzu developed during the eighteenth century in Japan as a combination of acupuncture and the traditional amma form of Oriental massage. Am (press) ma (stroke) was a simple pressing and rubbing of painful spots on the body by the fingers and palms of the hands. It was determined that instead of needles, direct thumb and finger pressure on the acupuncture meridian points would gain similar results. The points are, in effect, the floodgates which when stimulated with steady direct pressure keep the energy systems in motion. This innovation is regarded as the beginnings of shiatzu as we know it, although it was nearly two hundred years later, in the 1920s, that the name shiatzu became part of the Japanese language. Today there are over 20,000 licensed shiatzu therapists in Japan, and the art itself is a part of nearly every Japanese life.

Although shiatzu is closely allied to acupuncture and shares its effects on the body, I strongly favor shiatzu as an individual discipline for a normally healthy person. Acupuncture is primarily a way to treat ailments, while shiatzu's main function is to maintain health and well-being—although it does overcome many ailments and aches. Shiatzu is free of the risks of infection or rupture that are inherent in needle therapy. While it is not possible for a layman to give acupuncture, virtually anyone can learn the basic shiatzu techniques. And you can apply shiatzu to yourself easily.

The fundamental philosophy of my work with shiatzu is giving, to ease another's pain, to make another feel better.

We often take our hands and fingers for granted, but they serve us as a means of communication and a way to ease pain. When in love, people hold hands or touch each other. When one is in pain, one's hands reach directly to the area of the pain. Being at one with your hands is the essence of shiatzu. Whether you are giving to another or practicing self-shiatzu, energy is transmitted from your hands.

Specifically, shiatzu is given with the thumbs, fingers and palms, but these serve only as the outlet for your energy. In fact, you give shiatzu with your entire body, focusing your weight and consciousness at your fingers.

When giving shiatzu to a partner, you soon develop an ability to sense the degree of pressure which should be exerted. You should be on the thin line between pleasure and mild pain. The more tension you sense, the greater the pressure you should offer.

One way to become familiar with the various pressures is to practice your touch on a bathroom scale. Place the flats, or the bulbs, of both of your thumbs on the scale. Straighten your arms and press straight down with your arms bearing your body weight until the scale indicator reaches twenty pounds. This is the amount of maximum pressure which should be applied to the strong-muscled portions of the body. Count to three and raise your thumbs from the scale, pause, and again press down for a three count. Repeat this a few times until you are familiar with the amount of pressure which you must exert to reach the twenty-pound level. Do the same exercise at fifteen pounds and at ten pounds. Fifteen pounds is approximately the pressure you should use on the head and stomach. Ten pounds is the level for the front and sides of the neck and the lower abdomen. ☼

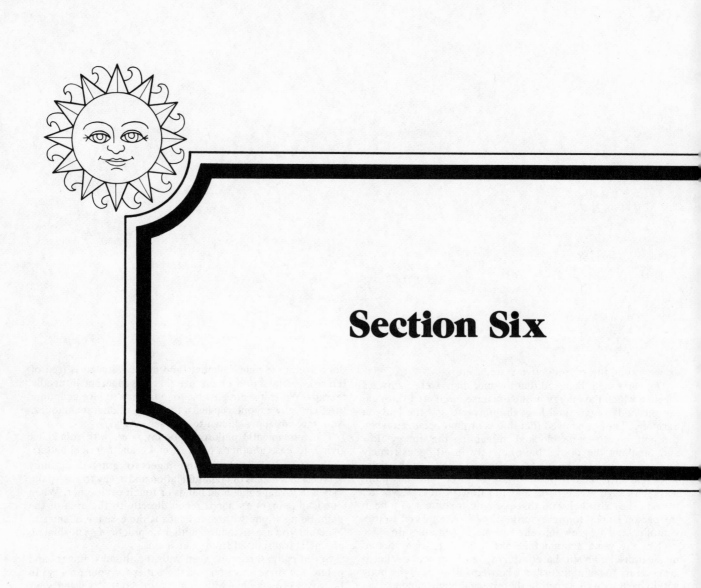

Section Six

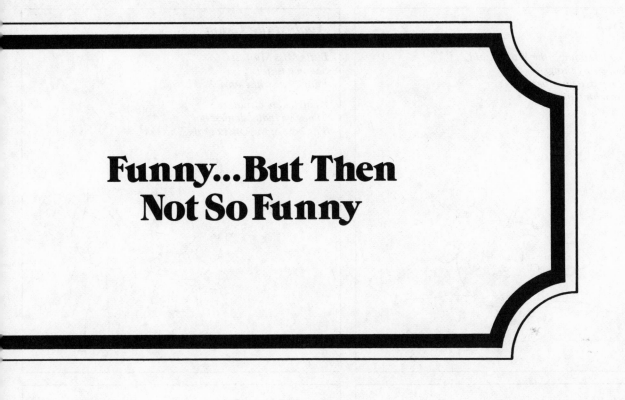

Funny...But Then
Not So Funny

A Polluter's Garden Of Verses

by Barbara Jurgensen and Murray Goodwin

Illustrations by Jerry McLaughlin

Why Dye

"The time has come," the Walrus said,
"To ask of many things—
Of why they dye potatoes, nuts
And maraschino bings."

Against the Grain

Little Miss Muffett
Sat on a tuffet
Eating her white enriched bread.

Along came a spider.
"They've really denied her
The best of the wheat grain," he said.

City Noise

Tell me not in mournful numbers
Who creates our city's din,
Ruining work, disturbing slumbers,
What a raucous fix we're in.

Won't someone kindly pass a law
To cut the ceaseless clatters?
We beg you do it soon, before
We all go mad as hatters.

Let Me Eat Cake

Pat-a-cake, pat-a-cake, baker's man,
Bake me a cake as free as you can
Of lethal preservatives, for goodness sake,
I need preserving more than the cake.

Unripe at Any Price

One a quarter, two a quarter, three a quarter, four
We pay enough for fruit we should hope to get much more.
They're picked so green, so hard, so raw,
They'd make a lovely marble floor.

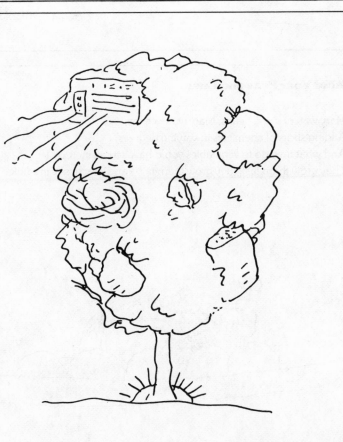

It's Cool

I think that I shall never see
An air conditioner like a tree.
A tree can do the work of ten,
Give fruit or nuts, then cool again.

Give leaves for mulch or figs for newtons
Or birds' nests—great for soup and croutons.
A tree does so much, as a rule,
Besides just making sure we're cool.

And More Pollution from Our Garden

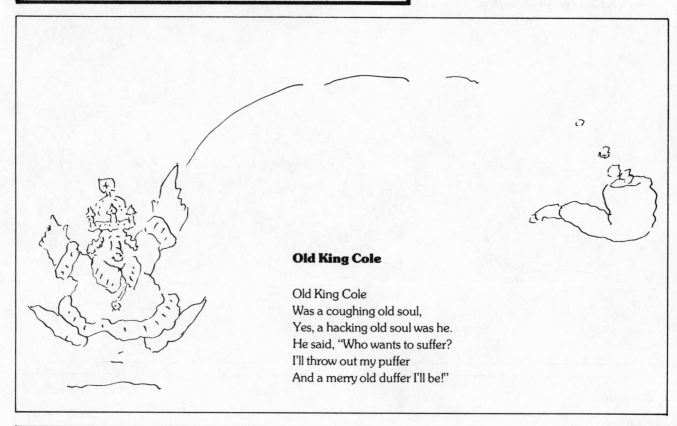

Old King Cole

Old King Cole
Was a coughing old soul,
Yes, a hacking old soul was he.
He said, "Who wants to suffer?
I'll throw out my puffer
And a merry old duffer I'll be!"

Mind Your Peas and Cues

Mary waters string beans, Mary waters peas,
Adding shots of chemicals in varying degrees.
And what they do to vegetables you'd have to call incredible.
They grow them fast, they grow them tall—and practically inedible.

Well-Bread Singer

Little Tommy Tucker sings for his supper.
What does he eat? Good bread and butter.
Little Tommy Tucker sings by the hour
For bread made of unbleached spring-wheat flour.

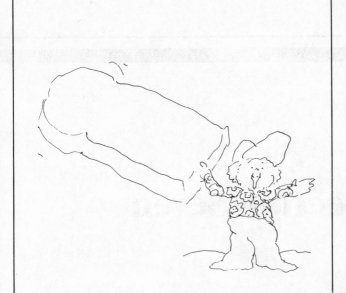

The Spider and the Fly

"Won't you come into my parlor?"
Said the spider to the fly.
"I'm a little short on protein
And just now you caught my eye."
Said the fly, "Have you considered
Eggs and seafood, beans and peas?
Milk and nuts have proteins also.
I'm off duty. Try them, please."

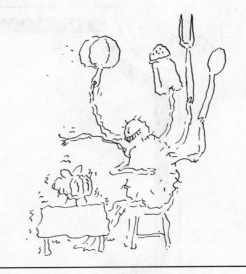

Twas Brillig

Twas brillig, and the compost pile
 Made vegetables feel lucky,
It brought them up to taste worthwhile,
And that's no Jabberwocky!

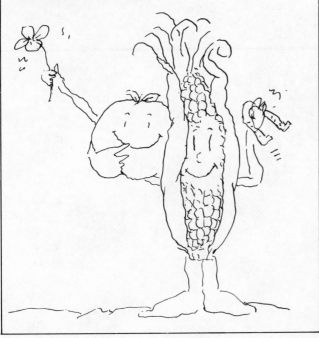

Thought

It would be very nice to think
The world was full of meat and drink
So children small in every place
Could have some food to follow grace.

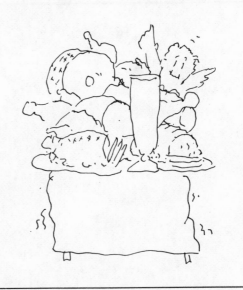

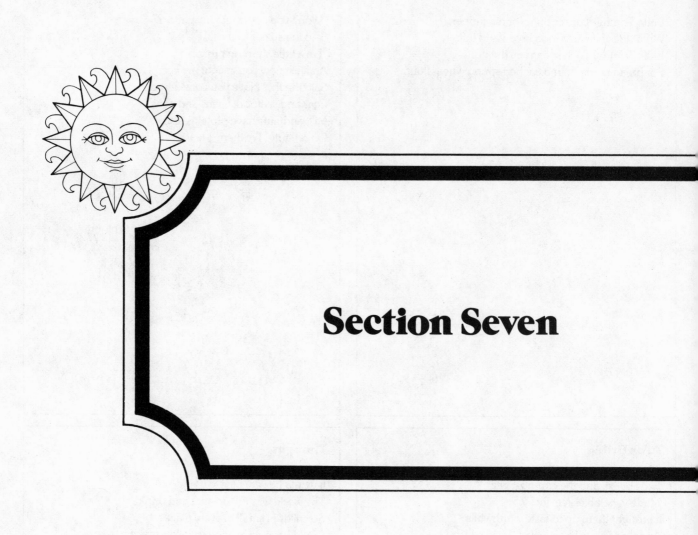

Section Seven

Caution: No Junk Foods or Empty Calories Allowed

Oh, How You'll Love to Get Up in the Morning! - for Those Marvelous Breakfasts, of Course.

by Nikki and David Goldbeck

We Need a Good Breakfast

No matter how much food you consumed yesterday, you still must eat today. Each day your body has certain food needs — calories (for energy), protein (for the building and maintenance of muscles, bones, blood, and all the bodily organs), minerals (which act along with the proteins), and vitamins (which serve as catalysts to keep the work of the other food elements in progress). Once the daily requisite for calories and protein has been satisfied *any excess is stored as fat*; the body cannot put away protein from one day to fill a deficiency in the coming days. While you can store some of the minerals in small quantities, and the vitamins A, D, E and K, all other unassimilated vitamins and minerals are excreted.

Consequently, when you begin a new day it is important to give your body a fresh source of nutrients to run on. Those who become cranky, inattentive, nervous, and prone to headaches in the early part of the day, seemingly for no reason, may find that there is a reason after all — too little morning nourishment.

Poor breakfasts have also contributed to many of our national ills, both physical and economic. Low blood sugar, obesity, diabetes, heart conditions, hyperactivity, chronic constipation, and many other ailments could all be controlled more effectively with a nourishing breakfast.

With a good breakfast under your belt you can eat smaller, more evenly balanced meals. You no longer have to stuff yourself in the evening after starving yourself during the day. Thus you can eliminate the strain on your heart from overindulging and the nighttime stress on the digestive organs. By choosing less-processed breakfast foods — like fresh and dried fruits and whole-grain cereals and baked goods — you will receive more roughage in your meal. For many this means improved regularity without resorting to laxatives.

A good breakfast, one balanced with protein, fat, carbohydrates, vitamins, and minerals, also makes it easier to resist the pastry wagon at coffee-break time. You can enjoy a shorter, lighter meal at noon and spend the remainder of the hour in a stroll through the neighborhood rather than shuttling from the chair behind your desk to the chair behind the lunch counter. At the same time you are conserving calories and getting some good exercise, you will also be saving money — the expense of lunch being one of the biggest salary-eaters.

Many people who swear by a morning "meal" of a cigarette and a cup of coffee would not need the "coffee kick" if they would accustom their systems to some real *food energizing* instead.

Moreover, work efficiency and learning ability can be enhanced by a satisfied stomach. Your brain, like all your body organs, is dependent on food for nourishment. Unless the blood, which feeds all the cells, is supplied with fresh fuel in the morning your mind will remain as empty as your stomach. As one UNESCO official succinctly phrased it, "If you want to have democracy in education, you have to feed the children first."

What Constitutes a Good Breakfast?

Everyone has his or her own opinion of what foods qualify as breakfast fare. While eggs, cereals and sweet rolls are popular in this country, in Egypt, Fuul Mudammas (a cooked bean dish) is the morning staple. In Japan, the traditional breakfast includes rice and miso (fermented soybean soup), while in Israel a huge buffet including yogurt, fish, radishes, turnips, other vegetables, eggs, and cheese is set out each morning.

The fact is, most foods that are good for you are good for you at any time of day. Thus, food selection at breakfast time is limited only by your imagination. Of course, for some, time may be a consideration, but this too can be easily surmounted with a little advance planning. Many families that are out all day still enjoy dinners of stews, casseroles, and roasts, which demand lengthy preparation or cooking time. They are able to do this because they prepare in advance. There is no reason why some of this time cannot be spent planning breakfast, for actually, if given a choice between a substantial morning meal or a substantial evening meal, you would be better off opting for the former.

Although there are no hard and fast rules about what to serve for breakfast, rich sauces, heavy spices, and the use of alcoholic beverages in cooking are generally avoided. These all tax the digestive system and serve to weigh you down rather than invigorate you. Though some fat is important to prolong digestion and keep you satisfied longer, too much fat also has a depressing effect on the body systems.

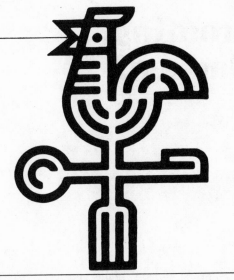

Here are several essential dietary factors that should be met at breakfast:
* A good supply of protein
* Foods besides protein to furnish energy
* The fat-soluble and water-soluble vitamins
* An abundance of minerals, including calcium, iron, and phosphorus
* Roughage or bulk-forming foods
* Appetizing foods, sometimes referred to as pan-peptogenic, to stimulate the appetite

Serve Breakfast To Suit Your Situation
How you present these essential foods at breakfast time will depend on your life style. If you are rushed in the morning

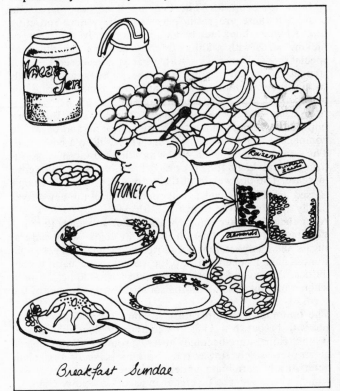

Breakfast Sundae

it might speed things up if you lay out your breakfast in the evening, setting the table with nonperishables and placing other necessary ingredients in a prominent spot in the refrigerator. This is not an uncommon habit.

If there are several people to feed in your household, weekend breakfasts can be served buffet or cafeteria style, set up in the kitchen where food can be piled onto plates and taken to the table by each person as needed. The Kibbutz Breakfast and Breakfast Sundaes are good examples of meals that work well with large families, as are hot cooked cereals or soups that can be held warm until served.

When you have more time in the morning, or when the entire family sits down together, you can choose foods that have to be served immediately. For even more leisurely breakfasts, you can look forward to more elaborate dishes such as Baked Apple Pancake, Cheese Pudding, French Toast Fondue, or even the "Gothic" Brunch.

Breakfast Sundae
A great breakfast that lets everyone be creative and select the foods he or she likes best; requires no cooking, just getting it together. All you have to do is assemble yogurt, nuts, and fresh and dried fruits on the table and let everyone make his or her own combination. Elders can concoct sundaes for those too young to handle food themselves. You can even simulate a soda fountain frappé to tantalize troublesome eaters.
* Place your storage containers or bowls full of peanuts, walnuts, raw cashews, almonds, and sunflower and pumpkin seeds on the table (protein and minerals).
* Do the same with dried fruits, including raisins, dates, apricots, and figs (vitamins and minerals).
* Give each person a container or bowl of unflavored yogurt (protein).
* Provide a platter of fresh fruits in season, offering bananas, pears, oranges, and apples in the winter and adding strawberries, melons, peaches, apricots, cherries, and so forth, in the summer (vitamins).
* Have honey or pure maple syrup and wheat germ in easy reach (more vitamins and minerals).

Now let everyone mix and match to create a breakfast sundae to his or her own taste. Or even a banana split.

Kibbutz Breakfast
The Kibbutz Breakfast is another breakfast where everyone can pick and choose what they like. A meal such as this is served each morning (and each evening as well) at every Israeli kibbutz.

Place any or all of the following foods on the table:

sliced tomatoes	scallions
sliced cucumbers	kohlrabi
strips of green pepper	olives
radishes	carrot sticks
shredded cabbage	sardines
sprigs of parsley	sliced cheeses
and dill	butter, nut butters
oil, lemon, and vinegar	honey
sour cream	assorted breads
yogurt	and crackers
cottage cheese	a pot of coffee,
hard-cooked eggs	tea, and a
herring	pitcher of milk

Give each person a plate and let everyone pile it on according to taste. Forget the formalities like peeling the eggs

(continued on page 276)

The Magic of Sprouting... How Does It Happen?

by Martha H. Oliver

Seeds in their dormant state are hard, dry bundles of starch surrounding a tiny embryo. Their metabolism, for they are alive, is so slow as to be almost unmeasurable; their respiration is minute. In this state, seeds can remain for years and still be viable (able to sprout when given the proper conditions). Tests on some legumes show that they can germinate after 200 years of storage under favorable conditions. (I should pause here to note, somewhat regretfully, that the stories of viable wheat seeds taken from Egyptian pyramids are all false. Wheat is quite short-lived, and all seeds from ancient tombs have been found to be entirely broken down to carbon husks.) The oldest viable seeds on record were found in a lemming burrow deeply buried in permanently frozen silt of the Pleistocene age in unglaciated central Yukon. They turned out to be a legume, the arctic tundra lupine, and when taken to the laboratory, they germinated and produced healthy plants. Carbon dating of skulls and other objects found near them in the burrow established their age as at least 10,000 years. Probably only the frozen conditions kept them viable all that time.

Yet the question of what kept them alive is not nearly as difficult to answer as the question of what kept them from sprouting at all during those centuries. Dormancy is still a puzzle to plant biochemists. Is it a quiescent period that requires a triggering action to break its sleep? Or is there an actual *block* to growth that must be removed before vital processes can take place? Are dormant seeds sleeping beauties waiting for a prince's kiss or Gullivers tied down while they strain to escape?

If we leave the dynamics out of it, however, dormancy is easy to explain from the evolutionary point of view. It is the seed's way of waiting out a period when conditions are unfavorable to the growth of the new plant. It may wait several seasons until the weather is just right, or, in the case of desert plants, years, until sufficient rain falls to ensure the seedling's survival. In this particular case, germination-inhibiting substances in the seeds may require at least an inch of rain to leach away their restricting action; otherwise, premature sprouting after a light shower, which is quickly evaporated, could be fatal. Many seeds, (and, as gardeners know, some early spring blooming bulbs) require a period of cold weather to start them growing again, or even a hard frost to crack the seed coat. Apple seeds rarely if ever germinate within the apple; a cyanide-releasing compound, which is found in the seeds

of peaches, pears, apricots, plums and roses, may function as a germinating inhibitor. (It does inhibit the germination of other seeds when they are treated with it prior to sprouting). If the apple rots, or passes through the gut of a horse, these substances are washed away, and the seed can germinate. Most seeds with which we are familiar are of the cultivated, garden variety; these have been bred to germinate easily. The vast majority of seeds in the wild, however, employ these elegant and complex protective devices to ensure that they will begin life as a plant under the most favorable conditions possible.

Seeds that are sprouted for food are almost all from two highly cultivated families, the *Leguminoseae* (beans, peas, alfalfa) and the *Gramineae* (grasses: wheat, rye, oats, barley), both of which have been domesticated, and consequently bred, for centuries. The Leguminoseae have hard seed coats, but these are easily permeated by water. Sprouting in the home, then, luckily requires no involved process of nicking seeds with a knife, freezing and thawing them, or special aging. One begins with what is considered the first step in the actual germination process: soaking the seeds so that they can take up water into their tissues. During this period of eight to twelve hours, referred to as the "imbibition phase," the dry seeds double or triple in size. But more important, enzymes in the seeds are activated, and begin the complicated series of changes that will result in a new plant. The same enzymes which, in the mouth, degrade starches into sugars and begin the process of digestion, show an intense increase. The dry weight of the seed is decreased as energy is used up. These changes will continue until the new leaves finally appear, on the fourth or fifth day.

After the seeds have imbibed, the water in which they are standing is found to be rich in amino acids, some natural sugars and a large number of inorganic elements. These substances have leached out into the water; under natural conditions, they would return to the soil surrounding the seed when rains and moisture in the soil dissolved them out of the seeds.

The optimum air temperature for rapid sprout growth appears to be between 25-35° Centigrade (77-95° Fahrenheit). As the temperature becomes lower, sprouting will take place at an increasingly slower rate. Sprouts of seeds that characteristically germinate under very low temperatures, like winter wheat, seem to be higher in ascorbic acid (vitamin C)

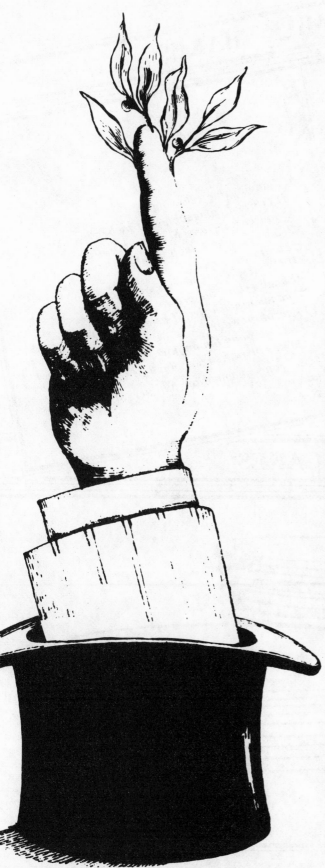

content than those that germinate under warmer conditions (e.g., spring wheat). Frost-resistant varieties contain even more vitamin C; wheat germinated at 5-8° C. (41-46° F.) contains two to three times that found in wheat germinated at 18-22° C. (65-72° F.). In humans, vitamin C helps prevent capillary fragility (easily broken blood vessels); it is possible that similar action in growing plant tissue could help a plant resist the expansion-contraction effect of freezing and thawing.

Sprouts will continue to grow under severe conditions; their requirements of moisture, air and a favorable temperature range are not narrowly limited, but quite adaptable to a large variety of situations. Yet the elaborate chemical changes that accompany germination are intricate, simultaneous and interrelated metabolic reactions: storage protein is hydrolyzed (broken down into its component amino acids); many vitamins, especially the water-soluble B-complex and vitamin C, are synthesized; fats and carbohydrates are degraded into simple sugars; and some food energy, in the form of calories, is lost. These processes have been intensely studied from the point of view of the use of seeds as a source of human food; the following discussion will view these changes from a similar standpoint.

The intense rise in metabolic activity in a seed that is beginning to germinate is responsible for the phenomenal increase of the water-soluble vitamins; vitamin C and most of the B-complex factor are found in almost all growing plant tissues, and the more active the growth, the higher the concentration of these vitamins. They are essential in the formation of certain enzymes, and therefore vital in cell metabolism. Since sprouting seeds are highly active, increasing to several times their original size in a few days, one might expect to find in them a rich source of vitamins.

Much of the research on vitamin incrementation in germinating seeds as a source of human food has been done in the past two decades by a group of Indian investigators. Faced with staggering nutritional as well as caloric deficiencies, Indian researchers have explored this source, but so far the government has not attempted to exploit sprouting on a major scale. Dr. Sachchidananda Banerjee and others have investigated nearly all of the B-vitamin complex now identified and isolated, and they report rises in every one except

(continued on page 277)

TIGER MILK SHAKES

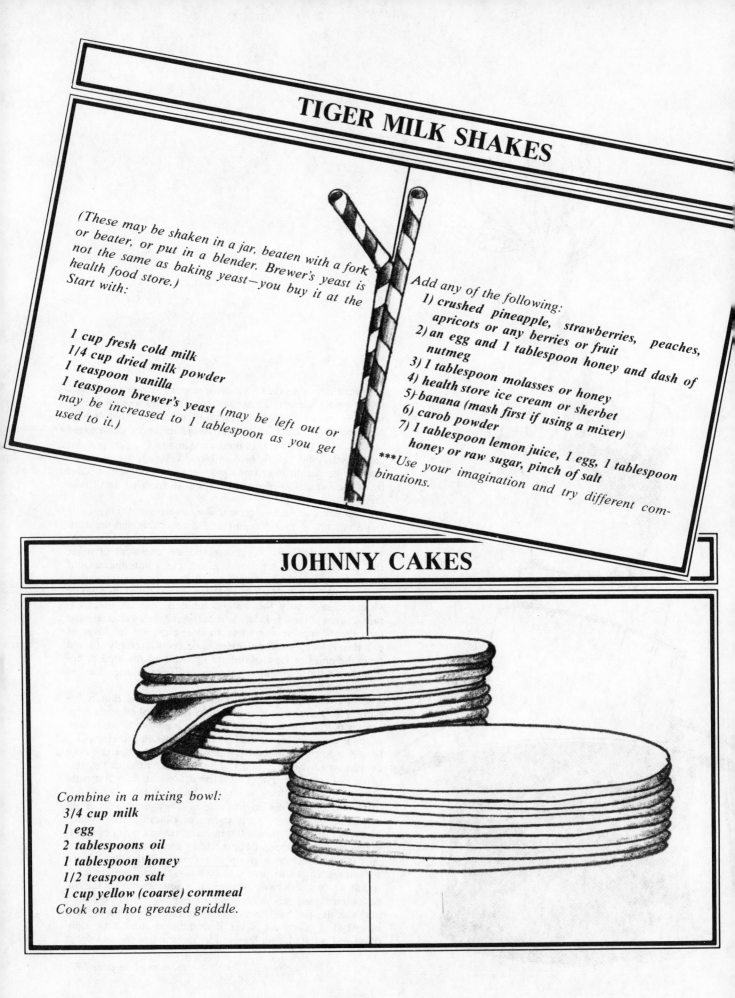

(These may be shaken in a jar, beaten with a fork or beater, or put in a blender. Brewer's yeast is not the same as baking yeast—you buy it at the health food store.)
Start with:

1 cup fresh cold milk
1/4 cup dried milk powder
1 teaspoon vanilla
1 teaspoon brewer's yeast (may be left out or may be increased to 1 tablespoon as you get used to it.)

Add any of the following:
1) crushed pineapple, strawberries, peaches, apricots or any berries or fruit
2) an egg and 1 tablespoon honey and dash of nutmeg
3) 1 tablespoon molasses or honey
4) health store ice cream or sherbet
5) banana (mash first if using a mixer)
6) carob powder
7) 1 tablespoon lemon juice, 1 egg, 1 tablespoon honey or raw sugar, pinch of salt
***Use your imagination and try different combinations.

JOHNNY CAKES

Combine in a mixing bowl:
3/4 cup milk
1 egg
2 tablespoons oil
1 tablespoon honey
1/2 teaspoon salt
1 cup yellow (coarse) cornmeal
Cook on a hot greased griddle.

Some Treats From Aunt Tilda

by Karen Kelly and Joan Hopkins

KANGAROO COOKIES
(OATMEAL)

Preheat oven to 350°. Mix together:

1/2 cup oil or 2/3 cup butter or margarine
1-1/4 cup brown sugar
2 tablespoons molasses
1 egg
1/4 cup water
1 teaspoon baking powder
1 teaspoon salt
1/2 teaspoon cinnamon
1 teaspoon vanilla

Then mix:

1 cup flour (unbleached white flour or half whole wheat and half unbleached)
1/2 cup raisins or currants
1/2 cup chopped nuts, or any combination of seeds: pumpkin seeds, sunflower seeds, sesame seeds, etc.

Add flour mixture to liquid, and then add:

3 cups rolled oats

Spoon out on greased cookie sheets and bake in the oven 12 to 15 minutes. Makes about 50 cookies. Let cool.

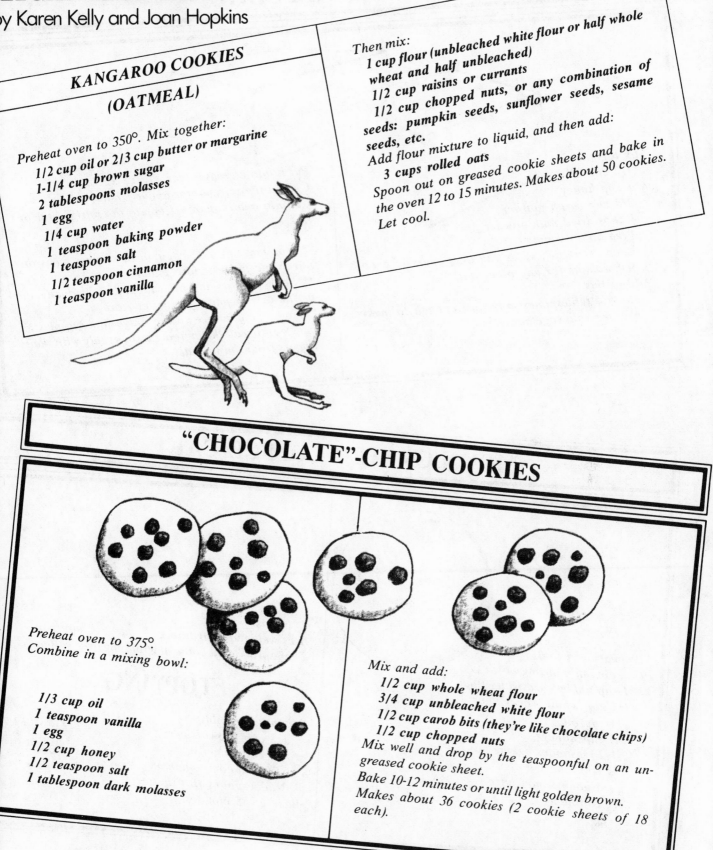

"CHOCOLATE"-CHIP COOKIES

Preheat oven to 375°.
Combine in a mixing bowl:

1/3 cup oil
1 teaspoon vanilla
1 egg
1/2 cup honey
1/2 teaspoon salt
1 tablespoon dark molasses

Mix and add:

1/2 cup whole wheat flour
3/4 cup unbleached white flour
1/2 cup carob bits (they're like chocolate chips)
1/2 cup chopped nuts

Mix well and drop by the teaspoonful on an ungreased cookie sheet.
Bake 10-12 minutes or until light golden brown.
Makes about 36 cookies (2 cookie sheets of 18 each).

NO-COOK FUDGE

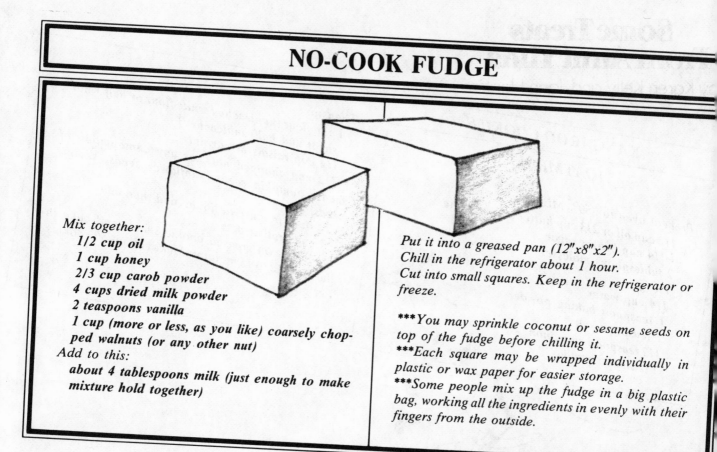

Mix together:
- 1/2 cup oil
- 1 cup honey
- 2/3 cup carob powder
- 4 cups dried milk powder
- 2 teaspoons vanilla
- 1 cup (more or less, as you like) coarsely chopped walnuts (or any other nut)

Add to this:
- about 4 tablespoons milk (just enough to make mixture hold together)

Put it into a greased pan (12"x8"x2").
Chill in the refrigerator about 1 hour.
Cut into small squares. Keep in the refrigerator or freeze.

***You may sprinkle coconut or sesame seeds on top of the fudge before chilling it.
***Each square may be wrapped individually in plastic or wax paper for easier storage.
***Some people mix up the fudge in a big plastic bag, working all the ingredients in evenly with their fingers from the outside.

MOON CRATER COFFEE CAKE

Preheat oven to 375°.
Combine in a mixing bowl:
- 1 cup unbleached white flour
- 1/2 cup whole wheat flour
- 1/4 cup oil
- 2/3 cup honey
- 2-1/2 teaspoons baking powder
- 1/2 teaspoon salt
- 1 teaspoon lemon juice
- 1/2 cup milk
- 1 egg

Beat well and pour into greased 8" square pan.
Then sprinkle the following topping over batter:

TOPPING

Mix until crumbly:
- 1/3 cup brown sugar
- 1/4 cup flour
- 1/2 teaspoon cinnamon
- 3 tablespoons firm butter

Bake 25-35 minutes.

And Still More Treats from Tilda

SANDWICHES:

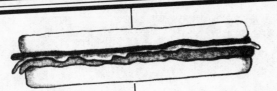

Ham, chicken, turkey, left-over meat loaf or roast beef, even ground **liver** and minced onions.

Cheeses—unprocessed; grated cheese with a little mayonnaise or salad dressing, or sliced with raw vegetables.

Cream cheese or **cottage cheese:** with chopped nuts, crumbled bits of bacon; chipped beef, bacon bits, olives, raisins, or chopped dates and walnuts, chopped celery, cucumbers, tomatoes, chives or green peppers, sunflower seeds or honey.

Peanut butter: with chopped dates and a bit of orange rind, crumbled bits of bacon, chipped beef, raisins and walnuts, cream cheese, honey or pickle.

Egg sandwiches: fried or omelet style or egg salad, with bits of ham, bacon, pickle, onion, relish, cheese or celery.

Honey: with butter, cinnamon, chopped dates or nuts.

Bacon and lettuce: with tomato, peanut butter or banana.

Tuna fish, salmon, sardines.

Grated **carrot:** with mayonnaise and raisins, dates or nuts. Or grated **cucumber** with mayonnaise and tomato.

***Most important of all—use good, nutritious bread.

WARM-UP PUNCH *(for cold evenings)*

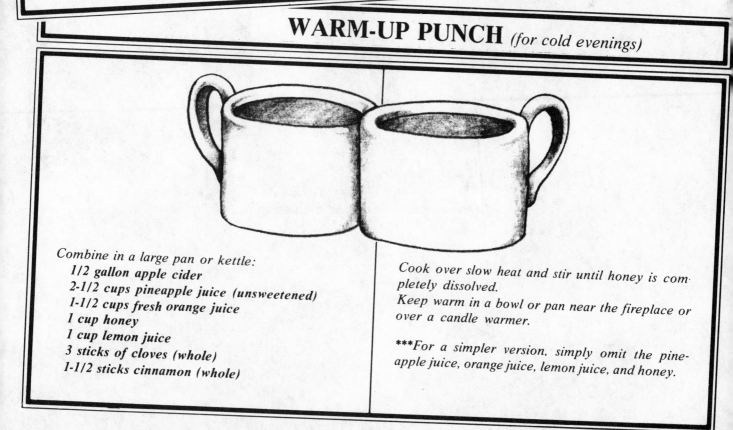

Combine in a large pan or kettle:
 1/2 gallon apple cider
 2-1/2 cups pineapple juice (unsweetened)
 1-1/2 cups fresh orange juice
 1 cup honey
 1 cup lemon juice
 3 sticks of cloves (whole)
 1-1/2 sticks cinnamon (whole)

Cook over slow heat and stir until honey is completely dissolved.

Keep warm in a bowl or pan near the fireplace or over a candle warmer.

***For a simpler version, simply omit the pineapple juice, orange juice, lemon juice, and honey.

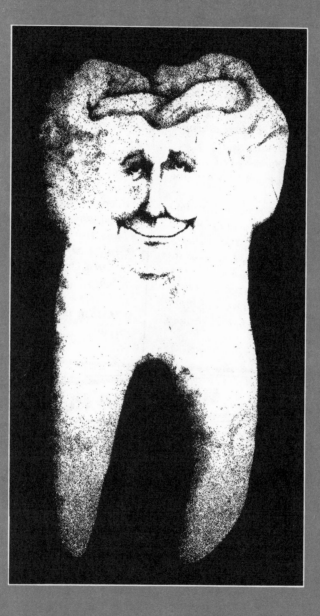

How To Sweet Talk That Sweet Tooth

by

Eunice Farmilant

About five years ago my father and brother introduced my family to the concept of eating whole, natural foods. However, it took several months before my father's enthusiasm became so contagious that I, too, was bitten by the bug and followed his footsteps to the health food stores seeking out many new varieties of foods.

Struggling with a rigid diet and eating foods I didn't really enjoy had never appealed to me. As a teen-ager I had gone on many crash diets and had even experimented with being a vegetarian for almost a year, but I always regained the weight I lost in a matter of months. But this new approach to eating, which involved eliminating all kinds of refined foods (including sugar), not only made me feel better, but I also lost thirty pounds that I have not regained.

I had always loved to cook and experiment with new recipes, so it wasn't long before I discovered that many favorite dishes — especially desserts and snack foods — could be successfully created by using whole, natural foods in place of refined products.

I started out originally by using wholewheat flour wherever white flour was called for in recipes, and replaced butter and margarine with vegetable oils. In place of cow's milk, I would use soy milk or soybean flour and water. But for sweetening certain desserts, finding a good substitute became a problem. Artificial sweetening agents were definitely out of the question because they are coal-tar derivatives and are not metabolized as food.

I discovered that fruit juices were great natural sweeteners, and besides, an eight-ounce portion of apple juice is only eighty calories, compared to 180 in an equal amount of milk. I would add protein-rich nuts and seeds as well as soybean flour to replace the nutrients found in milk.

As you can well imagine, my search for new ways of making desserts often led me out of the kitchen and into library reference books to research the nutritional value of foods. I also talked to many doctors and my own dentist, who hasn't used any sugar in his own house in years. Most of the doctors I met agreed that our diet, the typical American fare, that is, had become too rich; we were eating large amounts of empty foods that supplied lots of calories but not enough nutrients (like those gooey but deadly triple-layer frosted cakes that tempt us in magazines and bakery windows).

Milk is a wholesome food from a technical point of view, but many doctors have come to discover that it is not the best food for humans and not a perfect substitute for mother's milk. Besides being high in calories and fat content, it does contain valuable vitamins and minerals as well as protein. Contrary to its original intention pasteurization destroys much of the value contained in milk. Vitamins C, E, K, B_1 and riboflavin are altered along with enzymes. Pasteurized milk also lacks lactobacilli, which are destroyed by preservatives found in milk. Lactobacilli decompose sugar and produce lactic acid; they produce vitamins B_1, B_2, and B_{12}; they produce a growth factor that enables children to develop and are good for the prevention of food poisoning. However, raw milk does contain all the known vitamins, but it is extremely difficult to obtain today. But most of these nutrients can be obtained from other sources. Sesame seeds for instance, contain 1,600 milligrams of calcium in ¼ pound versus 590 milligrams in 2 cups of whole milk, and a quarter pound of carob flour contains 352 milligrams.

Preparing desserts with the aid of natural sweeteners is not a new concept in cooking. Refined sugar has been available on a large scale for only the past several hundred years, and there have been many times in modern man's history when he simply couldn't obtain it. During World War II, for instance, when there was an acute shortage of many foods, people throughout Europe had very little sugar or butter and were forced to use wholewheat flour. Government documents from Great Britain and other European countries prove that the incidence of many diseases actually decreased during these times of hardship — lack of many of our so called "luxury foods" actually improved people's health!

Today there are many things we take for granted including the endless variety of foods available in our supermarkets. Often we overindulge in foods that satisfy our desire and need for sweets but don't satisfy our nutritional needs.

Well, you may ask yourself, what's wrong with using a little sugar now and then to make foods taste sweet? The problem today is that we are almost constantly surrounded by foods that already contain sugar. Statistics indicate that the average person's intake of sugar is rapidly approaching almost two hundred pounds a year.

We have become a nation of weight-watchers, yet we are notoriously attracted to sweets. Sugar consumption in America is among the highest per capita in the world. Dr. John Yudkin, a distinguished professor of nutrition at London University, in England, describes in detail many of the serious effects excessive sugar consumption has had on our health. (*Sweet and Dangerous*, Peter H. Wyden, Inc., 1972.) In addition to tooth decay, he relates many major diseases, including heart disease, to sugar consump-

(continued on page 279)

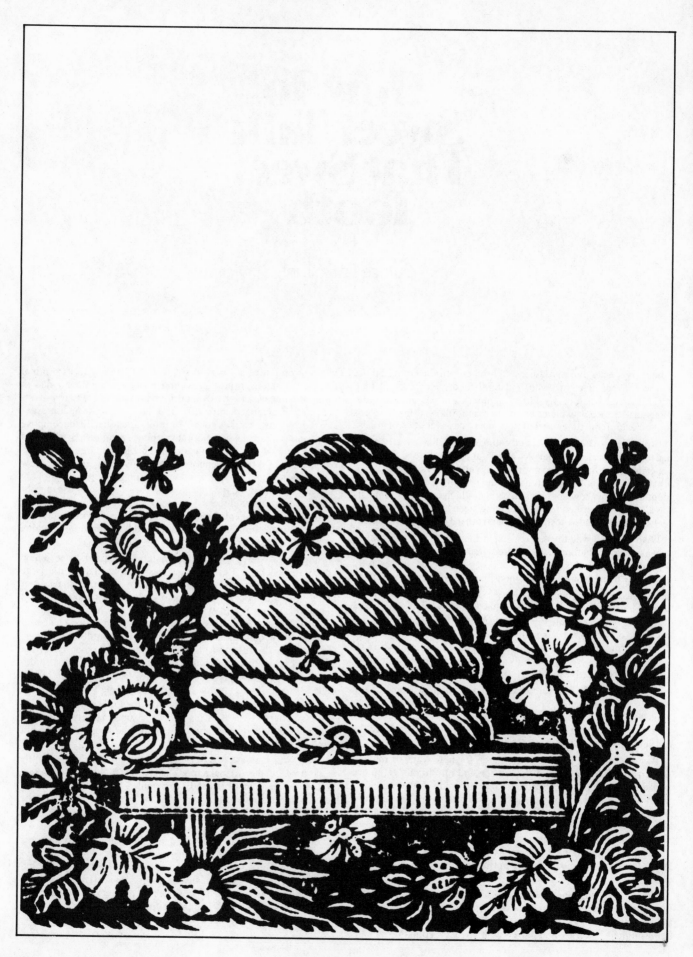

HONEY: SWEETHEART OF THE KITCHEN

by Agnes Toms

☐ Honey is one of nature's sweetest products and incredibly versatile when it comes to uses in the kitchen. It comes in a great variety of flavors because bees are so well-traveled (they frequently travel as far as 400 miles from one pollinating location to another). Often flavors are blended; they are called Wild, or Mountain Flowers instead of Buckwheat or Clover or Alfalfa. Whatever the flavor, honey is extremely durable, not needing refrigeration nor does it spoil for a long time.

☐ In addition to its sugars, honey contains as its minor components a number of minerals, seven members of the B-vitamin complex, ascorbic acid (vitamin C), dextrins, plant pigments, amino acids, other organic acids, traces of protein, esters and other aromatic compounds and several enzymes.

☐ Substituting honey for sugar in recipes is easy. Replace equal amounts up to one cup and decrease liquid ¼ cup for each cup of honey used. Also reduce baking temperatures 25 degrees to prevent overbrowning. When using honey in cooking, measure the oil or liquid first, then measure the honey in the same cup or spoon. It will slide off with ease.

Orange Buttermilk Molds

1 envelope
unflavored
gelatin
½ cup orange
juice
1 egg, separated
½ cup honey
⅛ teaspoon salt
¾ teaspoon
grated orange
peel
1¼ cups
buttermilk

Soften gelatin in orange juice in top of double boiler. Beat egg yolk lightly. Combine with gelatin and cook, stirring constantly, until gelatin dissolves and egg yolk thickens mixture slightly. Set aside 2 tablespoons of the honey for the egg white. Stir remaining honey, salt, orange peel and buttermilk into gelatin mixture. Cool until gelatin thickens and begins to jell. Beat egg white stiff. Gradually beat in remaining honey. Fold into gelatin. Turn into individual molds and chill until firm. Serves 4 or 5.

Apricot Cream

1 cup sieved cooked dried apricots
⅓ cup honey
½ teaspoon salt
2 cups dairy sour cream

Blend apricots, honey and salt into the sour cream. Chill for several hours or overnight before serving. Serve in sherbet glasses, garnished with toasted almonds or coconut. Serves 6.

Honey Syrup

Honey syrup may be made in quantity and stored in refrigerator ready for use.

Syrup for 6 large glass containers: Bring 1 quart water to boil, remove from heat, stir in about 1½ cups honey, according to sweetness desired, into water until well mixed. Allow to cool before refrigerating.

Freezing Peaches Or Apricots

Set up freezer containers in assembly-line order. Pour ¾ cup cold honey syrup into each container. Wash peaches quickly in cold water. Peel 1 peach at a time and slice directly into prepared syrup. Fill to 1 inch of top and be sure fruit is blended with syrup. Cover with piece of crumbled freezer wrap to keep fruit under syrup while freezing. Seal tightly with cover and freeze.

Apricots, if ripe, need not be peeled, only seeded and sliced.

Fluffy Honey Dressing

2 eggs
½ cup honey
¼ cup lemon
juice
2 tablespoons
frozen
orange-juice
concentrate
⅛ teaspoon
salt
½ cup yogurt
or whipped
cream
2 teaspoons
lemon peel

Beat eggs. Stir in honey, lemon juice, orange concentrate and salt. Cook over low heat until thickened. Cool. Fold in yogurt or whipped cream and lemon peel. Serve with fresh fruit. Serves 4.

Honey French Dressing

1 can (8 ounces)
tomato sauce
1⅓ cups salad oil
½ cup cider
vinegar
¼ cup lemon
juice
⅓ cup honey
1½ teaspoons
salt
2 teaspoons
paprika

Combine all ingredients in glass jar with tight-fitting lid and shake until well blended. Chill. Shake well before serving. Makes about 3 cups. ☼

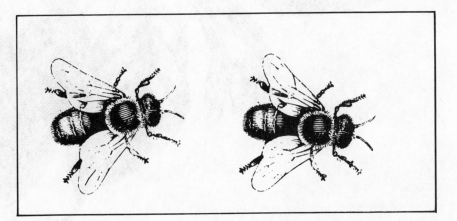

Liquid Lunches For Better Health

by Ed Flynn

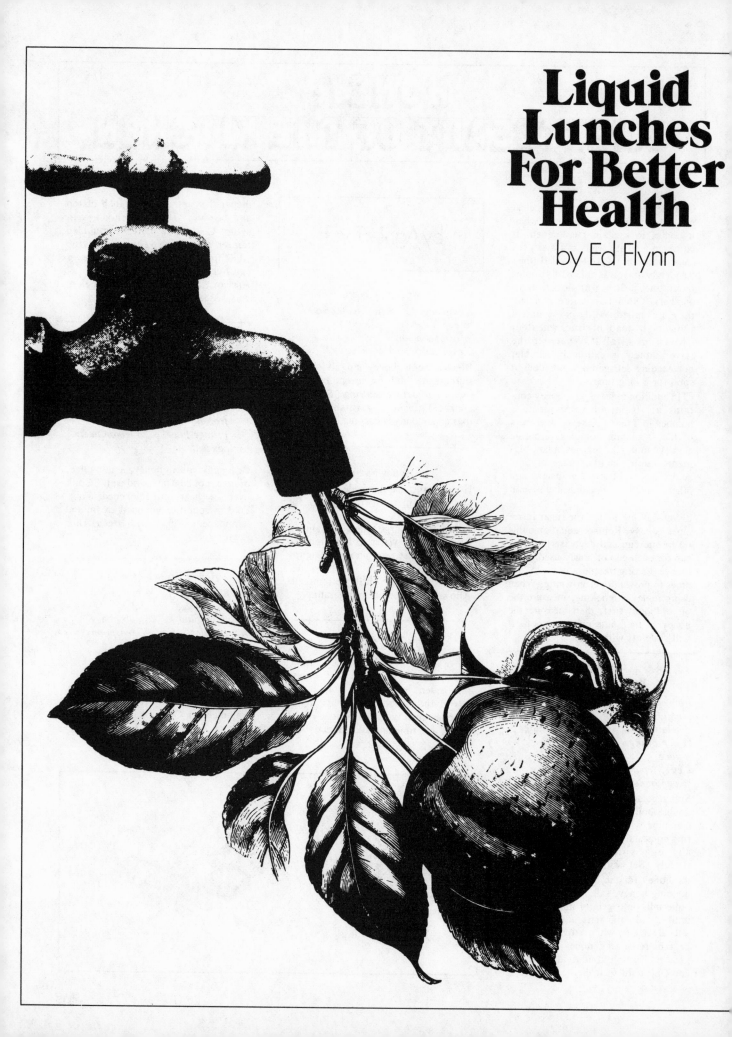

Trying to lose weight? Got digestive problems? An ulcer? High blood pressure? Worried about your heart? Try drinking your lunch.

☐ Now you may rush to point out that that's how you got in such sad shape in the first place so let me explain that I'm not talking about a martini at your favorite cocktail lounge but an elixir of health concocted in the seclusion of your own kitchen and consumed with secrecy at your office desk.

☐ Lost your appetite already, eh? Well hang in there a minute and give this idea a chance.

☐ Let's start with the premise that diets are no fun under any circumstances. For example, consider this noon-time delight:

3 oz. of chopped sirloin	2 pads of butter
1 baked potato, *no* sour cream	Black coffee
Salad with vinegar and oil dressing	No dessert
2 slices of bread	

☐ Not very exciting but it still adds up to approximately 800 calories, hardly a starvation diet for someone trying to take off weight.

☐ Now consider what I call my "Witches Brew." I take it to the office in a one pint thermos and each serving—about 2 full glasses—contains *less* calories than that dieter's snack listed above, at least *twice as much* protein, an abundance of the energy-giving B vitamins plus numerous other nutrients. This incidentally, isn't something I have dreamed up all on my own. Such noted nutritionists as Adelle Davis, Linda Clark and Carlton Fredericks are profuse in their praise of the individual ingredients. What I've done is simply stir them up with a little of my own imagination in an attempt to create some lunch-time excitement.

So here goes:

The Witches' Brew

This is the basic formula. It might be compared to the stock of a good soup, except that there's no cooking involved. All you need is a blender. The recipe which follows provides for a one-quart batch of Witches' Brew which in turn is extended to make 4 individual one-pint drinks.

First a few words of introduction concerning the ingredients:

☐ **Yogurt**—If you think yogurt is only for your secretary you're wrong. It's been around for centuries but it most recently gained prominence when it was credited with giving long life to Bulgarian shepherds who seemed to thrive on it. Yogurt is a soured-milk culture high in protein and calcium and it is believed to aid your digestion by introducing "friendly" bacteria to your system.

☐ **Brewer's Yeast**—You might have to go to a health food store for this and a few other ingredients although a number of supermarket chains now have health food departments. Brewer's yeast is so-named because it is a by-product of the beer-making process. However, it is also available under the name of primary or nutritional yeast. Brewer's yeast is considered by many to be a "miracle food." It is a complete protein. That means it contains all the amino acids considered essential for good health. It is also a rich source of the B vitamins. Specify instant, debittered.

☐ One word of caution. Brewer's yeast is by far the least tempting of the ingredients from a taste standpoint. Your taste buds may require a period of adjustment. Accordingly, it might be advisable to reduce the quantity of brewer's yeast in your first batch of Witches' Brew. You can increase it gradually.

☐ **Protein Powder**—Protein powder is a relatively new product, again available at any health food store. It can be derived either from natural vegetable or meat sources and provides a highly concentrated source of vital protein. The most commonly featured protein powder is based on soy flour, the soy bean being another of the "complete" proteins.

☐ **Lecithin**—Again, you may have to go to a health food store for this one. There appears to be considerable evidence that lecithin serves as a homogenizing agent which breaks down fat and cholesterol into minute particles which can more easily pass through your arteries.

☐ **Instant Non-Fat Dry Milk**—This is a readily available powdered form of skimmed milk. It is high in protein and calcium, generally has vitamins A and D added and, most importantly, has the cholesterol-producing fat removed.

☐ **Honey**—You know about the bees and the flowers, of course. I use honey in my Witches' Brew because its sweetness comes from glucose, a form of sugar which many experts believe to be less harmful than sucrose which is found in ordinary table sugar.

The Basic Formula

2 cups plain, unflavored yogurt	1 cup instant non-fat dry milk
8 T. brewer's or nutritional yeast*	2 T. lecithin
8 T. protein powder	4 T. honey
	Water

You can begin with considerably less brewer's yeast and gradually build quantity as your taste adjusts.

☐ Put all ingredients in a blender, mixing first with a spoon. Add just enough water to bring measure to a full quart. Blend only long enough to thoroughly mix ingredients into what will be a liquid of rather thick consistency. Store in the refrigerator. This amount is ample as a basis for 4 individual one-pint liquid lunches.

☐ The "Witches' Brew" formula might put hair on your chest if not on your head but by itself it's not exactly a taste sensation. However, neither is concentrated lemon juice. It's what you do with the concentrate that counts. Try these variations:

The Top Banana

1 cup of Witches' Brew	1 banana
1 t. vanilla flavoring	
1 raw egg	½ cup apple juice

Mix all ingredients in a blender. Store in refrigerator. Makes approximately 2 glasses or enough for a one-pint thermos.
Nutritional values: (Including Witches' Brew)*
Calories: 650 Grams of protein: 68**

☐ *Each of these recipes for individual drinks includes Witches' Brew as its base. The Witches' Brew brings to each all of the Vitamin B complex including 4 times the minimum daily requirement of B-1, 3 times the minimum daily requirement of B-2 and 4 times the minimum daily requirement of niacin. Assuming that the non-fat dry milk used in your Witches' Brew has been fortified (consult label of product used) your drink will also contain generous amounts of vitamins A and D. In addition, the ingredients in the Witches' Brew include such other nutrients as all essential amino acids, iron, calcium, phosphorus, potassium and other minerals.*

☐ **The Food and Nutritional Board of the National Research Council has set 70 grams of protein daily as a minimum requirement. Many consider this low. One gram for each two pounds of body weight is another acceptable approach for determining minimum requirement. Either way, The Top Banana goes a long way towards meeting the daily requirement.*

(continued on page 280)

Boy Scouts at Treasure Valley have tied a knot in the high cost of living. Scout chefs of Troop 165 cooked up a 5 course supper last night for the 12 members of the troop. It cost nothing. The only expenditure was time spent scouting the fields and forests of the mile-square reservation in search of edible plants and roots.

□ *Housewives wishing to prepare such a non-cost meal have the following recipes to guide them.*

□ *Cow Lily Potatoes: These are roots of cow lily plants. Wash off much before burying in live coals. Cook thoroughly to deaden marsh taste and serve hot.*

□ *Nettle Spinach: Leaves of stinging nettle plant cook quickly, like spinach, and make excellent green vegetable. Cook in boiling water and drain to get rid of poison from nettles. Rinse in hot water twice before eating.*

□ *Primrose Salad: Leaves should be thoroughly washed to avoid bugs in the salad.*

□ *Fruit Compote: Mix freshly-picked blueberries and wild raspberries. Add crushed wild mint leaves, 15 minutes before serving, stirring mixture.*

□ *Birch Tea: Made by steeping birch twigs and leaves in hot water.*

□ *Chicory Coffee: Roasted chicory roots are ground and boiled. Makes rather strong beverage.*

□ *Sumac Lemonade: Boil sumac twigs and leaves, then cool.*

–News Report

Whenever friends mention to me that their gardens get so cluttered up with such ''weeds'' as Dandelion, Burdock or Lambsquarters, I say to them: ''These weedy nondescripts may truly get on your horticultural nerves, and may become a bit rampant and take due advantage of the soil's richness or unmulched rows; but to discard as valueless many of these garden 'guests' or to avoid using them as a source of food or vegetables substitutes, is as unwise and uneconomical as depositing in the garbage disposal can a pound each of fresh Carrots and Celery.''

□ Such native edibles may well boast of their food values, possessing in many instances far more health-fortifying, nutritive, mineral-vitamin principles than many garden vegetables: Watercress contains three times as much vitamin E as Lettuce and almost three times as much calcium as Spinach. Dandelion offers six times the quantity of vitamin A and more than twice that of calcium, phosphorus and iron contained in garden Lettuce. Throughout medical history, friend Burdock has well earned its reputation as a ''blood purifier'' and today this property is ascertained by its much needed blood-fortifying minerals of calcium, silicon and sulfur.

□ Occasionally we may read in the newspapers and magazines thrilling articles and feature stories describing the practicability of employing as food many of the ubiquitous never-say-die herbs. Here are a few examples: ''Wild Berries Only Food Until Man Found. J.B. was exhausted and hungry, but had been eating wild Strawberries . . . .'' ''Plants with Edible Roots: Psoralea still is a favorite food of the plains Indians who dry it for a flour.'' (It is mentioned in the account of Lewis and Clark's and Fremont's travels) . . . .''Making Use of Native Shrub Fruits: The fruits of the High Bush Cranberry, Hawthorn and Rose are here recommended as ingredients for a syrup, sauce and jelly,'' which three are later described in the text . . . . ''Boy Lives Five Days on Diet of Grass: An 11 year-old boy picked up by a car halfway between Jerusalem and Tel Aviv declared that he had lived for five days on nothing but grass.''

□ Does the eating of grass or weeds or herbs seem strange to those accustomed to store-bought produce? Does the writer's habit of drinking a warm tea of freshly cut and quick-dried grass also seem strange to the uninitiated? Then do remember that young grass is one of Nature's richest sources of composite food nutrients. There is besides that much ballyhooed chlorophyll, a high content of vitamin A and C, five factors of vitamin B complex, K and G. It has been estimated that 12 pounds of powdered grass contain more vitamins than 340 pounds of vegetables and fruits—more vegetables and fruits than the average person can eat a year. (Please note that although vitamins per se were unknown in biblical days, the prophet Jeremiah observed that certain organic diseases were due to mineral-vitamin deficiency: ''Their eyes did fail, because there was no grass'' (14:6).

□ Dr. Charles F. Schnabel, formerly of Rockhurst College, Kansas City, believed that ''the time is not far off when we'll be consuming a daily portion of grass in butter, bread, milkshakes, candy bars, breakfast foods, pancakes, and even ice cream and cookies.'' He stated that by mixing dried grass to the daily diet, the annual food bill could be cut at least 25 percent and place a rounded-out diet in reach of everyone's pocketbook.

□ Had Dr. Schnabel's job as a mill feed chemist held out in the depression, grass as a human diet supplement might not be a scientific factor today. But 1931 found him hard hit for money to feed his family. He yielded to an urge to try his family on the grass that had put his small flock of chickens to producing eggs on an almost 100 percent basis for five months. By adding dehydrated grass to the family's menu he nourished the eight on a dollar a day—12 cents apiece. Today his children all are proportionately larger than their father. To have a constant supply of grass at the right stage, he space-planted his two acre plot at the edge of town on a two-week interval plan. Four o'clock every morning found him cutting grass. He quick-dried it over the hot air registers of his home. Then the grass was ground in a sausage grinder and put in the family's milk. Sometimes when the temperature was 80 degrees outside, the Schnabel furnace was running full blast. Mrs. Schnabel admits now she wouldn't like to go through the hot register process again but she adds, ''every woman who marries a scientist must expect such things.''

□ ''They are living proof,'' Schnabel says of his children, ''of the benefits of grass as a food. I've fed them grass for 11 years. Look at them. Not a decayed tooth in their heads. The only sicknesses they've known have been a few common child diseases.''

Winter Garden
□ To provide a fairly constant supply of herb greens throughout the Winter months, I will suggest that you first gather the fully ripened seeds of such everpresent stalwarts as Burdock, Shepherd's Purse, Dandelion and Peppergrass, and after allowing them to dry a few days, plant them in soil typical of their natural surroundings. It is important that the window where you place the flower pots have full sun. In a short time you will be presented with a dish of fresh salad greens. Any sprouted Onions and Garlic should also be potted too, to provide tangy, edible nutriment, as well as Chives, Parsley, and the culinaries Sage, Thyme, and Lemon Balm.

☼

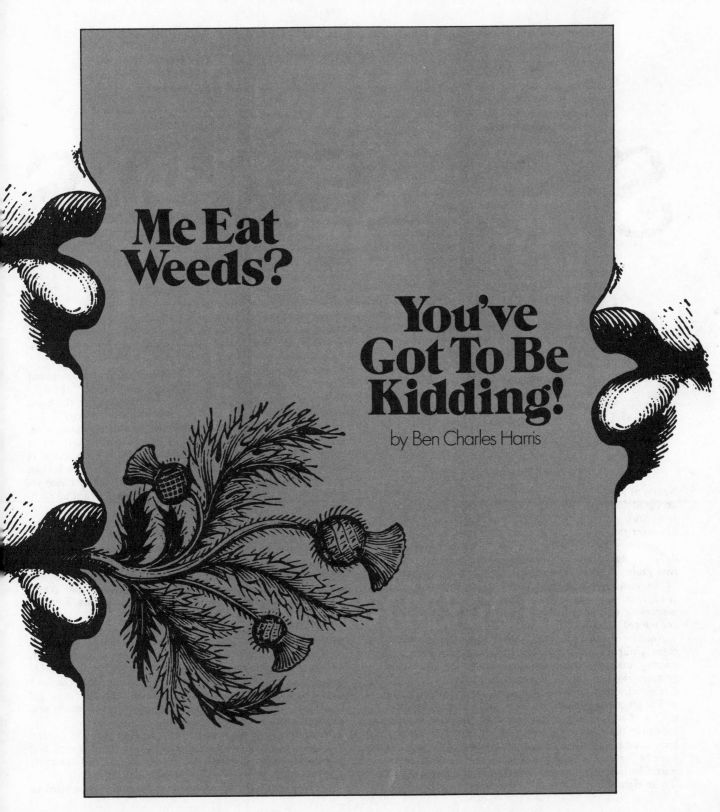

Me Eat Weeds?

You've Got To Be Kidding!

by Ben Charles Harris

SOYBEANS

by Barbara Farr

Nearly all of us learned in school that there are four generally accepted food groups. These are the meat group, the vegetable-fruit group, the milk group, and the bread-cereal group. We were taught that we should eat several foods from each group every day. While it is true that the growing infant definitely needs milk every day—mother's milk—it is also true that grains, legumes and cereals can adequately supply most of the needs provided by the meat and milk groups. Vitamin B-12 must be supplemented in an all-vegetable diet, and sources of calcium, minerals and other vitamins should be considered.

Another meaningful grouping of foods would consist of three groups: protein, carbohydrate and fats. These groups overlap, many foods containing all three. The body must ingest certain fats and oils; these are "essential fatty acids." Carbohydrate is broken down into simple sugars, one of which, glucose, is the brain's *only* "fuel." Protein is the actual matter of which body cells are formed. Proteins are also responsible for various functions which take place within the body. Certain proteins are manufactured in the body; others must be ingested. There are eight amino acids (proteins) which *must* be ingested and are therefore considered "essential." These eight are tryptophan, threonine, phenylalanine, lysine,

valine, isoleucine, methionine-cystine and leucine. They function in a specific ratio, so that if a food is deficient in any one of the eight, the value of the remaining seven is lowered proportionately.

This deficiency must be remedied immediately. You cannot eat a food deficient in lysine at lunch and "correct" the deficiency two hours later. This corrective balancing of the eight essential amino acids is "protein complementarity." For example, soybeans are somewhat low in methionine-cystine. Cereals and grains are rich in methionine-cystine but low in lysine, which is abundant in soybeans. Thus, soybeans plus cereals and grains in the same meal provide more protein than either could if eaten separately. In planning meals based on soybeans, remember to include wheat, sesame, peanuts, corn, brown rice, eggs or milk products.

Recently FDA (Food and Drug Administration) recommended daily allowances call for 45 to 65 grams of protein daily for an adult. (Needs of growing children, pregnant or lactating women differ.) One can attain that much protein in a pound of lean steak, or 8 eggs or a quart of milk. Soybean granules provide almost 50 grams of protein in 100 grams while steak provides 20 to 30 grams per 100 grams. Soybean curd is equivalent in calcium to cow's milk.

Certain minerals, such as iodine and zinc, should be supplemented on a vegetarian diet. Iodine occurs in sea vegetables such as kelp and nori, or one can use iodized salt or sea salt. Zinc is present in vegetables grown on zinc-rich soil. We were once subject to a zinc deficiency when we moved from one state to another that had zinc-poor soil, on which we grew our vegetables. We corrected it both by dietary supplements and adding zinc to the soil.

Vitamin B-12 is manufactured by animals, but the human body seems unable to manufacture its own. Unless eggs and dairy products are included in a vegetarian diet, B-12 must be supplemented.

Another factor in the diet which is becoming recognized as

increasingly important is dietary fiber, which is basically indigestible carbohydrate. Soybeans, legumes, whole grains, nuts, seeds and vegetables all contain significant amounts of fiber. Meats, poultry, seafood, eggs and dairy products contain *none*. The fiber may be finely ground as in flours and powders, for it is an indigestible molecule which gives the bulk, "roughage" and absorbency to food waste traveling through the body.

Our "magic" bean, then, contains fat (essential fatty acids), carbohydrates (including dietary fiber but no starch), and a lot of protein. It also contains calcium, iron, potassium and phosphorous and has an alkaline ash, which makes it valuable in a diet containing acid-forming grains and meats. Soybeans also contain vitamin A and vitamins of the B complex. When the

muscular. It's rather like the caterpillar's mushroom in *Alice in Wonderland:* too many calories will make you fat, too few calories will make you thin. Protein is another matter. The human body tissue is mainly composed of protein, some of which can be synthesized by the body, some of which must be ingested. Gayelord Hauser suggests 1 gram of protein for each 2.2 pounds of ideal body weight. That is for a normal adult. Special needs may increase the need for protein.

It is not too difficult to learn to balance your protein needs with the proper number of calories. The first and easiest step is to eliminate those foods that offer only empty calories, such as sugar and highly-refined foods. Sliced bread, for example, averages about 70 calories per slice. Protein content varies

&NUTRITION

beans are sprouted, they contain all of the above nutrients as well as vitamin C.

Dieting is one of the most popular national pastimes. People who are not actually dieting are usually regretting their last diet, or planning their next one. Thin is healthy, but dieting is boring, at best. Eating is one of the most basic necessities of life, and should be a pleasure. In fact, studies have shown that people who are relaxed and happy while eating have fewer digestive problems than those who are tense and unhappy.

It is possible to diet very happily. The trick is to diet constantly, which really means not dieting at all, just eating rationally. That means getting the necessary amount of vitamins, minerals, fats, carbohydrates, and protein. Fats and carbohydrates are relatively easy to obtain. Vitamins and minerals can be supplemented when not readily available in the foods one eats. Protein, however, is traditionally obtained from meats, fish, and poultry. Vegetarian sources of protein are plentiful, but not as well known or understood as animal protein. Even so, it is possible to get the proper nutrients. The trick is to obtain all of the necessary nutrients *without* getting too many calories. Excess calories are fattening. Period. Even if the excess calories are derived from protein, if they are in excess of the body's need, they will eventually become fatty tissue.

Nearly all foods contain some protein, but it is important to seek out those foods that offer the most protein with the fewest calories. Soybeans, cheese, seeds, eggs, nuts, milk, wheat germ and nutritional yeast are excellent sources of protein. Tofu is also an excellent source, providing about 69 calories and 7.5 grams of protein in a 4-ounce cake. Brewer's yeast contains 4 grams of protein in a 23-calorie tablespoonful. Soy powders and granules can be used in many dishes to boost protein at a relatively low cost in calories.

Your need for calories is variable, depending on your weight, rate of physical activity, etc. Obese and sedentary persons need fewer calories than do those who are active and

from about 2 grams to about 9 grams per slice. Obviously, the 9-gram slice gives you more for your calories.

WHY WE DO NOT USE
TEXTURED VEGETABLE PROTEIN

Textured vegetable protein (TVP) appears in many products, from meat analogs to extenders for processed meats. Because it is basically soy protein, it has been hailed as a solution to high meat consumption. However, it has many disadvantages which are not as widely touted.

First, most methods for producing TVP require isoelectrically precipitated soy protein. The drawbacks in isoelectric precipitation are that the resulting globulins combine with phytates and other low-molecular-weight compounds which decrease the availability of zinc and other essential minerals and that some of the proteins become insoluble.

The spinning method for producing TVP requires dispersion of the soy protein isolate in a 14 to 18 percent concentrated solution of sodium hydroxide, a pH of 10 to 11 and aging at 40° to 50° C. until the dispersion (called "spinning dope") reaches a spinnable state. It is then forced through a spinnerette into a coagulating bath containing acid and salts. Flavor is "improved" by treatment with sulfur dioxide.

Heat gelation adds the soy protein isolate to hot solution of trisodium phosphate, then mixing it with fat, emulsifier, color, smoke and other flavorings. Another method calls for granular particles of the isolate to be soaked in water containing calcium hydroxide or trisodium phosphate.

The extrusion method uses soy flour. (About 80 percent of the soy flour produced in this country is processed with hexane.) The flour is mixed with fat, flavorings, carbohydrates, colorings and sulfur or sulfur compounds. The mixture is then passed through an extruder under set conditions of moisture, temperature, pressure and time. The resulting mixture expands as it is extruded, and is cut to size by revolving knives. TVP is a chemical feast indeed! ☼

Those

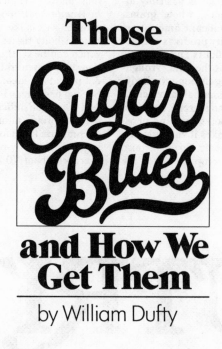

and How We Get Them

by William Dufty

I'll buy a huge piece of meat, cook it up for dinner, and then right before it's done, I'll break down and have what I wanted for dinner in the first place—bread and jam ... all I ever really want is sugar.

Andy Warhol, **New York Magazine,** *March 31, 1975*

So many of us have such heavy sugar habits today, it's hard for us to imagine the reaction of a sugarfree Crusader languishing in the land of the Infidel, taking his first sweet trip. In *Beyond the Chindwin,* Bernard Fergusson tells how men too exhausted even to speak were given a kind of sugar fudge to eat. "... the immediate result was astonishing, like a modern Pentecost. The string of our tongues loosed, and we spake plain." A substance that could produce this potent reaction on the brains of brawny men would hardly be what one would offer as a Christmas treat to the kiddies. Here was something more intoxicating than beer or wine and more potent than many drugs and potions then known to man. No wonder Arab and Jewish physicians used refined sugar carefully in minuscule amounts, adding it to their prescriptions with great care. It was a brain boggler. It could cause the human body and brain to run the gamut in no time at all from exhaustion to hallucination.

Today, the endocrinologists can tell us how it happens.

The difference between life and death is, in chemical terms, slighter than the difference between distilled water and that stuff from the tap. The brain is probably the most sensitive organ in the body. The difference between feeling up or down, sane or insane, calm or freaked out, inspired or depressed depends in large measure upon what we put in our mouth. For maximum efficiency of the whole body—of which the brain is merely a part—the amount of glucose in the blood must balance with the amount of blood oxygen. As Dr. E. M. Abrahamson and A. W. Pezet note in *Body, Mind, and Sugar,* "... a condition in which the blood sugar level is

relatively low ... tends to starve the body's cells, especially the brain cells. It is treated by diet. ... What happens to us when the cells of our bodies and especially our brains are chronically undernourished? The weakest, most vulnerable cells ... *suffer first.*" (Emphasis added.) When all is working well, this balance is maintained with fine precision under the supervision of our adrenal glands. When we take refined sugar (sucrose), it is the next thing to being glucose so it largely escapes chemical processing in our bodies. The sucrose passes directly to the intestines, where it becomes "predigested" glucose. This in turn is absorbed into the blood *where the glucose level has already been established in precise balance with oxygen.* The glucose level in the blood is thus drastically increased. Balance is destroyed. The body is in crisis.

The brain registers it first. Hormones pour from the adrenal casings and marshal every chemical resource for dealing with sugar: insulin from the endocrine "islets" of the pancreas works specifically to hold down the glucose level in the blood in complementary antagonism to the adrenal hormones concerned with keeping the glucose level up. All this proceeds at emergency pace, with predictable results. Going too fast, it goes too far. The bottom drops out of the blood glucose level and a second crisis comes out of the first. Pancreatic islets have to shut down; so do some departments of the adrenal casings. Other adrenal hormones must be produced to regulate the reversing of the chemical direction and bring the blood glucose level up again.

All this is reflected in how we feel. While the glucose is being absorbed into the blood, we feel "up." A quick pick-up. However, this surge of mortgaged energy is succeeded by the downs, when the bottom drops out of the blood glucose level. We are listless, tired; it requires effort to move or even think until the blood glucose level is brought up again. Our poor brain is vulnerable to suspicion, hallucinations. We can be irritable, all nerves, jumpy. The severity of the crisis on top of crisis depends on the glucose overload. If we continue taking sugar, a new double crisis is always beginning before the old one ends. The accumulative crisis at the end of the day can be a lulu.

After years of such days, the end result is damaged adrenals. They are worn out not from overwork but from continual whiplash. Overall production of hormones is low, amounts don't dovetail. This disturbed function, out of balance, is reflected all around the endocrine circuit. The brain may soon have trouble telling the unreal from the real; we're likely to go off half cocked. When stress comes our way, we go to pieces because we no longer have a healthy endocrine system to cope with it. Day-to-day efficiency lags, we're always tired, never seem to get anything done. We've really got the sugar blues.

Members of the medical profession who have studied this note that "since the cells of the brain are those that depend wholly upon the moment-to-moment blood sugar level for nourishment, they are perhaps the most susceptible to damage. The disturbingly large and ever-increasing number of neurotics in our population makes this clearly evident." Not everyone goes all the way. Some people start out with strong adrenals; others, like the late President Kennedy, don't. Degrees of sugar abuse and sugar blues vary. However, the body does not lie. If you take sugar, you feel the consequences.

The late endocrinologist John W. Tintera was quite emphatic in an interview in *Woman's Day,* February, 1958: "It is quite possible to improve your disposition, increase your efficiency, and change your personality for the better. The way to do it is to avoid cane and beet sugar in all forms and guises."

What the avant garde of endocrinology tells us today, the sorceress in what we call the Dark Ages knew by instinct or learned by experiment.

In the eyes of the sorceress, refined sugar was not a whole food. The words holy, whole, healthy, and hale all stemmed from the same root. A whole food was holy, blessed by the nature spirits, and intended to protect the health of man. Sugar was obviously not a whole food like a green plant or an amber grain. Sugar cane grew in tropical and warm regions. The average peasant, certainly those in Europe, would not refine sugar cane at home like bread, cheese, wine, and beer. Sugar was a foreign substance, imported from afar, made by unseen hands from a tropical plant that the sorceress had never studied with the dowser. If it had any history, it was an alien history. Judgment was therefore suspended unless and until a sorceress from Cheltenham could consult with a sorceress from Barbados. Meanwhile, it was brought from afar by lackeys of church and state who—in the eyes of the natural healers—had an unblemished record for having brought nothing but death and taxes, toil and trouble, wars and pestilence.

People learned from the sorceress or knew in their own veins that sugar was much too sweet not to be bad for them. But, like Eve in the Garden, they were tempted. They hoped to get away with it. Some people seemed to. Or thought they did. Or thought they did right up until the point—months or years later—when they found out differently. Especially the high and mighty. Sooner or later there were signs. Occurrences. Warnings. Their bodies were telling them something.

Soldiers and sailors, freighting precious cargoes of expensive sugar across thousands of miles, found that the stuff had a way of sticking to their fingers. They began to have more trouble with their teeth. Servants in the homes of the rich, where precious sugar was kept under lock and key, began to notice that the urine in the slop jars of the high and mighty started smelling exceptionally sweet. It was not something that could be talked about with anyone but the sorceress. Sailors shipwrecked at sea on sugar cargo ships tried to survive on a diet of sugar and rum. They went bonkers and often died. There was some talk about that. Men who worked in the new cities in sugar depots and refineries seemed to develop galloping consumption in great numbers. Sometimes they talked about it. Other times, when they'd been pinching bits of sugar here and there, it was not something one could talk about.

Ancient civilizations such as those of the Orientals believed that all disorders of body and mind proceed from what we eat. As the Oriental sages phrased it, the mind and the body are not two. The sorceress . . . wise woman . . . natural healer believed this too. However, by the time sugar was introduced widely in Europe, the natural healers were uncovered—practically overnight—as a declared enemy of church and state. Ailing people consulted them at very real peril. One literally risked life and limb having any truck with them. In turn, they risked life and limb to aid you.

In the age of witch hunts, the disorders, occurrences, and signs were divided into two categories: Those thought to be your own fault (physical) and those thought to be the work of the devil (mental). The milksick, a stomachache, galloping consumption, and other obvious signs and warnings were clearly physical. Invisible symptoms, however, from melancholy to migraine to madness were bewitchment.

For centuries, uninformed and unskilled physicians would continue to relegate signs of sugar blues—the simple remedy for which they overlooked—to bewitchment. Three centuries of medical mischief would produce a veritable babel of Greek and Latin symptoma: Schizophrenia, paranoia, catatonia, dementia praecox, neuroses, psychoses, psychoneuroses, chronic urticaria, neurodermatitis, cephalaigia, hermicrania, paraxysmal tachycardia—all as scarifying as the devil himself.

(continued on page 281)

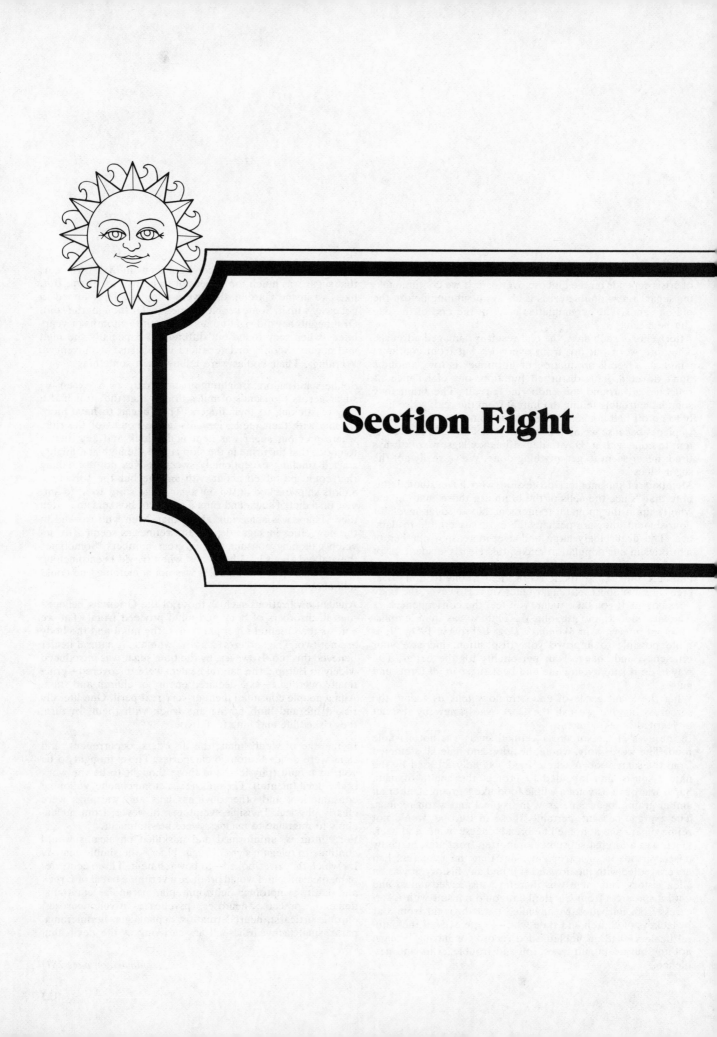

Section Eight

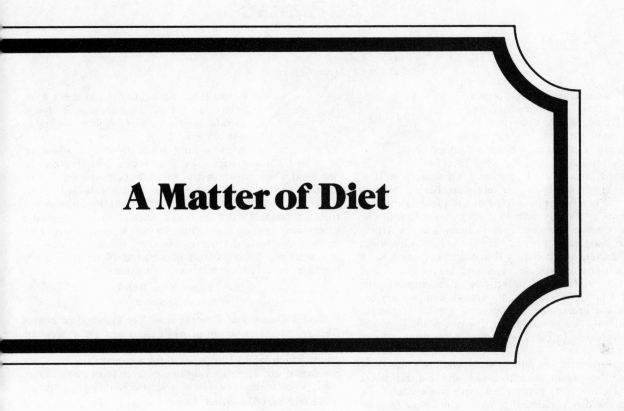

A Matter of Diet

If You Don't Want It, Don't Eat It!

The Famous Natural Diet To Prevent All Manifestations of the Saccharine Disease

by T.L. Cleave, Fellow Royal College of Physicians

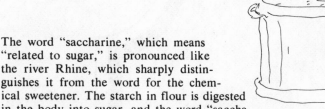

The word "saccharine," which means "related to sugar," is pronounced like the river Rhine, which sharply distinguishes it from the word for the chemical sweetener. The starch in flour is digested in the body into sugar, and the word "saccharine," as used here, means related to white flour as well as to white or brown sugar; and the term "saccharine disease" covers all the conditions held to be due to the consumption of these two artificially refined carbohydrate foods. The saccharine disease includes dental decay and pyorrhea; gastric and duodenal ulcer and other forms of indigestion; obesity, diabetes, and coronary disease; constipation, with its complications of varicose veins and hemorrhoids; and primary *Escherichia coli* infections, like appendicitis, cholecystitis (with or without gall-stones), and primary infections of the urinary tract. The same applies to certain skin conditions. Not one of these diseases is for practical purposes ever seen in races who do not consume refined carbohydrates.

The simple instructions in this diet prohibit white flour and sugar, but permit natural bread and natural sweet things (and also nearly every other type of foodstuff). By this means the diet is reduced to the evolutionary level to which man is adapted and reflects the principles of natural feeding seen in all living organisms. That is why this is entitled "The Natural Diet for Health," since the diet concerned is not really a medical diet at all. For the same reason it is not harsh, nor is it liable to change.

Needless to say, although the diet is aimed at the prevention and arrest of all the conditions listed above, other medical measures may be indicated for damage already inflicted by the consumption of these refined foods. For example, the prevention of dental decay will not reduce the necessity of dental treatment for decay already present.

Rules

The diet is based on two rules only, which may be summarized as follows:

1. Do not eat any food unless you definitely want it. — Eating food that is not wanted is a most unnatural act, yet frequently takes place today. One reason lies in eating routinely, especially when one is overtired or worried and does not really fancy any food at the time; another reason lies in eating a meal because someone has taken the trouble to prepare it, or in eating food to avoid wasting it; whilst yet another reason lies in eating food on social or business occasions, when it is taken for motives of politeness or policy. On all these occasions "if you don't want it, don't eat it." *This decision is always made most accurately before coming to the table.*

2. Avoid eating white flour and white or brown sugar. — This means avoiding on the one hand white bread, pastry, cakes, biscuits and other confectionery; and on the other hand white or brown sugar, jams, ices, chocolates, sweets, and sweet drinks. Substitute a true wholemeal bread and wholemeal flour for the first group, and raw or dried fruit for the second group. This restores the natural fiber to the diet, which will now be shown to be of the greatest importance. Notes on the application of this rule will be given later.

How These Two Rules Prevent Disease

Dental Decay and Pyorrhea. — The removal of coarse fiber in the manufacture of white flour and sugar prevents the natural cleansing of the teeth, and hardening of the gums, which take place when the unrefined original foods are consumed. The shocking loss of teeth from these causes today, even in the very young, is most certainly preventable.

Gastric and Duodenal Ulcer. — In treating these and other forms of indigestion the aim should be to *prevent* an excess of acid forming in the stomach, which is the main cause of the trouble, and not to neutralize the excess of acid with alkaline drugs (except in the presence of actual pain, under medical supervision).

There are two unnatural factors in the production of this excess acid, and both must be removed. One factor is eating food that is not wanted. Under these circumstances the food stagnates in the stomach and excess acidity results, which can often be felt in the back of the throat. Rule I is therefore most important, especially in times of worry. Note also that this rule prohibits the taking of unwanted food merely to relieve gastric pain. It is true that food may temporarily relieve such pain, but this unnatural food intake is not the right answer. Pain calls for alkaline drugs, under medical supervision, and probably treatment in bed.

The other factor in the production of excess acidity is the eating of white flour, or sugar. In the refining processes employed in the manufacture of these substances the protein component in the wheat is considerably reduced, and in the sugar-cane and sugar-beet is removed altogether. Since protein is the only food-stuff that neutralizes the gastric acid, the eating of white flour or sugar exposes the stomach mem-

(continued on page 282)

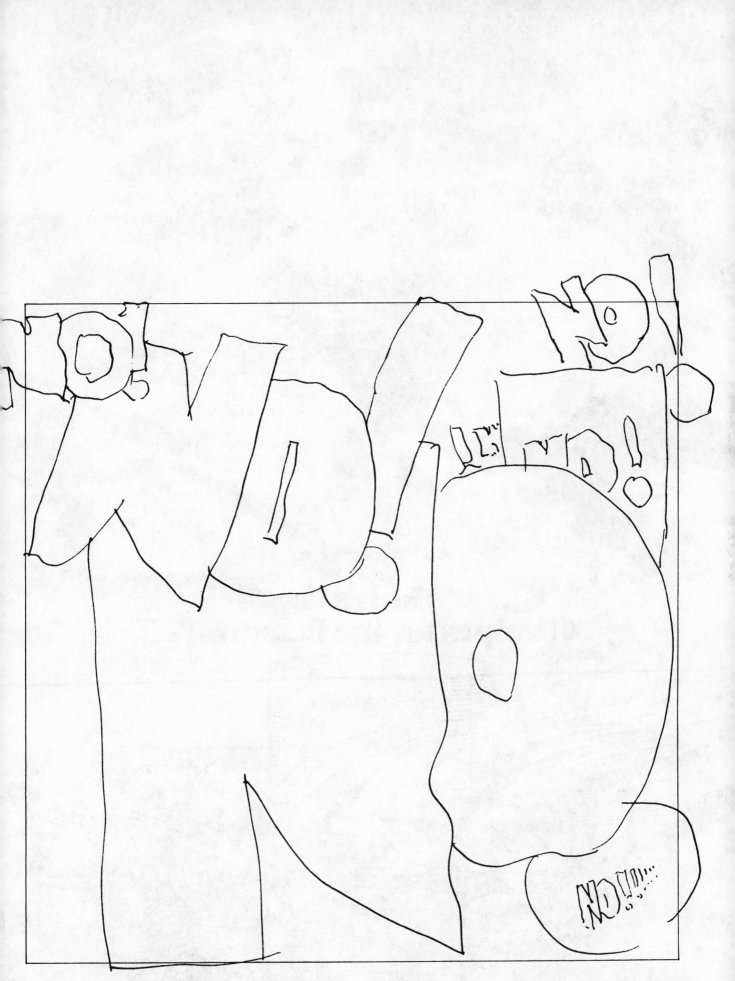

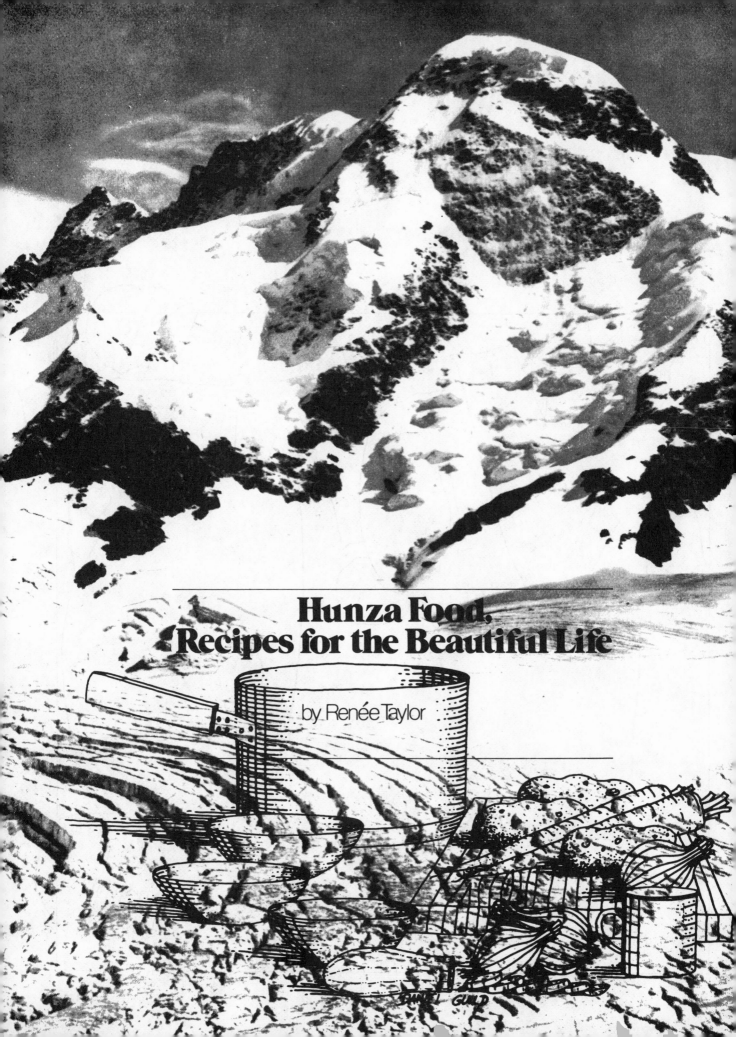

Hunza Food,
Recipes for the Beautiful Life

by Renée Taylor

LUNCH

Salad — consisting of fresh vegetables, cut up. Apricot oil and grape vinegar served separately as a dressing.
Cheese
Chapatti
A beverage — milk or lassi, or yogurt.

DINNER

A vegetable stew with millet, barley, or rice added to it.
Chapatti
A dessert or fresh fruit.

The Hunza people eat two meals a day. There isn't enough food for them to partake of more meals. But in between the meals and in the morning they drink water which they call "Glacier Milk," as it is of a grayish color. It comes from the melting snow from the glaciers, and brings the rich minerals with it. They are very lucky. The daily supply of fresh minerals nourishes their bodies, and apparently the body requires a great amount of minerals to be well. These minerals cannot be stored in the body; a fresh supply every day is essential.

Recently, I lectured at San Diego College, in National City in California, discussing the Hunza people and their health habits. After the program, Doctor C. S. Hansen came to meet me, to tell me that research is being conducted to determine the value of minerals in the human body, and that important findings might soon be revealed to the public.

The water which is served at the palace in Hunza comes directly from the glaciers and is full of sand which one feels under the teeth. But it tastes very good, so one gets used to it in no time at all. However, for the guests at the palace, if they prefer, the water is filtered and served clear. Obviously, the muddy water has more nutritional value — if one can overlook the sand.

Bread — Chapatti

Since the Hunzakuts have no mechanized farm equipment, all grains are harvested by hand. After being threshed, the grain is stored in a dry place, ready to be ground into flour as it is needed. The grain is ground in an ancient gristmill, operated by water from the irrigation system. By this method, the flour retains all of the natural nutrients found in wheat, including the bran and wheat germ.

Out of this flour "chapattis" are baked over an open fire by using a flat rock or a piece of metal. Chappatis are an example of the unleavened "staff of life" that is referred to in our Bible. The preparation of chapattis is quite complicated, an art that has been handed down from mother to daughter for centuries. They are made from wheat, barley, buckwheat, or millet; occasionally the flours are mixed together and baked in several shapes, small or large, according to the occasion.

This Hunza bread is wholesome, unrefined, maybe even coarse, but full of good nourishment. The part of the grain from which the new plant grows is called the germ. This germ is actually the most nourishing portion of the grain. The outer covering of the grain is known as bran. This gives the flour a brownish coloring. The Hunza people don't eat white flour; they have never seen it or tasted it. So by leaving in the germ and the bran, they make their flour full of excellent nourishment. This germ is known to us as "wheat germ" which supplies Vitamin E. It is also the part

of the grain which seems to assist the sexual powers of the animal who eats it, according to H. A. Mattill, M.D., who conducted an experiment and reported it in the *American Journal of Physiology* as far back as 1927. And then Dr. Evan Shute, of Canada, reported, in the *Urological and Cutaneous Review*, Volume 48, 1944, of using vitamin E extensively in therapy for productive disorders.

Hunza bread consists of all the nutrients of the grain. Maybe it accounts for the Hunzakuts' strong nerves and vigor into old age, as well as for the fact that their men are capable of fathering children at very old ages. Having lived for generations on sturdy brown bread, white bread doesn't appeal to them. Besides, coarse brown bread is chewy and exercises the gums.

Milk

Milk is a complete food. In Hunza it is used in various ways. The cream is separated and made into ghee, a sort of butter. Cottage cheese is made from the remains, and is a vital source of protein in their diet. Most of these products are made from goat's milk. Fresh, raw milk is nourishing and rich in protein. The Hunzakuts have no pasteurization system and drink the milk raw.

Vegetables

Vegetables play a great part in the Hunzakuts' diet, and since they don't cook too much, heat doesn't destroy the valuable nutrients stored in the plant. Every food consists of minerals, vitamins, enzymes and proteins, and when its values are diminished by extreme heat, there is little left to nourish our bodies.

The Hunzakuts don't grow too many vegetables, due to lack of tillable soil, but what they have has obviously been a wise choice. They grow leafy vegetables, such as spinach and lettuce, and cucumbers, radishes, carrots, turnips, and potatoes and a variety of herbs, which are used in cooking and also in beverages.

Cooking is done in covered vessels over a very low fire. If the vegetables are cooked in water, this liquid is served with them. Nothing is discarded or thrown away. All the minerals, such as phosphorus, calcium, iron, iodine, and many other valuable nutrients are consumed as food available in these tasty vegetables.

In Hunza, vegetables come directly from the gardens; they are fresh, and they are not sprayed with any chemicals, as it is forbidden by law to attempt to spray gardens. These vegetables and fruits can be eaten raw with the skin, which contains many valuable mineral salts, most of which are lost in soaking, vigorous scrubbing, peeling, and cooking.

Fruits

Apples, pears, peaches, mulberries, black and red cherries, and grapes are grown in moderate quantities. The Hunzas' favorite fruit is apricot. Apricots are eaten raw in summer and are sun-dried for the winter. The Hunzas have learned to extract from the kernel of the apricot a very rich oil which they use for cooking, salad dressing, even as a cosmetic on their skins and hair.

We always hear that a diet should be balanced and complete — consisting of proteins, carbohydrates, fats, minerals, vitamins, water, and oxygen. I sometimes wonder whether the Hunzakuts were aware of this factor, but maybe by instinct they realized that food without fat doesn't taste good, that something is lacking. A long search to find fat in some of their foods led them to discover it in the seed of the apricot. It is not simple to prepare, but nothing seems too much for them when it means their good health and survival. Since they don't eat pork, being Moslems, and very little other animal fat is available, they have no other choice

(continued on page 283)

Vegetarianism– From Ben Franklin To Dick Gregory

by Janet Barkas

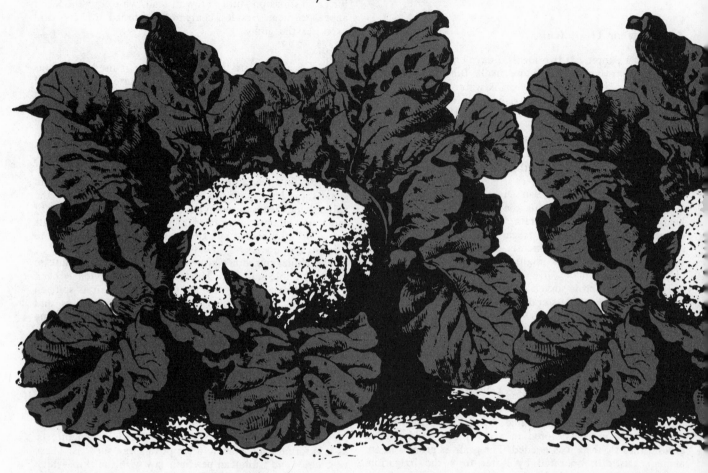

Throughout American history, there has been an epicurean clash between ethical convictions, nutritional fads, and positive advances, on the one hand, and the growing industrialization of food production, removing consumers even further from the land, on the other. To many persons, vegetarianism showed a way to rebel against the desensitization of nature and feelings as the god of Mammon overtook numerous aspects of life in the new land of promise and capitalization.

The first notable American vegetarian was Benjamin Franklin. At sixteen he read *Thomas Tyron's The Way to Health, Long Life and Happiness, Or A Discourse of Temperance.* That British publication inspired him to try a meatless diet. He was pleased by the two immediate results of his experiment: he saved money and since he began eating separately from his meat-eating brother James, he found extra time to devote to his favorite pastime, reading.

Until his first voyage from Boston, Franklin continued to be a vegetarian. Then, since the boat was stranded off Block Island, the travelers caught cod fish. Franklin had always loved the taste of fish and the aroma of freshly-caught cod was irresistible. He rationalized that since within the stomach of a large fish one would find a smaller fish, for the larger to eat the smaller was really the natural order of life. Thus he dined "very heartily" on the cod and began to eat with other people, "returning only now and then occasionally to a vegetable diet." Franklin, an open-minded, all-seeing thinker, realized he could endorse either action, depending on his momentary point of view.

Almost one hundred years passed from Franklin's conversion to the development of a vegetarian movement in America. Reverend William Metcalfe, an English clergyman and homeopathic doctor, interpreted the Bible in terms of vegetarianism and vehemently denounced meat-eating and alcohol. An essay, "Abstinence from the Flesh of Animals," was published in 1821 although his major achievement was the conversion in 1830 of Sylvester Graham and Dr. William Alcott.

Sylvester Graham, who had been a sickly child, became a Presbyterian minister in 1826 and traveled around the eastern states, developing into a fanatical prohibitionist while an agent for the Pennsylvania Society for the Suppression of the Use of Ardent Spirits. As the result of his meetings with Metcalfe, Graham added other platforms to his temperance lectures: sexual restraint, fresh air, baths and vegetarianism.

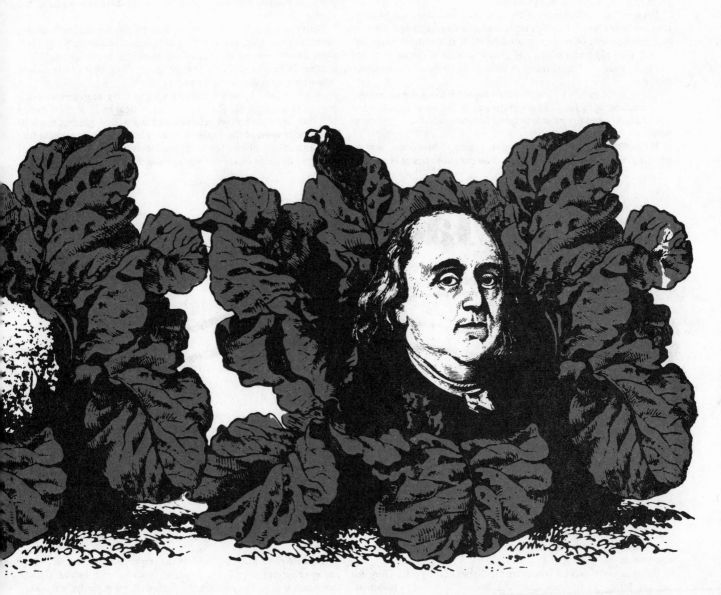

Followers, called Grahamites, began to apply his principles and hundreds started a regimen of Saturday night bathing, exercises before open windows, and sleeping on hard beds. *The Graham Journal of Health and Longevity* appeared, reiterating the diverse health principles of a man who was by now rich as well as famous. Sylvester Graham, known, of course, for Graham crackers, is now considered the founder of the modern health movement in America.

Horace Greeley, founder of the *New York Herald Tribune,* was an early convert to vegetarianism but his interest eventually waned, although he concluded that "a strict vegetarian will live ten years longer than a habitual flesh-eater, while suffering, on the average, less than half so much from sickness as the carnivorous must."

The Alcott family (Bronson, the teacher, William the doctor and writer Louisa May, author of *Little Women*) were thoroughly enmeshed in vegetarian dogma. The cousins, William and Bronson, shared a close childhood, exchanging books and ideas. William came under the influence of Graham in Boston. His major work in the field of vegetarianism was *The Vegetable Diet As Sanctioned by Medical Men and by Experience in All Ages,* which gives the unedited

statements of one hundred physicians about their experiences on a vegetable regimen, with Alcott's comments after each entry. There is not one completely negative reply, which somewhat decreases the credibility of the study. At the conclusion of the letters, Alcott gives seven reasons for his own preference for vegetarianism: anatomical, physiological, medical, political, economical, experimental and moral.

Bronson began following William's dicta in 1835, when he completely eliminated meat from his diet. With William and several other persons, they founded the Fruitlands, the vegetarian commune in Massachusetts that lasted only seven months because of conflict over the issues of marriage and the family.

Of the 500 American communes founded during the nineteenth century, others were far more successful than Fruitlands. One of the most intriguing was the Oneida Community, founded by John Humphrey Noyes in upstate New York.

This controversial experiment, begun in 1834, continued actively until 1881. The basic principles were a Perfectionist religion, continence, and after twenty years, a scientific system of eugenic procreation to improve future generations. It operated on vegetarian lines for health rather than ethical reasons. This is made clear by the astounding fact that the

(continued on page 285)

Nothing is more inspiring and beautiful on a kitchen shelf than a bag of grain. One partakes of its simplicity and is rendered safe from the complexities of the world.

Brown Rice is the staple of the cerealian who does not wish to involve himself in the difficult process of balancing food. Brown rice assures him of proper nourishment. It is the most balanced cereal, the only grain which contains nearly all of the ingredients our body needs, either directly or through the process of transmutation.

There are a number of varieties of brown rice — the short, the long and the very long. Short-grain rice is the most suitable for cold climates and the most satisfying for those who have given up meat.

Wheat is the grain of my native country, Morocco, where people prepare it in different ways. You eat couscous at Hassan's and spirit of the American Indian. Meanwhile, the French fed it to pigs, fattening them for the fair. Corn is the grain that accompanies a smaller amount of rice during the hottest months of the year.

Oats are eaten by horses as well as by the Scotch, who find it better to draw nigh the stable than to neigh in the freezing cold. Oats can be served as creams or soups for breakfast, lunch or dinner, in breads and cookies, or in anything that needs a little something to make it fluffy and crisp.

A grain-eater is like a jeweler who artfully prepares and displays a rare diamond. The man of rice, wheat and corn sets grains off with condiments, vegetables and black and green seaweeds from the bottom of the Japanese seas. He has numerous teas, fine oils and salted plums for vinegar. He is an artisan not only of flowers, but also of roots. Nor are sauces forgotten in his craft.

Macrobiotics:

the Cerealian's Dictionary

By Michel Abehsera

Restaurant and memories of exotic nights surround you like a bouquet.

Bulghur and Cracked Wheat are the dishes of the poor. They do not catch the eye like couscous, but appeal to a more elemental level. They are the most nourishing and faithful companions of Oriental travellers, who cook them during brief stopovers, for they are quickly prepared and require no seasoning.

In taste and form, **Barley** is the young prince, son of its king, Father Wheat. In digestibility it is a cousin to rice. Although not often used, it should be, for it is perhaps the noblest of the grains. In Morocco it is a common alternative to wheat, and in Korea and Japan monks mix it with white rice when the brown variety is unavailable.

Buckwheat is to Russians what rice is to Japanese. It is sometimes called "kasha."

Millet is an underrated grain whose light bitterness makes it as masculine as a cerealian could wish. It has been used in almost every civilization in history, from China to Africa, where it is cooked with onions and other vegetables. Some people prepare it with scallions and flavor it with dill. A multi-purpose grain, millet is very alkaline and makes deliciously sweet croquettes.

The word **Rye** has a magical sound. It has made me dream more than once of the bread my mother used to make in Morocco. I have eaten all kinds of rye bread in the U.S.A., but none matches the Moroccan.

Corn is the sacred grain whose kernels satisfied stomach, eye

Beans

Aduki Beans are small red beans imported from Japan. They are appropriate anywhere, anytime, cooked with brown rice or any other grain. They enhance a dish with their earthy red color, and make excellent soups and pies.

Black Beans, twin brothers of the red aduki in size, are sold in Chinese, Japanese and natural-food stores. They are the milk and honey of the bean family, and their flavor and texture impart a delightful sweetness and richness to any soup or vegetable dish.

Chick-peas, or Garbanzo Beans, are the bread of the "pulse"-eater. I have a great-uncle, eighty-five years old, whose sole food consists of dried chick-peas and lentils. Additionally, he eats couscous on Friday nights, with nothing but chick-peas and vegetables on the side. Some scientists have recently reported that whole-wheat and chick-peas are sufficient to fulfill a man's dietary requirements. Combined, they equal the properties of brown rice. If those same scientists would like living proof, I'll be happy to introduce them to my great-uncle.

The chick-pea is the Middle-Eastern aduki. It adapts perfectly well to couscous and vegetables. The unhappy and frustrated vegetarian, who craves a bit of meat, should try it as a beef-substitute.

Seaweeds

Seaweeds everyone remembers, having been alarmed by the unpleasantness of their touch while swimming. As children, we thought they might be sea-monsters.

Hijiki resembles thick black hair and tastes like noodles soaked in sea-water. A grain without hijiki on the side is like a pie-dough without filling. It is excellent for the heavy meat-eater who needs a cleansing.

Kombu looks like dark green ribbons. We often use it in soups and as a condiment. It is a delight when deep-fried in oil or toasted in a very hot oven. It has a taste unlike anything you've ever had before.

Wakame is a very tender seaweed especially good when cooked with onions or scallions. We use it in Miso soup, which we enjoy almost every day. Excellent for a healthy growth of hair.

Nori has the advantage of being in many ways the most practical. It comes in pressed, paper-thin sheets with which the Japanese prepare their famous Nori Maki. The sheet is dark brown, but when passed rapidly over a flame it turns a crisp, toasted green. We use it for rice balls or simply, when reduced to crumbs, over rice and noodles.

Dulse looks like chopped nori. It has such a strong taste and is so naturally spicy, that serving it to a friend runs the risk of alienating him.

Agar-Agar makes a firm jelly for desserts. Its uses are unlimited. When diluted in water, heated, mixed with vegetables or

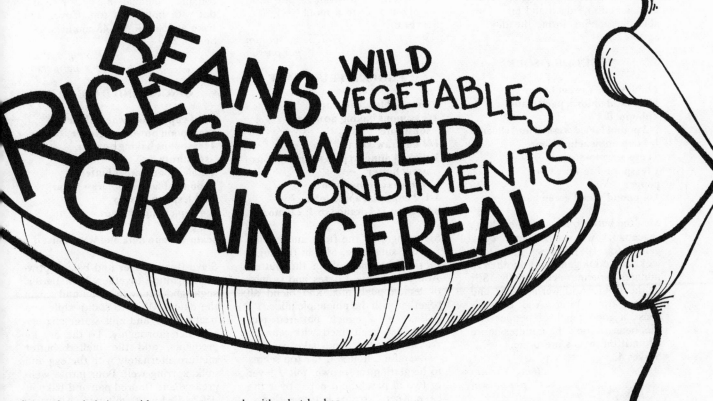

fish and cooled, it provides an amateur cook with what he has previously seen only in photographs — a true aquarium-like aspic with carrots, parsley and striped bass all caught in dramatic stop-action.

The Wild Vegetables

Japanese stores and some natural-food stores and vegetable stands sell the following roots. Be sure to learn their uses.

Burdock grows wild in fields and gardens and is very difficult to unearth, so deep is its root. It is a cousin of the dandelion, whose struggle for survival in the spring is nonetheless legendary despite its ill fate. Gardeners dislike them both. Burdock, however, receives special attention from root-eaters, who prize it for its taste and food value.

Ginger Root: A tiny bit of ginger, grated and boiled with bancha tea and soya sauce, is an excellent diaphoretic in cases of cold. Sometimes we add a tablespoon of grated daikon to make the remedy more palatable.

(continued on page 287)

LOW-SODIUM RECIPES

by
Gena Larson

MUESLI

6 tablespoons rolled oats
pineapple juice
juice of 1 lemon
4 teaspoons honey
2 teaspoons cream
2 apples, grated
nuts, chopped and unsalted
sunflower seeds

Soak the oats in pineapple juice overnight. The next morning add the rest of the ingredients, using nuts and sunflower seeds to taste. For a sharper muesli, use yogurt instead of cream and water instead of pineapple juice. This provides enough for two people, and is a good breakfast or bedtime dish, and an invaluable pick-me-up during the day. Serves 2.

VEGETABLE SOUP

2 tablespoons sweet butter
1/2 pound onions, peeled and
  chopped
1/2 pound leeks, washed and sliced
1/4 cup unbleached flour
6 cups warm water
1 teaspoon brewer's yeast
pepper
1/4 pound sliced green beans

Melt the butter on low heat in a large saucepan. Add onions and cook gently for 10 minutes. Then add leeks and cook gently for another 10 minutes, stirring occasionally. Stir in the flour. Add warm water and simmer for 1 hour. Add brewer's yeast, a good pinch of pepper and the beans. Cook 10 minutes more or until the beans are done. Serves 4.

80 mg. sodium
per person

BEEF MOLD

1/2 pound round steak cubed
1 small white onion, chopped very
  fine
4 cloves
12 peppercorns
1 bayleaf
water to cover
3 teaspoons powdered gelatin
2 tablespoons red wine vinegar
2 tablespoons sherry (optional)
1 tablespoon fresh parsley, chopped

1 tablespoon fresh chives, chopped
kelp or salt substitute if allowed

Choose a pot with a close-fitting lid. Put in beef cubes and the onion. Tie the cloves, peppercorns and bay leaf in a cheesecloth bag and add. Cover with water, cover the pot, and simmer for 2-1/2 hours. Remove the spice bag and flake the meat in the broth with a fork. Stir in the gelatin until it dissolves. Add vinegar, sherry, parsley, chives and the salt substitute if wished. Stir thoroughly and set in a mold. Serves 6.

175 mg. sodium
per person

EGGLESS FRUIT CAKE

3 cups unbleached flour
4 teaspoons baking powder
  substitute
1/4 cup raw sugar
1 stick (4 ounces) plus 4 tablespoons
  sweet butter
12 ounces chopped dates
1-1/2 cups pineapple juice
peel from 1/2 orange or 1/2 lemon

Sieve together the flour and baking powder substitute. Mix in the sugar thoroughly, and rub in the butter. Add the chopped dates and orange or lemon peel, mix, and blend all together with the pineapple juice.

Bake in a 6-inch buttered pan which has been lined with wax or parchment paper, and bake in a 350° F. oven for 2 hours. If the top seems to be getting too brown, put a layer or two of parchment paper over the cake. Keep two days before eating.

50 mg. sodium
per person

STUFFED CABBAGE LEAVES

1 medium onion, chopped fine
2 tablespoons sweet butter
pinch of thyme
1 medium tomato, chopped
1 teaspoon raw sugar
1 tablespoon wine vinegar
pinch of white pepper
pinch of cayenne pepper

1/2 pound chopped beef
1/4 cup wholewheat breadcrumbs,
  salt-free
8 cabbage leaves

Cook onion in butter for 5 minutes. Add thyme and tomato and cook another 5 minutes. Add sugar, vinegar, both peppers, chopped meat and breadcrumbs and cook 10 minutes. Meanwhile, immerse the cabbage leaves in boiling water for 5 minutes, and drain.

Divide the mixture into four parts, and pile each part onto a cabbage leaf and fold the leaf over the stuffing. Wrap a second leaf around each roll, place them all in a casserole and dot with butter on top. Cover and bake at 350° F. for 45 minutes. Serves 2.

185 mg. sodium
per person

GINGER AND DATE CAKE

1-3/4 cups whole wheat flour
1 teaspoon powdered ginger
4 teaspoons baking powder
  substitute
4 tablespoons sweet butter
1 rounded tablespoon raw sugar
2 tablespoons honey
1/4 cup chopped dates
1 egg
scant 1/2 cup milk and water mixed

Sieve flour, ginger and baking powder substitute together. Melt butter, sugar and honey in a pan and stir in the dates. Allow to stand while you beat the egg and milk-water mixture together thoroughly. To the dry ingredients, add the melted butter mixture alternately with the egg and milk, stirring well. Pour into a well-greased and floured pan and bake at 350° F. for 50 minutes. Allow to cool in the pan for about 20 minutes before turning out onto a rack.

60 mg. sodium
per person

Baking Powder Substitute for
Low-Sodium Baking Recipes

Ask your druggist to put together **28** grams of cornstarch, **39.8** grams of potassium bicarbonate, **7.5** grams of tartaric acid and **56.1** grams of potassium bitartrate. ☼

GOOD FOOD-GLUTEN FREE!

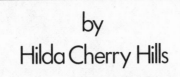
by
Hilda Cherry Hills

MILLET AND CHEESE DROPPIES

1 cup cracked millet
1 tablespoon soya flour
3 cups stock or salted water
1 cup cheese, grated
1 egg, beaten

Blend millet and soya flour with 1/2 cup of liquid. Heat rest of liquid. When boiling pour over mixture, add cheese and stir till smooth. Cook covered, over gentle heat, in basin in pan of hot water (or top of double boiler) till all liquid is absorbed. Remove and cool. Beat in egg and drop spoonfuls on oiled baking tin. Broil till brown. Turn and broil other side. Eat hot with butter.

FISH AND ONION PIE

1 pound flat fish fillets
2 tablespoons finely chopped parsley
1/2 cup finely chopped onion
salt to taste
1 pound potatoes (3 or 4 medium)
1/2 cup milk
2 tablespoons butter or soft margarine

Wash fillets and cut in pieces. Lay a few pieces in oiled pie pan, sprinkle with chopped parsley and onion, and salt lightly. Continue with similar layers till all are used. Steam potatoes, rub through sieve, beat in butter, season to taste, and make a soft paste with the milk. Spread over the fish, ripple with back of fork, dot with remainder of butter and bake about 20 minutes at 375º F.

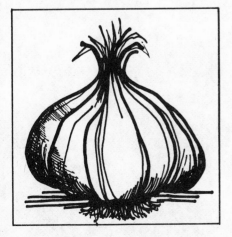

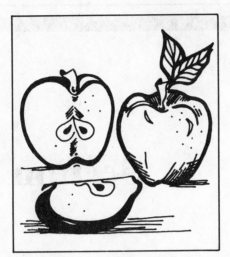

INSTANT CHUTNEY (1)

2 medium-sized tomatoes, chopped
2-1/2 cups freshly shredded coconut
1 finely chopped or grated onion
pinch of salt
grated nutmeg
1 cooking apple, grated
1 tablespoon finely chopped raisins
1/2 teaspoon lemon juice and grated rind of 1/2 lemon
pinch raw sugar

Mix thoroughly in a bowl. Serve with cold meats or rice dishes.

INSTANT CHUTNEY (2)

2 raw cooking apples, finely chopped
2 tablespoons chopped sweet peppers, seeded
2 tablespoons onion, grated
2 tablespoons raisins, pitted and quartered
1 teaspoon salt
2 tablespoons lemon juice
2 tablespoons sugar
1 teaspoon ground ginger (optional)
1 clove garlic, finely chopped (optional)

Mix thoroughly and serve with rice dishes or cold meats.

GOLDEN RICE AND LEFTOVERS

1 cup raw rice
2 tablespoons oil
2-3 cups water (boiling)
pinch of basil
1 teaspoon salt
3 pieces onion outer skin
1 minced garlic clove (optional)
1 cup diced cooked beef, heart, tongue, kidney, sweetbread, lamb or flaked fish, etc.

Wash rice rapidly. Pat thoroughly dry and fry in oil at high heat, stirring often, and cook till golden brown. Add slowly the salted boiling water, seasoning, outer skin of onion and garlic and simmer about 20 minutes or till tender, but not mushy. Just before ready, remove onion skin and stir in 1 cup of diced meat. Serve when heated through, with tossed green salad or plain watercress in bowl. If liked, garnish with ripe olives or toasted peanuts or almonds.

UNBAKED FRUIT CAKE

1 cup seedless raisins, chopped
1 cup coconut, grated
2 tablespoons lemon juice
grated rind of 1/2 lemon
1 cup nuts, chopped
1 cup chopped, pitted dates
1/2 cup chopped, dried bananas
enough non-instant powdered milk to absorb moisture

Mix thoroughly all ingredients except powdered milk. Add the powdered milk as required. Press mixture into lightly oiled loaf pan. Chill. Turn out on plate and slice very thinly with sharp knife dipped in hot water. ☼

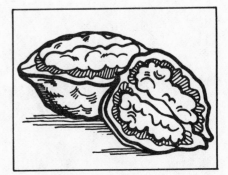

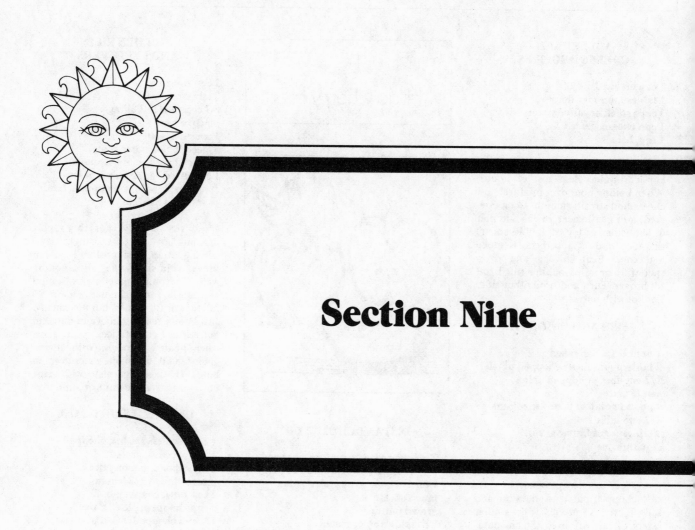

Section Nine

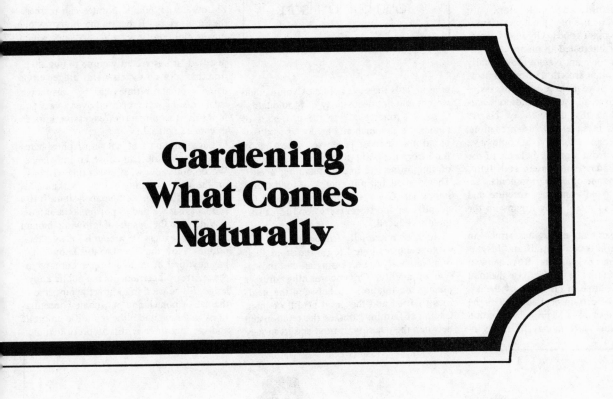

Gardening
What Comes
Naturally

ABC'S OF ORGANIC FARMING

□ Organic farming is a term used to denote the nourishing of plants with organic materials—barnyard manure, green crops, which are crops specially grown to nourish the soil, or any material that was once living or its byproduct; as such it is opposed to chemical farming in which plants are nourished by the use of synthetic or chemically treated plant foods. Organic farmers are naturally interested in plants and animals as food for man. Nature too is vitally interested in plant growth. Her experiments over millions of years have been successful in keeping alive all the multitudinous animals and plants that thrive today. Nature has done this in spite of the depredations practised by man. This survival could have resulted only from a proper balance of the processes of adaption between soil, light, heat, moisture and other environmental factors on one hand—and the structure and functions of various bodily organs on the other.

□ Natural man, left alone, has struck an even balance between himself and his animal and plant environment. But chemical man has found that he can increase the total weight and volume of his crops by the administration of certain chemicals. This he has proceeded to do—the primary intention being to obtain more money from the in-

Garden Talk
by
John B. Harrison

crease. This increase is one of volume and weight and not necessarily of food quality. Organic farmers look to the processes of nature for guidance and try as far as possible to imitate these processes. They regard food from the point of view of its functions of supporting life and maintaining health. They realize that it is quality of food that is important. Given the proper qualities, the quantity of food necessary for life can be greatly reduced.

□ Such commercially important attributes as appearance, long life on the store shelf or adaptability to processing are not indicative of quality. Organic farming stresses mainly the relationship between the qualities of food and the good health of man. Chemical farming stresses the relationship between the quantity of food and its money

value. These two philosophies differ widely. Which should we adopt as the more important? Healthy Man or Healthy Money?

Cost

□ Low-cost synthetic nitrates can increase the crop yield. Because the higher yield means more profit per acre any steps which can increase the yield consequently seem justified. It has recently come to our attention that spinach which yields bigger crops using synthetic nitrates can be poisonous. Infant deaths were reported over a year ago in the East as a result of excessive nitrates in canned spinach.

□ Large amounts of potash or phosphates added to the soil can cause an imbalance. We do not know what effect this will have on the plant system, nor do we know its ultimate effect on the human system. It is a sad fact that we had to poison some infants to find out the result of growing human food with excessive amounts of synthetic nitrates. Now that we have this knowledge, has anything been done to prevent a recurrence? If so, it certainly is not public knowledge. Since we don't know the outcome of the use of potash and phosphate concentrations we crawl under the scientific umbrella and say that there is still no proof that any-

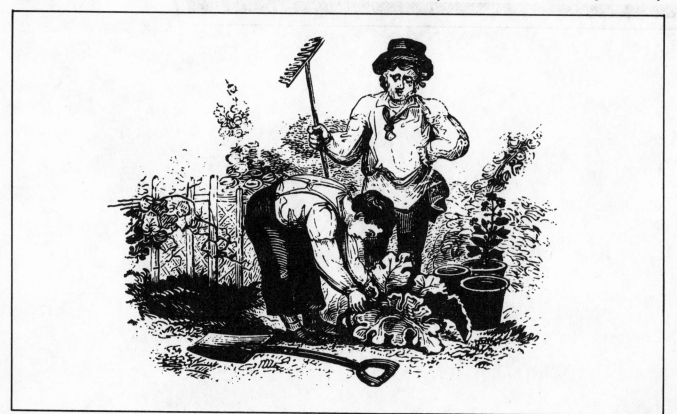

one has been harmed. But has there been no proof because thorough, exhaustive longterm tests were skillfully and impartially conducted in an attempt to determine whether anyone suffered, or has there been no proof merely because there has been no thorough investigation?

☐ We do know that plants forced with concentrated chemicals are more susceptible to insects and diseases. Under such conditions of growth, plants require pesticides to prevent them from total destruction. While appearing to solve an immediate problem and save the plants, pesticides create difficulties for the future. Insects develop resistance to them and the relationship between the predator and prey is upset. The effect of pesticides on the biosphere has reached the point where many thinking people are expressing concern about the ill-effects which are now becoming so obvious. A recent financial publication states: "It is imperative to his survival that man should recognize his animal nature and live within the boundaries set by his organic world."

☐ Eventually the amount of pesticides necessary to control an insect or disease in a particular plant will exceed the so-called safe amount.

☐ An even worse situation is that in at least one area the amount of pesticide left in the soil, as a result of repeated applications, is so great that human food cannot safely be produced on that soil for many years. Estimates of the time the soil remains toxic have ranged from ten to fifteen years. This estimated period may prove to be only a fraction of the time necessary for the toxicity to disappear. We can imagine what would happen if much of our soil were ruined in this way. There may even now be areas, where the agricultural chemical production is intense, which are already nearing this danger point. Some soils may already have excessive amounts of chemicals which may not yet have been discovered. Such soil could be producing unrecognized, unsuitable food going undetected onto the tables of our nation. Such a happening could easily occur accidentally, as for instance when a farm changes owners, should the second owner be unaware of the amount of pesticide already in the soil and use chemicals lavishly. Many unfortunate people could suffer quite innocently. The organic farmer creates no such risk. His method of farming avoids it.

Food Value

☐ It seems strange that in our highly developed technological era absolutely no criteria exist for the value of food in terms of its capacity to nourish, as distinct from its chemical constitution. This nutritional factor is commonly ignored. It did reach the point of scientific research some decades ago but was not popular. No board of governors or other ruling body ever made any decision to use the taxpayers' money to determine the true value of his daily bread. Yet the same authorities read papers by other scientists who analyzed and found that the mineral compositions of apparently identical vegetables can vary as much as hundreds percent. In spite of this not even a scientist, for fear of being scorned, may suggest that one of these apparently identical vegetables might be better than the other.

☐ Existing criteria of the quality of producers are mainly those which are of help in marketing: size, shape, color or absence of defects. The vitamin, protein and mineral content are only useful in a negative way. They can only indicate deficiencies or excesses. The optimum amount of each constituent is yet to be determined. We can imagine the ensuing tragedy if the nitrogen content was used as an indicator of the protein content in spinach which was to be fed to a very sickly infant; more nitrogen—more protein—but greater toxicity.

Organic Food vs. Ordinary Food

☐ The most noticeable difference is flavor. If the plant has all the biological chemical and physical requirements, it will grow to be a complete plant having all its constituents in the correct proportions. Such a plant can now attain full flavor. Should the plant not have all the foods necessary for its complete development, it becomes deficient in flavor. Flavor-revealing deficiencies can be recognized by very young children and by animals. This intangible quality called flavor attracts the consumer, and guided solely by flavor the consumer will tend to be properly nourished. Modern man's sense of taste and therefore his appreciation of flavor suffers from the use of highly seasoned foods. He easily loses his ability to differentiate between foods.

☐ What are the relative values of organic food free from pesticides and chemically produced food carrying so-called safe amounts of pesticides? What is the difference between salt water and fresh water to a person dying of thirst? Are such differences calculated in dollars and cents?

Pests

☐ Provided the growing plant has all its requirements it will be healthy and vigorous, and will have resistance to insects and disease. On the other hand should the plant not receive its requirements, insects and other diseases are attracted to it and can more easily destroy it. Nature has doomed such plants since they would not make good food for the higher forms of life. The insects and diseases, in destroying such plants, do a service: the remains of the plant fall to the earth and enrich it, thus making space for better plants to grow in its place. It would seem that insects and disease are really nature's censors. They point out that all is not well with the growing procedure. Killing such pests is only an expedient and doesn't attack the cause of the problem. So we have just another example of the common erroneous practice of attempting to cure the symptom rather than trying to eradicate the cause.

Pesticides

☐ Pesticides are a major source of agricultural pollution. These long-lived synthetic chemicals cripple, maim, deform and destroy as they move down and up and down the bioscale, eventually finding their way to the ocean where they continue their destruction for the life of the pesticide.

Health from the Soil to the Plant and to the Consumer:

☐ Sir Albert Howard, who was successful in salvaging the tea industry in India, discovered the relationship between the health of the soil and the health of the plants growing in it, and thus was led to develop a sound, permanent agricultural system.

☐ The relationship between the quality of food and the health of the consumer was adequately documented by the late Dr. Robert McCarrison. Dr. McCarrison conducted his famous experiment with caged rats at Coonoor, India. He fed the rats the diet of a sickly tribe and they were sickly. He could change the health of the rats at will, merely by switching diets.

☐ The works of these two great scientists have been largely ignored until the present. The theories they recommended are not in keeping with the times. They involve ideas to be promoted instead of materials to be sold and therefore are not popular.

☐ Scientific advances in agriculture are causing as many new problems as they are providing solutions to present difficulties. Over a quarter of a century of personal practical experience in growing crops of many different kinds on a commercial scale have convinced the writer, and I am sure too, that thousands of others have been convinced, as a result of their work, that agricultural practices must follow that of Nature instead of fighting her. Nature wins in the end!

☼

STARTING AN ORGANIC GARDEN

Before we go into some of what you need to start a natural or organic garden let us tell you how to make a midget instant organic garden. You can even do it in a window box.

First dig a little trench with a trowel, about as wide as your hand and a little deeper, say 4″ wide and 6″ deep. Then stuff a 3″-deep layer of vegetable trimmings from the kitchen into it and chop this coarsely with the trowel. On top of it sprinkle a little blood meal, about 1 tablespoon per square foot of surface. Then refill the trench to ground level with earth, patting lightly. Make a row by pressing the edge of a board ½″ deep into the middle of the fill, dampen with water, drop radish seeds 1″ apart into it and refill the row with earth, patting it down firmly. This will quickly give you a flourishing sample organic garden nourished largely by vegetable wastes that in most households end up in the garbage can. We mention this right away because it is nice and simple, and so natural. Organic gardening needn't be complicated.

Now, for the garden itself.

Because we have lived here and there about the country a good deal during our lives we have made a lot of gardens, and this experience has helped us to think in pretty basic garden terms. So we can tell you in two words what we look for whenever we start to make a garden: convenience and climate. Convenience means such things as having the garden easily accessible from the house, near a tool shed, and so on. Climate covers sun, air, and water.

Here are the points to consider:

Site

Close to the house. Try to have the garden near enough to the house so you can treat it as a living pantry. That way, you can whisk out for a handful of herbs or stalk of celery any time you need them, and can put off harvesting vegetables for a meal until the last minute, to keep all the sweetness and vitamins and tenderness intact.

Nearness to the house also makes for better attention to the garden by you. If you don't have to walk a country mile to get to it, you'll know what is going on in the garden nearly all the time. You can nip a lot of problems before they get well started, keep an eye on new plantings, harvest crops at their peaks of perfection. A garden is a living thing, changing every day and even every hour.

Sunshine. Try to locate your garden where it will have all-day sun. Impossible? It will settle for less. The practical minimum is 6 hours of sun. If you live in a

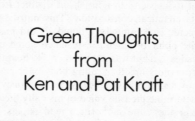

Green Thoughts from Ken and Pat Kraft

canyon and don't have even 6 sunny hours per day, try planting leafy vegetables such as lettuce, cress, chard, mustard. The fruiting vegetables, such as tomatoes and peppers, are pretty hopeless if they don't get plenty of sun, and most root crops are somewhere in between. In a canyon garden that we had a few years ago we managed to grow a good variety of crops despite scanty sun. The vegetables included most of the leafy greens, nearly all the root crops including Jerusalem artichokes (which grew 12′ tall reaching for more sunshine), squash, leeks, and so on. By putting some planters on a deck that received an extra hour or two of sun, we grew bush beans and midget tomatoes.

Trees. Locate the garden far enough from trees to prevent their competing with it for food and water. Tree roots usually extend out at least as far as the branches reach, sometimes twice as far. One way to keep them in their place is to dig a trench 2′ to 4′ deep between tree and garden, line it with galvanized sheet steel, and refill it. The digging will prune the tree roots too.

Air. Most plants do not grow well if the movement of air about them is much hindered, as by buildings or thick shrubbery. A slope is a help here since cooler air will move down it, setting up a circulation. If the slope is a gentle one, run plant rows crosswise to the direction of the slope to keep water from rushing downward and eroding your soil. A steep slope, say one of 10 degrees or more, should be terraced into a series of broad steplike beds to control erosion. Set a board on edge to serve as the rise of each step, and fill in earth behind it. Two or three stakes will hold the board in place and it can be left there permanently. Don't use creosoted boards. Plants cannot survive close to them.

Underground drainage. Most plants hate wet feet, as gardeners put it, and if your site is soggy, wet feet are what they'll have. Instead of laying a tile drainage line—the classic, expensive, and fairly permanent remedy when properly done and maintained—we suggest you plant in raised beds. This usually means bringing in earth and raising the level of the whole garden by

about 2′. You can build bottomless boxes and fill them with earth, or simply make a flat-topped pile of earth to cover the entire site. If you had a vast amount of raw plant material you could build a giant compost pile over the entire garden site and raise the level in that way. More realistically, bring in earth and keep adding to it the compost you make year in and year out.

Access to deliveries. If you do bring in earth, or anything else, you'll need a way to get it in. If your garden is so located that a truckload can be deposited alongside it, this will save hours of hard work.

Soil. Most gardeners must get along with whatever soil they have. This means you usually must keep on adding organic matter to your garden, as the great majority of soils need it and plants keep using it up.

Mostly for purposes of comparison with whatever soil you happen to have, here is what you'd have if you had a perfect garden soil: a loamy combination of sand, silt, clay, and a lot of organic matter; good structure, neither sticky nor loose, but rather spongy; high in all plant nutrients, earthworms, and micro-organisms; neutral or slightly acid; and, finally, plenty of depth so that roots could go down to 4′ in it.

Don't be discouraged by poor soil. You can do something about it. It takes Mother Nature a thousand years to make a single inch of topsoil, but her organic gardening children know some shortcuts.

Non-organic residues. If there had been a garden where you are now about to start your garden, you may be worried about the residual effect of chemical fertilizers and poisons used against pests by the previous gardener.

Keep in mind that most chemical insecticides and pesticides are decidedly short-lived. By and large, they lose potency within from a few hours to three weeks after application.

As to chemical fertilizers, there is still less to concern yourself with. Nearly all of them leach away rapidly. The thing to do is to rebuild the soil with additions of organic matter.

Water

Next to a good site, water is the most important thing your garden needs. Mulching will help here, but you'll still need *some* water. We worked out a system we recommend to you, to wit:

Sprinkler. When we decide where the garden is to go, we put a sprinkler in the middle of the site and turn it on. The area it covers is where we make the garden. By setting the sprinkler a few feet above ground level we can cover a larger area, and if we have space for still larger garden we set two sprinklers. After that, all we have to do to water the garden is to turn a handle.

A general rule for the amount of water a garden needs is, 1″ per week. If you have a 1″ rain, that takes care of it. You can measure how much a sprinkler is raining down by placing a few empty tin cans here and there in the garden to catch the water. After the sprinkler has run for 30 minutes, measure the water in the cans with a dip stick and you'll learn how long the sprinkler has to run to give the garden 1″ of water.

Additives in water. Gardeners who distrust the purifying materials in city water sometimes worry about their effect on the garden. We agree that rain is the best water, if it doesn't absorb pollutants on the way down. The earth itself is an excellent filter, and by the time water gets down to the roots, it has passed through a good deal of earth.

Tools

Some gardeners seem to attract tools. You need very few, really, and if you haven't gardened before, try getting along with the essentials at first. Here are the essentials: a spade, a fork, a trowel, a knife, a 3-pronged cultivator, a rake, a hoe, and a file to keep edges sharp.

You do big digging with the spade and little digging with the trowel. The knife is mainly for cutting when you harvest and for transplanting in cutting out blocks of earth with each plant in flats. The fork is for some digging and to turn compost. The cultivator can be a small hand tool for a small garden, or one on the end of a long handle for a larger garden, or a wheel hoe for a still larger garden. We find we use a small one 90 percent of the time. The hand hoe is for weeding and some cultivating, and the rake is for smoothing seedbeds and for general garden grooming.

If you can call them tools, there are a few other conveniences we keep on hand. One is an old kitchen fork for tiny cultivating and for hunting cutworms just below the soil surface. We keep a small board in the garden for making seed rows in flats, and another board 3′ long for making rows in beds, for a straight edge, and for leveling and hilling up earth. It is marked off with crayon into feet and inches for convenient measuring. A soft pencil for marking labels and seed packets with planting dates is kept in the garden, and so is a pair of scissors and an old spoon or two, for harvesting and for transplanting small things.

You need a place near the garden where you can keep tools. Otherwise you'll walk needless miles every season. If we find it impossible to locate a garden near tool storage, we compromise by installing a small storage place inside the garden for trowels and the other small tools. A rustic weatherproof box set on bricks serves nicely, and so does a parcel post rural mailbox, painted dark green, set on a post, and with a vine running up the post.

Garden Plan

Even if you don't follow it faithfully, making a garden plan is a good idea because it tells you things you ought to know ahead of time, such as what you don't have one speck of room for at all.

Our taste is for a garden divided into beds of various sizes. A typical bed might be 10′ long and 4′ wide. Not very wide, you see, so we don't have to step into it to cultivate or harvest, or at least not very often. We could plant this whole bed with one crop, say beans, but we usually don't. More likely it will have quite an assortment. To give a for-instance, we have just checked on the occupants of one bed in our present garden. It covers about 60 square feet, and in it are: 18 celery plants, 2 catnips, a few Chinese cabbage seedlings, 6 small marigolds, a row of parsley, some oregano cuttings being rooted, a dozen basils, 3 garlics, and 2 dozen snap beans. Most of these plants are repeated elsewhere in the garden.

In the space most home gardeners have, the bedding garden is a flexible and attractive arrangement. We used to make wide paths between beds, but later narrowed them to save space.

A bedding garden is as easy to alter as a row garden, and by numbering the beds you can more easily keep track of where and when plantings are made. Which brings us to the matter of keeping track.

Garden Record

Climates differ, even the climates of your garden and your neighbor's garden. So the general rules you get from books on gardening must remain general. This is one of the best arguments for keeping a garden record.

From your record you will learn when you planted something too early or too late, how near the average maturity time a vegetable took to ripen, what problems befell it and what helped with them, and all sorts of other facts.

We keep a record like this in a loose-leaf notebook, one page for each variety of vegetable, fruit and herb. At the top of each page is the year, the name of the plant and the variety.

For some vegetables and fruits we keep a record of the total harvest by weight or count. Other items often jotted on the record are: transplanting dates, if any; when mulched and with what; any unusual fertilizing; comments on growth; any experimental procedures we may be trying; companion plantings used.

Using Your Experience

When we set up the sheets for the next season's garden we use the experience gained from past seasons and write at the tops of the pages the planting times that have seemed best, the actual maturity times, the days it takes to sprout seed, and any special requirements or problems. We may not write all of this on every page, as we know some of it by heart, but we mention it here to show the value of a personal garden record. It could be much more elaborate and detailed, perhaps including photographs as well as the sketch of the garden layout and some general comments that we do include, but a fairly brief record is more apt to be kept up to date. ☼

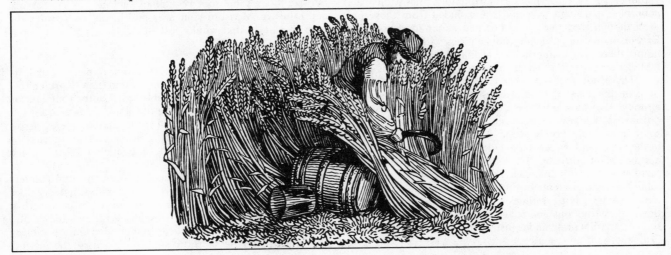

The Pleasures of Container Gardening

by Sharon Cadwallader

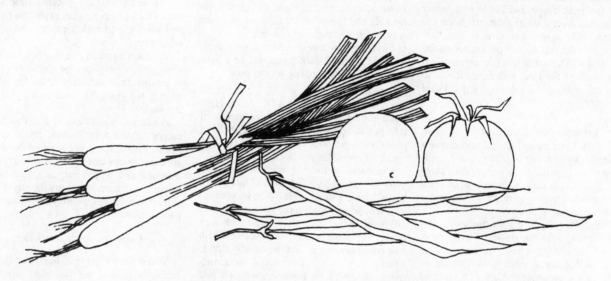

One satisfying activity in which people all over the country can participate is home gardening. In fact, the return to food gardening in the last few years in the United States is significant commentary on the interest in more resourceful living. Most gardeners of the organic method are part of the growing reaction to commercial, chemical gardening. Not since the Victory Gardens of the Second World War has so much collective spirit arisen for raising vegetables and fruit, and never before in this country have there been the community support and exchange of gardening ideas we see today.

A great deal has been published in recent years on the values and techniques of organic farming methods for the home gardener or small farmer. Unfortunately, many city and suburban apartment dwellers feel excluded from these projects though they may be concerned about food pollution. Except in special gardening publications with limited circulation, there is little information available on container vegetable gardening, although the interest in this activity is growing. Therefore, the vegetable gardening ideas and instructions in this article are addressed to those individuals who although they have not even a border of earth for cultivating, do have a balcony, an accessible rooftop, an atrium, or a sometimes-sunny porch. Roof gardens are not uncommon in the cities, and we see many balconies nowadays with flowers and plants thriving. The old-time window box is still a familiar sight in ethnic areas. Yet the possibility of making a salad from the contents of these container gardens is a new idea to many. I hope in time it will become a common practice. All instructions and suggestions given here are the result of experimenting under just such conditions with the adjustments that are required.

Planning Your Area

Summer vegetables and herbs need sun, although some require and benefit from less direct sun and cooler weather than others. Judge your area carefully in relation to size and light conditions. If you have a reasonably large porch, balcony, or rooftop area, you will be able to grow a good variety of vegetables, but if confined to a fairly small area with limited sun, you will get the best results by raising hearty greens and lettuce and perhaps pole beans and tomatoes. Each of these will give you a high yield for the space because you can cut back their outer leaves and the plants will continue to replenish themselves. If you have a limited amount of direct sunlight, but can create good soil conditions, it would be wise to try some root vegetables such as onions, carrots, and radishes. Measure your area and begin to consider the type of planter that would best fit.

Choosing Planters

There are a number of types of planters to make, round up, or buy that will work well for this garden plan. I prefer redwood planters as they are durable, pleasantly rough-hewn, cheap and easy to make, and the old standby terra-cotta pots which range in size from 2 to 14 inches in diameter. Narrow planters have two properties to consider: they are easy to build and they prevent creating a container of too much weight.

Nearly every nursery in the country carries redwood planters of different varieties and sizes. If your handiest nursery does not, it probably will order them for you or refer you to a place that does carry them. Considering the possibility of a lack of tools, the difficulty of carrying lumber on the subway or bus, and your having little skill in carpentry, the instructions for these planter boxes are designed to compete with the easiest "do-it-yourself kit" on the market.

FIVE-FOOT PLANTER *(Approximate cost: $4.00)*
Materials needed: 3 pieces 6-foot x 12-inch x 1-inch rough-
        sawn redwood
        1 pound 6d galvanized nails
        10-point hand saw
        hammer

1. Cut the lumber as shown.

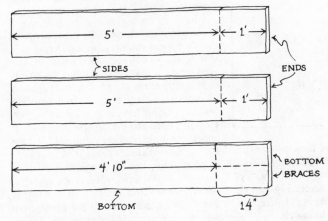

2. Cut three 1-inch triangular notches for drainage on each side of the 4-foot-10-inch piece. Avoid knots.

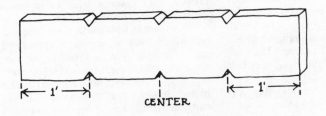

3. Square off one end piece to bottom piece and pound in three nails.

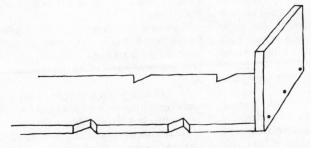

4. Attach side piece to end and bottom. Continue with other end and final side.

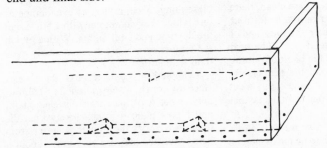

5. Nail 14-inch strips underneath to brace and elevate for drainage (or attach casters).
Don't nail over notches.

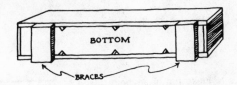

TWO-FOOT PLANTER *(Approximate cost: $2.00)*
Materials needed: 1 8-foot x 12-inch x 1-inch piece rough-
        sawn redwood
        6d galvanized nails
        10-point hand saw
        hammer

Cut as shown:

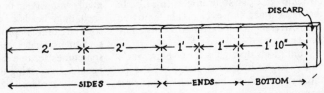

Notch bottom and follow same procedure as for larger planter. Use casters or bricks to elevate for drainage.

Drainage is a crucial factor for the apartment garden. Clay pots all have trays which work well for this purpose. With the redwood planters, the casters or wooden braces are to raise them for drainage and facilitate moving them in and out of the sun. Good soil will not drain like a sieve anyway, and the casters or braces will work well if you place ice cube trays, cut-off milk cartons, or any similar receptacle under all drainage holes. If the soil is good and you water more frequently and less intensely, drainage will not be profuse. Other receptacles will also work well for planting. Coffee cans and plastic cartons are fine if you punch good drainage holes. Bushel baskets, small barrels, or even most wooden crates or boxes are usable, but remember that they will need to be coated inside with creosote or an anti-rot preparation as they will not withstand moisture like redwood.

Soil Preparation
In my experiments, the best crops have come from soil combinations that are at least half good rich topsoil or garden loam. Most commercial planter mixes, while adequate for house plants already into their growing stage, do not contain enough nutrients to bring the vegetables to their final stage of development. I recommend finding a good source of natural soil to mix half and half with planter mix. If you are certain that your supply of natural soil is truly rich, you can lessen the total weight in the planter by mixing one-fourth vermiculite and one-fourth perlite. The first is a decomposition of rock and the other a light form of volcanic ash. It is difficult to prescribe an absolute soil combination to be used nationwide. Confer with a local nursery or vegetable gardener about the available soil and planter mixes in your area. Soil laboratories throughout the country are continuously experimenting with various mixes for nurseries and home gardeners.

(continued on page 287)

Secrets Revealed
by
Ruth Stout

I don't like to make fun of anybody, even including my betters, but I do have to smile sometimes at the mental convolutions the experts are going through in regard to compost piles. (Do this, don't do that, put on this, not too little, but be careful, not too much; wet it, but not too wet; now—no, we've changed our minds, this is better. *Now* we've got it—no, wait a minute—)

Don't misunderstand me; I am not against experimentation and attempts toward improvement in any field. I am sure that compost piles give you some mighty fine dirt. In the meantime, however, I am enjoying splendid compost all the time over my entire garden.

I didn't go through a lot of hard work, either, to put it there. I didn't have to go through the tedious hard work of carting it from where it was to where I wanted it. It was already there.

The dirt made by building a compost pile is a very desirable thing to have, but the man who goes through all the antics necessary to make this pile is like a man, let us say, who is suffering from a physical ailment and knows of a plant, growing on a far mountain, which will cure him. He makes the long, hard journey, finds the plant and is cured.

He is well satisfied until he returns home and finds that this plant also grows in his back yard. He had no way of knowing that until he saw the plant on the mountain and compared the two.

And so it is with those who build compost piles; they don't know any better way to make rich dirt. Now you are hearing of an easier, better way; you need no longer climb a mountain for your compost. It is yours for a small fraction of that labor.

My way is unscientific, but it has produced fine vegetables for eleven years. I simply spread mulch where I want the compost to be eventually. It rots and becomes rich dirt, with the valuable by-products of keeping down weeds, keeping the earth soft, holding moisture and eliminating plowing and spading, hoeing and cultivating.

I use lime, of course, to keep the soil from getting too acid and I put some cotton-seed meal on the strawberries, lettuce, spinach, corn and beets. This supplies the nitrogen they might otherwise lack.

The lettuce I grow now is crisp, fine flavored, solid and as big as your head with a sombrero on it. All the other crops are praiseworthy, not to say sensational: pepper plants with fifteen or more large peppers on each; huge heads of cauliflower; a ten-foot row of kohlrabi producing eighty perfect specimens; tender, crisp carrots, big enough sometimes for one to make a meal for five people. Everything else to match.

I have gardened like this for eleven years and I am satisfied with it. However, for those people who are so constituted that they must know by analysis rather than by results that they have an adequate soil for growing things, nothing could be easier than to have their soil analyzed and to add anything they may find lacking. They can still take advantage of this easy, effective way of building compost.

When I first heard of organic gardening (I was then already mulching) and read about its claims that this method eliminated pests, I muttered: ''Tut, tut! That is going a little far.'' And then forgot about it.

I had always hated the job of spraying poison on plants, but I had done it through the years pretty conscientiously. About the time I began to mulch I said to Art that I loathed fooling with poison sprays and he told me that someone he knew had controlled all pests effectively by keeping his plants covered with lime.

I tried that for awhile with fair success. Then, the third summer after I had started to mulch everything, it rained so frequently and washed off the lime so often that I gave up and didn't do anything about the bugs. And yet I saw almost none.

The following season I used neither lime nor poison. The tomatoes were clean; there was not one corn borer; only a handful of Mexican beetles instead of the thousands I had always had to contend with. The next year I boldly discarded the habit of putting little paper collars around the pepper and tomato plants. Not one was cut off by a cut worm. And I didn't see one bean beetle that second year.

Freedom from pests! For me that alone would have been enough to tie me to mulch-ing for life, without all of the bigger advantages.

I have, of course, told every gardener I know about mulching and a great many of them are doing it now. It appeals to the man who works all day and wants a garden, and who now can have one without the weeds constantly getting ahead of him. It appeals to mothers with young children who are glad they do not have to give up the vegetables they need and the flowers they love. It appeals to those who are getting old and are facing the unpleasant thought of being obliged to stop growing things. It appeals to people (like my nephew Roger and his wife, Gerry) who would rather read a book or have a swim than work in the garden, but who want their yard to be attractive. I spent a few weekends giving them a start; now they can read, swim, pick tulips, peonies, roses, chrysanthemums, and even to-matoes, with never a weed to reproach them.

Some people hesitate to adopt over-all mulching because they prefer the looks of a neatly cultivated garden. I used to, but now a garden with the earth exposed to the burning, baking sun looks helpless and pathetic to me. It looks fine if someone has just cultivated it after a good rain, but how often is that the case? At all other times an un-mulched garden looks to me like some naked thing which, for one reason or another, would be better off with a few clothes on.

Piecemeal mulching is nothing new. People have mulched strawberries for many years to keep them clean. Why are mulched peas and carrots uglier than mulched straw-berries?

A flourishing garden with clean hay spread neatly between the rows looks attractive to me, and comfortable.

I read somewhere recently the theory that corn and tomatoes should not be mulched because they need the heat of the sun around the roots. This has not been proven and I have another theory to present. Possibly these things need, rather, an even temperature which they do not get with a hot sun in the daytime and cool nights. With a mulch the temperature is much more nearly even than without it.

I can add this: only through these years since my corn has been mulched do I almost always get two fine ears from each stalk, and I now plant it more closely than the books advise. If the tomatoes suffer from being mulched they are very brave about it and keep it to themselves. I have never seen any indication that they mind at all.

I believe that growing old (and I don't mean from fifty to seventy, I mean from seventy to ninety) can well be the most delightful and exhilarating part of a person's life. I realize that those are almost fighting words and I am acquainted with many of the arguments against them. But my belief in them is a strong one and has a bearing on my present method of gardening.

One day last summer I faced the fact that if I did not die prematurely old age would eventually force me to slow up. This was a predicament; I come from two long-lived families, my health was perfect, and I hated to be forced. So I slowed up voluntarily.

I made out a plan of living, the keynote of which was enjoyment, for if there is one thing I thoroughly believe in, it is to enjoy the twenty-four hours of the day if you can possibly swing it.

I had to keep housework and cooking in my schedule, for those things are my con-tribution toward keeping Fred and me alive. I couldn't cut them down to a minimum, for they had been down there all of our married life. One more tiny cut and Fred would divorce me. That I wouldn't like.

Writing? I didn't have to give that up, for all of my other work was physical and a change of occupation is rest.

Growing vegetables and flowers. Can't you see exactly where I would have been heading if I had not thought up mulching? Who can turn over a compost pile at the age of ninety? Not I—not even at the age of seventy, and I wouldn't have enjoyed it at fifty. And who could hoe and cultivate and weed a garden of any size at that age?

With benefit of mulching I have set my-self a pleasant pace, which I can continue through my eighties if I don't break some bones. After ninety, from a wheelchair if necessary.

I have two rules: one is never to work after two o'clock in the afternoon except for a real emergency and to get dinner which, with a freezer to rely on, usually takes about twenty minutes. The other rule is never to do anything, even reading a novel or listen-ing to music, unless I feel enthusiastic about it. I am almost always buoyant until after lunch; then I often begin to run downhill. When I get to the point where I don't feel enthusiastic about anything at all it means I'm sleepy, so I go and take a nap.

I see no reason why I can't keep up this rhythm indefinitely, never realizing that old age has arrived until some well-meaning friend calls me "spry." Then, of course, I will know where I belong, and will make an effort to act my age.

It is clear that if I had not stumbled onto mulching I would have had to give up the work I love best.

And so, young or old, my friends, if for any reason you would like to grow things, throw away your spade and hoe and make your garden your compost pile. You will not be sorry, I promise you. ☼

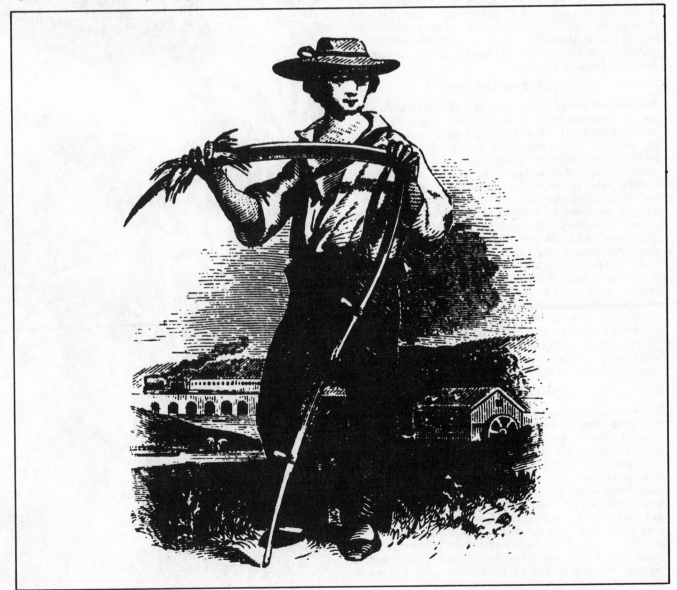

Companion Plants

by Helen Philbrick and Richard Gregg

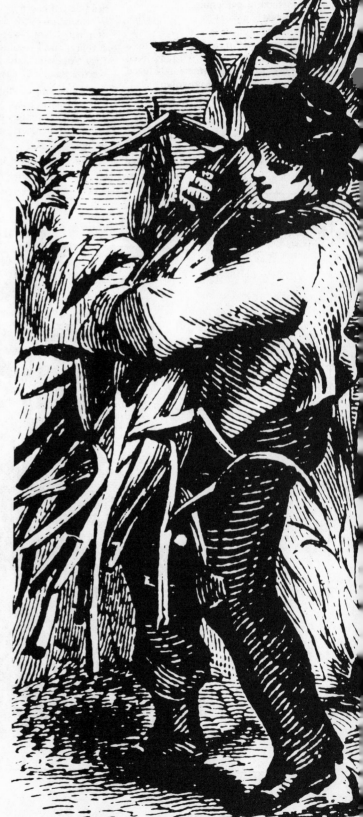

"The Bio-Dynamic Method of farming and gardening is based on the study of the mutual influences of living organisms."

Introduction, **Companion Plants**

BIO-DYNAMIC VEGETABLE GARDEN

A vegetable garden managed according to the Bio-Dynamic Method follows certain definite principles of plant symbiosis such as the use of a well-planned crop rotation, companionate plantings, juxtaposition of deep rooted plants with shallow rooted plants, and the generous use of summer-flowering shrubs and aromatic herbs all through the garden whether it be large or small. The observance of beneficial crop rotations and the careful use of companion plants, both in space (in one single year) and in time (from one year to another) make it possible to get maximum benefits from limited garden space with a minimum of labor without sacrificing the health-giving quality of the produce. Another most important factor of the Bio-Dynamic garden is that attention to all of these details insures that the garden soil is improved each year. Practice of the Bio-Dynamic Method cares for the soil and leaves it in improved biological condition by good cultural practices, especially in the return of soil nutrients each year through the use of Bio-Dynamic compost.

CROP ROTATION

Bio-Dynamic gardeners follow a system of crop rotation which can be described briefly as follows: The heavy feeders are planted immediately after fertilizing with a manure-containing compost. These include all of the cabbage varieties, cauliflower in particular, all leaf vegetables such as chard, head lettuce, endive and spinach, as well as celery and celeriac, leeks, cucumbers, squash and sweet corn. Rhubarb and tomatoes are also heavy feeders but are not included in the crop rotation since rhubarb is a perennial and tomatoes prefer to be retained in the same place year after year and fertilized with tomato compost. (However, there is a limit here; after 7-8 years one may find the tomatoes showing signs of blight. The best remedy is to move them somewhere else.)

The heavy feeders are followed by legumes or the soil improvers which add nitrogen to the soil through their root nodules. To this class belong beans and peas of all varieties.

The legumes should be followed by the light feeders which should be fertilized with a good compost, well-decomposed. They include the bulbs and all root vegetables such as carrots, beets, radishes, salsify, parsnips, turnips and rutabagas. For details, check on cultural practices in garden books.

COMPANION PLANTS

There are various reasons why certain plant combinations are successful. Plants having complementary physical demands are well suited to one another. For instance, a plant which needs plenty of light may be a good companion to another plant which can stand partial shade. Plants needing plenty of moisture may get along well with others which need less moisture. Deep-rooting plants open the ground for other species with less deep roots. Deep roots utilize a different part of the soil from shallow roots. Similarly, tall plants use a different part of the area above the garden from that filled with low-growing plants. Heavy feeders should be followed by light feeders, or plants that make the soil rich again, such as legumes. Plants that cannot stand the competition of weeds, should follow those that leave the soil free of weeds.

A Small Lexicon of Bio-Dynamic Gardening

Gardeners and biochemists are still investigating other less obvious factors in its environment which may influence plant health, such as aroma, leaf and root exudations, or influences from the roots of still other plants further out in the environment.

COMBINATIONS TO AVOID

Some plant combinations are bad. Among the herbs, Rue and Sweet Basil do not thrive near each other. Fennel seems to be of the most doubtful character; it hinders germination of Caraway and Coriander, disturbs the growth of bush beans and blights the growth of tomatoes. Tomatoes and kohlrabi do not like to grow together. In fact most of the cabbage family should not be grown near tomatoes. The tomato has such an antipathy for quack grass (*Agropyron repens*) that it can be used to suppress it.

COMPOST

One of the principles of making Bio-Dynamic compost is that plants, parts of plants, extracts and decoctions can influence the fermentation process that should go on in the compost heap. Plant preparations can be used on purpose to organize the complicated fermentation process as it occurs in the process of making compost. Even when added in tiny amounts to big masses of rotting materials, such plant preparations can influence the whole pile. Once the conditions of moisture, aeration, and temperature are satisfactory, a compost pile will soon be inhabited by myriads of earthworms, enchytraeids, and other small, mostly microscopic animals. These will carry the effects of the bacterial life, stimulated by the inoculants, all over the pile, thus promoting controlled fermentation.

There are a few simple rules to keep in mind when making Bio-Dynamic compost. Compost heaps should not be built under conifers because the turpentine substances retard proper fermentation. Do not build a compost heap on top of grass sod; dig out the sods and add them to the compost heap, but let the heap itself be built on the soil directly. Grass sods will impede fermentation. (For details on composting techniques, see the Bio-Dynamic literature.)

Professor A. Seiffert, who is a long time promoter of compost making on the old continent, says that the healing potentials in abundantly growing weeds can best be harnessed by putting them into the compost heap. This helps to combat what he calls "the exuberantly acting forces of nature." He reports that when he had to start a large vegetable garden some years ago on a heavy loam, he found the land completely overgrown with quack grass and Canada thistle. All the indicators of poorly drained, heavy soil, such as mint, buttercup, forgetmenot, knotweed and dock were also there. Large quantities of thistle and quack grass (*Agropyron*) were used to make compost. When this was turned back to the land, thistle and quack grass lost their vigor. The soil is now looser and the weeds can be controlled with ordinary means. He even says that by regular return of weed compost back to the land he was able to raise a sensitive variety of early potatoes on the same piece of land seventeen times. The weed composts had steadily rejuvenated the soil.

COMPOST PLANTS

In Bio-Dynamic composting a set of six herbs, each of which is specially prepared, is used to control and influence the fermentation of composts and manures. These herbs are:

Stinging Nettle (*Urtica dioica*) already known from everyday observation to be an excellent compost maker and soil builder, Dandelion (*Taraxacum officinale*), the bark of the oak tree (*Quercus alba* and *Q. rubra*), Yarrow (*Achillea millefolium*), Camomile (*Matricaria chamomilla*), and Valerian (*Valeriana officinalis*).

HERBS

Since time immemorial the various aromatic herbs have been planted as a border or in small patches in vegetable gardens where they are known to be beneficial to the more stolid vegetable plants. The one exception to this general rule is Fennel which has an adverse effect on several plants.

Many herbs have a good influence on plants in their vicinity. All vegetables are aided by most aromatic herbs, e.g. Borage (best grown in a nearby corner or in a separate bed), Lavender, Hyssop, Sage, Parsley, Chervil, Tarragon, Chives, Thyme, Marjoram, Dill, Camomile, Lovage; but *not* Wormwood or Fennel. If these are planted around the borders or at the ends of raised beds, they will sometimes help repel certain insects like the cabbage butterfly. Other herbs, including Santolina, Winter Savory, Blessed Thistle, Blue Hyssop (sometimes Pink and White), Lavender, and Marjoram are said to repel certain insects. Experiments are needed to make this information more exact, and records should be kept. Onions, shallots and garlic also repel insects.

Another beneficial effect of herbs is that they bring an aromatic scent into the atmosphere when planted amongst vegetables, in small proportion, as in a border or at the end of the row.

Stinging Nettle growing near any herb plant will increase the pungency and aroma of the herb itself. Stinging Nettle growing near Peppermint nearly doubles the quantity of essential oil in the Peppermint.

Yarrow also increases the aromatic quality of all herbs which grow nearby.

Mixed cultures of herbs make faster and closer growth than a single species. On a very poor stony soil the following species, when intercropped, formed a very good, close stand within a short time: Rue (*Ruta graveolens*), Hyssop (*Hyssopus officinalis*), Sage (*Salvia officinalis*), Lavender (*Lavendula spica*), Thyme (*Thymus vulgaris*), St. Johnswort (*Hypericum perforatum: H. vulgare*), and Southernwood (*Artemisia abrotanum*).

Another way in which herbs help build and maintain good gardens is by controlling biologically both insect pests and plant diseases. Here again prevention is better than cure. Not only individual plants but whole landscapes become diseased through monocultural practices, since nature, left to herself, never produces acre after acre of only one kind of plant. Usually the more variation the better, whether in general landscape development, a farm unit, or a garden. In medieval horticulture no lines were drawn between the flower, vegetable and herb gardens. All grew together to their mutual benefit. Now, in the plant residues, root excretions and leaf and flower emanations absorbed from one plant to another we can see a reason for these benefactions. They are connected with the delicate balances which normally exist in countless numbers in nature, and which man unwittingly disturbs.

The influence of one herb upon another is another aspect of conservation and good gardening which relates to the quality

(continued on page 289)

COMPOSTING IN YOUR LIVING ROOM

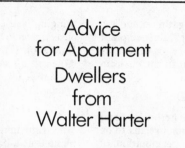

Advice
for Apartment
Dwellers
from
Walter Harter

You *can* grow vegetables and fruits in pots in your apartment or home, or in a patch of ground in the city; and grow them *organically,* free from the chemicals and pesticides that make so much commercially grown food tasteless and, in many cases, unhealthy.

But first you should know something about soil, and the things you can do with it and to it that will help it produce a pepper plant in your window or a row of tall corn in part of your backyard.

Although there are many variations of soils, they usually fall into four categories: sandy soils are near the seacoasts; clay soils are mostly in the interior; soil composed mostly of silt is at the mouths of rivers and creeks; loam is a dark soil found in forests. Each of these soils, to some degree, is alive with the bacteria of decayed and decaying plant and animal life. It is the action of these bacteria on even more organic material that releases the nutrients that are absorbed by seeds and roots.

Not all soils are rich in bacteria to begin with, and therefore are not capable of sustaining good plant growth. But all soils can be made rich by adding the elements they lack. Even the soil in a city playground that has been packed solid by pounding feet can, with the proper additives, grow flowers, fruits, and vegetables.

With poor soil, or soil that has been worn out by continuous plantings without returning natural elements to it, the practice has been to add chemical fertilizers to stimulate growth. These fertilizers are less expensive than organic fertilizers, but instead of replenishing the soil with natural nutrients, they continuously rob it of the remaining organic bacteria. The result is that more and more chemicals are added. Crops become tasteless, and sometimes are injurious to health. Organic fertilizers stimulate the growth of bacteria. They enrich the soil by returning to it the natural elements it lacks, or that have been taken from it.

Plants themselves help manufacture many of the elements they need. By a fantastic process called photosynthesis, plants convert water and carbons into some of the food necessary for their own growth. That is why various Federal, state, and local agencies are planting, where it is feasible, trees and grasses along our highways. The blades of grass and the leaves of trees gobble up the carbons spewed into the air by automobiles and convert them into oxygen. And that is why plants grown in pots in homes will purify the air in the rooms. Plants require oxygen too, but instead of getting it from the air, they obtain it from the water that sinks through the soil to their roots.

Plants need approximately fifteen different elements to enable them to reach full growth. Three of the most important are carbon, hydrogen, and oxygen, and are supplied to them in large degree by water and air. Other very important elements are nitrogen, potassium, phosphorus, calcium, magnesium, and sulphur, and these are supplied by the action of bacteria in the soil. Most of these bacteria are plentiful in rich soil, but where they are deficient they can be supplied by special organic fertilizers. Other nutrients, called secondary elements—copper, zinc, and manganese—are required in only minute quantities, and are usually included (from organic sources) in organic fertilizers.

All soils need help of some kind. There is no perfect soil. Most people think that "organic" gardening means beginning with a naturally rich earth. Not so, for there is no such thing. Even the most virgin forest loam will need help in some elements to grow our modern fruits and vegetables. A forest glen might be lush with ferns, but a radish or a tomato plant would die there for lack of the necessary food.

You can buy soil for your containers in most garden shops, or in the garden departments of many stores. This is usually called "potting soil," or some other misleading name. Misleading because, although it is dark and looks rich, it should never be put alone into a pot in which you hope to grow luxuriant plants. Even this soil needs help.

A good thing about this soil is that it usually has been sterilized to kill the various insidious insect larvae that might eventually hurt your young plants. But the sterilization process (baking at about 200 degrees for an hour) will kill any good bacteria in the soil, too. This isn't too unfortunate, because you will be adding all the needed bacteria to the medium.

Another reason for not using potting soil alone in containers is that this soil is fine, with hardly any texture, and will become like black cement after repeated waterings. The roots of plants need the oxygen in water and the soil must be kept loose so the water can sink rapidly. In a yard garden worms keep the ground loose. However, adding vermiculite (a powdered form of mica that has no nutrient value, but is excellent for keeping soil from packing and for giving tender roots something to hold on to) or coarse builders' sand to the potting mixture will serve the same purpose.

Potting soil costs about $2.00 for fifty pounds, enough to fill two dozen eight- or ten-inch pots or comparable containers. Vermiculite, bought wherever they sell potting soil, is very light, and a two-pound bag (costing about 75¢) will be almost the size of a fifty-pound bag of soil. Builders' sand can be purchased at any builders' supply company for a few cents. Use only rough builders' sand. Fine sand doesn't work as well. And never use sand from the seashore. A dozen washings won't remove all the salt, and salt will kill your plants. Several other ingredients are necessary to make commercial potting soil (or any other kind) ready for containers, or for that small patch of garden in your yard; peat and bone meal are two of them.

Peat is a partially decayed material found in bogs and swamps. It will add some organic elements to soil, but its principal use is to hold moisture. It is very absorbent and light in weight, and costs about the same as vermiculite. Bone meal (made from the skeletons of animals) is loaded with nitrogen and many of the trace elements needed for good plant growth. It breaks down very slowly in soil, and a little of it goes a long way.

A good basic mixture to use in containers is one-third potting soil, one-third peat, and one-third vermiculite or builders' sand. Add a spoonful of bone meal and mix thoroughly. This will supply the basic needs of any plant. However, there are organic fertilizers and combinations of organic fertilizers that will supply additional nutrients (if needed) and will speed the growth of

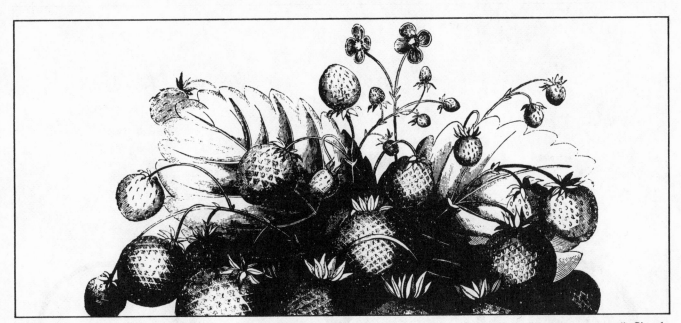

your plants. If you have made compost (described later), use one-quarter each of soil, compost, peat, and sand.

Organic fertilizers are made from natural materials; manures, mushroom (and other) composts, bone meal, cottonseed meal, and other organic substances. Their purpose is to return to the soil those *natural* nutrients that it lacked in the first place, or that have been taken from it by continuous use of chemicals. They are a concentrated form of compost, and will speed the propagation of active bacteria.

Each organic fertilizer is rich in some main nutrient, bone meal and manures are high in nitrogen, cottonseed meal is rich with phosphorus, and so on. Unless you are raising a plant whose needs are special (a camelia, for example, needs a very acid soil, and so sulphur is added to the container) the mixture of soil (and fresh compost, if you have it), peat, vermiculite or sand, with bone meal and a small amount of a general organic fertilizer, will take care of all the needs of most plants.

All fertilizers—organic and non-organic —are labeled with numbers that describe their contents: 6-6-6; 7-6-6; 10-5-5, for example. The first number always denotes the percentage of nitrogen in the mixture; the second number is the percentage of phosphorus; the third indicates the amount of potassium. The percentages of other nutrients in the mixture are listed elsewhere on the package. (Remember that three very essential elements—carbon, hydrogen, and oxygen—are obtained from the air and the water you feed your plants.) There is very little odor from organic fertilizers, even those that are almost one hundred percent manures.

They have been subjected to an aroma-destroying process that has no effect on the potency of the material.

Now about compost. You can grow luxuriant plants without it. Adding compost to those ingredients, however, will not only produce sturdier plants, but will be returning even more natural nutrients to the soil.

Compost is decayed and decaying plant life. It is amazing how much vegetable refuse is thrown away as useless garbage when, with a little effort, it can be made into a substance alive with elements needed for excellent plant growth. If you have no yard you can make compost this way. Get two or three large metal or plastic garbage cans and punch holes around the bases, several inches from the bottoms. (Compost needs air to aid in the decomposing process.) In one of the cans put in potato peeling, lettuce or any vegetable debris for two or three inches; then a layer of soil, a layer of manure (odorless) from a garden shop and start all over again. Keep it moist, but not wet, and covered.

When the first can is half full, turn the contents into the second can. In two weeks pour the mixture back into the first can. (You should be starting a series of layers in the third can.) After several turnings you will have a rich compost filling about a third of the first can. This will be more than enough to mix with the soil, vermiculite, or sand, and peat to fill dozens of containers. A good idea is to fill plastic garbage can liners with the surplus compost. For compost is like wine; the older it becomes the better it, is.

If you don't want to go to the bother of making compost there is still another way to make use of vegetable refuse.

It's called "instant compost." Simply place vegetable debris into a blender, add a little water, and mix. The result is an "organic soup." Used as a moistener in the basic mixture when you plant, or added occasionally to already potted plants, this will increase their growth tremendously. This soup can also be placed directly into your garden. Dig a hole large enough to contain the amount you have prepared and cover it with a layer of earth. By the next day it will have disappeared, leaving that patch of soil dark and moist. This isn't true compost, for bacteria hasn't had a chance to be produced, but it does quickly return to soil many of the nutrients it has lost.

Things To Watch

A word of warning, though. When making instant compost be sure to remove all the seeds in the vegetable refuse. Pepper and tomato seeds left in the mixture will begin to sprout in a few days after they are in the ground. That's fine if you are trying to grow peppers or tomatoes from seed, but you might have poured the soup around radishes or onions or begonias, and the new plants not only look strange popping up where they aren't wanted, but they will rob the older plants of needed nutrition.

This isn't the whole story of soils, fertilizers, or composts. But it's enough to help you to understand some of the wonders of the material you'll be working with.

With some care, and some common sense, you *can* have a fascinating hobby growing healthful vegetables and fruits in your own home, or in a small patch of earth in your back yard. ☼

Taking the Mystery Out of Mulching
by Malcolm Margolin

(Although the author is primarily interested in mulching trees, we feel that his mulching ideas are universal enough to be enjoyed and applied to any garden or deprived land as well. — The editors)

Stripped of its mystery, mulching is a very simple act. You locate a bunch of organic matter, like straw, leaves, lawn clippings, or wood chips; you collect it from where it's not wanted; and you spread it out someplace else where it will do some good.

Mulching is a very simple project — dull and repetitive if you take it too seriously or keep at it too long, but lots of fun for yourself or for groups of little kids who can roll in the mulch, horseplay in it, and throw it at each other while (incidentally, it seems) doing a piece of important work. Not only can it be fun, but if you think deeply about mulch, it can be a perceptually liberating experience as well.

These may sound like exaggerated claims, but there is something about mulching that generates fanatic devotion. Enthusiastic mulchers — and there is no other kind — insist that with the magic of mulching their gardens no longer need weeding, watering, or fertilizing as ordinary gardens do. Yet they grow king-sized cauliflowers, luxuriant lettuces, peas that ripen weeks before their neighbors', and squashes that stay firm long past the first frost. When I first heard about mulching, it sounded very interesting, very seductive, and very far-fetched. I didn't believe it!

In fact, for many years I had the vague idea that mulching was an exotic invention of organic gardeners. Or, to be more precise, the invention of a single organic gardener, an eccentric New York escapee named Ruth Stout who settled in Connecticut, wrote a book and several articles about mulching, and has become, so to speak, the *grande dame* of mulch.

But recently I have learned a lot more about mulching — especially about mulching on wild lands — and I've discovered that mulching was invented long before Ruth Stout. In fact, it was invented long before the human race. Mulching is a marvelous process invented by plants — a process by which wild plants have survived and prospered for eons. Without watering, without weeding, and without fertilizing.

The mulching process is actually very easy to understand. Every kid who has walked through the autumn woods, swishing and kicking the piles of dry leaves, knows something about mulch. Someday, attack one of those big piles of leaves, and as you scrape away at the various layers, your eyes, fingers and nose will tell you everything you have to know about mulch.

The topmost layer consists of dry, fresh-fallen leaves — whether the broad leaves of deciduous trees that fall all at one time or thin pine needles that drop throughout the year. Brush these dry leaves aside and beneath them you will find the older leaves — matted, moist, and half decomposed. Like an archeologist, keep digging down through time. The leaves will get more and more decayed until finally you reach the *leaf soil*, or *humus* — the thoroughly rotted leaves and twigs that earthworms and moles have already begun to mix with the mineral soil underneath.

There are more lessons to be learned from leafing through good soil than leafing through a good book. You can see how the area beneath a well-mulched tree lacks weeds and competing grasses, their seeds buried under tons of leaf litter. Dig your fingers under the humus and you can feel how the thick layer of leaves acts as a blanket, keeping the earth from freezing too deeply in the winter and from baking in the summer. Feel how squishy and spongelike the leaf mold is — a perfect texture for absorbing and holding water while allowing air to circulate. And you can easily understand how the leaf fall is actually a recycling of nutrients: the natural nitrates and other more exotic minerals that the roots have mined from the lower parts of the soil go into the leaves, and at the end of the growing season, they are returned to the soil for use again in the following years.

These are very important concepts, and they help one to understand that mulching is a natural process rather than some magic hocus-pocus piece of untidy mystification. But as you dig down into the leaf mold, I think you will discover something more amazing than just the physical properties of the mulch. This world of decaying leaves is, in itself, a marvelous thriving environment of incredible complexity and beauty. If you are lucky, you may stumble upon the giants of this environment: the salamanders, mice, and moles that tunnel through the humus. You are more likely to find the larger bugs, such as centipedes and pill bugs. But look closely, with a lens if possible, and you will *definitely* see a thriving, teeming world of creeping, crawling, humping, wiggling, thrashing, squirming beasties — thousands of them to the square foot. Some are barely visible motes gliding over a leaf edge; others are incredibly fierce and dramatic, like miniature dragons in a Chinese parade. This is a rich, full world — yet it is only a hint of the fantastic microscopic universe hidden to our eyes.

I feel that there is as much wonder, beauty, and mystery in this terribly alive environment as there is in the unexplored jungles of the Amazon. When I am with kids, I try to communicate this wonder to them, to make them realize that when we mulch a tree, we are not merely doing some mundane agricultural act that will benefit the tree and improve the soil. We are creating a natural environment that is very wonderful, very complicated, and forever beyond our understanding.

If you are dealing with kids, I urge you to get them to help you dig around in the humus. Most kids love to dig in dirt, and this is the most interesting dirt in the world — dirt crawling with decay, earthworms, and bugs. But some kids have been brainwashed by the Mr. Clean sterilize-the-world fanatics until they think that dirt and bugs are bad. This is tragic. Do your best to help them overcome it. If the kids are too uptight to dig around with you, try anyway. The knowledge that they have met some adult, however crazy, who likes dirt may someday help them in their quests to become healthy, accepting human animals.

To mulch or not to mulch? Before you run off madly from farm to farm begging for spoiled hay, rotten manure, and other such goodies, take a long, slow look at your forest

(continued on page 290)

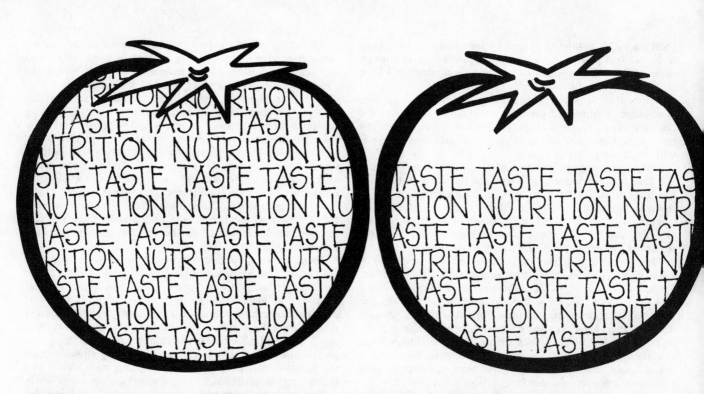

Whatever Happened to Tomatoes and

by Martha H. Oliver

There they lay, three or four perfectly round, pink, hard tennis-ball tomatoes in their tiny plastic coffin, serenely and sanitarily covered with a plastic wrap. Mrs. S, thinking of a tossed salad with her special garlic French, placed them carefully to the side in her shopping cart. She knew how easily the tender flesh bruised and spilled its sweet-acid juice, and treated them with respect.

Had she known what she was buying, she could have tossed her ten-pound roast on top of them. For these were Florida's MH-1, a new variety bred specially to be picked by machines in a "mature-green" state, commercially gassed in a process referred to by growers as "de-greening," and shipped a thousand miles by truck, without showing one bruise or dent. This marvel of the plant kingdom was recently demonstrated, and the results recorded in *The New Yorker* magazine, by being tossed six feet in the air and allowed to drop on a cement floor.

It did not even make a dent in the thick wall of the tomato.

The demonstration was made by its breeder, Dr. Bryan of the Florida Institute of Food and Agricultural Sciences. This newest example of the triumph of technology over conscience is just the latest step in a continuing breeding program which has only one object: food that travels well.

In the rush to develop the dentproof tomato, two other variables that used to be important have been discarded as merely "un-economic": taste and nutritional content.

It is difficult for me to assess which is the greater loss. C. E. Pantos and P. Markakis reported in the *Journal of Food Science* in 1973 that the six-and-a-half-million tons of tomatoes which are produced annually in the United States contain one third less vitamin C than, on the average, they should. The USDA gives 23 milligrams as the average value for 100 grams of fresh tomatoes. The researchers, working with two-pound samples from local food stores in December of 1972, found that they contained 14½ milligrams of vitamin C per 100 grams of fruit.

What could be the reason for the loss? Genetically, the variety may be an inferior one. When one characteristic is bred in (such as

thick walls to avoid bruising), others are sometimes lost. But it has been shown that tomatoes reach their peak value for vitamin C just before they are fully red. If picked mature-green, and stored ten days, they lose much vitamin C from enzyme activity, and this loss occurs *whatever the temperature*.

Tomatoes, in fact, are tropical fruits, originating in Peru, and as such, should not be ripened in the refrigerator but at room temperature. If allowed to stay in the refrigerator, they may become watery and spoil more easily without ripening at all.

The loss of flavor, of that true "tomato" taste, half sweet and half acid, is an equally devastating loss. Mrs. S's tomatoes, when she tried to eat them in the salad she had so carefully prepared, were tough, tasteless, and dry, nothing like her food memory told her tomatoes should taste. Mrs. S contemplated the problem. Even during the local tomato season, July to early October in her area, the produce available was just the same. When she had asked the manager where the local tomatoes were, he had explained that local tomatoes were too ripe when picked, they bruised and resulted in waste, and that they had a contract with a fruit supplier year-round for Florida tomatoes. She left, defeated by the logic of economics.

But not for long. Mrs. S was no fool, and she made a resolve to defeat the economics of hard tomatoes — by growing her own.

She is not alone. More Americans planted gardens, and experienced how vegetables should taste, in the summer of 1976, than in any year since the famous "Victory Gardens" of World War II. And the tomato is head and shoulders the most popular garden vegetable for the small home gardener. Why? They are easy to grow, almost foolproof, and guarantee a crop that will almost always exceed your expectations. Plants and seeds are available widely at the proper time. They have few insect pests and diseases. But the flavor of a warm, sun-ripened tomato, picked from the vine when deep red and eaten from the hand, is a memorable experience of summer, and the major reason for the popularity of the home-grown tomato.

Corn and Squash and, and, and ...?

If I had only a small lot in the city, or the suburbs, and could manage to keep a garden only eight feet in diameter, I would plant half a dozen good, hybrid tomato plants in a circle, and train them up a cylinder of stock fence seven feet tall, confident that by the end of the growing season I would have more tomatoes than my family could eat in salads and sandwiches, that I would have dozens to give away, and maybe even some for juice and canning. I would plant a ring of marigolds on the outside edge, to look pretty, and I would enjoy the finest tasting tomatoes that money couldn't buy.

Tomatoes aren't the only vegetable that has suffered from the "food to go" craze. In fact, if I were gardening for flavor alone, I would make a list of the worst casualties to technology, and as my garden increased in size, I would plant a few more kinds of vegetables, famous for taste alone.

Suppose I spaded under a few more feet of my lawn, which is a non-productive, energy-consuming green desert anyway. My next choice would be some lettuce — some really first-class varieties. In the winter and the summer, my supermarket stocks an unvarying selection of iceberg, romaine and leaf lettuce. This barely scratches the surface! The Burpee catalog (free for the asking from Burpee, Warminster, PA. 18974) lists twenty varieties of lettuce, including Buttercrunch and Bibb, Ruby, Salad Bowl, Deer Tongue, Oak Leaf and Endive, as well as nine varieties of spinach, and thirty-five varieties of tomatoes! All have mouth-watering pictures. And there are other seed houses as well, just as fine. My favorites are Buttercrunch, tender, thick and buttery, Green Ice, which lasts, tender, through the hottest weather, and the fragile, delicate Salad Bowl. Ruby makes an exquisite salad with cooked beets vinaigrette, since they look made for each other.

If I decided to do away with the lawn completely, I would then plant a few rows of peas. Peas, like corn, begin to lose sugar content as soon as they are picked. Enzymes begin to break down sweetness into starches. There is also the matter of maturity. Most commercial growers, interested in weight, allow peas to become too mature before harvest. If you like young, sweet peas, the only way is to grow them yourself. I feel that the extra early varieties, like Alaska, don't begin to compare with the ones that mature just a few days later, like Burpeeana Early and Lincoln. I have bought these since they were first introduced. They are worth the price.

As my garden grew, and my taste buds began to re-awaken to sensations they had forgotten, I would add two or three rows of beets, snap beans, lima beans and sugar peas. When I see these in the fresh-food departments of the supermarket, I wince, because, in my opinion, they have been allowed to get far too mature. Snap beans with bulges showing the location of every maturing seed, limas bursting the pods, beets the size of grapefruit, and never an edible pea pod at all! These are four vegetables I just couldn't do without, but to get them my way I have to grow my own.

I try to get the beets when they are the size of golf balls, and the snap beans when they are no longer than three inches. The limas must be filled out, and it is sometimes tricky to tell how big they are and catch them at the point of sweet flavor, but I find that the fingers do a better job than the eyes at judging readiness. Run your fingers lightly over the pods — don't squeeze. Our four-year-old loves these small limas, fresh and frozen, but I have noticed that she eats them starting with the smallest and working up to the biggest. She appreciates the flavor of the tender young ones. ("Eat the best first, and then you're always eating the best," as her great-grandfather always said.) That should tell us something about the taste buds of the young. Edible-pod, or sugar peas, are eaten pod and all, just as we eat the pods of snap beans. The peas *must* be very tiny! When I find filled-out pods I have missed when picking, I have eaten them, and the peas are starchy and flavorless. But the pods, when young, are sweet and tender and perfect in a stew, soup or Chinese stir-fry.

By this time, I may be renting land from a neighbor, or a community plot out of town, or perhaps have bought a tract of my

(continued on page 291)

PESTS ARE PESTS - MAN MADE THEM SO!

Recorded history shows that man's agricultural efforts have always been beset by pests. In ancient times serious outbreaks of pests were so rare as to be attributed to the wrath of gods because of some human offense. In the biblical recounting, plagues of locusts and crop failures in Greek and Roman vineyards are usually attributed to breaches of the moral code. It is only in the last century that we have come to recognize that agricultural pest problems are a breach of the natural law and are of man's own making.

"Multiplication of insects and their devastations are largely incited by the degeneracy in our plants and the badness of our culture," wrote Horace Greeley, the American journalist, in 1870. Approximately seventy years later, Sir Albert Howard had published his principles of natural plant growing in which he maintained that the plants themselves should be able to resist their natural enemies, insects and disease. Observant farmers recognize that pest problems can be traced usually to areas where the soil conditions are out of balance. Low spots with poor drainage can become breeding grounds for pests; fungi can flourish on plants grown where there are excessive amounts of organic materials, because the materials have not had time to change into a form of food that the plants can use.

Various Pests

Fungi

The fine filaments of some fungi inhabiting the soil are almost invisible, others, such as mushrooms, form fleshy, pulpy masses which grow on the earth's surface. A gourmet may balk at admitting that this exquisite delicacy is actually a parasite and a fungus, yet it is both.

An example of a "good guy" is the penicillium fungus which was accidentally found to interfere with the growth of bacteria.

Garden Talk
by
John B. Harrison

On the other side of the ledger are the fungi that attack our plants and our bodies too. Thus far, the fungus that causes "athlete's foot" has not proved to have one beneficial side effect for man, while the awful destructiveness of the common late blight fungus of potatoes has affected the history of mankind.

Bacteria

Some bacteria in the soil act as pests because they kill the living cells while others act on dead cells and convert them into substances which nourish plants thus completing nature's cycle.

Viruses

Scientists are still arguing about whether a virus is a living organism or not. We do know from bitter experience that viruses attack food plants, reduce their yields and cause extensive losses. The virus is transmitted by insects when they feed from a virus-infected plant and then move to healthy plants. If the plant is infected with a virus it may show symptoms of stunted growth, mottling, and yellowing or crinkling of leaves. A virus causing spotted wilt or curly top can kill tomatoes in a short time but most of the viruses cause degeneration of the plant only.

Weeds

When weeds do not compete with crop plants for light, moisture or plant nutrients, their role in soil regeneration is too valuable for us to dismiss them as pests. Deep-rooted weeds do the same important, soil-building jobs as the plants cultivated by man. They bring minerals from deep in the soil and

assist the moisture to rise by capillarity from the subsoil. By covering the earth between plantings, weeds protect the soil from being leached by the rain and dehydrated by the sun and wind. Turned over at the advent of a new growing season, weeds add to the organic content of the soil.

Why Insects Eat Certain Plants

It is not surprising that insects are drawn to the poorly grown plants with energy-rich carbohydrate levels, especially when one considers the distance a flea jumps in relation to its size. The energy equivalent in the animal kingdom might be that of the hair-raising sight of a horse jumping over the Empire State Building in a single bound. Man and animals are not only slower moving but their longer life span and great intelligence demand the body-building and repairing properties of protein more urgently than those of carbohydrates.

Weather conditions can temporarily favour a speedy multiplication of pests but not necessarily their predators. For example, in our area we know when the soil in the strawberry patch becomes too dry and the temperature too high the mites multiply seemingly unchecked and damage the crop. This problem is met by having an irrigation system ready to go into action during dry spells.

Chemical Pest Control

The chemical industry has made available to farmers an arsenal of modern pesticides and herbicides which are without a doubt very effective in killing. In order to build sales and subsequent profits, they have employed the talents of specialists in merchandising, marketing and advertising necessary to sustain and expand the industry. At the receiving end of this massive brain-washing is the ultimate buyer of the farmer's produce—the housewife. Trained by years of four-colour, glossy magazine illustrations to judge food by its appearance rather than by its nourishing quality, she will refuse to buy food that does not look like the magazine illustrations. So the wholesaler and retailer in turn refuse produce that does not have this "plastic" quality. And the grower is compelled to make certain that there are neither insects nor insect damage on the food he sends to market.

Unfortunately, few people realize that instead of containing insect damage which is obvious and can be cut out or washed off . . . chemically sprayed food contains unknown quantities of invisible, tasteless materials which can destroy our cells at random. Such materials may accumulate in

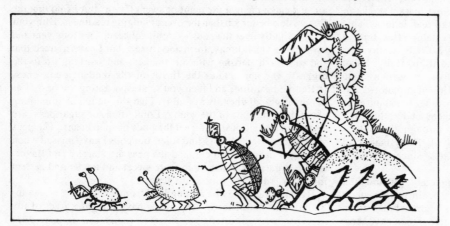

our bodies and injure us years later or affect our genetic cells and produce mutations in our children and our grandchildren such as those following the use of thalidomide. Were the earth to have a pesticide disaster millions of children could be victimized . . . yet we continue putting massive chemical dosages on food plants. In terms of human life modern pesticides are new; therefore we cannot know the effects of ingestion during a complete human life. Nor can we know their full impact on subsequent human generations because there has not yet been one complete generation, let alone the several generations which would be necessary to ensure that no damage occurred.

Natural Pest Control

Winter, the slack time in the grower's calendar, is the time for the organic grower to consider his pest control techniques for the coming season based on his successes and failures during the previous season. However serious or trivial a pest problem the grower may have had, its very existence indicates that one or more biological errors have been made. Some questions that would aid in pinpointing the source of the problem are:

Was the soil adequately drained the previous winter?

Was the soil properly prepared and adequately nourished?

Were the seeds or tubers planted, viable and of good quality?

Were the seeds planted at the right time of the year? and some might add, at the right phase of the moon?

Was the area planted to a single species so large that it was monocultural rather than polycultural?

Was a place provided, where beneficial predators could survive during their dormant period?

If such an area was provided, was it close enough to the growing area for the predator to reach its prey?

If any species of plant was pest-infested, was that species of plant suitable to the area?

Until a balanced nourishing soil is established, the incidence of insect and disease pests in crops is apt to be unpredictable. If one particular crop has attracted more pests than others, it would be wise to abandon growing it until the soil enrichment program has had a chance to work. If, however, economic necessity dictates a repeat planting of the previous year's troublesome crop, the farmer faces a difficult decision—either he uses natural but admittedly safe materials and salvages what can be only inferior plants or he loses a large percentage of his crop to the same pests or diseases that attacked the year before.

The serious organic grower will choose to assign the difficult-to-grow plants

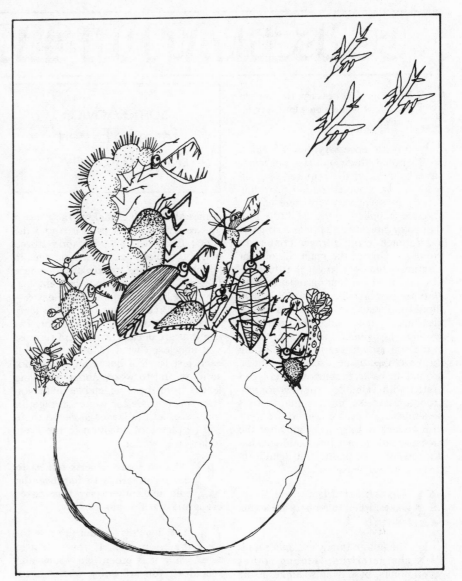

to those fields that present the healthiest soil conditions and will first try with small blocks of them set out among dissimilar plants.

Applied Biological Pest Control

Organic farming, or natural biological control, is the maintenance of a hospitable set of conditions in the area so that all forms of life, prey and predator alike, can live in harmony aiding one another; applied biological control on the other hand is the process of introducing predators, such as the lady bug and praying mantis which eat the insects that threaten a crop.

Sterilization of males is another method of biological pest control. It has been used successfully among herds of livestock infested with screw worms. Overall, the returns for each dollar spent for biological control are calculated to be about thirty dollars, while a dollar spent on chemical controls will yield a return of only five dollars, and even this diminishes as the immunity of the pest builds up.

The applied biological control has this disadvantage. Should a second pest for which there is no biological control require chemical control, the predators applied to control the first pest could be victimized by the chemical. Applied biological control involves the use of materials and organisms which are not destructive to the environment so that it is far preferable to chemical control. In unusual circumstances such as when a pest is accidentally imported into an area which lacks its natural predator or as in forests, rangelands or non-food producing areas it appears to be an ideal solution. But in commercial agriculture it is preferable to use sound organic practices and to maintain a natural environment which will harbour the predator type insect.

When the aphids attack the cabbages do not apply DDT. If you must, try washing them off with the garden hose or introducing lady bugs, but better still, for your next season correct any conditions that weakened the cabbages and made them attractive to the aphids. ✿

CONSERVATION GARDENING

Q Why is it necessary to use an inoculant when you plant any legume?

A It is not necessary, but it is safer. Should there not be sufficient bacteria of the required type already in the ground, you are providing them. The seeds will germinate and be at once supplied with the little rod-shaped organisms which make so great a difference in the nitrogen content of the plant. One of the main reasons for planting legumes is to get that high nitrogen, free. Now that an inoculant for *all* types of vegetables is available, you should inoculate all your seeds before planting, as these other bacteria also produce nitrogen compounds, but right in the soil around the roots, not inside the vegetable tissue itself. The region around the roots, the rhizosphere, is saturated with valuable materials for microorganisms—so much so that there is an almost rigid casing around the roots firm enough to keep its shape after the root dies and decays into nothing. That is a good place to find the nitrogen from these non-legume bacteria.

Q Why is it not alright to eat potato leaves, when the tubers are so nutritious?

A The potato family (Solanaceae) is characterized, among other points, by having solanine in the leaves, and solanine is a compound which is toxic to humans. You should not eat the leaves of related plants, either: eggplant, sweet pepper, tomato, nightshade. In fact, even the greened skin and eyes of the potato should not be eaten, although ordinarily the amount eaten at one meal is not likely to be dangerous. Bailey says that even the cooking water is used to kill insects on animals and should not be used in cooking other foods, but that is an extreme view. Many of us use potato cooking water in bread and gravy, etc.

Q Why is it alright to keep picking leaves from leafy crops such as spinach and lettuce and chard, and yet not right to cut off the asparagus tops?

A Asparagus has storage roots which provide the nutrition for sending up green shoots each spring. The leafy tops are the photosynthesis factories which make the sugar which be-

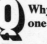

Some Advice from an Expert
Bargyla Rateaver

comes all the things making the root. If you remove those tops you starve the roots; there will be little food stored and you will not get much asparagus in spring. Leave the tops to die right where they are. If the messy look bothers you, cover the bed with manure and leaves—a good routine anyway. With other leafy vegetables, storage is not a factor. Exceptions are beets, carrots, and turnips; you may even want to have a row of each just for leaf harvesting. It is not so important to worry about removing leaves from these vegetables until you start saving some for winter storage; in that case, let the leaves alone so there will be plenty of nutrition in the roots to last over winter.

Q Why do some experts tell us to use cover crops to improve the soil, and others say that cover crops will not do that job?

A It all depends on your purpose for the cover crop. If you turn it in while it is green and young and succulent, you are doing what Cocannouer recommends because he says the microbes need and want that kind of tissue, which they readily break down. An advantage of that is that in the process, the microorganisms produce the polysaccharides which make soil particles cling together and make the desired crumbly structure and give the "velvety" feel. On the other hand, since this tender tissue is so quickly used up, there is not enough organic matter derived from it to build up the percentage of it in the soil. For adding a larger quantity of organic matter on a longer-term basis, a cover crop is incorporated much later in the season when the proportion of carbohydrates is much higher, the tissue coarser and maybe even partly woody. This is decomposed more slowly and leaves more of the longer-lasting material to make humus. Turning in a cover crop just before it begins to bloom gives a higher protein content in the green manure, because after the plant starts flowering it will alter its metabolism to produce seed.

Q Why is it that so many of the fruits one buys are watery?

A Experiments in this country as well as Europe showed that when large quantities of chemical fertilizer high in nitrogen were used, the percentage of water increased. If the land is poor, as it becomes where chemicals are used, plant parts will become watery—in fact, it has been recommended that irrigation not be used under such conditions. You can think of the plants as being thirsty, just as you are when you have eaten too-salty foods—all you want to do is drink and drink and drink!

Q Why does it take longer for a compost heap to decompose when it is made of heaps of grass clippings and sawdust than when it is made of a mixture of garden trash and garbage?

A Aeration is important in an aerobic pile. The microorganisms responsible for decay respire, and burn up the carbohydrate materials as they inhale and exhale. (This process gives off quite a bit of heat.) When tightly-packed stuff like matted grass clippings, stuck-together coffee grounds, finely-textured sawdust, etc. fill the compost pile, aeration is poor. Adding some source of nitrogen and water would perhaps fill even more air spaces, depending on what was used. Bacterial action is slowed down, but also it seems that microorganisms do better work when they work on a mixture of materials, but I am not aware that anyone knows just why. Not only that, but when you compost tightly-knit materials, you lose more nitrogen than when you heap the pile with supplies that are better aerated and ventilated, such as straw and weeds along with the garbage.

Q Why do organic growers claim that the source of nutrients makes a difference to the plant?

A There is evidence for this, and there would be more if research were done to add more data. Spinks in Canada showed with radioactive tracers that wheat took up almost 100 percent more nutrient when the source was manure than when it was chemicals. London's Agricultural Research Council has found that isotopes not only have the well-known differing optical properties (rotating the plane of polarized light) but also differing energy properties. According to Hainsworth, certain plants have a distinct preference for certain isotopes. He cites Sudan grass as accumulating "heavy" carbon and nitrogen, and willows "heavy" hydrogen. There are many bits of data scattered here and there in the technical literature, which need to be assembled.

Q Why are the trace elements in seaweed so valuable just because they are chelated?

A Because it has been shown that chelation permits absorption of the elements under certain conditions where absorption would otherwise be impossible. For instance, in chlorotic plants, where simple ionized minerals are not absorbed and the leaves of the plant turn yellow with only the veins remaining green, seaweed will green the leaves quickly because the organically tied-up minerals (usually iron) then can be taken into the plant and utilized. In the case of plants which are thought to demand acid soil, seaweed permits them to grow in alkaline soil because the minerals are absorbed regardless of the pH. In other cases it is the use of the mineral in enzymes that becomes important. An enzyme is a protein type of structure with an atom or two of mineral tucked inside it —what could be called a chelated structure. For example, legumes need molybdenum to form nodules of bacteria on the roots. Here again the mineral, along with iron, is part of a chelated formation as an enzyme which catalyzes the production of useable nitrogen forms. Additionally, the chelate molecule enters the plant and continues all the way to the site where it is needed, in spite of the demands which may be made for the mineral on the way up. That kind of "responsible action" can be important. Chelating turns the mineral into an organic form, which is what the plant wants.

Q Why do weeds keep coming up even after they are apparently completely weeded out?

A Weeds have many seeds, some in astronomical numbers. Mullein may have a quarter of a million per plant, witchweed half a million. Their longevity is phenomenal. Seeds of dock, evening primrose and mullein can stick it out almost a hundred years. They can put up with practically any bad conditions. Bindweed will germi-

nate even after being immersed in water for almost five years. The seeds are programmed to germinate at different times, so some may come up many years after the original plant has been pulled out. Russian pigweed is said to germinate in ice and on frozen terrain. For some, low temperatures induce dormancy; for others it is high temperature that does it. Some wait for alternating cold and heat. Some are smart enough to have a special kind of dormancy which lets them wait for just the right conditions. Some will ripen on the plant even after the plant has been uprooted and dried. Some seeds are still viable after they have been in silage for four years. How can a mere human hope to outsmart them?

Q Why is the caterpillar pest remedy effective?

A Because it is specific for caterpillars—or what many call worms. It is a bacterial disease (Bacillus thuringiensis) which forms a toxin in the stomach cells of caterpillars only, not any other pest. A crystal forms in the cells and paralyzes, so the poor thing has to stop eating. Although the crop damage stops almost at once, the pest may not die for a couple of days or so. It is not claimed to be effective on all caterpillars, but does work on almost anything likely to be found in a garden.

Q Why are pine needles such a good mulch for strawberries?

A Partly because in decay they give an acid reaction, and strawberries like to grow in a slightly acid soil. Also, there is some compound in the needles which is of value to the berries. Then, too, the mulch is loose and dry, well-aerated, and spongy enough to hold the berries off the soil except for only small points of contact, so that the berries do not rest against a moist surface to rot.

Q What is salt hay and how is it used?

A According to Webster, salt hay refers to any herbage of salt meadows or alkaline areas. Some of the genera are Distichlis and Spartina. D. spicata is common, and a perennial grass with rhizomes is S. patens. Sometimes such plants are called feather grass. They are often found in brackish water areas or on salt flats. People use such grasses or weeds for mulch because they do not reseed themselves and become a nuisance.

Q What does bonemeal do for plants and what kind should be bought?

A Bonemeal is merely ground up bone and contains the values of bone: a protein base, calcium and phosphorus. Usually sold as steamed bonemeal, the marrow fat is steamed out of the bone before the bone is ground, so that it is not attractive to ants. Dogs are wild about it and will gobble it even if they have to push out of the way a very strong man. It is heavily supplied to bulbs planted in fall, often to roses, to legumes and even to blueberries.

Q Should planting be regulated by the moon phases?

A I have never known for sure about that. Some believers have their data so confused with astrology that one cannot make any scientifically accurate conclusions from them. However, Dr. Pfeiffer said that when the moon pulls the tides, it pulls all the water in the earth, which would raise the water table. A Dr. Panzer at Tulane has found some apparently definite effects on seeds, which she thinks may be electrical effects, or magnetic ones. Evidently there is much practical experience behind the routine, but no overwhelming scientific basis.

Q Why should corn and cucumbers be planted in mounds?

A No reason why they should. Any level surface is good. Corn, as it grows tall, acquires adventitious roots which grow out of the base to support the tall stem. People like to cover them by hilling the soil, but it is not necessary. All squash family seeds are often planted in "hills." Although originally this may have literally meant a hill, it no longer means anything but a small group of seeds. The reason is that, as all seeds germinate, some will be huskier and are kept, while the ones appearing weaker are discarded. I think, myself, this is a cruelty. There is no need to mound soil around cucumber seedlings. The important thing in both cases cited is that the soil be very fertile, and that there be plenty of water: for corn because it grows so huge, and for cucumbers because they are the thirstiest of all and almost 99 percent water. Those who want record crops dig out a large basin and fill it with superior materials: manure, seaweed, rock phosphate, granite dust, etc., before planting, then mulch, then spray a foliar feed. ☼

157

RESIS

How to Resist the...

by
Catharine Osgood Foster

In spite of what we have known in the past and in spite of what biochemists and plant physiologists are discovering every day now, there are still pockets of deep-seated reluctance to avowing oneself an organic gardener or farmer. There is even a tendency in certain quarters to be suspicious of those who do.

There seems to be quite an array of reasons for this resistance. One is a typical human combination of ignorance and prejudice. Some who know very little about organic gardening methods do know about rumors reporting that no one but "a food faddist" practices those methods.

As a matter of fact, the people called "food faddists" have several million more people in their fold than they did when they hit the scene twenty or thirty years ago. Back then these particular people objected to DDT. They warned, early, what the results now are known to be: every average American has right this minute twelve parts per million of DDT in his own system. It has been found even in newborn babies.

You can grow your own food and fend off a goodly percentage of that twelve parts per million. Some people have resisted doing this; some could not do it—so preferred not to think of the possible results. The easiest thing to do is to say: "No one has yet died from having had twelve parts per million of DDT in his system, so why worry?"

Few people learned in school that one of the main causes of the decline and fall of the Roman Empire was their continued perennial use of lead mugs to drink out of, lead pipes to bring in their water from the hills, cosmetics with lead in them, and lead in their cooking utensils and plates.

Few people are aware that the largest percentage of funds now being expended for the study of pest control at federal biological research stations is being spent for biological control experiments. Many people disregard the biological advances already made and believe that if we in the United States do not use the powerful hard pesticides and chemical fertilizers, we shall not be able to feed the world.

They do know, that the federal and state centers of agricultural advice to farmers are usually focused on methods economically feasible—judging cultivation practices not on the basis of what is best for the crop, the people who will eat it, and the soil itself, but on which dollar return will make it worthwhile to do what. Obviously there is a certain check—for out-and-out ruination of the soil is economically brainless. For years farmers ruined American soils and moved on to another location when they no longer could survive where they were.

I think one reason why so many people today are rallying to Earth Day calls and ecology action groups is a deep and persistent wish to make up for past devastation of the land.

This movement to make up for old ills by returning to the land what we take from it was started in a very small way—with such people as Louis Bromfield and the Friends of the Land who met at his farm in the early forties. His books and his followers popularized his efforts to bring back the old exhausted Ohio farmland where he lived to a new bloom of fertility, by organic methods. Edward H. Faulkner, who wrote *Plowman's Folly,* was another who recovered ruined land. His own family had devastated several farms for one generation after another, and he vowed to atone.

But the majority, feeling no such drive, called the Bromfields and the Faulkners of the period nuts. Many preferred not to use compost and the natural sources of fertilizer, as the organic gardeners did. There are lots of odd little reasons why people resist composting. One is a dislike of having things secondhand; along with this is a dislike of manure. We are so store-oriented that we have a continual craving to buy new materials and resist what nature provides so easily. Even city people can use their garbage for a garden, not to mention the dumpings from the kitty pan.

You have to remember that the farmer who recently ar-

158

TERS

rived at an affluence which enabled him to buy fertilizer was glad enough to give up shoveling manure. New social and financial gains would be hard to break. Moreover, various sources of information that influence farmers keep preaching that commercial fertilizers are the way to get affluent. They also preach that nitrogen is nitrogen no matter where it comes from and no matter in what complex pattern it exists and moves.

Unfortunately, most of us never get beyond first-year chemistry, or inorganic chemistry. The mysteries of the organic world and its chemistry and its other interrelationships often remain closed to us. People are all too likely to interpret in terms of lifeless, not living, criteria—because they are simple and clear. It is all so much easier that way.

It is also easier, and of course more satisfying to our love of using the brute-strength way of solving things, to approach a system going wrong by getting up and attacking. When monoculture, farm mechanization, and commercially fertilized crops in monoculture attracted pests to the feast, as it was only natural they would, we invented the attack of hard pesticide poisons. Now, of course, we have hybrid corn crops in the Midwest that won't respond and the encephalitis or sleeping sickness mosquito that won't respond.

There are two ironies. With a typical faith that our flying machines and powerful spraying techniques will get every single mosquito (or other pest), we overlook the fact that a few escape. Those who have survived have turned out to be very rugged individuals capable of propagating huge colonies of resistant offspring. The other irony is that after discovering this answer, we make up new ones which lead us back to exactly the same error as the one we made in the first place.

Another odd factor is the appeal of gigantism to Americans. We love big things, big operations, big machines to do them with. Those who like them resist the warnings and pleas of those who do not fall for it. During World War II the standard for measuring foods was switched from quantity to weight. One result of this has been that the bigger the peas or beans or corn per unit that the farmer can put on the market, the better the financial return for him. Customers no longer can shop for the best quality per peck. Now we blow up plants and fruits to big size, even as we blow up bread with air and fluffy, almost lifeless starch and turkeys with stilbestrol and water. The fact that proteins are lost and carbohydrates increased in older vegetables doesn't bother many housewives any more because we have been conditioned to like something (almost anything) bright green and have forgotten that the protein value of good young peas is what we really want for our families. When we do not know these things—and thus do not care—we become unwitting resisters to organic home gardening.

Resisters include many commercial growers who want to produce the big vegetables fastest, and who therefore use large quantities of nitrogen fertilizers. Overnitrated, fast-grown spinach, lettuce, and Swiss chard can distort the food value of plants and, when combined with certain amino acids, can form substances of dubious safety to eat. Nitrates in infant food have been challenged by biologists as dangerous. Their effect, when combined with food preservatives for long shelf life, is suspected of being toxic. But these are vague unknowns to resisters, and they tend to brush such things off.

A sad group of resisters is the generation of hamburger eaters, whose craving for more and more hot dogs, hamburgers, white buns, bags of crackers and popcorn, and gallons of imitation, gelatinized dairy ices is never satisfied because they are simply not getting the nutrition their body needs. Eventually they do not like fresh fruits and vegetables, unprocessed and without additives. They are unconscious resisters to organic foods and organic methods.

(continued on page 292)

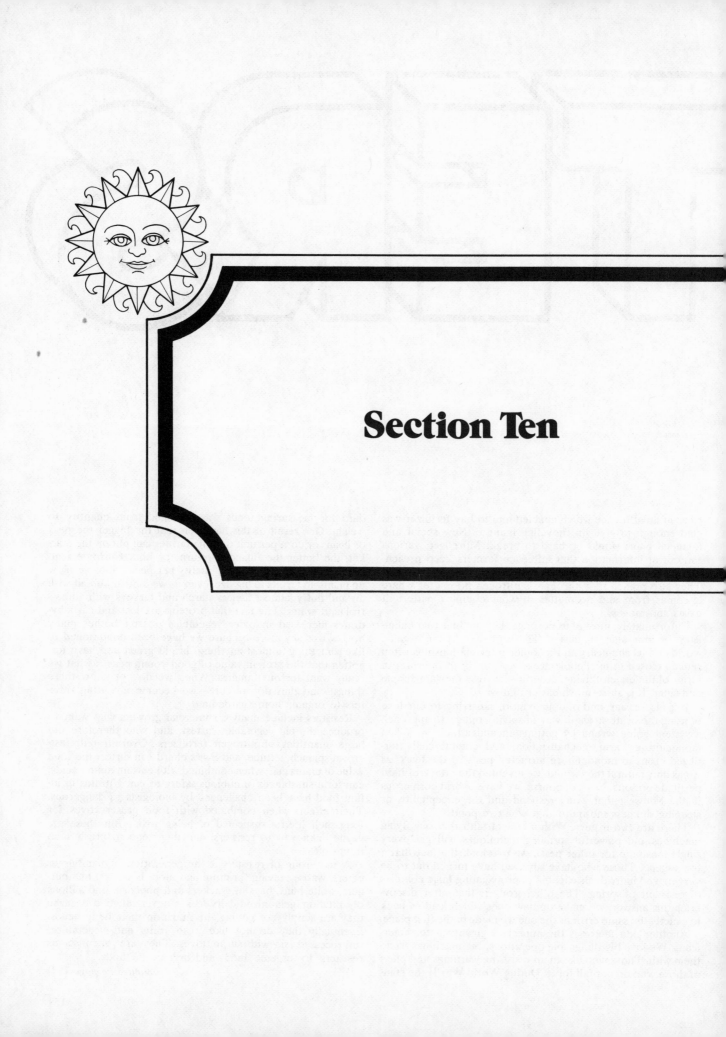

Section Ten

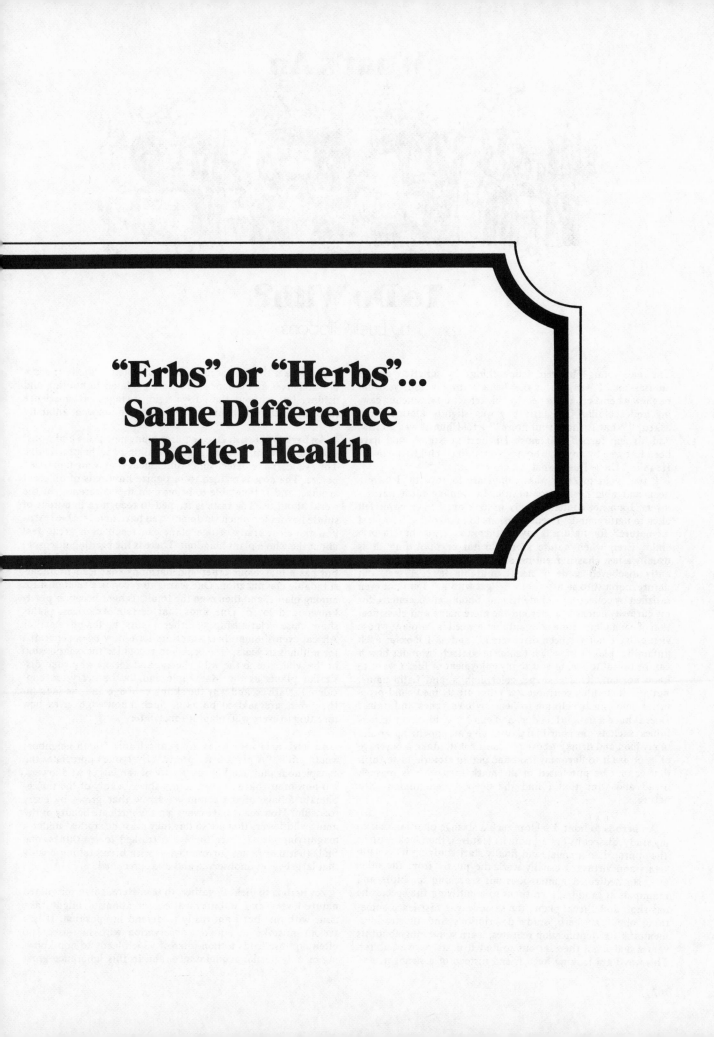

"Erbs" or "Herbs"...
Same Difference
...Better Health

What's An

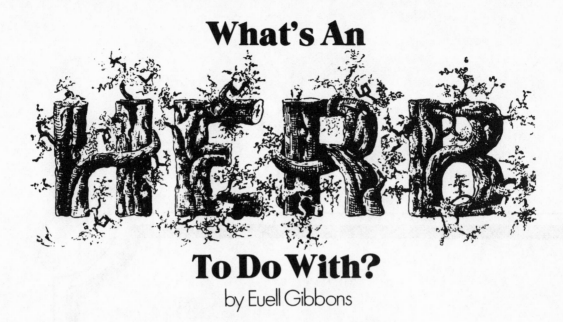

HERB

To Do With?

by Euell Gibbons

The way young children define things by function always amuses me. I was out in the fields with my four-year-old nephew when a crow in a nearby thicket set up a raucous cawing and scolding. The little boy was slightly alarmed and asked, "What is that awful noise?" I told him it was a crow, and his fear turned to interest. His next question could have been foreseen by anyone who has ever studied children closely. He said, "Uncle Euell, what is a crow to do with?"

I, too, want to know what things are to do with. I have a deep and abiding love for nature, but unlike most nature-lovers, I am not content merely to look on. I have never felt alien to nature, and I resent allusions to mankind's "conquest of nature," for nature is my mother and I am her favorite child. Even when nature seems brutal or punishing, it is usually a just chastisement because we have willfully or ignorantly disobeyed some of her immutable laws. I seek out nature, not just to sightsee, but to "get with it." I am not even satisfied by collecting and identifying botanical specimens, for my curiosity extends far beyond the mere name and classification of each plant. Emerson said that a weed is "a plant whose virtues have not yet been discovered," and as I look at each unfamiliar plant with which I come in contact, I wonder how it can be useful to me, or add to my enjoyment of life. I want to know not only its size, shape, color, habits, and Latin name, but also its hidden constituents. What are its medicinal properties, and can it help me to heal my own aches and pains? Does it have a delightful odor, and can I use this scent in perfumes, sachets, potpourri jars, or to give an appetizing aroma to my food and drink? Above all, can I eat it, make a beverage of it, or use it to flavor my food and get an esoteric taste thrill that cannot be purchased in the marketplace? It is in such bread and wine that I find the deepest communion with nature.

An herb is to hunt. I seldom pick a strange plant, take it to my study, dissect its flower, note its features, then look it up in the appropriate manual, and finally start studying its constituents and virtues. I usually work the puzzle from the other end. No dedicated hunter goes out searching for birds and mammals at random, then turns to identifying the species he has shot, and I treat plants the same way. I first learn something about an herb, study descriptions and illustrations, memorize its identification features, learn something about its values and uses, then set out to find it in its native habitat. This way I am looking for a friend instead of a stranger, and

experience a thrill of accomplishment when I finally track it down. This is an outdoor sport closely related to hunting and fishing, but without the gut-wringing twinges of conscience that always come to haunt me when I kill an innocent animal.

An herb is to learn. One acquires many new skills and a vast store of interesting knowledge in stalking the helpful herbs. The eye learns to detect small differences that went unnoticed before. The nose is trained to recognize hundreds of different aromas, and is then able to bring us a new awareness of the world about us. The taste is trained to recognize hundreds of subtle flavors for which we do not even have names. One learns how the close study of one plant can teach us a great deal about the whole plant kingdom. There is the exciting discovery that nature is not the chaos that it seems to the uninitiated, but has a marvelous order and harmony that lead to understandable classification. One learns to recognize relationships among plants, and then even the total stranger becomes partly known and loved. One finds that certain American plants show close relationship to other plants in far-off Asia or Africa, even though their ancestors have now been separated for millions of years. One begins to recognize the relationship of the wild rose to the wild cherry, and learns why such dissimilar plants as the May apple and the barberry are considered relatives, and why the skunk cabbage and the Jack-in-the-pulpit are said to be akin. Such knowledge gives new meaning to every wild plant we encounter.

An herb is to see. Or, as my Pennsylvania Dutch neighbors would put it, "A plant is for pretty." Everyone appreciates the conspicuous and flamboyant beauty of the larger wildflowers, but how many have thrilled to the sheer beauty of the thrice-pinnate foliage of the common yarrow that grows by every roadside? How many have ever seen the intricate beauty of the many wildflowers that are so tiny they must be studied under a magnifying glass? Once the eye is trained to see things, one finds that nature has surrounded us with breathtaking beauty that largely goes unobserved and unappreciated.

An herb is to pick, to gather, to use. Here, some misguided nature-lovers and uninformed conservationists might take issue with me, but I am ready to defend my position. It is a serious mistake to equate conservation with non-use. Too often non-use leads to non-interest which leads to non-knowing or only partial acquaintance, and in this ignorance great destruction is wrought. Sometimes it is the conservationists who want to eradicate certain plants for which they can see no immediate use, even though they might have a thousand virtues of which they never dreamed. It is the forager, the lover of wild foods and the culler of herbs and simples who is most interested in the protection and preservation of these products of untamed nature, and he will learn to gather and use without destroying. He will not only know when and how to pick and use, but when to refrain from picking, so these simple wayside plants can be preserved for future generations to experience the joys they offer; sometimes an herb is to leave alone.

An herb is to taste. A great many of the wild plants have delightful flavors that can add new interest to salads, confections or other culinary preparations, lifting them from the humdrum class to that of gourmet products. Food should never be merely nourishment, a means of keeping us alive, but should be one of the amenities that make life a joy. The sheer enjoyment of food contributes to its digestibility and healthfulness, and a great many wild herbs have delicious and appropriate flavors that they stand ready to contribute—free—to this cause.

An herb is to smell. Most people know that many wildflowers have sweet and pleasant odors, but how many know that many wild plants also have fruit, foliage, and even roots, that exude delightful perfume? These joyful scents can not only be enjoyed out in the fields and woods, but can be captured in various ways to perfume our houses, clothes, and bodies, giving them the sweet, clean aromas of nature, rather than the cloying and powerful scents of the perfumers' art. Delightful smells not only give present enjoyment, but have a subtle effect on memory, and to introduce a child to the woodland odors is to give him the ability, in later years, to recapture the joys of childhood merely by smelling of a wild plant or fruit or a crushed leaf.

An herb is to cure our illnesses. There is simply no doubt that many herbs have weapons they stand ready to contribute to mankind's battle against disease and sickness. Although most of these will be administered by professional doctors, the home remedy has always been with us, and in some areas is here to stay. I know that home preparations can contribute to my comfort during certain minor illnesses and can relieve my minor aches and pains. Such home remedies have a further value in enabling the well members of the family to express their concern and love for the sick person by gathering and preparing a wild herb remedy and tenderly administering it to the patient. Such things also have value.

An herb is to eat. Some wild herbs successfully make the leap from mere condiments to hearty foods that can be served in ample helpings, and many of these are better vegetables than some that come regularly to our tables from commercial markets. The health benefits of herbs can often be better utilized and assimilated if the herb is eaten as food rather than taken as medicine, and some of these wild herbs are delicious. Wild plants can contribute variety and many new and delightful flavors to our diets.

An herb is to nourish our bodies. I had long suspected that a great many of the astonishing cures attributed to herbal medicines by the ancient practitioners of this art were due neither to magic nor to medicinal properties, but to the vitamins, minerals, and other nutrients contained in these plants. When one reads that an herb will cure such diverse complaints as poor vision; dull or inflamed and itching eyes; styes; pimples on the face; blackheads; dry, rough, and itching skin; boils and carbuncles; dull hair and dandruff; dry, rough throat; superficial tubercles about the neck and throat; cysts; and many kinds of infections, one is apt to dismiss such claims as nonsense, or to ascribe the results to psychological effect on the patient. But look again. All these complaints, thought of as different illnesses by the ancient herbalists, could be symptoms arising from a single cause, an acute deficiency of vitamin A.

Similarly, when one reads that a certain herb or plant will cure scurvy, poisoning, all manner of infections, pink toothbrush, and the tendency to bruise easily, and will even aid in healing battle wounds and broken bones, one suspects that what the plant really will do is correct a vitamin C shortage. Often, I have seen the above lists of complaints and herbal or plant cures combined, giving a clue that here are wild things rich in both vitamins A and C.

I approached the Food and Nutrition Department of Pennsylvania State University with this idea, and they became interested. We searched the literature and found that quite a number of the wild plants most commonly used as food had been thoroughly explored for their nutritional properties. We assembled this data and then plunged into the unknown. Because of limited time, personnel, and funds, our research project was necessarily small in scope and modest in its goals. By kitchen research I had determined that certain unusual and nutritionally unexplored plants were eminently edible, so we limited ourselves to finding the vitamin A and C content of these, with a few side excursions into their mineral and protein contents. I gathered the material and delivered it to the University, and a staff lab technician made the analyses. Even this almost superficial examination of only a few herbs yielded some exciting results and opened a field of great promise to some future and more ambitious researcher. We found that a small helping of cooked violet leaves, which are delicious when prepared and served like spinach, could furnish all one's daily minimum requirements of vitamins A and C, and are probably good sources of other nutrients. Even violet flowers were found to be a good food, rich in protective vitamins. The common nettle, a favorite potherb of many foragers, not only proved an excellent source of vitamins A and C, but also is exceedingly rich in protein. Wild mint, besides its ability to contribute an almost universally liked flavor and fragrance, proved to be very rich in vitamins A and C, and should be eaten—not merely used as a seasoning and garnish.

After engaging in this research, I understood why the children of my Pennsylvania Dutch neighbors ate violet blossoms and chewed on catnip and mint. Their wise little bodies were informing these children what was needed. I also understood how they could maintain glowing health on a seemingly inadequate diet. They were getting their vitamins, minerals, and other food supplements from the wild plants they were consuming between meals. If we are ever cut off from our present sources of fresh food and diet supplements, we need never suffer from malnutrition if only we know which wild plants to reach for. The malnourished poor of some depressed rural areas could achieve glowing and abundant health, if only one could persuade them to eat the vitamin-rich wild plants that grow all about them.

And finally, an herb is to enjoy. Exploring the possible uses of wild plants has furnished me with a fascinating, lifelong hobby that has brought me more hours of pleasant recreation than anything else on God's green earth. I have found that children are easily interested in this sport and when properly guided will spend many pleasant and highly educational hours in pursuit of knowledge about wild vegetation. A child will probably be bored stiff by any attempt to teach him formal botany, but the whole picture changes when he knows what a plant is to do with. Anyone who plunges into this hobby with diligence and enthusiasm will soon learn that an herb is to love. ☼

ABC eginner's uide to Herbs,

ALLSPICE symbolizes compassion. It is the dried, unripe berry of a West Indian tree. It is available both whole and powdered. Allspice is used mainly in marinades, curries, pickling, and in cakes, cookies and pies. Its flavor is like a combination of cinnamon, nutmeg and cloves.

ANISE is a fragrant herb whose seeds have been used for flavoring since classical times. It is used in the manufacture of liqueurs and as a flavoring in cookies, breads and cakes.

BASIL is named from the Greek word for "king," and is a treasured flavoring in all of the Mediterranean region. It also occurs in tropical Asia, Africa and the Pacific islands. It is sometimes regarded as a symbol of love, and is a marvelous complement to tomato flavor. The fresh or dried leaves are used in salads, sauces, soups and stews.

BAY LEAF or bay laurel is the leaf of a Mediterranean evergreen. The leaf symbolizes constancy. Bay is one of the principal flavorings in French cuisine, but a little goes a long way. One dried leaf to a marinade, court bouillon, or stew pot is usual.

CAPERS are the unopened flower bud of a shrub that grows wild in the Mediterranean region. The pungent, tender buds are packed in salt or vinegar and are used to flavor sauces, fish dishes, and tomato and eggplant dishes such as *caponata*.

CARAWAY SEED is actually the fruit of the attractive caraway plant. It grows in Europe and ranges as far as Siberia, Persia and the Himalayas. Caraway seeds are used to flavor cakes, breads, sauerkraut, cheese, cookies and soups.

CARDAMOM seeds are the fruits of a perennial plant native to India and Ceylon. The seed-containing capsules are carefully harvested before they are fully ripe, then dried with care to prevent the thin outer shell from splitting. Purchased in the pod, the seeds are removed and crushed to flavor pastries (especially those from Scandinavia), curries and spiced coffees, or chewed to sweeten the breath.

CAYENNE is a fiery powder made from the dried pods of various peppers of the genus *Capsicum frutescens*. Strength of the powder is variable, from rather hot to inferno. A small amount can be used to add sparkle to most savory foods. Heat enhances the flavor.

CELERY SEED is an aromatic seed used to flavor salads, roasts, sauces and stews. It adds an excellent pungency to chili con carne. Seeds are produced in the second year by the celery plant.

CHERVIL symbolizes sincerity. Planted in the fall and harvested in the spring, chervil resembles parsley, but has a more delicate flavor. It is used in soups, salads, omelets, cottage cheese and to season fish as well as a garnish. Usually purchased in dried flakes.

CHIVES are a delicate member of the onion family and have been used as a seasoning for over five thousand years, according to one source. Freshly chopped chives are delicious in salads, omelets, vichyssoise, and cottage cheese. Fresh chives are easily grown, but dried or frozen chopped chives are also available.

fruit or "seed" is ground and used extensively to flavor Mexican and Indian dishes.

DILL SEED and **DILL WEED** are both used in cooking. The "weed" or leaf of fresh dill may be used fresh or dried in fish dishes, with eggs, cream cheeses, Scandinavian open-faced sandwiches, and is delightful with cucumbers with sour cream or yogurt. Dill seeds have been used as a medicinal since ancient times, and are used in pickling.

FENNEL grows wild in a Mediterranean climate, and is abundant along California roadsides. Symbolizing flattery, nearly all of the plant is used. The bulb and stalk are a delicious vegetable, and the leaves and seeds are used for seasoning. The fresh or dried leaves flavor soups, salads, sauces and fish dishes with a mild anise-like flavor. The stronger flavored seeds are used in breads, Italian sausage and pickles. They also help flatulence. Try a few in a pot of beans!

FENUGREEK has been known since ancient times in India and the Mediterranean area. Fenugreek, mentioned in a first century Roman cookbook, is an ingredient in Indian curries.

FINES HERBES is a classic French combination of chervil, tarragon, parsley and chives. The freshly chopped herbs are used in equal proportions in such dishes as "omelet fines herbes" which calls for 2 teaspoons of the mix per omelet.

GARLIC has been used in medicine and cooking since Babylonian times. It is reputed to perform all sorts of wonders from relieving bronchitis to repelling werewolves. Garlic is used lovingly in many dishes from salads to soups and stews, and is the basis of a Provencal garlic mayonnaise and joins basil in an Italian sauce for pasta.

GINGER is the root or rhizome of a tropical plant. It is one of the world's most versatile and popular spices. It gives its name and flavor to gingersnaps, gingerbread, and ginger ale and beer. The powdered root is widely available and can be used in

Spices and Seasonings by Barbara Farr

CINNAMON, the bark of the cinnamon tree, is one of the most ancient spices known to man. Bark, removed from the tropical tree during the rainy season, is scraped into long strips which dry into semi-tubular "quills." As a spice, cinnamon is used in curries and a wide variety of dishes ranging from moussaka to rice pudding. Cinnamon may be purchased as quills or sticks, and in powder. The powder may sometimes be adulterated with cheaper cassia.

CLOVES are the dried flower buds of a tropical tree, native to Indonesia. The buds are picked by hand and dried in the sun. Symbolizing dignity, cloves are strongly pungent and flavor a great range of dishes from savories to sweets. The Dutch once had a monopoly on cloves, and an onion studded with 2 or 3 cloves adds an ineffable flavor to Dutch pea soup.

CORIANDER is used in the United States mainly as a dried seed. Coriander seeds are used in sausages, soups, stews, chili dishes and curries. The fresh leaves have a very pungent taste and are used extensively in the cuisines of India, China, Mexico and South America.

CUMIN was used in Roman times to allay nausea, and symbolizes greed. It is also native to India and China. The dried

many dishes. Fresh ginger root is a most important ingredient in Indian, Chinese and Caribbean cuisine.

HORSERADISH is the root of a perennial herb. Its distinctively hot flavor adds piquancy to sauces for meats and seafoods. Freshly grated horseradish is mixed with vinegar and salt, or prepared as sauce. Commercially prepared horseradish sauce is also available.

MACE is the outer coating, or aril, of the nutmeg seed. The bright red aril turns brown as it dries, and is sold as a powder. It has a mild flavor similar to nutmeg and is used in baked goods, pickles and seafood sauces.

MARJORAM's name derives from Greek words meaning "joy of the mountain." Native to the Mediterranean region, marjoram belongs to the aromatic mint family. Versatile marjoram is used in soups, sauces, stews, stuffings, salads, savory pies, etc. and is a favorite with lamb.

MINT includes an enormous family of herbs, symbolizing virtue. The most commonly used varieties are peppermint and spearmint. Mint is delightful in vegetable dishes, cold soups, yogurt dishes, lamb dishes, beverages and desserts.

(continued on page 292)

Some Culinary Herbs

Angelica
Basil
Bay
Chicory
The Chives
Chervil
Coriander
Curry Plant
Dill
Fennel
Garlic
Leek
Lemon Balm
Lemon Verbena
Lovage
Marjoram
The Mints
Oregano
Parsley
Sage
Savory Burnet
Sorrel
Tarragon
The Thymes
Watercress
Welsh Onion

Some Medicinal Herbs

Acanthus
Balsam
Boneset
Catmint
Celandine
Chamomile
Comfrey
Dandelion
Eyebright
Feverfew

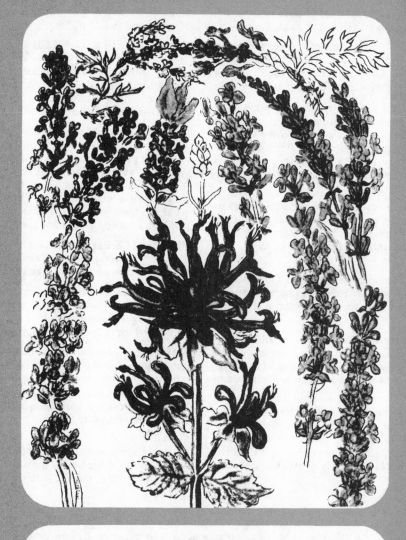

Herbal Glossary

alternative	healing, beneficial, improving an ailment
anticolic	digestive, helps stomach complaints
anti-lithic	gravel-removing
aromatic	having a distinctive fragrance
astringent	substance that draws together or binds
bitter	tonic produced from some aromatic herbs
carminative	gas expellent
decoction	an extract obtained by boiling a substance down to a concentrated form
demulcent	a soothing, usually oily or viscous substance
diaphoretic	induces perspiration
diuretic	stimulates kidneys and bladder to excrete urine
dyspepsia	indigestion
herb	a plant or plant part valued for its medicinal, culinary or aromatic qualities. Webster places parentheses around the (h) to indicate that some people pronounce the letter and others do not. In "Dos and Don'ts" the h is pronounced.
infusion	a liquid resulting from steeping without boiling
stimulant	increases activity or function
stomachic	stimulates the action of the stomach
tisane	an infusion, as tea
tonic	a stimulant, activator or refresher

Fleabane
Gentian
Heartsease
Horehound
Hound's Tongue
Lady's Mantle
Linseed
Licorice
Lungwort
The Mallows
Meadowsweet
Melilot
Motherwort
Mullein
Nettle
Poke-root
Rue
Sea Holly
Tansy
Thistle
Vervain
Wild Carrot
(Queen Anne's Lace)
Yarrow

Some Aromatic Herbs

Dittany-of-Crete
Geranium
Heliotrope
The Lavenders
The Mints
Old Lady
Pelargonium
Rosemary
Southernwood
The Thymes
Woodruff
Wormwood

Herbs: Dos and Don'ts

by Ben Charles Harris, R. Ph., N.D.

1—Do remember that a teaspoonful of dried herbs has the equivalent aromatic or therapeutic potency of a tablespoonful of fresh herbs.

2—Do add aromatics *sparingly* to season your foods until you're sure of their true flavoring power. Use a scant two-finger pinch at first and even less than suggested by a recipe. Unless designated as "fines herbes," food-seasoning herbs are added near the end of the cooking period. Remember: not every dish requires aromatics.

3—Do raise herbs, sprouts, and vegetables during the fall-winter months. Use all spare windowsills of every sunny room *and* window boxes, jars, flower pots, and old cookware. (See #47.)

4—Do use fresh herbs for every new cup of herb tea (infusion, tisane). Stir a given amount at least thirty-five times and cover seven to ten minutes. To such natives as Boneset, Burdock, Yarrow, Clovers, and Linden, always flavor with aromatics such as Mints, Chamomile, Catnip, and food-seasoners like Marjoram, Thyme, Basil, et al. A tea of each aromatic helps you to appreciate its taste and savory qualities.

5—Do include citrus rinds and then some kitchen wastes in the category of herbs. The peels of Oranges, Lemons, Tangerines, and Limes are invaluable aromatizers of meat and fish mixtures, soups, stews, jellies, preserves, turkey stuffing, pastry, breads, and wine or fruit punch; and of herb teas and sachets.

The dried seeds of Squash and Pumpkin make a nice wintertime nibble and a worm expellent for young children. Watermelon seeds and Corn silk serve in kidney problems, used tea bags in an eye lotion and poison antidote, Pomegranate rinds as another worm expellent remedy, Quince seeds in hand lotions, etc.

6—Do record all your happenings and experiences with which herbs and their many uses, i.e., as food, tea, remedy, dye, etc. Note the who, what, where, when and how of every event. Occasionally review your dated statements and make up-to-date comparisons, the better to note your progress and to improve a harmonious relationship with herbs.

7—Do use the following powdered herbs to make an acceptable salt substitute: the leaves and seeds of Wild and cultivated Carrot, the leaves and/or fruits of Shepherd's Purse, Peppergrass, Lamb's-quarters, Yellow Dock, Parsley, Watercress, Goldenrod, Mints, early Tansy, and Sassafras. Add equal amounts of powdered aromatics—Dill, Basil, Marjoram, Savory and others of your choice, and of Kelp. Mix well. Use in all warm foods, even on toast.

8—Do use *all* parts of Wild Carrot (Queen Anne's Lace): the early fresh greens in salads, soups, omelets, etc., the maturing seeds as a substitute for Caraway in food recipes and in remedies (colic, griping, and other mild stomach discomforts), and the summer leaf tops with broiled or baked fish or chicken. The older leaves, dried, powdered and sifted, become an ingredient of a herb powder (salt-substitute). The late-summer roots serve as a mild, stimulating diuretic in kidney problems.

9—Do have a herb garden. You can grow ten or twelve herbs in a space of five by eight feet in your sunful backyard. At first grow the easy ones: Sage, Basil, Mints, Marjoram and Summer Savory.

Thin your regular garden soil with sand, a few small stones, and bits of charcoal. Refrain from enriching the soil; otherwise you may obtain larger foliage and plant growth but a poor quality of the desired fragrance.

10—Do gather seeds of wild or cultivated herbs at the time of their ripening. Cut the herb below the seeds, let dry thoroughly, shake and sort (use the remainder in herb teas) and label the date of collection. And do plant them during the wintertime, as indicated under #3.

11—Do include the much neglected Sheep Sorrel, Shepherd's Purse and Peppergrass in your foods and remedies: the early fresh leaves and fruits in salads and assorted food mixtures and dried, powdered, in a salt substitute. An infusion of all summer-gathered parts, dried and coarsely ground, helps to remove gravel from the urinary tract.

12—Do learn to remember the true aroma and savor of the food-seasoning herbs you generally use. Every day during a herb's growing stage, taste or chew a leaf of Basil, Sage and/or Thyme and learn the difference between each herb. To supplement this test, do drink a warm infusion of each herb on separate days.

Study and practice the therapeutics and healing properties of food seasoners: Marjoram, Fennel, and Caraway for the stomach and intestines, Thyme and Anise for the bronchial area, and Sage for all organs.

13—Do use Chamomile not only for a pleasantly flavored tea. Its anticolic, carminative and quieting properties are quite useful in all gastrointestinal disturbances—for all, from infants to grandparents. The herb is also good for nervousness and sleeplessness. For tired or inflamed eyes, use a carefully strained *weak* infusion of Chamomile and Fennel seeds. It is well named the "plant's physician;" grown among Wheat, it helps to produce larger ears. Grow it also among Garlic and Onions and Cabbage, and use it to flavor the latter and its relatives.

Used as a rinse, Chamomile turns blond hair into pure gold.

14—Do save and use two of the best known garden weed-residents: Dandelion's early leaves are a nutrient-rich food, the dried summer leaves are coarsely ground and incorporated in most herb teas, and the finely ground roots enter into kidney and stomach/liver remedies. A suitable spring-tonic and blood purifier is rendered by decocting equal parts of Dandelion, Burdock, Yellow Dock, Sassafras and Sarsaparilla. Dandelion wine is made from yellow Dandelions.

Do use all of dried and finely cut Quackgrass or Witchgrass as an excellent demulcent, anti-lithic and diuretic in all genito-urinary affections.

15—Do use small amounts of the leaves of all Gentians in

(continued on page 293)

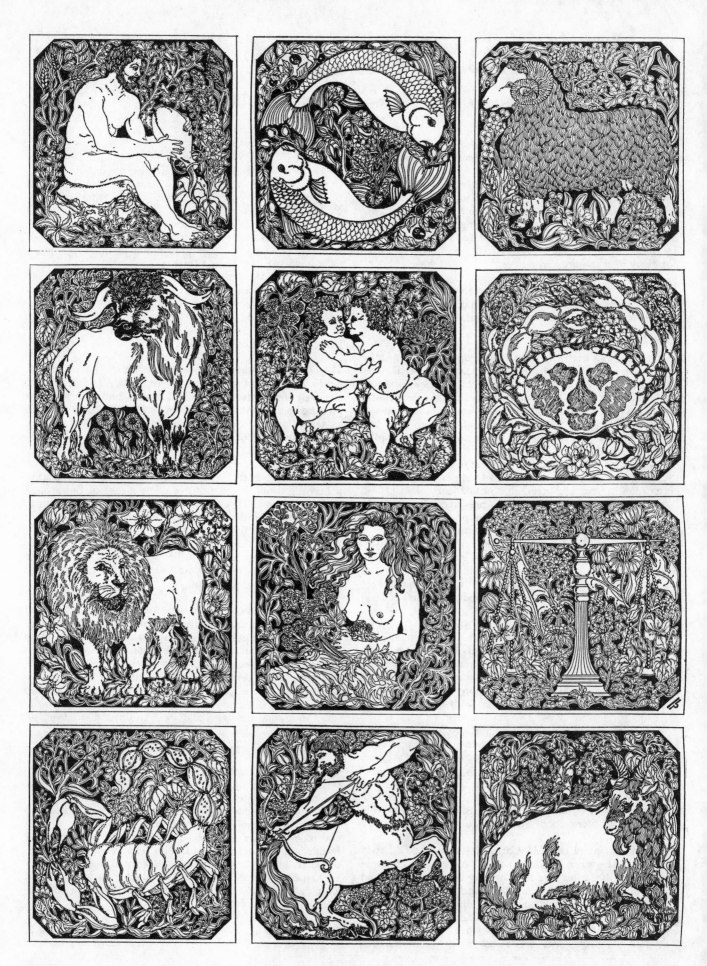

It was my grandmother, Anyeta, from faraway Romania, who first introduced me to the mysteries of herbal remedies as the Romanies know them. Her wise, lined face would crinkle in a smile as she recited the qualities of her favourite herbs, lingering lovingly over their fragrance and texture, and ruminating on their ancient powers.

"Stand on any hill," she would tell me, "and look for miles around at the view. There will you see God's bounty growing, just for the taking . . . plentiful. In everything that grows we find the mystery of life a million times."

She was right, of course, Why there is such variety in life remains a complete and eternal mystery. Why a thousand species of insect? Why a million species of grasses? A billion kinds of green growing things? Why did not the eternal One grow just one "herb" on his planet Earth—a green stuff like spinach—and say: "That's your lot. Sufficient unto the day . . . !"

admit that they were not uttering mumbo-jumbo—but were infinitely wise before their time.

Culpeper, the seventeenth century astrologer and herbalist, believed this to be the true philosophy of life. He not only assigned each herb its ruling planet, but treated each subject of the Zodiac—the hot-headed Arien, the stubborn Taurean, the mercurial Geminian—according to their lights, their planet, their "stars."

His advice to the readers of his *Complete Herbal* on when to gather herbs for treatment was as follows: "Such as are astrologers (and indeed none else are fit to make physicians) such I advise; let the planet that governs the herb be angular, and the stronger the better; if they can, in herbs of Saturn, let Saturn be in the ascendant; in the herbs of Mars, let Mars be in the Mid-heaven, for in those houses they delight; let the Moon apply to them by good aspect, and let her not be in the houses of her enemies; if you cannot well stay

Herbs, Astrology and the Rhythm of Life

by
Leon Petulengro

Instead, we have this wonderful variety from which to choose, each green growing thing, from a humble grass trodden underfoot to a giant redwood tree scraping the sky, with its own use in life, its place in nature, its history and background enough to fill a book.

And through all this abundant life there is a pulse beating which we Romanies and the wise ones of old—the astrologers—believe to be a rhythm which is generated in the universe. As the planets in their courses whirl and pulsate, so their rhythm is one with the herbs that grow on earth, all life that breathes, the tides that beat our shores.

If the scientists have gone a million miles towards knowing the secrets of this life, then by all means let us applaud them. But there is one way in which they could be deemed less wise than their predecessors—the alchemists who laid the groundwork for the chemists, the herbalists who went before the doctors, above all, the astrologers who led the way into astronomy (how many know today that the first Astronomer Royal, Flamsteed, was also an astrologer?). They have taken so long to acknowledge the rhythm of life that is everywhere and which is set down in the philosophy we call Astrology.

Now, however, it has been discovered, by scientific means, and recorded by the Nutritional Science Research Institute of England, that *each individual food or material or disease radiates energy of a radiation-type characteristic via a unique pattern or wave field. This is an extended force field that exists around all forms of matter, whether animate or inanimate.* So, knowing as we do that planets and stars emit their own individual signals or vibrations, how can we disbelieve that ancient lore was right and that herbs and plants, and indeed humans, are ruled by these various vibrations or force fields. The cosmic influence at last seems to be acknowledged by the white-coated men of science. What better time than now, on the threshold of the New Aquarian age, to re-examine those ancient beliefs of the Wise Men and

till she apply them, let her apply to a planet of the same triplicity; if you cannot wait that time neither, let her be with a fixed star of their nature."

To anyone with an ear for English that passage reads like poetry; to an astrologer it also contains precise instructions, as does the following advice from Culpeper on *"The way of mixing Medicines according to the cause of the Disease, and part of the body afflicted.* To such as study astrology (who are the only men I know that are fit to study physic, physic, without astrology, being like a lamp without oil) you are the men I exceedingly respect, and such documents as my brain can give you at present, being absent from my study, I shall give you.

1. Fortify the body with herbs of the nature of the Lord of the Ascendant, 'tis no matter whether he be a Fortune or Infortunate in this case.

2. Let your medicine be something anti-pathetical to the Lord of the Sixth.

3. Let your medicine be something of the nature of his sign Ascending.

4. If the Lord of the Tenth be strong, make use of his medicines.

5. If this cannot well be, make use of the medicines of the Light of Time.

6. Be sure always to fortify the grieved part of the body by sympathetical remedies.

7. Regard the heart, keep that upon the wheels, because the sun is the foundation of life, and therefore those universal remedies Aarum Potabile, and the Philosopher's stone cure all diseases by fortifying the heart."

Whether this early form of treatment stands up against modern medicine with all its "advanced" drugs, is not my argument here, but let us admit it sounds more enchanting to the philosophical ear than "Keep on taking the tablets." As I have said so often before, a man who will not give some

(continued on page 299)

Harvesting, Drying

Domestic Drying

A natural and simple method of preserving herbs is drying. In this way they can be used in the kitchen all the year round. In order to retain the green colour and all their qualities, the herbs have to be picked at the right moment, mostly before blossoming, and dried immediately afterwards. This can be done at home in a heated airing cupboard, in an oven with low temperature, or with a home-made drying cabinet.

The principle of drying, once the herb is harvested, is to dry without any delay in the dark and not allow sun or wind to reduce its valuable properties such as the volatile oils.

Airing cupboard: Spread the herbs thinly on trays covered with nylon net or stainless steel wire mesh, then stack them, leaving some space between for the warm air to circulate, at the same time allowing for ventilation. You must decide when the herbs are dry by your own judgment for they are all different in thickness of leaves and stalks. Generally speaking, when the herbs are really brittle in leaf and stalk but still green in colour, they can be considered dry. If the herbs turn brown, they are burnt.

Oven drying: A less satisfactory method as the temperature of the oven should not exceed 90°F. (32°C.). Herbs are inclined to lose their colour when dried in higher temperatures but if you can achieve this low temperature, spread the herbs on trays in the same way as for the airing cupboard and leave the oven door ajar for ventilation.

A simple domestic herb drying cabinet can be made at home, consisting of a wood-framed cupboard lined with hardboard approximately 3 feet 6 inches (116 centimeters) high and with an inside measurement of 12 inches (30 centimeters) square, or to suit the size of a small heater. Trays should be made to fit the inside diameter and wooden batten supports fixed to the sides to carry them. The height of the lowest tray should be 12 inches (30 centimeters) from the floor. A small greenhouse-type heater can be used or any suitable electric convector or blown air heater which fits the area. It may be advisable to reverse the top and bottom trays after some time of drying, which should be done without interruption. The herbs when dry, are rubbed by hand, discarding the hard stalks, then sieved and stored.

Storing Herbs—Where to Keep Them

Herbs, once dried, are best kept in airtight glass containers in a dark cupboard. This is advice against the herb racks which are so often displayed by shops selling herbs. Nothing

and Storing Herbs

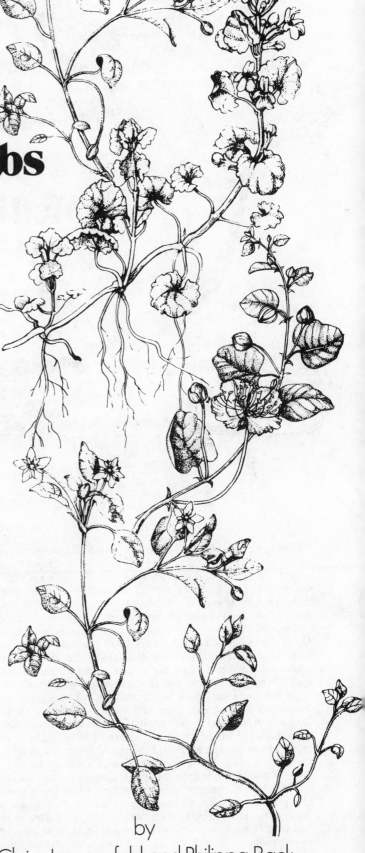

is more detrimental for dried herbs than to keep them in a place where light has access to them, fading their colour and spoiling their special qualities. Glass is the best material, being clean and lasting, and if the container is well closed by a plastic screwtop lid or even a glass stopper, the scent cannot escape. If it is not possible to find space in a dark cupboard, a large label round the container will help to keep out the light. If harvesting very large quantities of herbs for drying, these can be kept satisfactorily in any kind of bin or container, provided the herbs are first put into linen or cotton bags, and the container well closed.

Fresh herbs can be stored for some time in the refrigerator in large glass jars with airtight closures and parsley and chives packed tightly in such a jar—a preserving jar or empty honey jar will do—will keep for several weeks without losing much colour or crispness.

Deep Freezing

A good method for keeping herbs in their original condition is to deep freeze them. Although they will not be crisp enough when thawed to sprinkle over a dish, they are perfect for adding to a variety of recipes, either singly or as mixed bouquets of herbs such as bouquet garni.

How to do it: Cut the herbs when the dew has evaporated, wash and shake free of excess water and harden for a few minutes by putting them on a plate in the deep-freeze. Make individual bunches of the herb, tie with thread, put into small cellophane bags and close with deep-freeze wire closures. Six or more of these bunches can then be put into a large bag, closed and labelled. It is important to get the air out of the bags before closing.

Frozen herb bouquets can be stored in the same way except that the individual bunches will consist of a mixture of herbs.

Frozen herb cubes—a good way to freeze small quantities of single herbs. Chop up the herbs after washing them, ladle into ice cube trays with small divisions. Then fill each division with concentrated stock made from a cube and ¼ pint (5 fluid ounces) water. When frozen remove cubes carefully, wrap in foil and deep-freeze in the usual way in cellophane bags. This method is especially good for making chervil soup when fresh chervil is not available. Make a roux of 2 tablespoons butter and 2 tablespoons flour. Gradually smooth in 1½ pints (30 fluid ounces) cold stock. Then add 3 frozen cubes and cook for 20 minutes, adding salt if necessary and a little cream at the end.

by
Claire Loewenfeld and Philippa Back

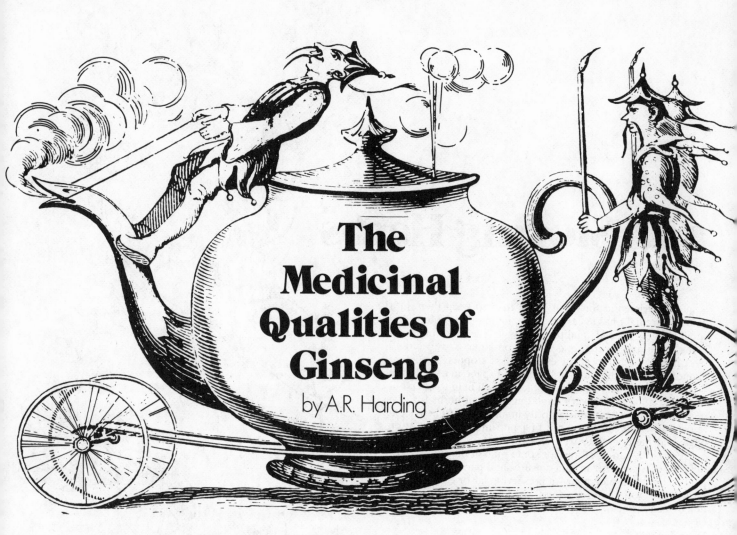

The Medicinal Qualities of Ginseng

by A.R. Harding

I will suggest this way to use Ginseng as a medicine for a general homemade use, says a writer in *Special Crops:* Take very dry root, break it up with a hammer and grind it thru a coffee mill three or four times till reduced to a fine powder. Then take three ounces of powder and one ounce of milk sugar. To the milk sugar add sixty drops of oil of wintergreen and mix all the powders by rubbing them together and bottle. Dose one teaspoonful, put into a small teacupful of boiling water. Let it stay a little short of boiling point ten minutes. Then cool and drink it all, hot as can be borne, before each meal. It may be filtered and the tea served with cream and sugar with the meal. Made as directed this is a high grade and a most pleasant aromatic tea and has a good effect on the stomach, brain and nervous system. To those who have chronic constipation, I would advise one fourth of aloin, taken every night, or just enough to control the constipation, while taking the Ginseng tea. If the evening dose of Ginseng be much larger it is a good safe hypnotic, producing good natural sleep.

The writer prefers the above treatment to all the whiskey and patent medicine made. To those who are damaged or made nervous by drinking coffee or tea, quit the coffee or tea and take Ginseng tea as above directed. It is most pleasant tasted and a good medicine for your stomach. I do not know just how the Chinese prepare it into medicine, but I suppose much of it is used in a tea form as well as a tincture. As it is so valuable a medicine their mode of administration has been kept a secret for thousands of years. There must be some medical value about it of great power or the Chinese could not pay the price for it. It has been thought heretofore that the Chinese were a superstitious people and used Ginseng thru ignorance, but as we get more light on the medical value of the plant the plainer it gets that it is us fellows—the Americans—that have been and are yet in the "shade" and in a dark shade, too. We think the time not far off when it will be recognized as a medical plant and a good one, too, and its great medical value be made known to the world.

For several years past I have been experimenting with Ginseng as a medical agent and of late I have prescribed, or rather added it, to the treatment of some cases of rheumatism. I remember one instance in particular of a middle-aged man who had gone the rounds of the neighborhood doctors and failed of relief, when he employed me. After treating him for several weeks and failing to entirely relieve him, more especially the distress in bowels and back, I concluded to add Ginseng to his treatment. After using the medicine he returned, saying the last bottle had served him so well that he wanted it filled with the same medicine as before. I attribute the curative properties of Ginseng in rheumatism to stimulating to healthy action of the gastric juices; causing a healthy flow of the digestive fluids of the stomach, thereby neutralizing the extra secretion of acid that is carried to the nervous membranes of the body and joints, causing the inflammatory condition incident to rheumatism.

Ginseng combined with the juices of a good ripe pineapple is par excellent as a treatment for indigestion. It stimulates the healthy secretion of pepsin, thereby insuring good digestion without incurring the habit of taking pepsin or after-dinner pills to relieve the fullness and distress so common to the American people. The above compound prepared with good wine in the proper way will relieve many aches and pains of a rebellious stomach.

Ginseng has been used to some extent as a domestic medicine in the United States for many years. As far as I can learn, the home use is along the line of tonic and stimulant to the digestive and the nervous system. Many people have great faith in the power of the Ginseng root to increase the general strength and appetite as well as to relieve eructations from the stomach. As long ago as Bigelow's time, some wonderful effects are recorded of the uses of half a root in the increase of the general strength and the removal of fatigue. Only the other day a young farmer told me that Ginseng tea was a good thing to break up an acute cold and I think you will find it used for rheumatism and skin diseases. It undoubtedly has some effect on the circulation, perhaps thru its action on the nervous system and to this action is probably due its ascribed anti-spasmodic properties.

The use of Ginseng has largely increased within the last few years and several favorable reports have been published in the medical journals. One physician, whose name and medium of publication I cannot now recall, speaks highly of its anti-spasmodic action in relieving certain forms of hiccough. If this is true, it places it at once among the important and powerful anti-spasmodics and suggests its use in other spasmodic and reflex nervous diseases as whooping cough, asthma, etc.

I have practiced medicine for eight years. I sold my practice one year ago and since have devoted my entire attention to the cultivation of Ginseng and experimenting with Ginseng in diseases and am satisfied that it is all that the Chinese claim for it; and, if the people of the United States were educated as to its use, our supply would be consumed in our own country and it would be a hard blow to the medical profession.

It would make too long an article for me to enumerate the cases that I have cured; but, I think it will suffice to say that I have cured every case where I have used it with one exception and that was a case of consumption in its last stages; but the lady and her husband both told me that it was the only medicine that she took during her illness that did her any good. The good it did her was by loosening her cough; she could give one cough and expectorate from the lungs without any exertion. I believe it is the best medicine for consumption in its first stages and will probably cure.

I wish the readers of *Special Crops* to try it in their own families—no difference what the disease is. Make a tea of it. A good way is to grate it in a nutmeg grater. Grate what would make about 15 grains, or about one-fourth to one-half teaspoonful and add half a pint or less of boiling water. The dose to be taken at meal times and between meals. In a cold on the lungs it will cure in two or three days, if care is taken and the patient is not exposed.

I will cite one case; a neighbor lady had been treated by two different physicians for a year for a chronic cough. I gave her some Ginseng and told her to make a tea of it and take it at meal times and between meals; in two weeks I saw her and she told me that she was cured and that she never took medicine that did her so much good, saying that it acted as a mild cathartic and made her feel good. She keeps Ginseng in her house now all the time and takes a dose or two when she does not feel well.

I am satisfied that wonderful cures can be made with Ginseng and am making them myself, curing patients that doctors have given up; and if handled properly our supply will not equal the demand at home in the course of five or six years, thus increasing the price.

At the last annual meeting of the Michigan Ginseng Association, Dr. H.S. McMaster of Cass Co. presented a paper on the uses of this plant, which appeared in the *Michigan Farmer*. He spoke in part as follows:

"Ginseng is a mild, non-poisonous plant, well adapted to domestic as well as professional uses. In this respect it may be classed with such herbs as boneset, oxbalm, rhubarb and dandelion. The medicinal qualities are known to be a mild tonic, stimulant, nervine and stomachic. It is especially a remedy for ills incident to old age.

"For home or domestic use we would suggest the following methods of preparing this drug:

"1st. The simplest preparation and one formerly used to some extent by the pioneers of our forest lands, is to dig, wash and eat the green root, or to pluck and chew the green leaves. Ginseng, like boneset, aconite and lobelia, has medicinal qualities in the leaf.

"To get the best effect, like any other medicine it should be taken regularly from three to six times a day and in medicinal quantities. In using the green root we would suggest as a dose a piece not larger than one to two inches of a lead pencil, and of green leaves one to three leaflets. These, however, would be pleasanter and better taken in infusion with a little milk and sweetened and used as a warm drink as other teas are.

"2nd. The next simplest form of use is the dried root carried in the pocket, and a portion as large as a kernel of corn, well chewed, may be taken every two or three hours. Good results come from this mode of using, and it is well known that the Chinese use much of the root in this way.

"3d. Make a tincture of the dried root, or leaves. The dried root should be grated fine, then the root, fiber or leaves, separately or together, may be put into a fruit jar and barely covered with equal parts of alcohol and water. If the Ginseng swells, add a little more alcohol and water to keep it covered. Screw top on to keep from evaporating. Macerate in this way 10 to 14 days, strain off and press all fluid out, and you have a tincture of Ginseng. The dose would be 10 to 15 drops for adults.

"Put an ounce of this tincture in a six-ounce vial, fill the vial with a simple elixir obtained at any drug store, and you have an elixir of Ginseng, a pleasant medicine to take. The dose is one teaspoonful three or four times a day.

"The tincture may be combined with the extracted juice of a ripe pineapple for digestion, or combined with other remedies for rheumatism or other maladies.

"4th. Lastly I will mention Ginseng tea, made from the dry leaves or blossom umbels. After the berries are gathered, select the brightest, cleanest leaves from mature plants. Dry them slowly about the kitchen stove in thick bunches, turning and mixing them until quite dry, then put away in paper sacks.

"Tea from these leaves is steeped as you would ordinary teas, and may be used with cream and sugar. It is excellent for nervous indigestion.

"These home preparations are efficacious in neuralgia, rheumatism, gout, irritation of bronchi or lungs from cold, gastro-enteric indigestion, weak heart, cerebro-spinal and other nervous affections, and is especially adapted to the treatment of young children as well as the aged. Ginseng is a hypnotic, producing sleep, an anodyne, stimulant, nerve tonic and slightly laxative."

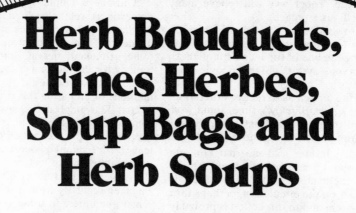

Herb Bouquets, Fines Herbes, Soup Bags and Herb Soups

by Irene Botsford Hoffman

The **Herb Bouquet** is in such frequent demand, for soups, for stews, in the cooking of vegetables, that it is important to understand just what is meant by the term. It is a bunch of three or four fresh herbs tied together, which is removed after cooking. It may be varied, but the classic combination, unless otherwise specified, consists of parsley, celery leaves, an onion, and a sprig of thyme.

Some good combinations for special purposes are as follows:

Cut fine herbs with a small pair of scissors kept solely for that purpose.

If the dried herbs are used, the amount should be much less, as they are stronger and more concentrated than the fresh. One teaspoon of the dried or one tablespoon of the fresh herbs is a good rule to follow.

Ravigote (good with beef)
Burnet
Chervil
Chives
Tarragon

For Lamb Stew

Parsley		Rosemary
Thyme	or	Parsley
Clove		Celery

For Veal Stew
Sweet Marjoram
Parsley
Onion

For Pea Soups

Rosemary		Thyme		Mint
Celery	or	Celery	or	Parsley
Parsley		Parsley		

For Tomato Soup
Basil
Parsley
Onion
Bay Leaf

Fine Herbs *(fines herbes):* a mixture, finely ·minced, of four or five herbs in different combinations, but always including chives and either parsley or chervil.
Chives, parsley, burnet, tarragon, chervil (ravigote).
Chives, chervil, basil, burnet, thyme.
Chives, burnet, tarragon, marjoram, parsley.
Chives, chervil, savory, burnet.
Tarragon, although an ingredient of ravigote and other fine-herb combinations, has such a distinctive and individual flavor that it is really better used alone, or at any rate not with other herbs of strong flavor such as thyme, summer savory, basil, or rosemary. Nor should thyme and summer savory be used together, as they are both of strong individual flavors. The beginner should err on the side of too little rather than too much. It is as easy to over-flavor as to over-season, and one flavor should never be allowed to kill another. Tarragon should never be allowed to cook more than a few minutes in soups or sauces; it should be added at the last.

Soup Bags: The following directions for making soup bags are taken from Mrs. Hollis Webster's excellent *Bulletin on Herbs.*

Make small cheesecloth bags about 2 inches square and fill with a bouquet of dried herbs. The quantity given in the following recipes will fill three bags, and in each is enough seasoning for about two quarts of liquid. The bags are dropped into the boiling soup toward the end of cooking, and should not be left in more than an hour or according to taste. Long cooking makes herbs bitter and destroys the fine essence of distinction between the different kinds in the "bouquet." The little sack of herbs should not be used again.

For Consomme
1/4 teaspoon peppercorns
3 cloves (1 in each bag)
2 teaspoons thyme
1 teaspoon marjoram
5 teaspoons parsley
1/2 teaspoon savory
3 tablespoons celery

For Tomato Soup
1 small bay leaf
3 cloves (1 in each bag)
1 teaspoon thyme
1 teaspoon basil
2 tablespoons celery
1 tablespoon parsley

For Fish Stock (or to boil with salmon, halibut, etc.)
1 small bay leaf
1/2 teaspoon sage
1 teaspoon savory
3 cloves (1 in each bag)
3 peppercorns
2 tablespoons celery
1/4 teaspoon basil
1/2 teaspoon fennel

For Flavoring Meat Gravies, Beef Stock, and Baked Liver
1 teaspoon dried parsley
1 teaspoon dried thyme
1 teaspoon dried marjoram
1/4 teaspoon dried sage
1/2 teaspoon savory
1/4 teaspoon bay leaf
2 teaspoons dried celery (leaf and
   stem tips or the grated root of this herb)

(continued on page 300)

The Wonderful World

by Barbara Farr
with Kathy Cranor,
Dan Moon,
Jaime and Kids

Herb Teas cover a wide range of variety and function. From ancient times, the leaves, stems, flowers, roots or bark of plants have been steeped to provide beverages that were delicious to drink and used for medicinal purposes as well. Since many vitamins and minerals are water-soluble, the teas may provide some nutritional value. Herb teas are increasingly popular as alternatives to caffeine-containing tea and coffee, or sugar-laden soft drinks. Herb teas should be drunk without milk or sugar, although a bit of honey may sometimes be added, and a squeeze of fresh lemon. Curative powers are accorded to some teas but we make no claims for their effectiveness.

According to our friends from pipsissewa, the proper way to make an herbal tea is to use an earthenware or china teapot. Boil water in a non-metal container and pour over tea. Use about 1 teaspoon of tea per cup. Ten minutes of steeping will produce a fairly strong tea. Sweeten your tea with mountain honey, or spice with a bit of cinnamon bark, clove, orange, lemon, cardamom, etc. Teas, incidentally, should be stored in tightly closed containers, away from the light, then used as desired.

Single Teas

ALFALFA LEAF TEA mixes well with mint, and is rich in minerals. Steep 1 teaspoon of dried leaves in 2 cups of boiling water for 10 minutes.

BALM (MELISSA) TEA is reputed to ward off aging, reduce fever and act as a tranquillizer. It is sometimes flavored with rosemary or lavender. Steep 1 teaspoon dried balm in 2 cups boiling water for 10 minutes.

BASIL TEA is delicious. Step 1 heaping teaspoon of fresh or dried leaves in 1 cup boiling water for 15 minutes.

BLUEBERRY LEAF TEA is said to be effective against fatigue and diabetes.

CATNIP TEA has a reputation as an aid in relaxing, reducing fever and infant colic. Steep 1 teaspoon dried or fresh leaves in 2 cups boiling water for 10 minutes.

CHAMOMILE TEA is soothing, and often drunk as a nightcap. Some say it is helpful against nervous conditions, neuralgia, menstrual cramps and indigestion. Steep 1 teaspoon of blossoms in 1 cup boiling water for 10 minutes. Chamomile is good cold, and an old recipe calls for 2 parts chamomile to 1 part crushed fennel seed for an after-dinner tea. A strong solution makes a fine rinse for blond hair.

# of Herb Teas

COMFREY TEA, or boneset tea has long been a popular medicinal. It is reputed to be useful in speeding the healing of bones (obviously), and for chest problems, ulcers and diarrhea. Steep 1 teaspoon leaves or root in 1 cup boiling water for 30 minutes. Comfrey tea is often flavored with mint.

DAMIANA TEA, from Mexico makes a fragrant, pleasantly bitter brew that is reputed to be mildly aphrodisiac.

DILL TEA is said to be slightly sedative, and an aid to digestion. Steep 1/2 teaspoon dill seeds in 1 cup boiling water 10 minutes.

ELDER TEA has long been used to soothe nerves and cleanse the blood. Teas can be made from either the flowers or berries.

FENNEL TEA is also reputed to help the digestion, increase mother's milk, and be sedative. Steep 1 teaspoon seeds in 1 cup boiling water.

FENUGREEK TEA has been used since ancient times, and is supposed to be good for the digestion, colds, sinus troubles and fevers. Steep 1 teaspoon seeds in 2 cups boiling water.

GINGER TEA is made by steeping fresh or dried ginger root in boiling water for a pleasant spicy brew which is supposed to be useful for nausea and indigestion. It warms in cool or damp weather, too.

GOLDENROD TEA made from the dried flowers is recommended for ulcers, kidney problems, exhaustion, colds and fatigue. Boil 1 teaspoon dried flowers for 1 minute, steep for 15 and strain.

HOREHOUND TEA is a remedy for colds, coughs and asthma. When brewed very strong it can be laxative. 1 teaspoon leaves should be steeped in 2 cups boiling water for 20 minutes. One recipe for a bedtime tea calls for 1 cup horehound tea with a dash of cayenne and a teaspoon of vinegar, sweetened to taste with honey.

LEMON GRASS TEA is a delightful drink hot or iced. West Indian natives spice their brew with a clove or two.

(continued on page 300)

How Herbs Can Make You Sleep Better

by Dian Dincin Buchman

"I often think this insomnia business is about 90 per cent nonsense," said Stephen Leacock. "When I was a young man living in a boarding house in Toronto, my brother George came to visit me, and since there was no spare room, we had to share my bed. In the morning, after daylight, I said to George, 'Did you get much sleep?' 'Not a damn minute,' said he. 'Neither did I,' I rejoined. 'I could hear every sound all night.' Then we put our heads up from the bedclothes and saw that the bed was covered with plaster. The ceiling had fallen on us in the night, but we hadn't noticed it. We had 'insomnia.' "

□ Leacock was one of the many people who only think they don't sleep; but for people who actually toss and turn the whole night through, there are true physical manifestations. The skin on the face feels saggy and heavy, and lacks tone. Their eyes are bleary and baggy, and their entire body feels dull. On the other hand a good night's sleep produces a feeling of well-being, freshness and physical energy.

□ Many people have excellent sleeping habits and only stay awake on the rare occasions when they have something profoundly worrying on their mind, or have eaten too late or overeaten. Anxiety, cold feet, poor breathing habits and bad circulation are specific causes of sleeplessness. I number quite a few insomniacs among my closest friends, and if they have a single common denominator it is that they are all clever and creative people who cannot, or will not, let their minds stop working. They all say they hate not sleeping, but they won't give up the pleasures of staying up late into the night talking, reading or thinking. Basically they are night people, and they actually wake up physically and psychologically later in the day than other people. I suppose none of them would go along with the adage that "one hour's sleep before midnight is worth three after."

Physical and Mental Relaxers

□ There is no reason for this sort of insomnia, for there are ways to retrain the too active mind. Before going to bed, do a little bit of exercise—some stretching at least; get into a full warm tub, or for a real surprise, a cold foot bath, or sitz bath; and pop into bed *without drying*. Take any one of the nightcap herbal teas in the next section, and start breathing deeply. Deep breathing or deep yawning will make your body feel heavy and languid.

□ Breathe deeply 3 or 4 times and then hold in the last breath as long as you possibly can, and repeat this action several times. Then, as your body and mind begin to feel drowsy, a touch of autosuggestion. Lie down on your back; slowly and precisely concentrate on your feet, and say to yourself, "My feet are heavy, they feel heavy." Slowly think of each part of your body in the same way. Your legs are heavy, your thighs are heavy, your stomach, your chest, your arms are heavy, heavy, heavy. You feel as if you are floating on water, but now your body is too heavy for you even to lift your arms, your fingers, your wrists. Then mentally make your neck heavy—and then your lips, your nose, your eyes, your head. If you have thoroughly concentrated (and learning this intense concentration sometimes takes a little time), you

can fall asleep immediately. But if you find that you are even slightly awake, lie in a comfortable position, preferably with your entire body serenely relaxed, and lift your right foot. Tense it and relax it suddenly. Do the same with your left foot. Lift your right hand. Clench it. Drop it suddenly. Do the same with your left hand. Now tighten your face in a grimace—make an ugly face. Relax it. Give in to the heaviness of your body, if necessary making each part of your body heavy again.

□ If you are still resisting—and it *is* a matter of resisting—try mentally writing the number 3—*slowly*. Do this as slowly as you can 3 times, and you should be fast asleep seconds later.

Relaxing Baths

□ Since relaxed sleep is one of the keys to good health and good looks, all the great herbalist-healers are preoccupied with sleeping aids. Father Kneipp tells of his successful water cures.

□ Take a cold, 1-to-3-minute foot bath with water up to the calves. According to Father Kneipp, this will "cure fatigue and produce sound and wholesome sleep."

□ Another suggested bath is the cold 3-to-5 minute semi-bath, either kneeling in the water so that the thighs are covered, or sitting in cold water which reaches to the pit of the stomach. Father Kneipp claims that these last two semi-baths are valuable and useful in that they have a great effect on the digestion and intestines. "It serves to regulate circulation, expel unhealthy gases, and make the body impervious to catching colds." These two baths will not only help you to fall asleep, but can be taken to advantage after a bad night's rest.

□ Father Kneipp insists that the body should *not* be dried with a towel. Just get straight into a warm bed and dry in your night clothes, or if the idea of that upsets you, jump into bed with a lot of towels wrapped round you. If bathing in the early morning, put your clothes on straight away and exercise until your body temperature returns to normal.

Aids to Sleep

Foods

□ Calcium and vitamin D are nature's most readily available nightcaps. Warm a glass of whole or skim milk and add a tablespoon of honey and you have an old-fashioned sleeping potion. The calcium tranquillizes and the honey helps the body to retain fluids, thus keeping the kidneys from alerting you during the night. Honey can be used in any herbal tea. Nutritionists also suggest taking 2 tablets of calcium. Personally, I like calcium with magnesium.

Herbs

□ Most of the following herbs can be used as nightcap teas. Add 1 teaspoon to a glass of boiling water, steep and strain. Add honey if you like, particularly if getting up frequently to pass water is a problem. Most tea herbs can be extracted with 15 minutes of steeping, but if the time is longer it will be noted.

(continued on page 301)

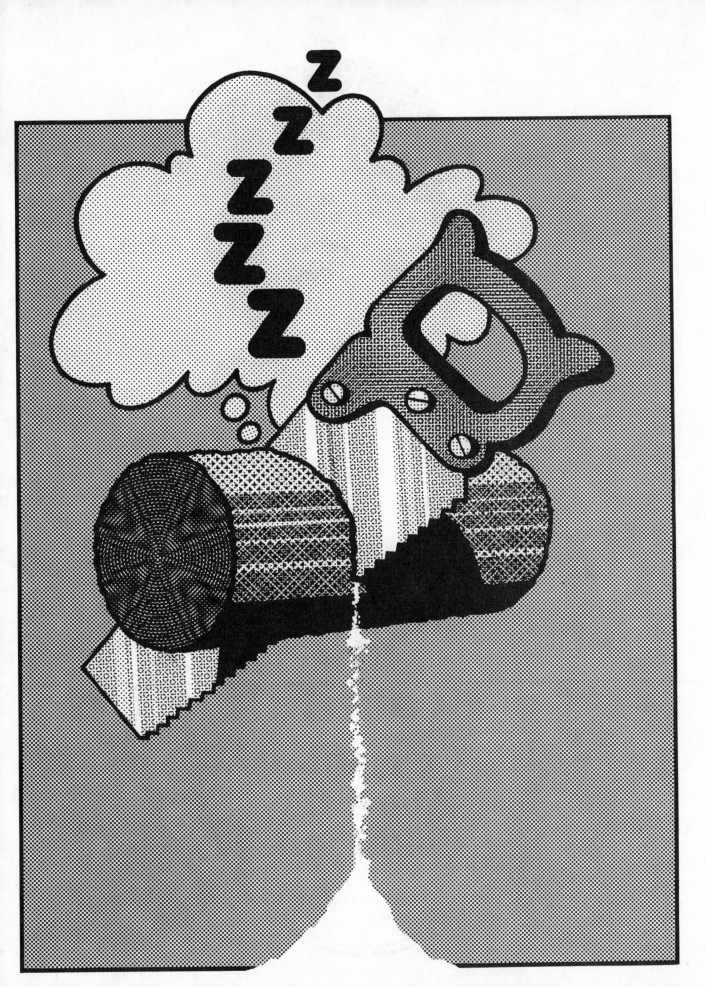

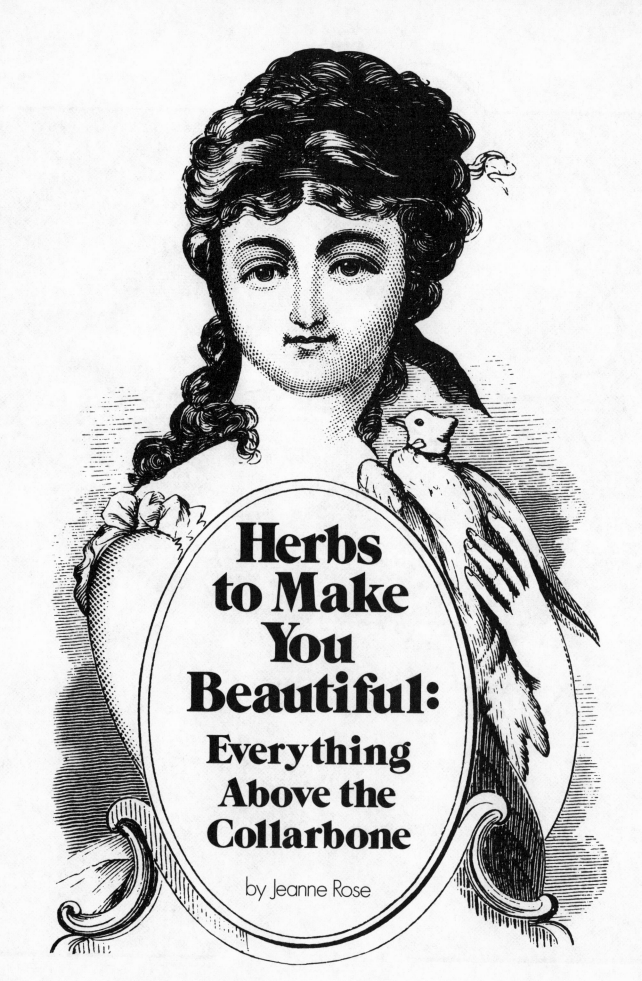

Herbs to Make You Beautiful:
Everything Above the Collarbone

by Jeanne Rose

Do your *eyebrows* stick up, act unruly, and need shine? Make a little southernwood oil and use it twice a day as a gloss and strengthener. You can also use this oil to stimulate your *eyelashes* to grow thick and long. But put the oil only on the eyelash and not the eyelids. Try applying it with a cotton-wrapped toothpick. A long-standing folk remedy to stimulate eyelashes to grow is to rub them daily with castor oil or olive oil and use a thick decoction of Sage to darken them and make them less unruly.

Ice cold milk is used in many ways in herbal cosmetics, as an ingredient in more complicated formulas and also by itself. Lie down, dip cotton balls in icy milk and apply the balls to *swollen eyelids*. For *tired eyes, red eyes, puffy eyes* try different herbal concoctions. Some of the best are: for toning, a compress of Comfrey leaf followed by a vitamin E eye pat; for refreshing, soak Cucumber slices in fresh raw milk, lie down, and apply the slices to your eyes; to reduce puffiness, make some ordinary tea extra strong, refrigerate it (add honey if you like), chill the tea bags, and apply them as a compress and drink the tea, the tannin in the tea is nicely astringent; for reducing bags and dark circles try a thin slice of Casaba Melon or Pear under each eye while taking a ten-minute rest, or juice some Parsley in a juicer, add a teaspoon of instant Ginseng to a tablespoon of the Parsley and a bit of mucilage or jello to hold it together and apply this to the eye area while taking a rest. Do it whenever and how often you deem necessary; *puffy eyes* can also be greatly helped by raising the head of your bed a few inches off the floor; this prevents excess body fluid from accumulating in the loose tissue around the eye. Sleep on your back with a small pillow only under the neck and start your mornings with a compress of milk, tea, Lavender, or Cucumber. For *watering eyes,* wash them often with decoctions of Fennel roots, Parsley, Betony, Comfrey root or leaves, honey and Rue or Chervil. Fennel seed water is also good for *tired eyes* as a compress, wash, or drops. For nourishing *tired eyes* try Apple compress; fresh raw sliced Potatoes are terrific for *circles* and *bags*. Whenever using herbal remedies, do make and use your ingredients as quickly as possible; it wouldn't be good at all to introduce any infection where there had been none before by using herbal waters made the day before yesterday. So make Fennel seed water now and use it now or, at best, refrigerate it only overnight. *Eyes* are also benefited by a decoction of Golden Seal and Eyebright as an eyewash or compress.

As for those store-bought eye creams that cost a fortune, the very finest are made at home. Formulate an eye cream for that fragile thin skin around the eye. Try

Super Emollient Cream

1 ounce lanolin	enough vitamin E capsules
1/2 ounce Almond oil	to supply 2500
1/2 ounce Apricot kernel oil	units

Melt the lanolin in a tiny pan, add the oils and put up in a tiny jar. Gently massage this cream into the area around the eyes to reduce those lines and wrinkles. Remember that persistence will pay off here, so don't give up after a week has elapsed saying that it didn't work for you. If you are lazy, pierce a vitamin E capsule and use the oil directly on the wrinkles.

For *sty in the eye,* wash with California poppy water or warm buttermilk or very weak salted water.

Tiny *broken veins* or *thread veins* will respond well to various herbs. There is absolutely no substitute for good food, rest, and exercise for encouraging a handsome complexion, so first increase vitamins P (permeability) and C; eat and drink lots of Violet leaf tea plus Orange peel (Violet leaf contains more C than Oranges), and then, when you eat the Oranges,

eat the white part under the skin also. Compresses of Marigolds, Coltsfoot, Witch Hazel, Parsley, Arnica, and Comfrey work well, especially combinations of these herbs such as Marigold and Comfrey or Parsley juice and Violet leaves. Use these latter combinations both inside as a tea and outside as a compress.

Your *nose* is often neglected and usually has enlarged dirty pores around the nostrils. Make an egg white mask with a drop or two of Lemon juice to tighten the pores of the nose and degrease the oily areas on the face. Naturally you will start with a facial steam or at least a clean face. Apply the egg white/Lemon juice with a small clean paint brush and let the mask dry on the nose. Rinse with warm water, then splash with seltzer or mineral water and pat dry. You can also use the gritty insides of an Avocado peel as a cleansing exfoliant. The water from boiled Lemon and Orange peels is useful for a *red nose*.

Freckles and blemishes are considerably diminished with a Horseradish-buttermilk wash. Just grate 1 tablespoon of Horseradish into 2 or 3 tablespoons of buttermilk and let it infuse for 2 or 3 hours, then strain and apply.

Upper lip wrinkles and upper lip lines can be helped with a Papaya "milk" exfoliation followed by an application of vitamin E as a moisturizer.

Cold sores are soothed with an astringent mixture of Alum root water that has had tincture of Camphor added to it.

Lips are tender and delicate, and mixtures of vitamins C, E, lanolin, and Camphor work well on them if they are dry or chapped.

Chapped Lips

Melt 2 teaspoons beeswax with 4 teaspoons of Apricot oil and ½ teaspoon of Camphor. Stir until the Camphor is dissolved and pour into a small jar. Use whenever necessary. Most chapped lips recipes are just variations on this same theme.

Chapped Lips #2

Beeswax 4 ounces, Camphor 2 tablespoons, melted together with 5 ounces Olive oil and 1 tablespoon glycerin. Beat until cold.

Chapped Lips #3,
More Complicated

Macerate together with the back of a wooden spoon in a small nonmetal pan ¼ ounce each of gum Benzoin, Storax, a chopped red Apple, a small bunch of black Grapes, 4 ounces sweet butter. Add 2½ ounces beeswax and simmer until the wax is melted, and everything is well mixed. Strain out the solids and discard them and beat the remainder until cool. Grease a muffin tin and spoon the mixture into the tin. Then store away for future use.

Cinnamon Toothpowder

1/2 ounce chalk	2 teaspoons powdered
1/2 ounce cuttlefish bone	Peruvian bark
	2 teaspoons Orris root

Mix all together and sift through a fine sieve. This may be colored with Beet juice and scented with a few drops oil of Cinnamon.

A Receipt to Clean the Teeth and Gums,
and Make the Flesh Grow Close
to the Root of the Enamel

Take an ounce of Myrrh in fine powder, two spoonfuls of the best white Honey, and a little green Sage in fine powder; mix them well together, and rub the teeth and gums with a little of this Balsam every night and morning.

—*The Toilet of Flora, 1779*

(continued on page 302)

Herbs are in fashion, as evidenced by the many new books and articles written about them, by the increase of specialist herb shops, and even by the new concern for more natural medicines to avoid the over-use of modern drugs. The demand for herbs of every kind is growing—so why not grow herbs for profit?

Nearly everyone who has a garden, however small, grows some parsley, mint and chives for the kitchen, but even if you have never grown any herbs, they are easy to cultivate and make few demands on your time or available space.

Growing herbs to sell could become a profitable occupation or side line for the amateur gardener or the complete beginner, and especially for retired people keen on gardening, who could combine the pleasures with the added incentive of some income from the sales.

Herb growing and selling can be an all-the-year-round business if you own a greenhouse; the herbs can be sold either cut fresh in season, in pots for other growers and gardeners, green-dried in jars or bags. This means that surplus crops can always be used, for herbs must be cut at the right time, usually before flowering.

Herbs in winter
Some herbs are suitable for growing indoors or in a green-house to give a fresh supply in winter.
Parsley
Chives
Chervil (seeds to be sown in autumn)
Dill (seeds to be sown in autumn)

Fragrant herbs for gifts
Many specialist herb shops, gift shops and counters now sell a wide variety of fragrant products suitable for present giving; old-fashioned ideas revived such as lavender bags, herb sachets and pot-pourris. These two can be made at home then sold fresh or pre-dried:

Angelica	Costmary	Lemon Verbena
Anise	Dill	Peppermint
Basil	Eau de Cologne Mint	Rose Geranium
Bergamot	Lavender	Rosemary
Borage	Lemon Balm	Sage
Bowles Mint	Lemon Thyme	Tarragon
Coriander		

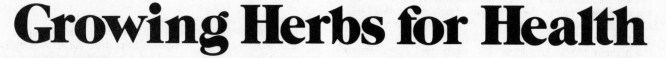

Growing Herbs for Health

You could succeed with more specialized sales such as large crops of thyme, sage or marjoram for supplying to local butchers and sausage makers, who use these herbs in fairly large quantities. Your best plan would be to dry the herbs at home and crush them for packing into containers, which should be made of glass or plastic with screw-top lids. You could then come to an arrangement with your buyer to return the empties for re-use.

Dried herbs keep best if not exposed to light, so the jars will need a large masking label and these can be an attractive selling feature, perhaps especially printed with your name on them.

There are herbs for many different purposes. The main group is for cooking. Some of them are known and used regularly by the public; others are seldom grown or sold but are nevertheless wonderful flavoring herbs, used for centuries on the continent.

Familiar kitchen herbs
Parsley	Thyme	Rosemary
Mint	Garlic	Marjoram
Chives	Basil	Tarragon
Sage	Dill	Fennel

Less known flavors
Chervil	Summer Savory	Caraway
Lemon Balm	Sweet Cicely	Coriander
Salad Burnet	Welsh Onion	Lovage

Herbs for special purposes
There are also herbs which can be used for summer drinks, cake decorations and jam making.
Angelica	Bowles Mint	Marigold
Anise	Coriander	Nasturtium
Borage	Peppermint	Rose Geranium

Pot-pourris
Some of the flowers needed for petals to provide scent and color to the mixtures will already be growing in the garden.
Chamomile flowers	Pansies
Cornflowers	Roses
Marigold petals	Verbascum flowers
Nasturtium flowers	

Should you decide to specialize in any of the suggested groups of herbs it is advisable to start by growing just a few of as many varieties as possible. In this way you will discover which herbs do best in your locality and in your garden, both from the selling and cultivation points of view. Once your herb plants and your reputation are established you can gradually start to specialise in the herb group of your choice.

Some herbs, the annuals, have to be sown and can be started in boxes or pots in the greenhouse, in cold frames or under cloches for later transplanting. Otherwise, the seeds are sown at the appropriate time in their permanent positions in the herb garden or beds, and thinned out.

Herbs for sowing
Anise	Chervil	Parsley
Basil	Coriander	Summer Savory
Borage	Dill	Sweet Marjoram
Caraway	Garlic (bulblets)	

Flowers for sowing
Chamomile	Nasturtium
Cornflowers	Pansies
Marigold	Verbascum

Herbs to be planted
Other herbs, the perennials and biennials, can be bought

(continued on page 303)

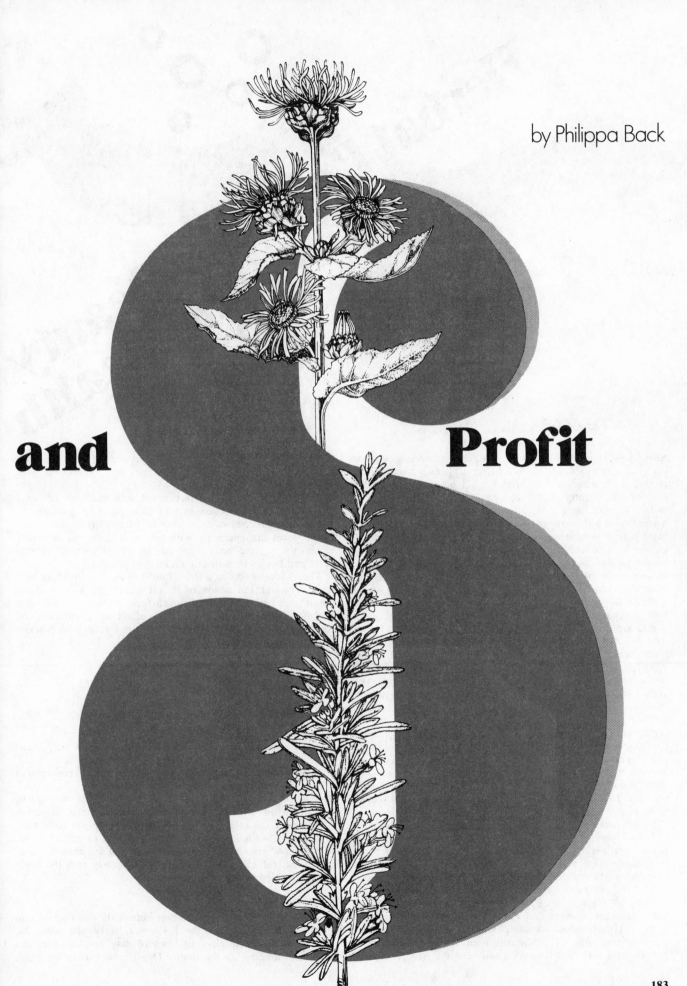

by Philippa Back

and Profit

Herbal Baths for Beauty and Health

by Jeanne Rose

Some years ago I had a lovely little house overlooking the ocean. Every month of the year different plants were in bloom around it. Electricity and plumbing had not yet reached that part of the country, but I did have gas and therefore hot water. My bathtub was outside overlooking the ocean next to a giant rock with moss growing on its side and a huge century plant acting as sentinel on top. The tub was painted purple on the outside and an old arbor of wild lilac overhung the whole bathing enclosure. I would attach the garden hose to the hot water heater and fill the tub full of hot water. Herbs from my garden and rose petals were added next. Ah, what a delightful sensuous experience, particularly when it was a little foggy or during a slight drizzle.

Bathing should be one of the most pleasurable acts of your day. What could be more relaxing than sitting in a tubful of warm water, full of the delicate aroma of healthful herbs. Keep some green growing plants in your bathroom. They inhale stale carbon dioxide and exhale oxygen, leaving you with a pleasant atmosphere for bathing. Turn on your stereo. Purchase a luffa and use it as a daily scrub for your body to remove old dried scales of skin. Keep several bottles of different kinds of herbs around for different kinds of experiences—pine if you like a forest; a combination of rosemary and lavender if the scent near the ocean is what you prefer; jasmine if you like the feel of a warm tropical evening. They smell beautiful and perform the important function of smoothing and hydrating the skin, leaving it looking and feeling younger.

Some botanicals act as astringents, tightening the poor old tired pores; others act as diaphoretics, opening up the pores to allow more perspiration and waste matter, from a particularly hard day, to escape. Some are used at spas to help in weight reduction. They are used to help one to sleep or to help one to wake; to relieve itchy skin; to nourish the bosom; to relax a tense back—to do just about anything that you want them to do. There are hundreds of combinations. Various scents stimulate various senses and various parts of the body. The Romans used mints for the arms, lemon grass for the sebaceous glands and the hair, camomile for the eyes, bergamot for sleep, and orange for the entire skin surface. Try some of my recipes and experiment with combinations of your own.

The surface of the skin is covered with hundreds of vents called pores that function as tiny little pipes or passages to allow accumulated waste matter to escape from the body. If the pores are encrusted with dirt or oil, the waste matter cannot escape; the body loses one of its main excretory surfaces and begins to suffocate on its own poisons.

The skin also acts as a line of defense against invading bacteria. Through the action of its oil glands the skin is lubricated and protected against surface bacteria. The skin breathes for us and has a salutary effect on circulation and metabolism. Thus it is important that one learn and practice the genteel art of bathing.

How to Take a Herbal Bath
Hot Baths are enervating.
Warm Baths are pleasant.
Cold Baths are stimulating.

Method 1. *The Longest and Most Luxurious Method*
1. Take a minimum of ½ cup herbs and simmer in 1 quart of water in a covered nonmetal pot for 10-20 minutes.
2. While the herbs are simmering take a quick shower or a soap and water bath to remove the surface dirt.
3. When you are through with your quick bath or shower, fill the tub with warm or hot water. Strain the decoction and pour the herb liquid into the tub. Wrap the solid residue in a washcloth and tie with a ribbon or rubber band.
4. Step into your tub and soak for at least 20 minutes, read a book, relax, and rub your body vigorously with the herbs that are tied in the washcloth.

Method 2.
Put a large handful of whatever botanicals you choose into the bathtub and turn on the hot water. Read and soak. Be careful of this method: your landlord may not like the idea of herbs clogging up the drain. This is not always the case,

however; usually they collect near the drain and can be scooped out when you are finished bathing.

Method 3. *This method is most useful to men who don't like the idea of soaking in a tub.*

Place a large handful of herbs in 2 cups of boiling water in a covered nonmetal container. Simmer for 10-20 minutes. Strain. Take a soap and water shower. When through, wrap the solid matter in a washcloth and rub the body vigorously. Use the liquid as a rinse after the shower and the rub. This is very invigorating and an easy method to use when you don't have much time.

Method 4.

Wrap a large handful of herbs in a cloth bag and tie securely. Place the bag right into the bath water, or tie it onto the spout of the bathtub or onto the head of the shower and let the hot water run through it.

Method 5. *Vapor Method*

1. Mix a little coconut oil, olive oil, or almond oil with water.
2. Plug an electric frying pan or vaporizer into a bathroom outlet.
3. Add the oil and water mixture to the pan and drop in some fresh flower petals and scented botanicals—roses, bay leaf, eucalyptus, lemon grass, or a little of any of the recipes that follow. (You can add a little of your favorite perfume instead of the herbs. Men might use rosemary, thyme, or mint.) Keep the bathroom door closed and sit in your warm bath. The steam will rise, perfuming the air and steaming your skin clean of impurities.

Some Recipes

Ninon Bath Herbs

Ninon de Lenclos, properly Anne de Lanclos, was born in 1620 and died eighty-five years later after having lived an exciting and scandalous life as a French courtesan, epicurean, and confidante to such literate men as Moliere. She was a celebrated beauty. Her body retained its youthful curves, her skin remained moist and smooth for all of her eighty-five years. Her beauty secrets were many and varied but the one she felt to be most important was her daily herbal bath:

Mix together thoroughly one handful each of dried or fresh lavender flowers, rosemary, mint, crushed comfrey root, and thyme. Pour a quart of boiling water over the mixture, cover, and steep for 20 minutes. Pour the entire contents into your bathtub and soak for at least 20 minutes. For a nice variation, add 1 handful of rosebuds or celandine.

Dawn Bath

This herbal preparation leaves the skin with an overall delicious smell. Mix together thoroughly all ingredients and add about 1 ounce to your bath.

3 large handfuls geranium leaf
1 handful strawberry leaf   ½ handful calamus
1 handful mint   1 T. benzoin
1 handful orange leaves   1 dropper rose geranium oil
1 handful camomile   1 dropper lemon oil

Milk Bath

This bath is for soaking, for smoothing dry, tired skin, and for general overall skin care. Simmer ½ cup barley in 1 quart of water for at least 3 hours. Mix together ¼ cup oatmeal, ¼ cup orris root, and ¼ cup almond meal and tie securely in a bag. Place the bag in your bath water and add to your tub 2-4 cups of milk and the cooking liquid from the barley.

A Sweet-Scented Bath

Take of Roses, Citron peel, Sweet flowers, Orange flowers, Jessamy, Bays, Rosemary, Lavender, Mint, Pennyroyal, of each a sufficient quantity, boil them together gently and make a Bath to which add Oyl of Spike six drops, musk five grains, Ambergris three grains.

—from *The Receipt Book of John Middleton,* 1734

Patchouli-Green Bath for Rejuvenation

3 ounces patchouli
3 ounces geranium leaf
2 ounces mint
2 ounces orange leaf
2 ounces sage
1 ounce strawberry leaf
1 ounce pennyroyal
1 ounce woodruff
1 ounce rosemary

Mix together all ingredients. Can be used as a sachet in your clothing or for 16 baths.

Green Bath I

Mix together ¼ cup of each: camomile, rosemary, verbena, white willow bark, geranium leaves, and lemon grass. This is enough for 2 baths. Very good for lazy, oily skin.

Green Bath II

For oily skin and for general aches and pains of the body. Mix together ¼ cup of each: strawberry leaves, mint, orange leaves, camomile, borage, pennyroyal, woodruff, passionflower herb, rosemary, patchouli. Add ½ cup geranium leaves and 1 dropper of rose geranium oil. Enough for 3-4 baths.

Field & Flower Bath

Mix together 1 cup lavender, ½ cup bitter orange peel, and ¼ cup of each of the following: thyme, raspberry leaf, wild rose leaf, white willow bark, borage, mint, woodruff, rosemary, sage. Add a few crushed cloves, some calamus, 1 dropper oil of petitgrain, and a little lemon. Enough for 4-5 baths.

(continued on page 303)

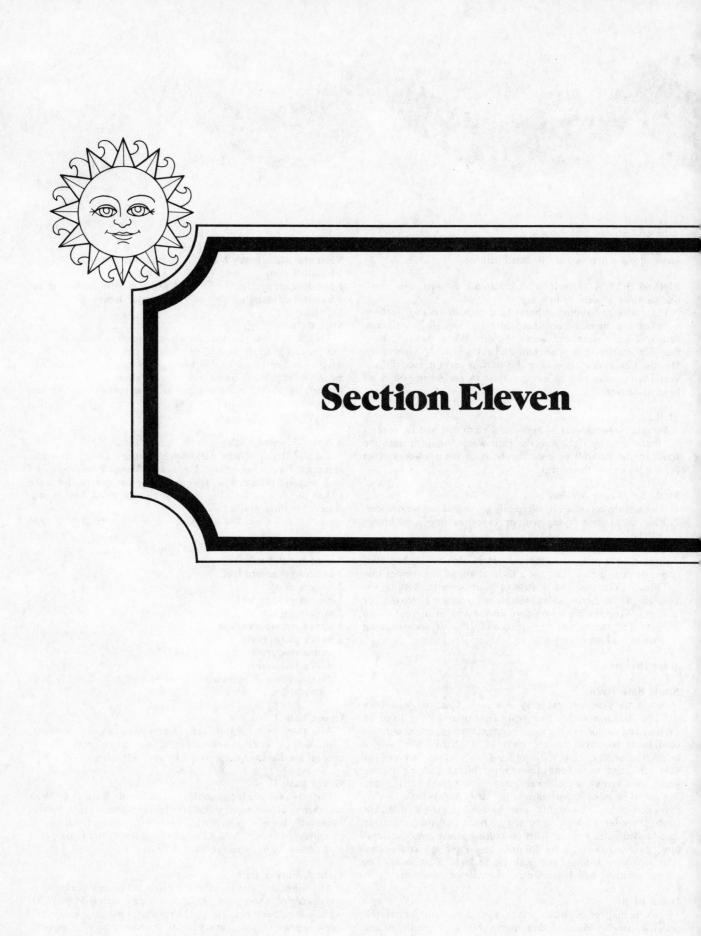

Section Eleven

Exercises
for the Serious
and
Not-So-Serious

For the sitting ducks: sedentary secretaries, tense typists and others

An eight to five sit-down job may be deleterious to health and body fitness. To spend many hours in a fixed sitting position can cause unused muscles to lose elasticity and tone. The body relaxes, muscles sag, bulges appear, the much talked about secretary spread develops. Women holding sedentary jobs, such as school teachers, telephone operators, secretaries, and executives are faced with a constant fitness problem. And the longer they hold down a job without some sort of activity, the more their bodies will soften. Working over a desk with improper posture is number one cause of round shoulders, dowager's hump (on the back of the neck), and double chins. Tenseness and fatigue develop as muscles become taut and strained. The internal organs also get their share of mistreatment; lungs are not fully utilized; digestion and bowel function are impaired. Tension headaches come with eye strain and bad fluorescent lighting. As a result of sitting on chairs where the feet do not touch the floor, varicosities may develop; blood circulation is cut off by the edge of the chair, causing the blood to pool in the veins. Sitting in a chair constantly, women also develop saddle-bag thighs, protruding abdomens, and flat, flabby buttocks. Once the muscles lose efficiency, one has to work twice as hard to restore strength and tone.

Taking your problems home
Most career women are not through work when the clock strikes five. Very few have the opportunity to come home and prop their feet up and relax. Some have families to feed and children to chauffeur, others housework and personal duties. It seems the circle never stops. The standard lament of the working girl seems to be that she is tired all the time. Faced with any physical or mental stress on the job, the ordinarily energetic woman finds that her energy wanes early in the day. For stress quickly depletes the body's natural store of vitamins and minerals. The end result may well be extreme fatigue or depression by the time she is ready to face her tasks at home. When she is in this condition, the only way to restore health and body fitness is through proper diet and exercise coupled with a good natural vitamin and mineral supply.

Exercises For The Career Girl or One Whose Day Is Sedentary
by Barbara Hegne, Illustrated by Lois Zener Amsler

Replenishing the body's store of nutrients
Start your day with a good breakfast. Skipping this particular meal is a common mistake of many dieters. The body has been fasting all night and needs energy foods to break-the-fast in the morning. Drinking coffee all morning stimulates the blood sugar level to super-high; then it falls sharply, leaving its victim in a weak, irritable mood. Replace the coffee habit with a hot nutritional drink available at most health food stores. Take your vitamins with breakfast, they will give you a powerful store of energy to draw from all day long. B-complex, calcium, and magnesium (dolomite) will calm your nerves and give you a boost of energy to rid you of the tired feeling at the end of the day. If you are a smoker you will need extra vitamin C. Smoking destroys vitamin C. If there are smokers around you, your intake of their exhaled smoke is about half as much as the actual smoker. So you will need extra C. It is wise to buy natural C chewables and keep them on your desk. At break time, instead of coffee, drink fruit juices: apple, grape or grapefruit. These natural drinks add to rather than take away from body substances.

Getting your body together
The ability to withstand stress and tension is greatly reduced by physical inactivity. A few specialized exercises daily will improve your figure, your mental attitude, and your general health.

Miracle Stretch 1
A good exercise that can be done at work sitting at your desk or home. This exercise should be done at the first sign of tenseness or fatigue. Lace your fingers together and stretch out in front of your body, stretch your legs out at the same time with toes pointed. Now stretch up toward the ceiling, separat-

ing each vertebra in the spine. Relax and stretch again. Think of yourself as a rubber band stretching and relaxing 10 times. The feeling derived from the Miracle Stretch is one of complete body rejuvenation head to toe. Circulation is greatly improved and energy stimulated.

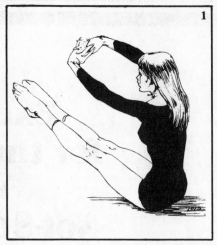

Spreading thighs and buttocks 2
Here is a wonderful exercise that slims hips, thighs and buttocks: Get down on your hands and knees, keep your hands in a direct line with your knees. Lift your bent knee up to the side (hip level). Then kick your leg to the rear (toe

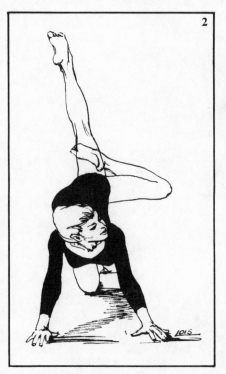

pointed). Bring it back to the side and down. Alternate each leg until you have completed 10 leg kicks to each side.

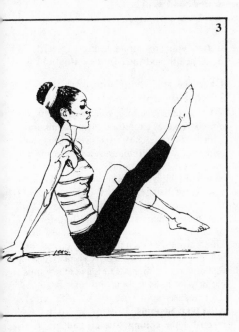

Firming flabby tummy muscles 3
This is a good tummy firmer you can do according to your own ability. Sit down and begin by extending both legs forward as you lean back slightly. Beginners or those with back problems should not lean way back. Veteran exercisers can really stretch the body out, putting maximum strain on the abdominal muscles. Do 10 stretches.

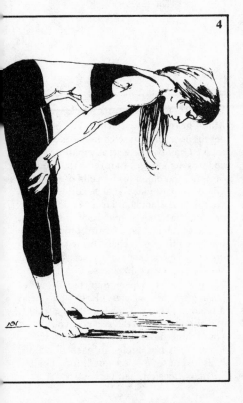

Digestion and elimination exercise 4
This exercise will gently massage internal organs so they can function properly on their own.
Bend over, place your hand on your knees and let all air out of your lungs in one big breath. Pull your tummy muscles in as far as possible. Think of pulling abdomen to spinal cord. Now move the abdominal muscles in and out 3 times while you are holding your breath out. Inhale deeply. Rest for 1 minute and repeat exercise 1 more time. It is very important that you exhale all air out before contracting abdominal muscle.

Waistline and midriff bulge 5
Get down on your knees, keep your back very straight. Lean directly over to the side and try to touch the floor beside your knee, then change to touch the opposite side. Repeat this movement rapidly side to side. If it is easy to touch fingers to the floor, make a fist and touch knuckles. Repeat 10 touches to each side.

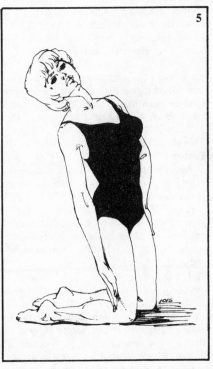

Heart, lungs and circulatory system
All sedentary workers should combine calisthenics with aerobics. Aerobics includes any activity employing the cardiovascular and cardiorespiratory systems. A person can be in top physical condition by exercising and become exhausted climbing stairs or hills when some sort of aerobics has not been added to the program. The main purpose of aerobics is to bring more oxygen into the body for utilization, which in turn increases stamina and endurance.

Some aerobics are:

Brisk walking
Brisk walking is good for persons of all ages since energy expenditure depends on your speed.
Benefits: improves breathing and blood circulation, and relieves tenseness.

Swimming
Swimming is one of the best forms of exercise; it greatly improves strength, endurance, and stamina. Swimming also burns many calories and improves lung and breathing capacity.

Tennis
Tennis increases muscular endurance, strengthens legs, improves coordination. The effect on heart and lungs will depend on the vigor with which you play.

Rope skipping
Rope skipping improves coordination and cardiovascular fitness along with firming arms, shoulders, back, and legs.

Bicycling
Bicycling is a good exercise both physically and mentally. A blend of body fitness and taking in the great outdoors, bicycling improves blood circulation, relieves tenseness, and strengthens back and leg muscles. Lung and heart functions are greatly improved.

Health and body tips for the office worker
Glance away from your work occasionally to reduce eye strain. If there is a window available, gaze out at the sky or horizon. A few seconds' change can eliminate the buildup of tension and headaches. Natural lighting is always the best when available. Change sitting positions regularly. Practice the Miracle Stretch often. Do not sit with one leg crossed over the other at the knee joint and take a chance of cutting off blood circulation. To cross at the ankles is better.
If your job requires many hours of writing or typing, stop and flick your fingers rapidly. Shrug your shoulders up and down. Drop your head to your chest and let it hang for a few seconds. Do not stifle a yawn. This is a natural facial relaxer and nature's way of helping you.

It's worth it
Health and fitness are a delicate combination easily lost through carelessness. But by making a modest effort you can retain your youthful figure and precious health. Be the first one to start a health campaign in your group. You will be greatly admired by fellow workers and happily surprised when they ask to join you. ☼

Exercise is for everyone. Of course aging is inevitable, but keeping the body fit and healthy will increase longevity and give an extra zest for living. Men and women regardless of age need some form of daily activity. With the passing years the body naturally slows down a little. Metabolic activity wanes along with other body functions. You may begin to notice a few aches and pains, decreased energy, numb fingers or cold toes from faulty circulation, and a distressingly sluggish system affecting digestive and bowel function. Some have a tendency to accept passively these changes as unavoidable consequences of aging. It seems easier to slip into a sedentary life style than bother with the vigorous tyranny of exercise. Perhaps a few good tries have ended up in disappointment for the senior citizen who shows up enthusiastically at the local gym and is met by stares from the younger generation. Yes, it may all seem pretty dire at that point and you may wonder, why bother?

Let's tackle the challenge of exercising and decide for ourselves if it is worth the effort. After all, we *are* interested in ourselves and our well-being.

Benefits

Statistics prove that persons who exercise have fewer heart attacks than do the inactive. Exercise reduces cholesterol levels, increases lung efficiency, helps prevent blood clots, improves circulation, tones and firms muscles, slims the body, alleviates tensions and helps produce sound sleep. The daily habit of activity can stimulate the brain and beautify the body and give you health in abundance.

Your doctor's check-up

These benefits are indeed inspiring. What more can we possibly hope for? Getting started is the first step and it is a must to have a doctor's check-up before starting any physical exercise program or sport. Your doctor will check your blood pressure, heart and probably do some lab work. Let him be the judge of how strenuous your program should be. After he gives you the go-ahead begin right away.

Take it easy

If you have not had previous body conditioning or you are a beginner to the wonderful world of exercise, start slowly and do only 2 or 3 repetitions of each exercise. Increase to 10 as your body becomes conditioned and strengthened.

Breathing

Proper breathing is of utmost importance through all of the exercises. You may think you are breathing correctly and find you are breathing shallow. Proper breathing and breath control will add years to your life.

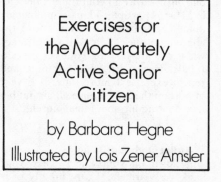

Exercises for the Moderately Active Senior Citizen

by Barbara Hegne
Illustrated by Lois Zener Amsler

Inhale deeply the air that purifies the blood circulating through your body. Learn to utilize all your lung space. Inhale through your nose, fill your diaphragm (located between the rib cage) and let it expand with fresh air. Then, exhale long and slowly, getting all the stale air out. If this seems hard for you or you have been used to incorrect breathing, it may be difficult to break the habit of shallow breathing. Try this simple technique to help acquaint you with your respiration muscles.

Lie down and relax your muscles. Now place a 2 or 3 pound weight or book on your diaphragm. As you inhale, concentrate on pushing out and lifting the weight up slightly. Fill all of your lungs. When exhaling, the weight will lower slowly. This should be a smooth controlled motion.

Posture

Another desirable preparation for exercising is good posture. Good posture creates more lung space, keeps the spine in perfect alignment and corrects sagging organs. Stand tall, chest forward, shoulders squared, back straight and chin lifted slightly. You will immediately notice a sense of well-being.

Don't overdo it

Anxious as you may be to start, a word of caution must prevail. To overdo will cause sore muscles and slow down or stop your exercise program before it gets underway. A sore muscle is theoretically caused when metabolic waste (lactic acid) stays in the muscles after exercise or heavy sport and causes pain. The pain may not show up until the second or even third day after activity. Muscle soreness is characterized by a tight, stiff painful feeling when you move. If through over-enthusiasm you unconsciously overdo it, you can alleviate muscle soreness by continued light activity coupled with hot water or sauna baths. It is a great temptation to remain stationary, but to "work out" the soreness is best.

Ready now!

Try these exercises, designed especially for the moderately active person. Once started you are bound to find rewards in body health and total fitness. Begin now.

Exercise #1 Stretching and Limbering up

Why stretch? Before you advance to the more strenuous exercises, always limber up with a few stretches first. Stretching will improve your circulation and warm the muscles, consequently lessening the chance of injury. Stretching also produces a sense of balance and co-ordination. Almost anyone can do a few stretches. And they can be done while doing housework, brushing your teeth or watching television. Don't sit idle: stretch those toes, circle your ankle, exercise your face. A wonderful and fast tension remover is to tense every muscle in your body tight as a rubber band and then release all at once. You'll feel great.

All Over Stretch. Lift up on your toes, reach for the ceiling, stretch and lift. Pretend you are climbing a ladder. Do this limbering-up exercise at least 1 to 3 minutes to get the circulation going.

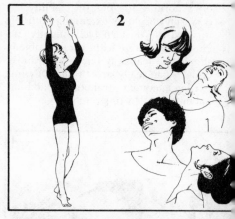

Exercise #2 Face and Neck

Make gravity your friend. The older we get the more the muscles in the facial area relax. Gravity is constantly pulling down and it is a good idea to reverse the process, bringing the blood to the cells of the face. One way is to place your head lower than your feet. A slant board is a wonderful aid, or place one end of your ironing board up on the couch and lie down feet higher than head. If sitting in a chair, bring your head down by your knees. Raise your head slowly to prevent dizziness.

Head Circles. Open your mouth wide, tensing facial muscles. Roll your head around slowly in a big circle to the left. When you come to the center, gently push your chin massagingly into your chest. Continue 5 big circles in each direction. This exercise is also good for shoulder stiffness, tension, and headaches.

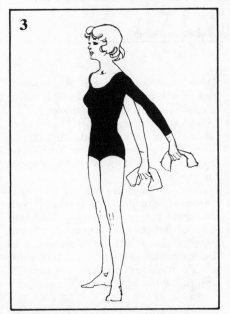

3

Exercise #3 Underarm Area

Source of embarrassment. Flabby underarms are a more common problem for women than for men, perhaps because of different occupations and muscle-building factors. Women have more adipose (fatty) tissue than men and generally do not build the muscles in their arms or elsewhere in their bodies as men do. At any rate, whatever the reason, a flabby, baggy underarm can be a source of concern and embarrassment.

A few of these magic exercises presented here will put you back into sleeveless dresses for summer. Of course, this area is hard to correct and perseverance is the only answer.

Correction. Hold 2 to 3 pound weights or books in your hands. Stand with your feet together, your palms facing backward. Action: lift your arms slowly to the rear. Do not lean forward. Hold 30 seconds, release and repeat 5 times. Immediately, you will feel the benefits of this powerful exercise.

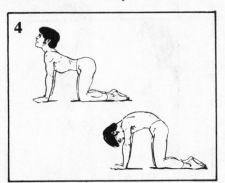

4

Exercise #4 The Back

Back problems. Many Americans develop back problems sometime in their lives. To some it is a temporary problem while others always suffer discomfort all their lives. Causes of back problems are numerous and individual causes vary. Lifting "too heavy" objects can throw the back

out of alignment as does poor posture and wearing extremely high-heeled shoes that tilt the body forward. Twisting rapidly to the side can cause unexpected injury and throw a vertebra out of place.

When exercising, always maintain smooth flowing movements, bend your knees while trying to touch your toes, and in doing sit-ups keep the knees bent to alleviate pressure on the lower spine. Remember your spine is the life bone of your body—protect it. The back arch presented here is an excellent exercise to keep the back limber and strengthen weak muscles.

Back Arch. Get down on your hands and knees. Action: arch your back up slowly toward the ceiling, drop your head down. Hold this position 30 seconds. Relax your back and look to the ceiling. Repeat entire exercise 8 times. Feel the warmth flood the spine as each vetebra is gently separated. This exercise is done smoothly and evenly.

Exercise #5 Mid-Section

Spare tire. Too many calorie-laden foods and not enough activity can cause a "spare tire" around the mid-section of your body. You may notice extra flab hanging over your trousers or skirt. That is the time to begin to firm sagging abdominal muscles. The "pot belly" detracts more from appearance than any other area. Wearing a girdle only pushes the fat somewhere else and pinches the organs.

Three-Fold Exercise. This three-fold exercise affecting abdomen, midriff, chest and arms requires light weights or books of approximately 2 to 3 pounds. You may hang your weights over a broomstick for extra leverage. Lie down flat, take your weights in each hand. Raise your arms slowly overhead until they almost touch the floor behind you. Now tighten the abdominal muscles and hold tight 30 seconds. Bring your arms to their original position. Relax for a few seconds, and repeat 5 times.

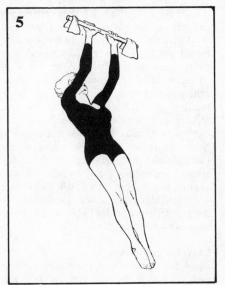

5

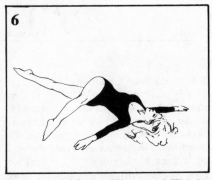

6

Exercise #6 Legs, Hips, and Thighs

Positive thinking helps. The mind can be a powerful tool to use while exercising. When you think of the area you are firming, you unconsciously work harder. Think small waistline, flat stomach, firm thighs. Think health and you will become healthy.

This exercise will slim the hips, improve circulation to the legs and massage internal organs. The digestive tract gets its exercise.

Leg Lifts. Lie down, arms outstretched for balance. Action: lift your right leg up and over trying to get as close to your left hand as possible. Keep hips on the floor. Lift left leg over to touch right hand. Repeat movements 6 times to each side.

Learn To Relax

It is a good idea to deliberately slow down on the last few exercises to normalize your breathing and pulse rate before continuing your day. Learn to relax after your exercise program as a delightful final touch. Take a few minutes to quiet your mind and bind together mind, spirit and body in perfect harmony. Revitalize your flow of energy, utilizing positive thinking in this ancient and proven method. Lie down on your back, stretch your arms above your head, tense your body tightly and then go limp all at once. Roll your head gently from side to side. Visualize each part of your body in your mind and relax it entirely. Begin with your toes, then ankles, calves, knees, thighs, even your spinal cord, picturing and relaxing each vertebra, your shoulder blades and finally your face. Be sure you do not create wrinkles on your face when you visualize. This should be an easy and effortless experience.

When you have relaxed your body, challenge your mind: disregard annoying thoughts flitting across your mental screen. Fashion your own scene, one of beauty that brings happiness and peace to you. A beautiful mountain, a picnic, clouds drifting overhead, happy thoughts. An easy example would be to think of your favorite flower. Picture it in detail. Smell its fragrance as you become oblivious to the outside world. Lie quietly for a few minutes. Then, while your eyes remain closed, stretch slowly like a cat, one arm, one leg, inhale deeply and open your eyes. You will feel completely refreshed. ☼

Why does your back ache?

Lower back pain seems to be as common as the cold, and just as miserable. Many persons from all walks of life are bothered with mild to severe back discomforts. Few are spared the ill-effects of a sore back caused by overstrain. Among the multitude of causes of lower back pain are improper posture, lack of activity, and weak abdominal and back supporting muscles. If you find yourself among the hordes of back sufferers who apply home remedies and find no relief, check with your doctor. After you have been examined and released with the diagnosis of having no serious medical ailment, take a close look at these three major causes of back pain.

Poor posture

Poor posture throws the spinal cord out of alignment with the rest of the body and places a tremendous strain on the back muscles. The muscles tense and tighten with the additional pressure causing muscle spasms and pain. Many people have poor posture and don't realize it. When they first experience a slight back pain, they distort their bodies to find immediate relief. The pain, usually a daily occurrence, leaves the unsuspecting victim in a quandary. Seemingly unaware, the poor back sufferer continues poor posture, hunched shoulders, spine curved, and head tilted, easy prey to re-occurring discomfort. The constant use of poor postural habits can ruin health, appearance, and happiness.

Weak muscles

The abdominal muscles help support the back. If they are flabby and weak, the whole load is thrown on the back. With this extra burden the back tenses and pains. Eventually, the back muscles lose strength and elasticity and chances of injury increase. Even a simple fall could result in permanent damage.

Lack of activity

Modern conveniences and easy living contribute to lessened activity. The backache syndrome is no respecter of age, and it is not uncommon to hear youngsters complain of back trouble. In school they might not begin sports or physical activity until later grades. Later, some allow the modern comforts throughout life to encourage inactivity. As they get older and take sedentary jobs, the back continues to suffer. It seems to be a life-time problem and

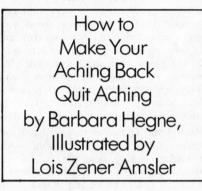

How to
Make Your
Aching Back
Quit Aching
by Barbara Hegne,
Illustrated by
Lois Zener Amsler

one that should be given special attention immediately.

Other causes

Obesity adds to back strain, especially when the person has a large protruding abdomen. This is why so many pregnant women complain constantly of lower back pain. As the baby develops, the mother tends to lean back and puts extra stress on the spinal cord.

Incorrect, tight-fitting shoes, including those with high heels cut off circulation and pinch nerves in the feet. They also tilt the body forward causing improper posture and strained back muscles.

Sleeping on a pillow and mattress too soft to support the body properly causes people to wake up in the morning with tension headaches, body aching and tired all over. A sad way to start the day.

Overstuffed chairs and deep soft sofas are luxurious to look at but detrimental to an already weakened back structure.

Detrimental exercises

It is indeed annoying to have a nagging backache regardless of the cause. To despair and concede that you are saddled with life-long back problems would be an unfortunate error. The best way to protect the health of your back is through daily exercise. Statistics prove athletes and sportsmen have less back trouble than the non-athletic person. Whether a person is athletic or not, exercises should be chosen carefully. Some exercises can be harmful. Exercise should not be competitive, nor should impossible goals be set. All programs should be based on individual abilities. Here are a few guidelines to help guard and protect your back while you are exercising.

Exercise guidelines

Bend the knees deeply when touching toes. No straight leg toe touches for back sufferers.

Do exercises, sports, and other activities slowly and with controlled movements. Avoid fast jerky motions.

Avoid straight leg sit ups. Bent knee sit ups are recommended. Leg raises from a lying down position can also be harmful. It is better to draw your knees to your chest first.

Your good judgment will tell you what exercises should not be done. If you feel great pain in your lower back, do not do that particular motion. Choose another that works the same area.

Be especially careful of twisting exercises to the side. This kind of movement can throw the back out faster than any other.

Back building and strengthening exercises

These exercises have been carefully chosen to help strengthen the stomach and back muscles. They are usually accepted by most physicians but, do check with your doctor for the O.K. to do any exercise. Your back is your life-line, guard it carefully. The exercises should be done slowly, gradually increasing speed as your condition improves and your back shows strength. If your back feels a slight discomfort when you first begin to exercise, don't give up; these annoyances should pass as your back muscles become stronger. Not only will exercise strengthen and tone muscles but circulation, energy, and endurance will be greatly improved. There is no time like the present to get started on the road to health and fitness.

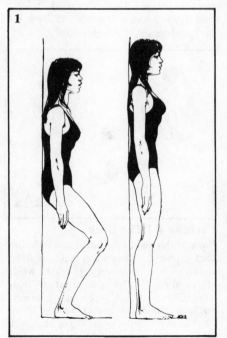

1

#1 Posture perfect

Here is a good posture exercise that will help train you to walk with spine straight, shoulders back, and head and neck directly over spinal cord. Walking with perfect posture relieves undue strain on internal and external muscles and organs. Your total health and well-being will be restored.

Stand with your back against a wall, bend the knees slightly. *Action:* push your back firmly into the wall and slide up to a standing position. Now, take 5 steps forward keeping your back in that straight position. Repeat the complete exercise 5 times. Try to walk with perfect posture at all times.

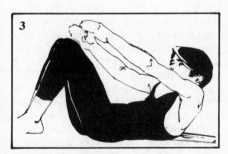

#2 The Spinal Stretch

You may have noticed how a cat stretches after a nap, one paw, then the other, then an all over body stretch. This is how the Spinal Stretch is done. Get down on all four's, begin stretching one arm out in front of you, then the other. Slide your hands out until your elbows touch the floor. Your buttocks will be lifted up high and your spine will be in a long body stretch. In this position each vertebra of the spine is expanded in a gentle manner. Hold position for 10 seconds, then slowly slide your hands back toward your body and sit up. Do the Spinal Stretch a couple of times a day.

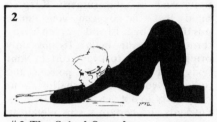

#3 The Semi-Sit-Up

The Semi-Sit-up will strengthen abdominal, upper back and neck muscles. This exercise should be done at your own level without force or strain. Lie down with knees bent and arms at your side. Lift your head and upper torso slowly off the floor. Try to touch your knees with your hands. Do not hold the up position, come down slowly but immediately. As your abdominal and upper back muscles toughen to this exercise, then you may hold the lifted position for 10 to 20 seconds. Repeat exercise 5 times.

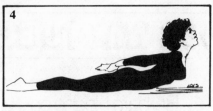

#4 Torso Lift

Torso Lift strengthens back, neck, head and buttocks. Abdominal muscles are also contracted and toned. Lie down on your tummy, lock your hands behind your back, contract buttock and abdominal muscles as you slowly lift your torso off the floor. Raise your body until you feel a stretch and a tightening, no higher. Lower down immediately and repeat 3 times. When your muscles are stronger, you may hold the lifted position for 8 seconds.

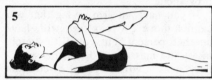

#5 Alternate knee to chest

A good upper hip and thigh flex. Lie down on your back. If you are a beginner at exercising, bend both knees, feet flat on the floor. If you have been exercising, you may straighten one leg, bend the other. Grab your knee with both hands and pull it tightly into your chest. At the same time try to press your back flat to the floor. Change legs and pull the opposite knee into the chest. Repeat alternate knee to chest 10 times each leg.

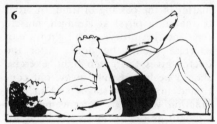

#6 Both knees to chest

A variation of the alternate knee to chest is bringing both knees to chest. Take the same position as for alternate knees to chest. Grab both knees with your hands and pull knees tightly into your chest. Try to push back gently into the floor. Hold 5 seconds. Repeat.

Your back and your diet

Your diet affects all body processes. If your diet is lacking in much-needed nutrients, the supply finally drains out. The body is left in a weakened state and easy victim to illness and disease. Muscles and bones deteriorate when the body is robbed of its valuable nutrients. Many things attack the body's supply, mainly chemicals in the food, and air and water pollutants. The important nutrients must be replaced daily or all body systems suffer. The muscles and bones of the back need special attention if they are weak. Vitamin C is needed in large quantities to maintain healthy tissues and help neutralize body toxins. The B-complex is for the nerves in the spinal cord, calcium for strong bones and to help prevent muscle spasms, vitamin D is noted to develop strong bones, vitamin E has been proved to help the muscles absorb oxygen. Vitamins, minerals, protein and amino acids share a close working relationship together to nourish and maintain strong body structures. Eat a balanced diet as one nutrient depends on another for best performance. Most health food stores carry an excellent supply of vitamin and mineral supplements to choose from. Add them to your diet.

Here are a few tips to make your daily living a little easier.

Do

1. *wear well-fitting shoes*
2. *sleep on a firm mattress*
3. *exercise daily*
4. *choose straight-backed chairs*
5. *maintain normal weight*
6. *eat nutritious foods*
7. *bend knees and squat down when picking up objects*
8. *take warm baths to sooth and relax tense muscles*
9. *let someone massage your tired back, it's good for you*
10. *buy a support cushion if you drive a lot*

Don't

1. *sit or stand for long periods of time*
2. *twist to the side rapidly*
3. *lift heavy objects: ask for assistance*
4. *reach way out in front of your body to open or close a window*
5. *throw your body out of alignment when walking*
6. *change directions suddenly*
7. *change temperatures quickly from hot to air-conditioned rooms; cold may settle in your back*
8. *slump while sitting*
9. *overstretch or tire back muscles*
10. *take drugstore drugs, they deplete body completely of vitamins and minerals.*

Take all things into consideration if you have back discomfort: your eating habits, your posture, and your exercise. If you have one or all three to improve upon, keep trying until it becomes automatic. Eventually, you will notice an improvement in your condition. As you take the opportunity to better your health, your body will respond. Posture will be perfect, muscles strong, and you will develop a respect for the proper exercise. Life will be easier to live in every way. ☼

EXERCISING YOUR WAY TO BETTER HEALTH

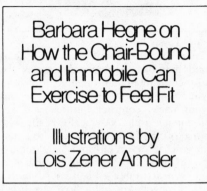

Barbara Hegne on How the Chair-Bound and Immobile Can Exercise to Feel Fit

Illustrations by Lois Zener Amsler

A person can be confined to a chair for many reasons — accident, handicap, surgery, or even because of the problems of advancing age. Such confinement amounts to a command performance of exercising, for although exercise is important in anyone's daily regimen in order to achieve and maintain a satisfactory standard of good health, it is absolutely vital for chairbound or partially immobilized people.

Exercise Restores Hope

An accident can cause mental as well as physical trauma when someone who is active is suddenly forced into a passive role, Shock is the first reaction, and very often depression and apathy follow. If the will to recovery fades, the combination of mental attitude and physical inactivity seriously affects the general health. Muscles quickly lose elasticity and tone, the joints become stiff and seem to congeal together, and mobility becomes increasingly limited. It may become difficult and painful to move any part of the body whether affected by the accident or not. To further complicate matters, loss of appetite and the ingestion of pain-killers and sleeping pills deplete the body's natural supply of vitamins and minerals.

Is this a hopeless situation? Of course not! With a little effort, the accident victim can retrieve the old feeling of vitality and zest for living. Exercise will improve circulation and help the joints keep limber and flexible. Vitamins and minerals can be replenished, particularly by wheat germ oil, vitamin E oil and cod liver oil to help keep the joints lubricated and make mobility easier. It is really possible to get back in touch with life before life gets out of touch with anyone who has suffered a traumatic accident and is confined to a chair.

Even Flicking Your Finger Can Help

Many handicapped people must be chair-bound a great deal of the time. Whether the handicap is one of mobility or involving sight, hearing or any form of communication, anyone limited in these ways can benefit greatly from a simple exercise program individually and specifically designed to suit each particular need. Many handicapped people are encouraged by their doctors and therapy attendants to exercise. This, of course, is indicative that exercise is most beneficial for improvement.

If you have an arm or leg that you cannot move by your own will, have another person help you lift, stretch, move and massage it. Even this secondary action will improve circulation and flexibility and keep nerves and muscles stimulated. There is nothing like exercise and activity to make the body feel refreshed and alive no matter what its condition. Many basic exercises can be done. Simple head circles, finger flicks, shoulder hunches and ankle circles — any movement, however slight, will benefit and improve health and fitness.

You Will Recover

Confinement from surgery is usually temporary and recuperation is only a matter of the passing of time. In order to maintain physical strength, muscle tone and flexibility, some light form of exercise should be done. After the doctor gives the green light, exercise should be begun right away, but continued in gradual stages and in conjunction with body improvement. As strength gradually increases, bring all the major muscles into action by doing the exercises presented here for chairbounders.

Surgery, coupled with super drugs and anesthetics has a way of completely draining your system. You may feel pained, depressed and irritable and completely sapped of your body strength. Of all the times in your life when you need the help of supplements, you need them now. You will need calcium, magnesium, vitamin C and the B-complex for nervousness and stress. Vitamin C, calcium, magnesium, zinc, vitamin D and protein for bone healing. Vitamin C and zinc for wound healing. Vitamin C for bruising, vitamin K for normal blood clotting and vitamin E to help dissolve any foreign blood clots. Calcium and vitamin D for muscle cramps. Vitamin E (internally and externally) for burns and scars. You may want to take more than is indicated for an average healthy body until your body returns to its normal state.

Take a Breather

A proper breathing exercise is a must for everyone, but particularly for anyone experiencing a decrease of activity such as after surgery. Keep in mind that the oxygen you inhale purifies the blood circulating throughout your body. It not only brings nutrients to every cell in your body, but carries away poisons and toxins. If your breath is shallow, your body cells do not get their fair share of nutrients and certain toxins remain in your system. Try this lung purifying exercise.

Sit with your spine very straight, chest forward and feet flat on the floor. Relax abdominal muscles so you are better able to completely fill the lower lungs. Begin inhaling to the count of 10 and as you do, bring your arms way over your head to really open and fill your lungs. Exhale slowly and lower your arms. Repeat as often as possible.

Your Age Is Showing

Many people think they are too old to shape up. They spend their time sitting, watching television, playing bridge, knitting or reading. They wonder why they have back aches, swollen ankles and varicose veins and why their muscles turn to flab, not realizing how their attitudes may be more at fault than age itself. They may believe that the retirement age is the time to forget all about exercise. After all, who wants to exercise with stiff joints and an aching back? But if they only knew it, their backs would stop aching with a gentle strengthening of their abdominal muscles and their stiff joints would limber up through activity. There is nothing better than exercise and proper nutrition to help increase vitality and longevity.

Exercise will massage the blood out of the veins and back to the heart, thus helping to eliminate pooling of the blood in the veins and increasing chances of varicosities. Exercise will also improve the abdominal muscles and correct overloads thrown on the back.

Basic body motions can be done while watching television or playing bridge. If you have to sit too long, call for a body-refresher by taking a break and shaking the lead out. Wiggle your toes, scissor your legs and stretch your tongue to work and tone face and neck muscles. You can be a totally healthy person and resist premature aging if you watch your diet and stay active.

Weight Control

Weight control is difficult for a sedentary person since it is important to keep food intake and activity output in balance. When one consumes more calories than one uses, fat develops. Choice of food is very important. Rich desserts, processed foods and foods containing chemical preservatives will only load down the system and add unused calories to the body. A person who is suffering body trauma and sitting most of the time, should take special care in choosing the right foods.

Choose fresh vegetables and fruits, whole grain bread, dairy products, wholesome meat, fish and poultry and a good mineral-vitamin supplement.

On to Exercise

All the exercises should be done with care and concentration on the area you desire to work. A gentle steady stretch is the best way to begin the exercises.

Some of the exercises will be easy, others more difficult depending on your body condition. Keep a specific number of repetitions in mind as your goal to try for. Begin the first day by doing only 5 or 6 repetitions, 7 or 8 the next day and so on until you reach your goal.

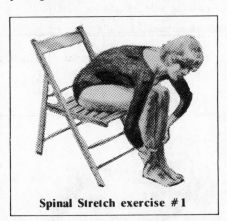

Spinal Stretch exercise #1

Sit with your back straight, chest forward. Begin leaning forward and round out your back as you slide your hands down your legs to your ankles. Drop your head forward and hold this position for 10 seconds. Come up

slowly, as the blood drains down to your head when you are bent forward and you need to normalize the flow gradually. Repeat this exercise when you feel tense muscles in your back, shoulders and neck area.

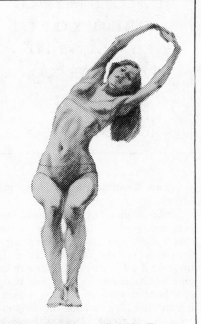

Waistline-Upper Midriff Toner exercise #2

Sit with your back straight and your hands locked together over your head, palms up toward the ceiling. Begin stretching slowly to the side, then over to the opposite side 10 times each. When your muscles become strong, you may bounce your arms twice to each side.

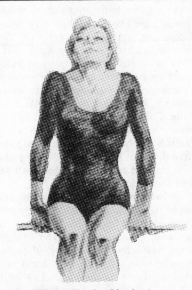

Shoulders, Back, Neck Area exercise #3

Sit tall and hold onto the edge of your chair. Look toward the ceiling and slowly lift your shoulders up toward your ears, really lift them high. Lower down and repeat 8 times.

This exercise is a wonderful tension reliever and can be done several times a day.

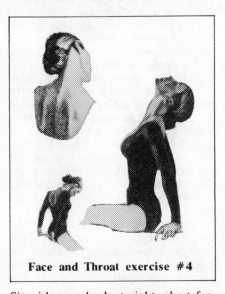

Face and Throat exercise #4

Sit with your back straight, chest forward and place your hands on the seat of the chair behind you. Tilt your head slowly side to side 5 times, then drop your chin forward to your chest and let it hang 10 counts, then look toward the ceiling and open your mouth. Hold 10 counts. These three motions will completely work the face and throat area.

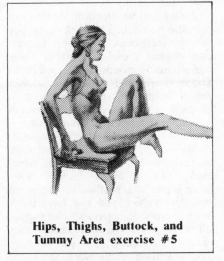

Hips, Thighs, Buttock, and Tummy Area exercise #5

This exercise is a little more advanced, be sure your body is in good condition before you attempt it.

Sit slightly forward on your chair and hold onto the sides of the chair tightly with both hands. Lift your legs up in front of you and slowly bicycle 5 times in each direction. ☼

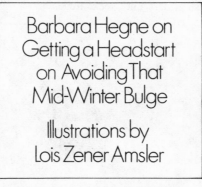

Barbara Hegne on Getting a Headstart on Avoiding That Mid-Winter Bulge

Illustrations by Lois Zener Amsler

Winter is the prime time to neglect exercise, and as is most obvious, abdominal muscles are among the first to lose their tone. A sagging, bulging abdomen detracts from the appearance more than any other flabby area. To disguise it, many women rely on a tight-fitting girdle, but this merely forces the fat into the wrong place and shape. A girdle also makes it easy to relax the abdomen, thus adding to the depletion of good muscle tone. Indeed, after wearing a girdle for some time, you can actually end up with a bigger sag than you started with. So don't let anyone tell you that lack of exercise is the *only* reason for the midriff bulge. But at winter's end, it bears most of the blame.

Overindulgence in food can be another cause. Snacking has become part of our lifestyle. Store displays, radio and TV commercials, and magazine articles and advertisements continually encourage all of us to have goodies on hand wherever we are. If you are susceptible to all of this propaganda and you also have been inactive, watch out down below! As the stomach expands, the abdomen has more weight to support, the back is thrown out of alignment; the body becomes sluggish; and various internal organs are projected forward or cramped together. When you get to this sad state, take quick action to save your health.

Abdominal muscles do more than support the stomach. They help keep posture perfect, back flat, chest forward and internal muscles in place. Three major muscle groups are located in the abdominal cavity: *transversus abdominis,* a flat muscle which helps hold abdominal contents and controls some involuntary functions; *obliquus (externus* and *internus)* located at an angle on either side of your body in the waistline area; and *rectus abdominis,* which runs down the middle of your body, from under the bustline to the groin. Needless to say, you will have to do several types of exercises to strengthen all these muscles in their various locations. For example, you will need sit-ups which especially work the *rectus abdominis,* and sit-ups coupled with waistline twists, which tone both *rectus abdominis* and *obliquus.* All the various types of exercises needed to build a strong, natural muscular corset are presented below. Included are leg lifts, sit-ups, stretches, contractions and tightening, holding and inverted positions to stimulate and tone inner organs.

Some of these exercises need mini-gym accessories. From three of these simple aids, you can get maximum results with even the easiest exercise. The first one is a *beauty pole.* This can be a mop or broom handle, or a pole bought at a lumber yard, measuring 4 feet in length and 1⅛ inches in diameter. Smooth any rough places with sandpaper. When you exercise, think of your beauty pole as an extension of yourself which enables you to stretch farther, pull in all directions more effectively and exercise some parts of your body otherwise difficult to work. For pennies, a beauty pole is one of the best investments you can make.

You will also need a *power ball:* a small, soft rubber ball 3 to 4 inches in diameter. It is a "power" tool for firming muscles, and a gentle massager.

Weight pouches give fantastic results when used for body contouring. Muscles that are used with weights work harder. Therefore, toning is much faster. Make light weights of 3 to 4 pounds out of sand or buckshot, or buy them from a sport shop. If you make your own, use upholstery material and cut it approximately 14 inches long by 10 inches wide. Fold material lengthwise and sew side edges and one end. Fill with 2 pounds of buckshot, then stitch end. (See diagram.) If you can't buy or make weights, use two socks filled with sand and then stitch or tie them.

To achieve a trim abdominal look, begin right now by standing sideways in front of a full-length mirror. Place one hand on your abdomen, the other on your buttocks. Push your abdominal muscles upward with one hand while pushing down on the buttocks with the other. Tuck your hips underneath your body. This exercise will give you the idea of how the tummy, chest and back should look. Your breathing will be deeper and your posture will be correct. Now go on to the exercises. Start them today. You will be on your way to membership in the "in" fashion crowd that can wear blouses tucked in, hip-huggers, tops that bare the midriff, even bikini bathing suits. Be all that you can be, for besides looking and feeling attractive, a comfortable, flab-free frontage is a sure sign of health and fitness.

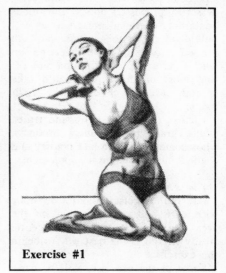

Exercise #1

Kneel down and then sit on the backs of your legs. Hold your weight pouches over your shoulders and behind your back. Lift your body up and over to the right side of your legs touching your buttocks down on the floor. Then lift up and all the way over to the left side. Continue side to side for 12 counts.

← 14 inches →		5 inches
2 pounds buckshot	2 pounds buckshot	

Weight Pouch — finished

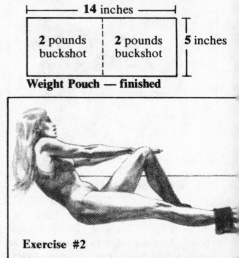

Exercise #2

To prepare for this exercise, sit down on the floor; bend one leg and extend the other. Place a weight pouch on each ankle and lower your back to the floor. Now you are ready.

Lift your body forward and touch both hands on the outside of the bent knee. Then lower your back to the floor. Repeat this lift 8 times. Change leg positions, and continue the exercise for 8 more times.

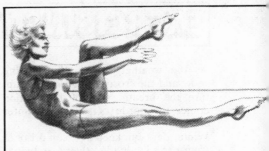

Exercise #6

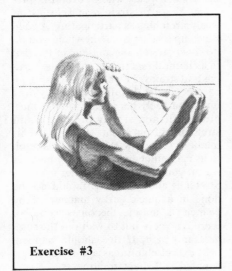

Exercise #3

Lie on your back and draw your knees in toward your chest. Spread your knees wide apart and hold them with your hands. Tighten buttocks and abdominal muscles as you lift your upper back (spine curved) off the floor and bring your head forward toward your knees. Then bring your knees in to touch each other as you resist with your hands. Repeat in-and-out knee action 10 times, rest and do 10 more.

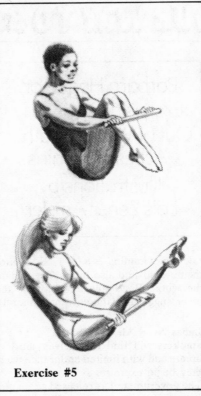

Exercise #5

Sit down on the floor and extend both legs. With hands wide apart, grasp your beauty pole. Lean back; lift your legs up and slip your beauty pole under them; then straighten your body. Now bend your knees, bring your beauty pole out from under your body, and lean back with your pole above your body. Aim for a smooth in-and-out rocking motion as you perform the entire exercise 10 times.

Lie on your back. Lift upper torso and one leg at the same time. Touch your hands together underneath the raised leg. Lie down again and repeat movement with opposite leg. Do exercise 5 times with each leg.

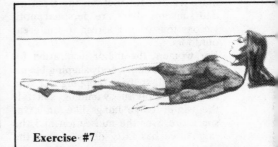

Exercise #7

An easy stomach exercise and one especially good for anyone with a back problem.

Lie down on your back, arms down by your sides. Lift your head and shoulders off the floor and look at your toes. Hold this position for 10 counts; return to starting position, and repeat exercise 5 times.

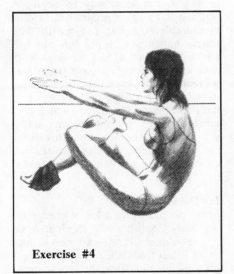

Exercise #4

Sit on the floor, knees bent, and place both weight pouches on the right ankle. Lie down and rest the left leg on the right knee. Hold your arms out to the side, then swing them forward and come to a sitting position. Lower, and repeat 5 times. Change leg positions and repeat.

Exercise #8

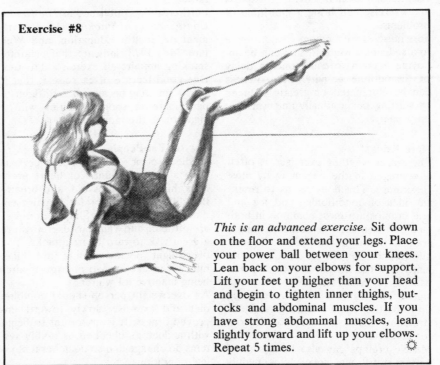

This is an advanced exercise. Sit down on the floor and extend your legs. Place your power ball between your knees. Lean back on your elbows for support. Lift your feet up higher than your head and begin to tighten inner thighs, buttocks and abdominal muscles. If you have strong abdominal muscles, lean slightly forward and lift up your elbows. Repeat 5 times. ☼

EXERCISING YOUR WAY TO BETTER HEALTH

As the weather warms, the melting snow and the frosty air no longer capture the breath. Out of hibernation comes the horde of sedentary winter athletes.

Winter days can keep a person prisoner from participating in athletic acitivities for three or four months at a time, barred from jogging, swimming in the creek, water skiing, horseback riding, and bicycling. All these sports are somewhat limited in the cold winter months. After all, who wants to take a chance on jogging on ice, or bicycling through mud puddles? Summer certainly has more advantages. Besides the fresh air and sunshine there are personal motivations that trigger a rush to the great outdoors.

For women, the major inspiration for spring and summer body shaping begins after the first trip shopping for the newest fashion in swimming suits. If the winter bulge hangs like an extra spare tire over the midsection and the thigh area has fatty deposits that the elastic pushes out even further, she heads for the gym.

Men too have their winter left-overs. With their heavy suits put away for the season, a tee shirt will not cover a pot belly.

Everyone from the grandmother of teens to the teenager himself hears the beckoning call to exercise.

The determined person's enthusiastic rush to summertime activities for sports and exercise can bring a multitude of problems.

Sore muscles are a common occurrence to a sedentary winterite and can be annoying enough to cause one to delay or discontinue activity. But soreness can be eliminated or greatly reduced by starting out gradually and warming up properly.

More Pains

The warm weather exerciser is often discouraged in the beginning by muscle cramps. The body seems to resent any idea of conditioning and leg and arm cramps are most common in both men and women. The cause of muscle cramps is not known, although it is known that the muscle contracts violently and the fastest way to stop the pain is to re-stretch the muscle out again. This can be done by pressing down on the foot if it is a leg cramp or stretching the back and shoulder out for arm cramps.

Muscle cramps can also be a sign of certain nutritional deficiencies, mainly

Barbara Hegne on Exercising Your Way Out of Warm Weather Aches and Pains Illustrations by Lois Zener Amsler

calcium, vitamins B-6, B-1, E, pantothenic acid and also biotin. Try adding the whole B complex along with the other suggested vitamins and minerals.

Lungs Need Air Not Smoke

Smokers will find themselves short of breath and with limited endurance when they begin exercise.

The government has released some new facts about cigarette smoking. Here's what the studies reveal about what happens with every cigarette smoked.

In just three seconds a cigarette makes the heart beat faster, shoots the blood pressure up, replaces oxygen in the blood with carbon monoxide and leaves cancer-causing chemicals to spread throughout the body. With all this happening with each cigarette, it's no wonder many smokers find exercise too difficult.

Further studies published in *The Health Consequences of Smoking,* U.S. Department of Health, Education, and Welfare, May 1973, indicate that cigarette smoking impairs all exercise activities. One good feature of exercise is that it delays smoking because it is difficult to participate in sport activities with a cigarette in the mouth.

Not for Fat People

Medical science tells us obese persons have a greater chance of heart problems, high blood pressure, and breathing difficulties. Extra fat impairs endurance and stamina. Simple exercises are difficult and vigorous exercises are a great risk toward heart attacks. The overweight person should not hike, hunt or engage in vigorous sports after being inactive all winter.

An overweight person should combine diet and exercise slowly toward improved fitness. It is important to begin with a doctor's checkup as bodily systems do change and so do general physical conditions.

Warm Up and Stretch First.

It is very important to warm up your cold muscles before attempting to exercise. *How* you stretch out and warm up affects your whole exercise program. You can strain a muscle just as easily stretching as participating. A good warm-up session is one in which you do not over-stretch the muscle so far that in its natural reaction it contracts, tightens and strains. The best type of stretches are gentle: bending the body first until you feel the stretch of the muscles, and then slowly bouncing and stretching from that position. This method will allow the body to stretch to its maximum and as the body muscles warm, you can stretch further.

Stretches and warm ups should not be done in a quick, jerky manner. If by chance a muscle becomes strained, there is no cure but to wait out the soreness and pain. If this should happen, light exercise and massage is suggested coupled with heat treatments.

Jogging is Good

Jogging is a good full body exercise, improving heart and lung function, blood circulation, stamina and endurance, and it also conditions major muscle groups. All this is wonderful, but jogging too vigorously can cause sore muscles and invite chances of lung and heart exhaustion.

A combination of brisk walking and jogging is the ideal way to begin. A walking and jogging program should be pleasurable. Gasping for breath with tongue hanging out is not fun, nor is it healthy. Jogging should be done with ease and comfort. To gasp for breath is creating an oxygen debt such as happens in fast sprinting, the opposite of the main reason for jogging which is to inhale more oxygen into the system. If you are just naturally out of breath or sort of breathless, you may have an iron deficiency and iron can easily be added to your diet.

Jog Correctly

Many people waste a lot of energy using body English while jogging. Arms fly, shoulders lift up and down, hips swing wildly from side to side and knees lift too high and cause the feet to come down too hard.

Body posture is very important. The head should be up, eyes straight ahead, back straight, shoulders level and the arms should swing naturally. Joggers have different ways of landing on their feet. Beginners usually run up on their toes and many times suffer sore muscles. Others run flat-footed, landing evenly on the bottom of the foot. There is a little controversy about this method, but some long distance runners use it quite successfully.

The most widely accepted method is to put down the heel first, then roll forward to the toe (or ball of foot). Striking the heel against the ground first seems to cushion the shock quite well.

Proper shoes are the only equipment jogging requires. Special jogging-style tennis shoes are recommended for full jogging benefit and protection.

When you jog, begin gradually and pick an area without automobiles, since carbon monoxide is readily absorbed through the lungs. And since jogging calls for deep breathing, only fresh air will suffice.

Be careful when jogging during high temperatures as the heat can quickly exhaust your energy levels and cause fainting.

Jog on a soft surface, to avoid the jarring that causes muscle pain and shin splints (a tenderness of the shin bone).

Jogging may be the most valuable total body exercise to do. An alternate jog and walk combination is a good way to begin the spring and summer. Fortunately, jogging can be carried through during the winter months by stationary running. This is a simple running and walk program timed by the minute. Begin at 30 seconds and increase 5 seconds daily until jogging steadily for up to 8 full minutes.

Swimming too can be compared to jogging and is a wonderful way to regain the vitality and fitness lost through the sedentary winter months.

Swimming is a total body sport and also requires previous body stretching and warming up before active participation.

Exercise #1

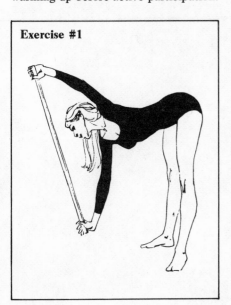

Exercise #1 Full Body Stretch
Use your broomstick or any slender pole over four feet long for a wonderful body-stretching aid. The pole will enable you to stretch farther, pull in all directions more effectively, and exercise and stretch some parts of your body otherwise difficult to work.

Stand tall with your pole up toward the ceiling, then slowly bend forward and touch your right hand to the floor by your right foot. Lift up to the ceiling and repeat to the opposite side. Repeat 10 times to each side.

Exercise #2

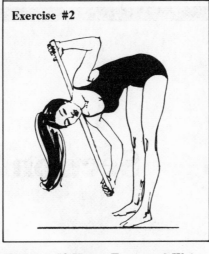

Exercise #2 Upper Torso and Waist-line Stretch
Use your broomstick or pole for this exercise.

Place the pole gently on your shoulders and be careful not to press the pole into your back vertebrae. Lean forward and begin to twist toward the center of the floor. When your muscles warm and stretch, try to twist and touch opposite hand to opposite foot. Repeat 10 times to each side.

Exercise #3

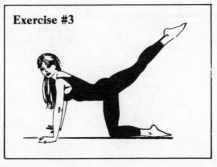

Exercise #3 Back, Thigh and Buttocks
Warm and stretch back thigh and buttocks muscles before fast-moving sports such as tennis or jogging.

Get down on all fours and raise your left leg behind you, then touch the floor and lift toward the ceiling 10 times. Do not jerk your leg up. This motion should be controlled. Repeat 8 times to each leg.

Exercise #4

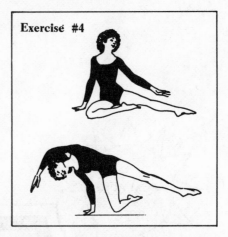

Exercise #4 Another All-Over Body-stretch
Sit down with one leg tucked in front of your body and the other extended out in front. Lift up on bent knee and bring opposite hand over your head as far as possible. Lower down and repeat 5 times and change leg positions.

Exercise #5

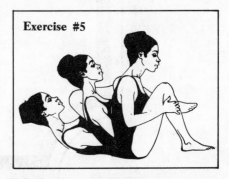

Exercise #5 Spinal Massage
Warm up the spine before any heavy body sports or exercise. Sit down on a soft mat or pillow, grab your knees and pull them in close to your chest. Begin to roll back and forth massaging each vertebra in your spine. Roll 10 times.

Exercise #6

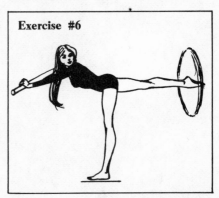

Exercise #6 Leg and Ankle Warmer
Hold onto your kitchen sink or chair and stretch out. Extend your leg behind you and begin to circle leg and ankle 10 times in each direction. Repeat to opposite leg. ☼

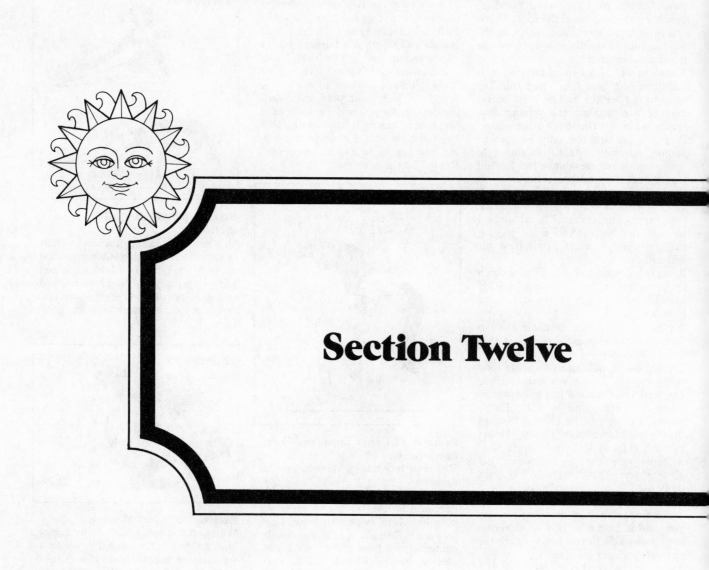

Section Twelve

If Better Health
Is the Answer,
What Is the Question?

HEALTH QUESTIONS ON YOUR MIND

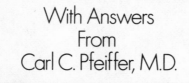

With Answers
From
Carl C. Pfeiffer, M.D.

Q What is the best way to take vitamin and mineral supplements —all at once in the morning, or spread out over the day? And should I take one concentration (in liquid or capsule form) of vitamins and another of minerals . . . or should I take each vitamin and mineral separately?

A Since supplements are a form of food, an ideal situation is to take them with food, while the digestive juices are at work. However, there are some extra rules to keep in mind. There are certain vitamins and minerals which should not be taken together: for instance, calcium with zinc or iron. The B vitamins are another special case. Vitamin B-6 should be taken twice daily. Some research scientists in clinical ecology rotate the B vitamins. But, in general, vitamins and minerals can be taken together, at a mealtime. For children, supplements in liquid form are best.

Q Can my mood swings be related to food?

A Yes, different reactions to certain foods can be related to mood swings. Common food sensitivities are: wheat, milk, beef, corn and egg whites. Many hyperactive children react to food additives (chemicals) such as food coloring, flavoring and preservatives.

To detect food sensitivities, an elimination diet, where foods are methodically eliminated from the diet, one at a time, with a pulse test (the normal pulse is 70—this will increase after ingestion of a food to which the system is sensitive) is recommended, along with consultation with a clinical ecologist who will study sensitivity to various foods by having you follow a rotating diet.

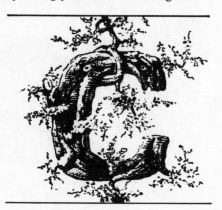

Q What nutrients help memory?

A Many elderly patients with memory impairments improve with zinc, folic acid and B-12 for reduction of copper in the tissues. A vitamin B-12 injection weekly also helps prevent senility. Without proper nutrients, proteins cannot be manufactured nor the nerve cells efficiently used to maintain desirable mental function, including memory. Faulty memory and bizarre thought patterns may be evident in someone whose biochemistry is inherently imbalanced or whose diet does not supply the brain with all the needed nutrients (both vitamins and minerals).

Through maximum dietary and supplementary doses of essential nutrients, an individual can usually ensure body fitness and maximum mental functioning, enabling him to cope with the stresses and demands of everyday life. Alcohol, sugar and junk food should be eliminated from the diet since they may lead to hypoglycemia and promote memory deterioration.

Q Can anything be taken to help heal broken bones?

A Vitamin C can aid the healing of wounds. Zinc gluconate also helps in wound healing. Specifically, dolomite and bonemeal help make bones stronger.

Q My brother and I have extreme difficulty in waking. Three alarm clocks won't wake me—and if no one is there I can sleep for over twenty hours. Can this be caused by a nutritional deficiency?

A This could be a symptom of hypoglycemia (low blood sugar). Hence, the difficulty in waking might be alleviated by following a high protein, low carbohydrate diet with frequent high protein snacks to keep the blood sugar level normalized. Many vitamins and trace minerals, including vitamin C, the B-complex vitamins, calcium, potassium, magnesium, zinc and phosphorus mediate glucose metabolism and control the activities of the endocrine glands, so the problem might be related to glandular malfunction. Anyone needing twenty hours of sleep should seek maximum nutritional advice.

Q Is there any nutrient that helps nearsightedness?

A Research studies are indicating that organic "myopia" might possibly benefit from vitamin D. The condition of nearsightedness may be related to calcium deficiency. Vitamin A (the traditional carrot) benefits the retina and cornea but will not affect nearsightedness. In general, good nutrition promotes *clear*sightedness!

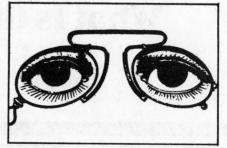

Q What causes those transitory pains like a "stitch" in the side?

A Running can cause transitory pains or a "stitch" in the side. Also, at the Brain Bio Center, we find that many of our pyroluric patients (a condition related to schizophrenia and treated with dosages of vitamin B-6 and zinc) have a symptom very similar to the runner's "stitch." This symptom responds to vitamin B-6 and zinc supplementation.

Q Can one obtain the same benefits from taking choline and inositol as from taking lecithin?

A Choline is a lipotropic agent which helps (with methionine and inositol) in preventing the deposition of fat in the body by promoting the utilization of fat. Lecithin is an emulsifier and helps to keep fats and esters suspended in the watery medium of the bloodstream, but is not necessarily ridding the body of those fats.

HEALTH QUESTIONS ON YOUR MIND

Q What do you recommend to help insomnia?

A Insomnia may be caused by various chemical imbalances and a stressful life style. We suggest controlling your copper/zinc balance. If insomnia is due to excess copper, a zinc supplement over many months will push this excess copper out of your body. We have found that vitamin B-6 and zinc help insomnia. The patients need enough B-6 to have dream recall. The dosage would be from 25 mg am and pm to 500 mg am and pm with a 15 mg zinc gluconate supplement. We suggest that the B-6 be taken am and pm not throughout the day and it should be taken with zinc because they work in the brain together. The B vitamin inositol has a calming effect and may promote prolonged natural sleep. Also, we recommend dolomite calcium, hot baths, yoga, deep breathing, warm milk and a lot of exercise during the day to relieve stress.

Q What are the basic rules for losing weight?

A The basic rules for losing weight are for most people:
A. eating less on a low salt high protein diet
B. eating carefully and taking suggested nutritional supplements
C. exercise
D. rotating whole foods
E. and a healthy water intake.
Ideal reducing diets must satisfy nutritional needs. By severely restricting kinds of foods which contain the body's basic requirements, (carbohydrates, proteins, fats) we deprive it of the essential vitamins and minerals needed to maintain optimal mental functions. Symptoms common to those who "crash diet" are dizziness, fatigue and even psychotic and neurotic behavior patterns.
Diet pills are disastrous to both the body and the mind.
Avoid all sweets, get lots of fiber in your diet such as whole grains, bran and leafy vegetables.

Q How is vitamin B-12 important? Can it be assimilated if taken orally?

Good Advice from the author of Mental and Elemental Nutrients

A Vitamin B-12 is needed for the actions of methionine (an amino acid) and RNA and DNA. Absence of B-12 in the body causes pernicious anemia which is an arrest of red blood cell growth. The actions of folic acid and B-12 are intertwined biochemically.
The most common findings in B-12 deficiency are motor and mental difficulties, i.e., poor memory, agitation, moodiness, depression, delusions, hallucinations and paranoia. However, B-12 deficiency is rare because daily requirement is so low, although B-12 deficiency does occur frequently in vegetarians.
In older patients we know that B-12 is not well absorbed orally, so an intramuscular injection is helpful. It is known that B-12 helps to prevent aging. There are two forms of B-12: the cyanocobalamin or regular, and the hydroxocobalamin, trade marked "alpha-redisol" whose effect is longer lasting.
Ellis and Nasser reported in the *British Journal of Nutrition* in 1973, a double blind study, involving 28 patients complaining of tiredness. Those receiving B-12 injections were reported to be happier and had a feeling of general well being.

Q If excess copper is prevalent and dangerous, how can it be controlled?

A Our bodies need some copper, as discovered by Hart/Steinbock in Wisconsin in 1928. The Princeton Group has published *frequently* that excess copper may cause insomnia, anxiety, nervousness and depression. It plays a role in premenstrual irritability and depression, headaches of various kinds, high blood pressure and possibly stuttering. The inability to eliminate copper can be a familial disorder.
Excess copper in our system can stem from copper water pipes, estrogen in

---

birth control pills, multivitamins with minerals which often contain 2 mg of copper sulfate and zinc deficient diets. (Some hospital diets have only 8-11 mg of zinc. The MDR is 15 mg.)
The best way to control high copper content is by avoiding multivitamins with copper, the birth control pill, high coppered water and by taking a daily zinc supplement with vitamin C.

Q How can a vegetarian be certain of balanced nutrition?

A The vegetarian must ensure an adequate protein intake for proper health. The diet should include proper amino acid combinations. Emphasis should be placed on quality not quantity of protein. Plant and animal sources (cereals and dairy products) can be combined in the same meal. Also, different plant foods which have mutually complementing amino acid proteins can be eaten together resulting in an increase of protein value in the meal. Protein is needed for growth, maintenance of tissue and bones for certain metabolic reactions. Eggs are recommended for their high zinc and protein content.
Vitamin B-12 is found only in animal products: Complete vegetarians need B-12 supplements. The consequences of B-12 deficiency are megaloblastic anemia and possible degeneration of the spinal cord.
Total vegetarians should substitute beans, legumes (rich in phytates) and grains for meat (a major source of zinc). These foods bind zinc, calcium and other minerals. It is recommended to sprout these vegetables. This neutralizes the phytates. A zinc supplement is a definite must! *Zinc* is the intelligent alternative to *iron*. Soybeans are high in copper and should be avoided in excess as too much copper in the body causes many physical and psychiatric disorders.
Philosophically, the fact that man's chemistry requires both *folic acid* from *vegetables* and *B-12* from *animals* may be a cogent argument for the omnivorous nature of Mankind! ✿

HEALTH QUESTIONS ON YOUR MIND

Q Our four-year-old son has been diagnosed as mildly hyperactive. Is there anything we can give him that would help?

A We introduced DMAE in 1957 as a biochemical stimulant under the trade name Deaner (generic name deanol). The compound has been used as a substitute for drug stimulants in the treatment of hyperactive children. Deanol has several advantages over Ritalin or the amphetamines in treating hyperactivity or learning disorders in children. Amphetamines produce lack of appetite or weight loss in hyperactive children who may have feeding problems already. A single dose of deanol usually lasts all day and carries no risk of abuse due to its slow biochemical effect. Oral doses of vitamin C and zinc get rid of excess copper and lead, both of which may cause hyperactivity in animals and children.

Q Is there a nutritional way to control migraine?

A Caffeine withdrawal headache: Caffeine intake should be carefully regulated by all who are susceptible to periodic headaches. Beverages which contain caffeine are coffee, tea and cola drinks, including some low-calorie ones such as "Tab." Foods which contain caffeine are coffee ice cream and chocolate. Liquors with caffeine are crème de cacao, kalua and possibly benedictine.

Hypoglycemic patients (hungry headache) need snack foods — a hard-boiled egg, a piece of cheese, or peanuts. Food allergy headache is most commonly precipitated by garlic, onions, green peppers, chocolate, watermelon, cabbage, cucumbers, parsley and radishes. Most of these foods contain sulfur or other compounds which lower blood pressure.

Most migraine patients are high in copper and the incidence and severity of their headaches is decreased when dietary zinc is given to reduce the copper level.

Migraine patients should regulate their hours of sleep; one nurse got a migraine on her day off because she slept more than her usual eight hours. She was advised by her doctor to set her alarm, wake at the usual time and

Dr. Pfeiffer
Directs the
Brain Bio-Center

catch up on extra sleep by napping later.

Q We have never heard of selenium until recently, but just lately it seems to be described as invaluable by experts. Why and how is it so beneficial?

A Selenium is an essential trace mineral for animals and man. Both selenium and zinc protect against the toxic effects of the pollutant cadmium. Tests on laboratory animals have shown that selenium increases the effectiveness of vitamin E and it appears to reduce the chances of getting any type of cancer. It is an antioxidant that helps prevent chromosomal breakage in tissue culture.

Human milk contains six times as much selenium as cow's milk and twice as much vitamin E. Selenium is necessary for protein synthesis.

Good food sources of selenium are brewer's yeast, garlic, liver and eggs. One disadvantage of selenium is its possible tendency to increase dental caries in children up to the age of ten. Heavy consumption of selenium seems to decrease the beneficial effect of fluoride, which helps prevent tooth decay.

One patient had scabs on his scalp that did not respond to standard medical treatment or vitamin E. Selenium supplementation was prescribed and the results were excellent.

Q Is milk a necessary part of a teen-ager's diet?

A Milk contains three solid components: protein, fats and carbohydrates. Milk's carbohydrate lactose is a disaccharide that must be split by the enzyme lactase into monosaccharides (glucose and galactose) in order to be absorbed by the body. The enzyme lactase breaks down lactose primarily in the upper gut. When the body is lacking the enzyme

lactase, the unabsorbed lactose passes to the lower gut where the milk sugar ferments and produces organic acids and gasses that irritate the intestine. This results in flatulence (gas), bloating, abdominal cramps and occasionally, diarrhea.

Usually lactose-intolerant people (15% of whites and 75% of blacks) can digest small amounts of milk without gastrointestinal symptoms.

Milk is a nutrient-rich food and for many people the daily drinking of milk supplies these nutritional benefits with no ill effects. Nevertheless, studies concerning lactose-intolerant subjects have resulted in the marketing of some lactose-free milk products.

Milk is a wonderful, nutritious food for teenagers if they aren't milk-sensitive. For those who can't tolerate milk, dolomite calcium could be considered.

Q What is the most effective nutritional treatment for alcoholism? Can it be cured?

A The alcoholic is usually suffering from dehydration, numerous nutritional deficiencies and hypoglycemia.

Niacin can help prevent the craving for alcohol. The nutrient program should include large doses of niacin and vitamin C, vitamin B-6, vitamin E and a super B-50 water-soluble vitamin complex. Zinc supplementation may be helpful as well. A high-protein, low-carbohydrate diet is also indicated.

Three recurring problems that can complicate the patient's recovery are concurrent drug use, previously undetected hypoglycemia (because low blood sugar creates nervousness) and perceptual distortions — distortions of taste, hearing, sight, personal awareness, time and space.

Social groups such as Alcoholics Anonymous (AA) or Recovery are very effective in boosting the morale of the alcoholic and thus preventing a recurrence.

It is in the literature that lithium carbonate is helpful in the treatment of alcoholism.

Alcoholism can be controlled by careful dietary habits, vitamin and mineral supplementation, and a strong willpower to abstain from the alcohol. ✧

HEALTH QUESTIONS ON YOUR MIND

Q Some diets are based on calorie amounts, some others are based on carbohydrates. I find this confusing, and wonder if you could tell me how these two measures can be interchanged.

A The diets that are based on carbohydrates usually restrict the amount of the carbohydrate in the diet and increase protein. This high protein, low carbohydrate combination is designed to induce ketosis — the presence in the body of excessive amounts of ketone (acetone). However, some carbohydrate is needed by the body to regulate protein and fat metabolism. Ketosis indicates an abnormal metabolic state due to lack of carbohydrates, which is very dangerous for some people.

The average weight loss should not exceed two pounds a week. A dieter needs sufficient calories to maintain physical vigor. An allowance of about 1,000 calories per day should be adequate for nutrition but low enough to permit weight loss.

Make those 1,000 calories nutritious. Use fats sparingly, avoid all refined sugar and junk foods, get lots of exercise, use roughage and take a multipurpose vitamin without copper. Brewer's yeast is the best source of the B-complex. If you are sensitive to brewer's yeast, it can cause some bloating when first started. You should be able to build up your dosage to 6 tablets daily. In addition, a source of zinc such as 20 mg. should be taken twice daily. Vitamin B-6 should be taken twice daily — enough for dream recall — as it aids in weight reduction.

Calorie conversion: 1 gram of carbohydrate = 4 calories

Q I have read conflicting reports on dolomite and whether or not it can be absorbed. If dolomite is able to be dissolved in the stomach, wouldn't it neutralize the needed stomach acids?

A An ideal calcium and magnesium supplement would include some bone meal for its phosphorus content.

Milk is ordinarily the best source of a balanced solution of calcium, magnesium and phosphorus. Two glasses of milk per day should be drunk by every growing individual. Dolomite (calcium and magnesium) can be used by the adult who is sensitive to milk. Since the magnesium makes the calcium soluble, the danger of

---

Practical Advice from an Authority on Orthomolecular Medicine

kidney stones which may occur with calcium alone is eliminated. Dolomite is usually well absorbed and can neutralize some stomach acid which would be a problem.

Q I have long been troubled with an "acid stomach" and want to know if commercial antacids are all right to take — since I do take them quite often. Also, is it this acid condition which causes me to get welts all over my body?

A The welts all over the body may be due to an allergic reaction to the antacids. Eliminate all antacids for a while and note any change. In the meantime, avoid any foods which may be acidic or irritating such as citrus fruits, tomatoes, onions, etc. You may want to check with your allergist for a food in your diet or something in your environment which may be causing symptoms.

Calcium carbonate is an acceptable antacid.

Q I suffer from extreme tiredness and intense depression. This has been diagnosed and treated as "adrenal exhaustion," but I am not being helped. Should I try treating myself for hypoglycemia; or should I keep changing doctors until I find one that helps me?

A Functional hypoglycemia can be one symptom of adrenal insufficiency; however, adrenal insufficiency itself is an uncommon condition and is rarely a cause of functional hypoglycemia.

For extreme fatigue and intense depression, a high protein, low carbohydrate diet with frequent feedings and no sugar or caffeine in the diet will be helpful. In addition to the hypoglycemic diet, combined vitamin and mineral supplements to correct faulty metabolism is found to be extremely effective in treatment of hypoglycemia. These may include a high potency multivitamin formula (without copper), choline for fat metabolism, calcium, and a good source of the trace elements zinc,

---

magnesium, chromium and manganese, and brewer's yeast and B-complex to assure adequate B vitamins. Also important are vitamin C, pantothenic acid, niacin, inositol, vitamin E, pyridoxine, B-12 and folic acid. If your blood pressure is low (as would be expected in adrenal exhaustion), manganese may be helpful. Generally it is best not to change doctors.

Q After a person has given up smoking, is there a way to help cleanse the body of tar and nicotine deposits on lung tissues?

A To cleanse the body of tar and nicotine after smoking has ceased, drink plenty of fluids such as water, juices, etc. Vitamin C helps detoxify and zinc and vitamin E speed healing.

Q It has been diagnosed that I have a "fast heart," and I am being treated with a tranquilizing drug. Can you recommend a nutritional treatment instead?

A A "fast heart" can be a symptom of a vast number of disorders. However, it could be an indication of an allergy. Evaluate your eating habits and determine foods that you use frequently in your diet. Common food allergies are wheat, corn, milk, egg whites, sugar and caffeine. Test for one food at a time by eliminating it from the diet for a period of four days and eating it by itself in its purest form on the fifth day. This should be done at the noon meal and eaten in a large quantity. Keep a food diary. Look for any symptoms during the testing and record them. If no symptoms occur, eat half of this portion a half hour later and note any symptoms. It would also be helpful to take your pulse before and after the food being tested is eaten. If the pulse increases after the food is ingested, this could indicate an allergy. Finding and eliminating from the diet the offending foods or food could slow the heart and eliminate the need for tranquilizers.

Q Can a change of climate really help someone's health, or is this just a plot device from a Victorian novel?

A A change of climate can help. One patient went to live in Santa Fe to avoid air pollution for her allergies. Arthritics do much better in a dry climate.

☼

HEALTHY SKIN AND HAIR FOR YOU

A Leading Dermatologist on the Role of Nutrition in Good Health

Q Do you routinely prescribe vitamins to your patients to help the condition of the skin and hair?

A Yes. I believe that the intake of daily vitamins acts beneficially and as a preventative to keep the skin and hair healthy. The daily vitamin intake I suggest is:
Vitamin A 25,000 units daily
Vitamin B complex 75 mgms. daily (high potency)
Vitamin C 500 mgms. daily
Vitamin E 200 units twice a day
Trace minerals 1 capsule daily
Of course the necessary medication is presented for each individual condition. Dietary requirements are discussed with each patient and each disorder.

Q What can I do about the large pores on my nose and cheeks?

A The large pores are dilated or enlarged openings of the terminal part of the sebaceous gland which pours its secretion on the skin to lubricate it. Occasionally, surface debris blocks the pores and they resemble blackheads. There is no known cosmetic which will cause contraction of the pores permanently. However, the use of an astringent, which usually contains alcohol, witch hazel, acetone, and water, will cleanse the pores and give the impression of contracted pores. Abrasive soaps, which contain pumice, polyethylene powder, and aluminum oxide particles, when used regularly with water may remove superficial layers of the skin and reduce the size of the openings of the pore.
A physician can prescribe salicylic acid in alcohol which, when applied to the surface of the pores, will exfoliate or peel the outer layers of skin to present an improved appearance.

Q What foods are the most likely to affect the skin adversely?

A Foods that are fried and foods that contain excessive amounts of iodide and saturated fatty acids may have a deleterious effect upon the skin. Therefore, I suggest to my patients with skin problems to abstain from nuts, chocolate, spices or heavily seasoned foods, iodized salt, spicy cheeses, and excessive amounts of shell fish. In cases with acne and seborrhea, I advise abstinence from hot coffee and tea. The use of cola drinks may adversely affect the greasy skin.
A simple balanced diet of protein, fats and carbohydrates, fortified with vegetables, salads, and fruits, is the sensible guide to follow.

Q Can anti-perspirants be harmful if used daily?

A The active ingredient of anti-perspirants or deodorants is aluminum chlorohydrate which causes constriction of the openings of the sweat ducts and thus diminishes the quantity of sweat produced daily. It is usually used in a concentration of about 20-25 percent.
In the majority of patients the use of this chemical in a stick, roll-on or spray is sufficient to reduce the perspiration to a comfortable degree.
In a small percentage of patients, a contact dermatitis of the armpit may be produced which causes an inflammatory reddened surface that is irritating and may become painful, uncomfortable and disabling. The proper treatment is to stop immediately the use of the anti-perspirant, use a boric acid compress several times a day, apply talcum powder, calamine lotion, or a cortisone cream.
Another chemical, a zirconium salt, is occasionally incorporated in an anti-perspirant and is known to produce bumps under the arm. These are known as granulomas. The Food and Drug Administration has ordered the discontinuance of this chemical in all anti-perspirants.

Q How can senior citizens guard against aging skin?

A The greatest danger in the production of aging skin is the continuous and frequent exposure to the ultraviolet rays of the sun. The exposure causes wrinkling, drying, and production of pigmentation and raised brownish spots which are usually irreversible.
The cellular layer of the skin grows upward and reaches the upper layer in 15-25 days. In certain diseased states, it is reduced to five days, as in psoriasis.
The rate of growth and normal appearance of the skin are influenced by hormones, vitamins, enzymes, and energy, which are secured from the intake of a balanced diet, rich in proteins and minerals, and low in fat and carbohydrates.
If sunburn is severe, consult a dermatologist. However, all of the damage due to sun exposure can be slowed down by the use of a sun-screening lotion containing para-aminobenzoic acid and its derivatives. After exposure use a moisturizing or emollient cream, or vegetable oils, to neutralize the painful effects. The sun-screen blocks the harmful ultraviolet rays and permits the tanning rays to increase the protective action of melanin.
As the individual ages, there is a lack of production of hormones which influences the formation of collagen, elastic fibers and fat tissues, and, as a result, the skin tissues become thin and flabby.
The use of external moisturizers containing vitamins A and D, panthenol, ribonucleic acid, aloe vera extract, and allantoin, may be helpful in reducing the lines of the skin and building up the weakening tissues. The value of hormone and steroid creams has not been established.

Q How can I keep from getting chapped lips?

A Chapped lips usually occur in the winter, but they may also develop any time of the year as an allergic reaction to certain lipsticks, or as the result of nervous biting or licking of lips. Never bite or suck lips, especially if they are dry and the tissue is beginning to crack! In this case, and during the winter as well, apply a lip softener and protector which contains emollients (lanolin is often the base), or externally apply vitamin A and vitamin E oils to the damaged lips. And finally, as is so often the case, a good internal supply of vitamins A, B, C, D, E and trace minerals is the best preventive measure of all.

HEALTHY SKIN AND HAIR FOR YOU

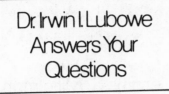

Dr. Irwin I. Lubowe
Answers Your
Questions

Q Will you please explain the physical structure of hair?

A A man and a woman each have about 100,000 hairs on their heads. A hair can grow for about six years, the length depending on the color. A cross section of the hair shows several layers. The outer layer is composed of a protective "horny" substance, akin in its chemical makeup to the scales of a fish. This layer is called the *cuticle,* a hardened outermost layer of the hairshaft. Next in the cross section comes the *cortex* or middle layer. This elastic material gives hair its amazing resilience and flexibility (manmade fibers would be really challenged in a competition with our own natural hair). The cortex contains the pigment which determines whether or not you will be a blonde, brunette, red- or black-haired lad or lass. Perhaps most important of all, the cortex also holds the bulk of amino acids, proteins and keratin.

The central core of a hair, called the *medulla,* resembles the marrow of a bone in that it is through this central shaft that the entire hair absorbs its nourishment. The medulla ends, in the scalp, with something that looks like a bulb. This bulb meets the *papilla* (a nipple-like projection) in the blood system, and through the papilla is supplied with vitamins and other nutrients—what happens at this juncture of the hair and head is the most important process for hair health. If this feeding is interfered with, the hair becomes dried out and thin, and splits. Just as with our bodies, we can apply all the external aids that we please, but if the inner support of oxygen and "fuel" is missing, then the entire structure suffers.

Q What can I do to solve my problem of dry skin?

A Some people naturally have only small amounts of water in their cutaneous layers (outer protective layers) of the skin, and therefore their skin tissues are always dry. This condition can be helped by using a superfatted soap or a cleansing cream which contains oil. After this, follow by applying a moisturizing cream containing 10 percent urea. A person who has dry skin should also take baths with bath oil added.

During the winter it is helpful to have a humidifier in your home, or to keep a shallow pan of water near your radiator, since indoor heating can be drying to the skin. Extra measures might need to be taken during the winter, such as an in-between-cleansings application to the skin surface of unsaturated fatty oils, such as sesame or avocado. Vaseline is also a good moisturizer since it keeps the natural water in the skin from evaporating.

Q Is there any way to thicken eyelashes and make them grow?

A Again, good health is the best insurance for beauty problems. But much of the determining factor in eyelashes is heredity, and the use of extra hormones or vitamins will not be able to make lashes any longer or thicker. To keep lashes healthy and to strengthen them against the drying onslaught of winter, you might try coating them with vegetable oil (especially castor oil). One great result of this treatment is that besides conditioning them, the oil can make lashes appear glossier and thicker.

Q What are some of the causes and types of baldness?

A Well, this is a difficult question to answer, for several reasons (one being that people are unwilling to talk about baldness or to listen to discussions on it). Often baldness is caused by a combination of factors. Let me just briefly list for you some common types of baldness:
1. Male Pattern Baldness is due basically to genetic coding or heredity.
2. Female Pattern Baldness is often due to hormone destruction or imbalance, such as too much male hormone.
3. *Alopecia aneata* is a spotty baldness.
4. Seborrheic Alopecia is the loss of hair due to a malfunction of the sebaceous glands (associated with the hair follicle) which secrete sebum, a mixture of fats and keratin.

5. Toxic Infections, such as caused by high fever, typhoid, measles, influenza or the poisoning influence of drugs can also lead to loss of hair.
6. Cicatrizing Alopecia refers to an infection of the hair follicle caused by bacteria and ringworm.
7. Postpartem Alopecia is a familiar case of hair loss which can occur from four to six months after giving birth. This is usually a disturbance of the telogen cycle, when a dead hair is held in the scalp for a certain amount of time before being released. During pregnancy these dead hairs may not be released, and are then lost all at once after birth.
8. Traction Baldness may follow after the use of curlers and rollers, or after teasing hair. It may also be caused by the tension on the scalp of certain hairstyles, such as a ponytail.
9. *Alopecia neurotica* is the formal term for baldness due to the nervous habit of pulling out hairs.
10. Cosmetic Abuse Alopecia is the baldness which can result after hair treatments such as dyeing, bleaching, straightening or permanent waving.

Q Can herbal treatments really do the hair some good?

A It is true that extracts of pine tar, balsam, lavender, thyme, rosemary and geranium are added to shampoos, conditioners and rinses. I would particularly recommend a balsam and hot oil treatment for damaged, dried-out, chemically or physically abused hair. (Note: balsam is a resinous substance which oozes from various plants.)

Q Are face masks helpful for the skin?

A They ususally consist of clay, bentonite and cleansing agents. There is also a peel-off mask which contains cleansing agents and a synthetic rubber compound.
The masks remove the dry, flaky skin and impurities, and produce a clean and smooth feeling. They also remove excessive oil, especially the clay mask. Their action is temporary. The same result can be secured more simply by using a neutral soap, astringent, and cleansing lotion at about half the cost.

☼

PREVENTIVE DENTAL CARE

Q My dentist says that I have periodontal disease, but my gums don't hurt and hardly ever bleed. Can you clear up my confusion about this?

A Patients are usually unaware when periodontal conditions are developing, because there is no pain or other warning in the early stages. Sore gums that bleed, food impaction, and bad breath are advanced signs. Progress is so insidious that symptoms are not often recognized by patients with much alarm, at least not until the opportunity for remedy has passed, and the teeth have to be sacrificed. If these symptoms are not attended to in time, the bone supporting the teeth becomes weakened and destroyed. Teeth loosen, and the disease progresses. When neighboring teeth are lost and are replaced, these loosened teeth are called upon to support new appliances. This further tends to weaken their support, and they are also soon condemned.

A survey by the U.S. Public Health Service showed that about three out of every four people who have natural teeth remaining showed some evidence of gingivitis or destructive periodontal disease.

The obvious answer is prevention, which means you must take the causes of gum disease into account. Treatment has to fail unless the factors that lead to the disease are considered. We must eliminate plaque (organized germ colonies growing on the teeth) and we must do it thoroughly once daily. We need to minimize and control stresses that can loosen teeth. These are mainly irregularities in the bite, and pressures of the tongue against the teeth which we find associated with abnormal swallowing habits. We need to raise our resistance level by adopting good health habits, including good nutrition. A recent observation by preventive periodontists suggests that a high protein breakfast is essential for healthy gums. People who skip breakfast or have a poor one appear to have periodontal difficulties, and they often actually lose their teeth, regardless of the in-office dental care they receive.

Q Which mouthwash is best to keep my breath clean?

A The most you can expect from a mouthwash is temporary freshening of the breath. The best way to solve a problem is to attack the cause,

Sound Advice on Good Oral Hygiene From Jerome S. Mittelman, D.D.S.

not the effect. The usual cause of bad breath, when it is due to conditions within the mouth, is plaque. Plaque is mainly composed of germ colonies organized around the necks of teeth, in between them, and under the gumline. Foul breath is caused by the waste products discharged by these germ growths. Mouthwash may flood away the surface accumulation of the waste products, but it will not seriously affect the plaque itself. We can take a smear, a sample of plaque from a tooth, place it on a microscope slide, add some "antiseptic" mouthwash, and look at it under a phase microscope. We see countless germs swimming and darting about unaffected by the mouthwash.

To protect your breath, you need to remove the plaque mechanically, using the Bass technique. The technique cannot be adequately taught in writing any more than you can teach someone to ride a bicycle with an essay. For the name of a preventive dentist in your area who can teach you the method, write to The American Society for Preventive Dentistry, 435 North Michigan Avenue, Chicago, Illinois 60611.

Sugar consumption encourages plaque formation, because the germs in the organized colonies that make up plaque thrive on it. On the other hand, some research indicates that vitamin C intake helps to diminish plaque formation. We suggest intake of 500 milligrams of vitamin C at least three times a day.

Q I'm told I grind my teeth at night. What causes me to do this? What can happen as a result? What can I do about it?

A Night clenching and grinding are common. Slight irregularities on the chewing surfaces of teeth trigger clenching. People clench on a high spot to grind it down, or to find a comfortable place to fit the jaws together. None of us are vegetables. We have nervous systems that respond to stress and tension. At night, when we think we are at peace with the world, many of us respond to the demands and tensions of the day. We grit our teeth in our sleep. Our jaw muscles clamp our teeth together with fantastic pressures—about 300 pounds per square inch, or about 68,000 pounds on the tip of a cusp. The muscles press upper and lower teeth together and from side to side. This pumping action can start disintegrating the bone that holds teeth, and the teeth loosen. One out of every four people in the United States has no teeth in one or both jaws, and the bone-weakening process is a major cause of this tragedy. The cure is to eliminate the cause. One can have his bite equilibrated to eliminate the trigger areas that set off clenching. Dentists sometimes construct plastic appliances with smooth, hard surfaces to cover any remaining trigger area. The appliance needs to be hard, because a soft, rubbery plastic would engage teeth in the opposing jaw and act as an orthodontic appliance, shifting and moving teeth. Nutritionally, we find that gritting teeth is associated with hypoglycemia, which can affect us even when we sleep. We therefore suggest a protein snack before retiring. Of course, if hypoglycemia is suspected—and it is common—then this should be checked by a nutritionally-oriented physician. Trace minerals calcium, magnesium and manganese are helpful to build resistance to the clenching and to protect the bone supporting the teeth.

Q What foods should a pregnant woman eat to assure healthy teeth for her baby?

A She should eat all the good foods that will provide for good health in general. But there are specific considerations. If the maternal diet contains much sugar, the teeth that are developing *in utero* will be more susceptible to decay. If the expectant mother avoids sugar, her child will have teeth that are more resistant to decay. During World War II there was little sugar eaten in Europe. Immediately after the war, sugar consumption increased rapidly, but the children whose teeth were formed when sugar was rare did not get the cavities that could be expected from the increased sugar intake. It is especially important to eat foods rich in calcium, phosphorus, and vitamins A, C, and D. ✿

BODY CHEMISTRY AND YOUR GLANDS

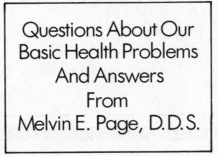

Questions About Our
Basic Health Problems
And Answers
From
Melvin E. Page, D.D.S.

Q Could you briefly explain some things that you do at your clinic, which a regular GP might not do.

A Our methods are to correct the body chemistry of a patient and to teach each patient about his dietary rules for they can be different for each individual. We stress his ancestral diet, for this diet served his ancestors very well for hundreds of generations. It is the diet to which his body has become adapted. The chief difference in our approach is that we want the patient to know about our methods and the reasons for his treatment and how to maintain the health of his body. We do not have a local practice. Our patients may live a long way from our city. The average stay with us as an out-patient is three weeks and we may not see the person again for a year or more but we try to keep in touch by requesting a yearly visit or by laboratory reports from his own vicinity. There is no mystery about our work that a person with fair intelligence cannot grasp in three weeks.

Q How do other doctors react to your work?

A About one-third of our patients are doctors or their families. We have no trouble with other doctors as we do not take medical cases. I like to say that other doctors (except for those whom we have trained), do not do our work and we do not do theirs. There is no conflict. We even hope that other doctors will learn how to do this work and give us some competition.

Q Are there any prevalent health dictates, as practiced by established medical treatment, that you have come to disagree with?

A When doctors try to tell their patients about nutrition, they are usually out of their field, as very little is taught about this subject in either the medical or dental schools. There are some that are quite knowledgeable about foods but they are self-taught. There are quite a few doctors that attempt to guide their patients as to diet but most do not know as much about the subject as the average housewife.

Q What kind of therapy do you prescribe for hormone and metabolism imbalances?

A For hormone and metabolism imbalances, we try to use the exocrines and endocrines in just the right amounts to compensate for the personal deficiency in the patient, in these substances. The glandular set-ups for each individual can be and usually are very different, for no two people are made alike.

Q Is diagnosis and treatment very different for males and females?

A There is very little, if any difference, in the diagnoses of male and female patients but there is a little difference in some of the hormones used and quite a lot of quantitative differences such as over-active anterior pituitaries being greater in the male and under-active posterior pituitaries being more than twice as great in the females.

Q Do you think that your kind of medical diagnosis and treatment, with body chemistry analysis, could be effectively used for animals as well as for humans?

A I think that hormone treatment is probably needed in other animals as well as man but how to diagnose deficiencies in an animal is the problem. I believe the individuality varies in all animals. This is due to the individual gene inheritance as well as in the food selected for them by man.

Q One hears increasingly of how diet can affect marriage. How do you feel that endocrinology affects married life and interpersonal relationships?

A This question deserves quite a lengthy answer. I have learned and have known for quite some time that when a couple has been married for a long time successfully, the graph of each couple is almost exactly opposite. What I have been unable to determine is how the graphs of couples differ, and in what respects, where they do not or have not gotten along and the marriage ends in divorce. This is because I have seen only one member of the couple when divorce occurred.

What I do not know is how successful marriages take place without a means of measuring compatibility before the marriage; but there are ways —as many marriages are successful. The miracle is that there are so many successful marriages—not that there are so many divorces.

When the measurements that I invented to determine the glandular pattern of a person are exactly opposite from the mate, the marriage is a good one and lasts. Both males and females have some ability to select the proper mate but this ability is greater in the female.

Q What do you find affects the body metabolism and chemistry besides food? For instance, is weather important, or psychological pressure? Or is the healthy body fairly impervious to such influences?

A The healthy body is practically impervious to the ordinary hazards of living. There are very few healthy Andrics that spend nearly all of their time sitting at a desk or at cocktail parties. This may be the main reason for the heart cases and for Americans to be in the twelfth place insofar as health goes.

Q To what degree is the body chemistry (the glandular balances) set at birth? Are there inescapable type-traits?

A The gene inheritance is set before birth but the gene inheritance determines the glandular pattern. We can't at present change the gene inheritance of a person, or the endocrine pattern, but by a good diet we can change the results of a bad pattern to a good chemistry. Our work is to change the bad results of a bad pattern to good body chemistry. We use minute amounts of hormones to do this quickly which otherwise might take many years to change by diet alone. ☼

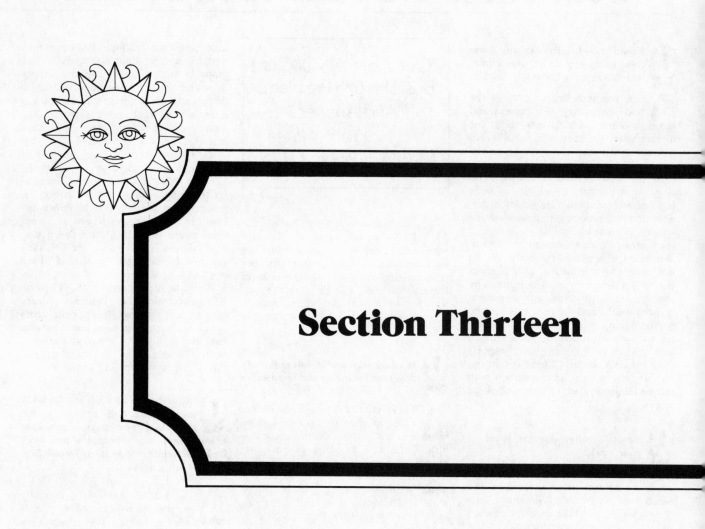

Section Thirteen

Recipes, Recipes and More Recipes

RICE AND NUT LOAF

3 cups cooked brown rice
1/2 cup chopped walnuts
1/4 cup chopped green pepper
2 eggs, separated
1/2 teaspoon salt
1/4 teaspoon paprika
pepper to taste

Preheat oven to 350° F.
Mix together all ingredients except the egg whites. Beat the egg whites until stiff. Fold the rice mixture into the egg whites and turn into casserole. Bake 30-45 minutes or until set. Serve with tomato sauce. Serves 4.

POTATO-CHEESE PIE

2 cups cottage cheese
2/3 cup sour cream
2 cups mashed potatoes
2 eggs, well beaten
1 teaspoon salt
1 medium chopped onion
3 tablespoons pimento or pimento-
   stuffed green olives
pepper to taste
1-1/2 tablespoons butter
1 9-inch pastry shell, unbaked

Preheat oven to 350° F.
Blend cottage cheese and sour cream, beat in the potatoes and then add all the rest of the ingredients except the butter. Pour into pastry shell, dot with butter and bake for 1 to 1-1/4 hours or until set. Serve hot or cold.
(Pie can be made with sweet potatoes.)
Serves 4.

EGGPLANT NIBBLER DIP

1 eggplant
3 tomatoes, peeled and chopped
4 tablespoons olive oil
1 tablespoon honey
1 tablespoon vinegar
salt and pepper

Preheat oven to 350° F.
Bake eggplant for 25 to 30 minutes. Cool, peel and chop into small cubes. Add tomatoes. Make a dressing of the remaining ingredients and pour over eggplant and tomatoes. Chill for 1 hour. Serve with crackers and a mild cheese such as cream or cottage cheese.
Serves 4 to 6.

Using Superfoods
in
Everyday dishes

HIGH-PROTEIN PANCAKES

Mix in blender:

3 eggs
1/2 cup cottage cheese
2 tablespoons oil
2 tablespoons milk
1/2 teaspoon vanilla (optional)

Combine and mix well:

1/4 cup whole wheat flour
1/2 teaspoon baking powder
1/2 teaspoon salt

Pour blended mixture over dry ingredients and stir thoroughly. Cook as usual for pancakes.
(Milk and flour can be adjusted for desired thickness: this recipe can be used for pancakes or crepes.)
Serves 2-3.

WHEAT GERM AND OATMEAL COOKIES

3/4 cup vegetable oil
1-1/4 cups honey or dark molasses
2 eggs, beaten
2 teaspoons vanilla
3/4 cup whole wheat or soy flour
1 cup raisins
1-1/2 cups wheat germ
2 cups rolled oats
1 teaspoon salt
1/2 cup powered milk

Preheat oven to 350° F.
Mix together all ingredients until the mixture is smooth. Drop from a teaspoon on to a baking sheet covered with foil or well-greased heavy brown paper. Keep cookies at least a cookie's distance apart. Bake for 10 to 12 minutes.

LECITHIN HONEY CANDY

12 ounce jar of creamed honey
3 tablespoons liquid lecithin
1 cup chopped nuts
2 tablespoons lemon juice

---

1 teaspoon bone meal
3 cups coconut, finely grated
1/2 cup soy powder
1/4 cup non-instant dry milk
1/4 cup sesame meal
1 tablespoon vanilla

Mix all ingredients very well. Place in an 8-inch by 8-inch pan. Sprinkle with extra chopped nuts and refrigerate for 2 hours or until firm. Cut into 1-inch squares or roll into balls and dip in grated coconut.

NUTRITIOUS SEED BREAD

2 cups unbleached white flour
1/4 cup wheat germ
1/2 teaspoon salt
2 teaspoons crushed sunflower
   seeds
3 teaspoons sesame seeds
1 teaspoon caraway seeds
1/2 cup raisins
2 teaspoons honey
2 eggs
1 cup milk

Preheat oven to 350° F.
Sift together flour, wheat germ and salt. Mix seeds and raisins and add to dry ingredients. Mix again and add honey. Beat eggs with milk and gradually stir into dry mixture. Stir until dough leaves the sides of the bowl. Dough will be slightly sticky. Bake in well-greased loaf pan for 45-55 minutes. Turn out and cool on wire rack.

HOT, HOT HORSERADISH FOR BEEF

3 tablespoons freshly grated
   horseradish
2 tablespoons lemon juice
¼ teaspoon sea salt
few grains cayenne
1 cup yogurt or sour cream or half
   and half

Grating horseradish cleans out every nasal, throat and even lung passage and may be well worth the weeping. This sauce is fine for any kind of roast beef or hamburger. Mix all ingredients thoroughly and chill for an hour or so before serving. ☼

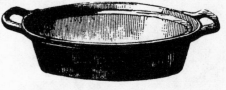

WONDERFUL WORLD OF SOYBEAN COOKERY

by
Barbara Farr

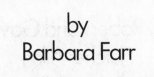

COOKING SOYBEANS

Method 1
Soak the soybeans 6 hours or overnight. 1/3 cup dry=1 cup soaked. Freeze the beans in soaking water, then cook for about 1 hour.

Method 2
Cook the soaked soybeans in a pressure cooker at 15 lbs. (standard) pressure for 45 minutes.

Method 3
Cook the soaked soybeans over low heat for several hours. Add water as needed. Skim foam from the beans when they reach a boil.

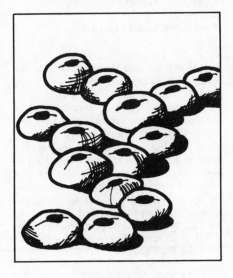

TOFU
(SOYA BEAN CURD)

4 cups water
1 cup soya powder
4 tablespoons lemon juice

Mix the soya powder and water together and let stand 20 minutes, stirring occasionally. Bring the mixture to a boil in a very large pot. Stir constantly. Reduce heat and simmer 5 minutes. Remove pan from heat and add lemon juice all at once, while stirring. Allow mixture to cool to room temperature. Drain mixture into a cheesecloth-lined colander. Wrap the drained curds in the cheesecloth and hang to drain for about an hour. Gently remove the cloth. Whole or sliced tofu may be stored in the refrigerator, covered with water, for several days.

CHILI SIN CARNE

1 cup dried soybeans
1 cup lentils
1/2 cup sesame seeds
2 green peppers, chopped fine
3 medium onions, chopped fine
2 tablespoons peanut oil
1 tablespoon salt
2 tablespoons chili powder
2 cloves garlic, crushed
1/2 teaspoon powdered cumin
1/2 teaspoon oregano

Cover the soybeans with cold water. Bring to a boil, remove from heat and let stand one hour. Drain the beans, cover with fresh cold water, bring to a boil and simmer over low heat 1 hour. Add the lentils and sesame seeds to the soybeans. Add enough cold water to cover. Bring to a simmer. Sauté the onions and peppers briefly in the peanut oil until they are barely limp. Add the vegetables and oil to the bean pot. Add

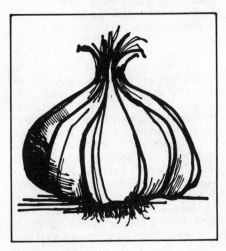

the remaining ingredients, and simmer for about 30 minutes or until everything is tender. Serve hot with brown rice. Serves 6.

Garnishes for chili dishes
Guacamole, grated cheese, diced tomato, minced onion, shredded lettuce, minced radish.

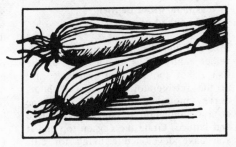

DIP JAPONAISE

2 scallions
2 tablespoons miso*
1 tablespoon tahini*
1/2 teaspoon fresh grated ginger (optional)
2/3 cup soy yogurt (or plain dairy yogurt)

Mince the scallions, keeping the green and white parts separate. Mix the miso, tahini, ginger and white part of scallion. Stir in the yogurt. Garnish with the green part of the scallion. Chill and serve as a dip with fresh vegetables, or heat in a double boiler and serve as a warm dip or sauce for cooked vegetables.

*Available in health stores

NEAR-EASTERN
TAHINI SPREAD

1 cup cooked soybeans
1/3 cup tahini
1-2 cloves garlic, crushed
2 tablespoons lemon juice
dash cayenne pepper
1/2 teaspoon sea salt
fresh parsley, chopped

Put all ingredients except parsley in a blender and blend until smooth. Pile in a bowl and garnish with lots of chopped parsley. Serve as a spread for thin crackers, or as a dip. ☼

NATURAL COOKERY FROM SCANDINAVIA

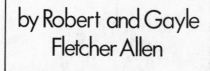

by Robert and Gayle
Fletcher Allen

FISH SALAD

2 cups cooked fish, deboned and flaked
1 cup sour cream
1 tablespoon grated horseradish
1 cup grated sweet onion
1 tablespoon lemon juice
1 tablespoon chopped fresh dill
1 teaspoon salt
¼ teaspoon white pepper
1 hard-cooked egg

Mix the ingredients except the egg together gently so as to not break up the fish flakes too much. Cover and chill in the refrigerator for about 1 hour. Serve, mounded on shredded lettuce or a combination of shredded cabbage and lettuce. Grate the egg on top and if you have developed a liking for dill, sprinkle a bit more on top. Serve with crisp-bread crackers with sweet butter or soft, spreadable cheese.

LAMB AND CABBAGE DINNER

2 tablespoons butter
2 pounds lamb shoulder, cut in 1-inch cubes
sea salt and pepper to taste
1 tablespoon lemon juice
1 onion, thinly sliced
1 cup chopped parsley
1 head firm cabbage

In a large Dutch oven melt the butter and quickly brown the lamb cubes. Add enough water to completely cover the lamb, about 2 cups. Season with salt, pepper and lemon juice. Cover and put into a preheated 325° F. oven for about 45 minutes. Add the onion and then the parsley. Cut the cabbage head into 8 wedges and add to the pot. Continue baking, covered, for an additional 45 minutes. Serve with boiled or steamed potatoes.

FINNISH HARDTACK

1 cake yeast or 1 tablespoon yeast granules
2 cups warm water
1 teaspoon salt
4 cups rye flour (approximate)

In a warm bowl dissolve the yeast in 2 cups water until it bubbles. Sift the salt into the rye flour and combine with yeast water. Mix well. Cover with a slightly damp towel and let rise in a warm place until doubled in bulk. Punch down and form into balls 3 inches in diameter. Use flour to prevent dough from sticking to your hands. Roll each ball out into a round, about 1/4 inch thick. Using a large spatula, lay each round out on a greased or teflon-surfaced cookie sheet. Cut a 2-inch diameter hole in the center of each round. Let rise about 30 minutes. Prick the top generously with the tines of a fork. Bake quickly in a preheated 450 oven for about 10 minutes.

You will want the rounds to be firm, but bendable when removed from the oven. Finnish housewives hang these rounds so they dry by themselves. We dry them by returning to a cool oven.

FRUIT SOUP

1½ quarts water (more if needed)
½ cup pitted dried prunes
½ cup dried apricots
½ cup dried peaches
½ cup raisins
½ cup tart apple slices
1 stick cinnamon
1 tablespoon lemon juice
1 teaspoon grated lemon rind
3 tablespoons quick tapioca
½ cup honey

Bring the water to a boil in a large kettle (the fruit volume will increase). Put in the prunes, apricots, peaches and raisins. Turn off the fire, cover, and let soak for 1 hour. If you prefer, soak fruit overnight in cold water. Cook with the apple, cinnamon stick, lemon juice, rind, tapioca and honey until thick and clear, stirring often with a wooden spoon to prevent sticking. If not sweet enough, add more honey. Cool and serve in clear glass dishes.

An interesting variation is to reduce the water to 5 cups and add 1 cup organic berry juice (grape, raspberry, boysenberry, blackberry or strawberry). Arrowroot flour may be substituted for the tapioca (use a scant 2 tablespoons).

For a creamier soup put the fruit in the blender and puree.

There are a number of good toppings for fruit soup, such as whipped cream, a few whole berries, sour cream or ice cream. But far and away the best is the one below.

SWEDISH CREAM

2 tablespoons butter
2 tablespoons unbleached flour
1 tablespoon honey
1 cup light cream
2 eggs
1 teaspoon vanilla extract

Melt the butter over low to medium heat. Add the flour and stir with a wire whisk until blended. Add the honey and cream, stirring constantly, until mixture thickens, about 5 minutes. *Do not let boil*. Remove from fire. Beat the eggs until light and lemon colored. Pour the hot mixture into the eggs a little at a time, stirring constantly. When thoroughly blended, put back over low heat and stir for an additional 2 minutes, or until thickened. If left too long the cream will appear curdled. If so, put in the blender. Add the vanilla last. Chill and serve for each guest to use over the fruit soup.

JANSSON'S TEMPTATION

4 medium-to-large potatoes
2 medium-to-large brown onions
8 anchovy fillets, well drained
¼ teaspoon white pepper
1 cup light cream
⅓ cup bread crumbs
2 tablespoons butter

Butter a casserole dish. Slice the potatoes, placing a layer on the bottom of the dish. Add the onions, sliced very thin, in a layer. Arrange the anchovies in a layer on top of the onions. Complete with a layer of potatoes. Sprinkle with white pepper and pour the cream over all. Top with the bread crumbs and dots of butter. Bake in a preheated 325° F. oven until the potatoes are tender. ☀

CARAWAY SEED CRESCENT ROLLS

1 tablespoon dry yeast granules
1/4 cup warm water
1/4 cup honey
1/3 cup oil
1 cup milk, scalded, and cooled to lukewarm
1-1/2 teaspoons sea salt or kelp
1/4 cup wheat germ
1/3 cup soy flour
3 cups unbleached white flour
3 cups oat flour (about)
2 tablespoons butter, melted
1/4 cup caraway seeds

Soften the yeast in the water. Measure into a large bowl the honey, oil, milk, and salt (or kelp). Mix thoroughly. When the yeast mixture has bubbled, combine the 2 mixtures. Gradually add the wheat germ and flours, using only enough oat flour to make a stiff dough. Turn the dough out onto a floured board, and knead until smooth and elastic. Place in a greased bowl, oil the top, cover, and set in a warm place to rise until double in bulk. Punch down, knead, and divide into 4 equal parts. Roll each part into a ball, and allow to rest for 10 minutes. Roll out each ball into a circle 1/4 inch thick. Cut each circle into 8 wedge-shaped pieces. Roll up each piece, starting with the wide end. Bend into a semi-circle. Place on greased cooky sheets, allowing space between. Brush with butter, and sprinkle with caraway seeds. Cover, and set in a warm place to rise until double in bulk. Bake at 425° F. for about 10 minutes. Yields 2-2/3 dozen crescent rolls.

HAMBURGER BUNS

2 tablespoons dry yeast granules
1/4 cup warm water
3 tablespoons honey
3 tablespoons oil
1 egg, beaten
1 teaspoon sea salt or kelp
3-1/2 cups whole wheat flour (about)
1/4 cup sesame seeds

Soften the yeast in the water. When the mixture bubbles, add the honey, oil, egg, and salt (or kelp). Blend thoroughly, and allow to rise for 10 minutes. Then add enough whole-

with
Beatrice Trum Hunter

wheat flour to make a soft dough. Turn the dough out onto a floured board, and knead until it is smooth and elastic. Shape into round, flat buns, and place on greased cooky sheets, allowing space between. Brush the tops of the buns with cold water, and sprinkle with sesame seeds. Cover the buns, and set in a warm place, to rise until double in bulk. Bake at 375° F. for 15 minutes. Yields 2 dozen buns.

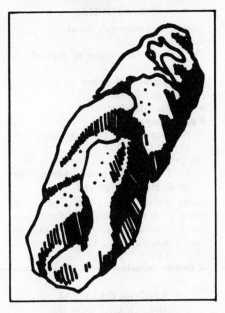

TANGY CHEESE BREAD

1 tablespoon dry yeast granules
3/4 cup warm water
2 tablespoons honey
2 tablespoons butter
2 eggs
1 cup milk
1 teaspoon sea salt or kelp
1/2 teaspoon sweet paprika, ground
1-1/4 cups sharp Cheddar cheese, grated
4-3/4 cups wholewheat flour (about)
1 egg yolk, beaten
1/3 cup sesame seeds

Soften the yeast in the water, with the honey added. When the mixture

bubbles, add the butter, eggs, milk, salt (or kelp), paprika, and cheese. Then add enough wholewheat flour to make a stiff dough. Turn the dough out onto a lightly floured board, and knead until smooth and elastic. Shape into a ball, place in a greased bowl, and brush the top with oil. Cover, and set in a warm place to rise until double in bulk. Turn the dough out onto the floured board again, and knead lightly for 1 minute. Divide the dough in half, and shape into loaves. Place in greased bread pans. Brush the tops with the beaten egg yolk, and then sprinkle them with the sesame seeds. Cover, and let rise in a warm place for about 40 minutes. Bake at 350° F. for 15 minutes, and then reduce the heat to 325° F. for 25 to 30 minutes longer. Yields 2 loaves.

SAND TARTS

In the days of early Christianity small heart-shaped cakes were baked on saints' days. They were called Life Cakes or Saints' Hearts. Later, these cakes were ornamented and bestowed as gifts on saints' days. The name became distorted from Saints' Hearts to Sand Tarts. The museum at Bath, England, has a collection of old cutters used in making these cakes.

1 cup honey
1 cup oil
1 teaspoon grated lemon rind, from organic fruit
3 egg whites
3-1/2 cups oat flour (about)
1/2 cup nutmeats, broken
cinnamon

Blend the honey, oil, lemon rind, and 2 of the egg whites. Add to this mixture enough oat flour to make a dough of a good consistency to hold together. Chill. Roll to 1/8-inch thickness, and cut into 2-inch rounds. Place the rounds on greased cooky sheets. Brush the tops with egg white, and then sprinkle with the nutmeats. Bake at 350° F. for 8 minutes. After removing the tarts from the oven, dust the tops with cinnamon. Then return the tarts to the oven for another minute. Yields 5 dozen tarts.

ONE-OF-A-KIND RECIPES TO LOVE

SOYCHEESE CASSEROLE

2 cups cottage cheese
2 cups presoaked soybeans
3 cups beef broth
3 garlic cloves
2 large onions, diced
3 large tomatoes
1 cup grated cheese (cheddar)
2 tablespoons butter
¾ teaspoon thyme
1 cup cooked brown rice
additional herbs and spices, to taste

Simmer soybeans in broth with thyme. In separate pan, brown garlic and onion in butter, add tomatoes, herbs and spices (basil, oregano, rosemary —whatever your preference). Simmer until onions are tender. Add cottage cheese and rice to cooked soybeans. Add ingredients of second pan to soybean pot, mix and pour entire mixture in casserole dish. Sprinkle with grated cheddar cheese, cover and bake 30 minutes at 350°.

Delicious!

SIMPLE SIMON PANCAKES

⅞ cup brown rice flour
⅛ cup unbleached white flour
1 level teaspoon baking soda
½ teaspoon sea salt

Combine with

1 tablespoon honey (more or less to taste)
2 eggs
1 cup kefir or thick buttermilk

Fry on very lightly greased griddle.

Note: Brown rice flour is sometimes grainy, hence the addition of the unbleached. If your brown rice flour is nice and smooth, the unbleached may be omitted and all rice flour used.

No shortening in the pancakes.

GLUTEN SOY BREAD

1 tablespoon dried yeast granules
1 tablespoon honey
1 tablespoon vegetable oil
1 teaspoon sea salt
1½ cups gluten flour
¾ cup soy flour
¼ cup wheat germ

Dissolve yeast in 1 cup plus 2 tablespoons warm water. Stir in honey and oil. Mix salt, gluten and soy flours and wheat germ, and stir very thoroughly into liquid. Spread ½ cup whole wheat or unbleached flour on kneading board. Knead dough for at least 10 minutes. The longer you knead, the lighter the

bread will be. Put in oiled covered bowl and let rise about 1¼ hours or until double in bulk. Punch down and place in 9 x 5 x 3 bread pan. Let rise again until dough is just a little higher than top of pan. Bake for 50-55 minutes at 325°.

I omit the salt for my own personal salt-free diet and you can't tell it is salt-free. This is a very high-protein, low starch loaf that is very light and very, very good.

RATATOUILLE

2 eggplants skinned, diced
6 zucchini, diced
1½ cups tomato sauce or stewed tomatoes
2 large onions, chopped
3 cloves garlic, minced
8 tablespoons olive oil
1 green pepper, diced
½ teaspoon each parsley, oregano, thyme
sea salt to taste
½ to 1 pound cheese, cheddar or jack, cubed or grated

Saute diced eggplant, zucchini and onion in garlic and olive oil for 10 minutes. Combine all ingredients in covered casserole and bake for 1 hour at 300°.

A family favorite

CHEWY OATMEAL MOLASSES COOKIES

1½ cups unbleached flour
1 teaspoon soda
½ teaspoon salt
½ teaspoon cloves
½ teaspoon ginger
½ cup brown sugar
½ cup raw sugar (pulverized in blender)
¾ cup soy margarine
⅓ cup dark molasses, or blackstrap
¾ cup oats (pulverized in blender)
1 cup walnuts, chopped fine

In a medium mixing bowl sift flour, soda, salt, cloves, ginger and sugar. Add margarine, egg and molasses. Beat until smooth—about 2 minutes. Add oats and walnuts.

Drop by level tablespoons, 2 inches

apart on an ungreased cooky sheet. I flatten them with a spoon. Bake 8 to 10 minutes at 375° or until brown. Let stand a minute or so before removing with a wide spatula. Store in a tightly covered container. Note: If you want to omit the walnuts, decrease molasses to ¼ cup. Almonds may be substituted, or any nuts you prefer.

CINDY'S PROTEIN CANDY

1 cup honey
1 cup peanut butter
½ cup soy grits (ground)
½ cup wheat germ
1 cup carob powder
1 cup sunflower seeds (ground)
1 cup sesame seeds (ground)
½ cup liquid lecithin

Mix together and form into small balls. Coat with nuts, coconut, or whatever you wish.

TREKIES

Combine:
⅜ cup soya oil
⅛ cup plus 1 tablespoon molasses
⅜ cup water
¼ cup peanut butter
½ cup powdered dry milk
1 egg
1 teaspoon vanilla (opt.)
1½ cups raw sugar
1-2 teaspoons brewer's yeast
¼-½ teaspoon kelp powder (opt.)
1 tablespoon bonemeal powder (opt.)

Mix well. In another bowl combine:
1½ cups brown rice flour or 2 cups whole wheat flour
½ cup soya flour
¾ teaspoon baking soda
½ teaspoon sea salt
⅓ cup sesame seeds
⅓ cup wheat germ

Combine with first mixture. Add about ⅓ cup rolled oats. Drop on greased cooky sheet. Flatten as much as possible with fork or palm. (The flatter the crispier!) Bake for 10-15 minutes at 325-350°. Makes about 4 dozen cookies. ☼

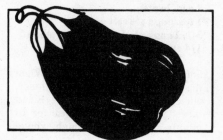

MEALS AND MENUS FOR BETTER HEALTH

SOUR DOUGH BREAD

3 cups hot water
1 cup milk
4 tablespoons oil
3 tablespoons honey or raw sugar
1 tablespoon sea salt
2 tablespoons dry granulated yeast
1-1/2 cups *Sour Dough Mix* (see below)
3 cups unbleached white flour
3 cups whole wheat flour
1 cup sunflower, pumpkin or sesame seeds (shelled)
1 cup sunflower, pumpkin or sesame meal
6 tablespoons wheat germ
3 tablespoons brewer's yeast
1 egg
2 tablespoons water
Sunflower kernels

Mix hot water, milk, oil and honey and let cool until lukewarm. Then add sea salt and yeast. Mix well and add Sour Dough Mix. Mix again and add unbleached white flour, whole wheat flour, sunflower seed, sunflower meal, wheat germ and brewer's yeast. Mix well and add enough unbleached white flour until mix is stiff enough to knead. Knead for about 20 to 30 minutes (until it no longer sticks to the hands). Put into greased large bowl and let rise until doubled in size. Knead down and again let rise until double. Then knead into loaves and put into bread pans so that they are half-filled. Mix egg and water and brush tops of loaves and sprinkle thickly with sunflower kernels. Bake loaves at 375 degrees for 40 minutes. Yield: 6 loaves.

SOUR DOUGH MIX

2 tablespoons dry yeast
2 cups lukewarm water (or potato water)
1 tablespoon honey
2 cups unbleached white flour

Mix above ingredients well and let stand 4 or 5 days, mixing occasionally. You will then have *Sour Dough Mix.*

Favorite Recipes to Share

Each time you bake, reactivate the Sour Dough the night before: Take the same ingredients as above, mix with leftover dough and let stand overnight. When you bake, take out 1 cup of the Sour Dough mix and save it in the refrigerator for the next time. Use 1½ cups of the mix for each six loaves of bread you bake.

BROWN EGGNOG

1 glass of milk
1 egg
3 teaspoons carob
Sprinkle of kelp powder

Mix all above ingredients in your blender; then serve with a sprinkle of wheat germ and drink with some solid food.

CARROT PRESERVES

1 pound carrots
12 ounces raw sugar (1 pound if desired)
1 cup fresh orange juice

Steam carrots in a small amount of water; then puree them in the remaining water. Add sugar and orange

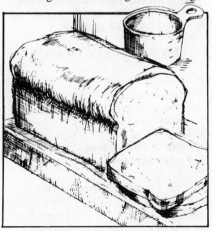

---

juice. Cook over low heat for approximately one and one-half hours or until it thickens to desired consistency. Stir often to prevent sticking or burning. Delicious on muffins or toast. Yield: one pint of preserves.

TUTTI FRUITTI BARS (PASSION BARS)

1/4 cup vegetable oil
1 tablespoon dark molasses
7/8 cup raw sugar
2 eggs
2 teaspoons vanilla
1 cup wheat germ or old fashioned rolled oats
1/4 teaspoon sea salt
1/2 cup milk
1/2 teaspoon baking powder
1/2 cup each of broken nut meats, raisins, dates
1/2 cup steamed dried prunes, diced

Blend all ingredients. Place in 8"x8" pan which has been oiled and sprinkled with wheat germ. Bake for 30 minutes (more or less) at 350 F. Watch carefully last ten minutes so as to not overbake. If doubling recipe, use 1 cup wheat germ and 1 cup oats.

OATMEAL PANCAKES/ WAFFLES

2 cups milk
2 cups oats (old fashioned rolled)
1/3 cup whole wheat flour
2 teaspoons baking powder
1 tablespoon raw sugar (optional)
1 teaspoon sea salt
2 eggs, separated
1/4 cup oil
1 apple (unpeeled), grated

Heat milk just to boiling. Pour over rolled oats in a 3-quart bowl. Stir until oats are moist. Cool until lukewarm. Sift flour with other dry ingredients. Separate eggs and add yolks and oil to oats. Add flour and dry ingredient mixture; then fold in egg whites and grated apple. Place in refrigerator if you are not ready then and there to try it. Serve with a syrup made with honey and oranges, and with homemade yogurt. ☼

RECIPES FOR SHARING

EDIBLE PLAY DOUGH

Mix together thoroughly:

1/2 cup peanut butter
1/4 cup honey
1/2 cup instant powdered milk
   (more if needed)

Be sure the children's hands are clean. Then let them mold or roll the dough into balls or shapes. When they tire of playing they can eat their creations.

FIBER COOKIES

3 to 4 tablespoons wheat bran
2/3 cup wheat germ
1/2 teaspoon baking soda
1/2 teaspoon baking powder
dash sea salt
1 tablespoon shortening
2-1/2 tablespoons raw sugar
4 tablespoons honey
2 eggs
carob-covered raisins
mixed nuts, sesame seeds and
   sesame-honey bars, chopped

Preheat oven to 375° F. Mix all ingredients together in a bowl. Drop by teaspoonfuls onto a greased cookie sheet and flatten. Bake for 10 minutes or until dark brown.

CHEESE BLINTZES

Batter:
3 eggs
2 tablespoons water

Beat eggs and water. Make thin pancakes, using 3 tablespoons of batter in a small, lightly greased skillet (6-inch). Tip pan in all directions to make an even layer of batter. Brown only one side and turn out on clean cloth or wax paper. (be sure that the pan is greased very lightly after each pancake or they will stick as they are very delicate.)

Filling:
2/3 cup cottage cheese
1 egg, beaten
1 small bunch green onions, chopped
1 tablespoon brewer's yeast
salt and pepper to taste

Combine filling ingredients and mash

**Taste + Nutrition
are part of
the new math**

---

well. Put 1 heaping tablespoon of filling on the edge of the browned side of pancake. Roll up, tuck in ends. Broil or bake in hot oven for 10 to 15 minutes. Serves 3.
Note: I double and triple this recipe successfully and store in the refrigerator, covered, for up to a week, using as needed. Sometimes I spread plain yogurt on top of the blintzes and sprinkle with sesame seeds.

BRAN-WHEAT GERM MUFFINS

1 cup whole wheat flour
1/2 cup bran
1/2 cup wheat germ
1/2 teaspoon sea salt
2-1/2 teaspoons baking powder
1 teaspoon cinnamon
1/2 teaspoon nutmeg
1/2 teaspoon allspice
4 tablespoons raw sugar
1 egg
1/2 cup safflower oil
1/2 cup chopped walnuts

Preheat oven to 450° F. Mix first 8 ingredients together in large bowl. Add next 4. Mix all ingredients until well blended. If you like raisins, add 1/2 cup. Fill muffin tins 2/3 full. Bake for 20 to 25 minutes at 425° F. Makes 12 muffins.

SUNSHINE RAISIN CANDY

1/2 cup honey
1/2 cup peanut butter
   (unhydrogenated)
1 cup powdered milk
1/2 cup raisins
1/4 cup sunflower seeds
1/4 cup wheat germ

Mix all ingredients well (I thin the honey a bit with water). Form balls a little smaller than a walnut. Roll in grated coconut or ground nuts.

GRANOLA

1 cup rolled wheat
1 cup rolled rye
1 cup rolled oats
1 cup millet meal
1/2 cup almonds
1/2 teaspoon sea salt
1/2 cup sesame seed
1/2 cup sunflower seed
1/2 cup coconut, grated
1/2 cup wheat grits
1/2 cup soy grits
1/3 cup soy oil
1 teaspoon vanilla
2 tablespoons honey
2 tablespoons apple cider
1/2 cup whey
1/2 cup chopped dates
1/2 cup raisins

Combine dry ingredients. Mix oil, vanilla, honey, cider and whey. Combine dry and wet ingredients and spread on cookie sheet. Bake at 325° F. for 40 minutes, turning every 10 to 15 minutes in order to brown evenly. When cereal is cool, add dates and raisins. Eat dry or with milk. Very little sweetening is needed because of the natural sweetness of whey, dates and raisins.

IMITATION STRAWBERRY COOLER

2 cups unsweetened pineapple juice
1 apple, cut up
3 small raw beets, grated
2 tablespoons honey
6 ice cubes
1 teaspoon vanilla (optional)

Put 1 cup pineapple juice in blender and add apple, beets and honey. Blend until smooth and add the rest of the pineapple juice, ice cubes and vanilla if wanted. Blend until thick. Makes 4 medium drinks.

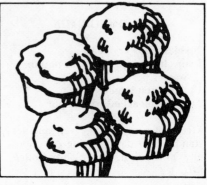

STUFFED EGGPLANT

2 eggplants
1 large onion, chopped
2 tablespoons, vegetable oil
2 cloves garlic, minced or pressed
1½ cups cooked beans (chopped or
    ground)—any beans will do—
    pinto, garbanzo, soy, or lima
1 cup cooked brown rice
½ cup chopped bell (green) pepper
1 tablespoon nutritional yeast
½ teaspoon each: basil, parsley,
    thyme
2 tablespoons soy sauce
1 egg, slightly beaten
1 large tomato, sliced
1 cup grated cheese

Cut eggplants lengthwise. Scoop out pulp, leaving ½″ thick shell. Set aside. Saute onion and garlic in oil until onion is transparent. Combine beans, rice, pepper, yeast, herbs, soy sauce and egg. Add onion and garlic. Mix well. Stuff eggplant shells with mixture. Place stuffed shells in a pan with 1 inch of hot water in the bottom. Bake 350° for 45 to 60 minutes. Check during baking to be sure water hasn't dried up. During last 5 minutes of baking top each portion with sliced tomatoes and grated cheese. Just before serving you may want to add a special touch and garnish with wheat germ and paprika.

MEATLESS MEATLOAF

3 cups cooked brown rice (1 cup
    rice to 3 cups water)
1½ cups cottage cheese
½ cup peanut butter
2 tablespoons butter, or oil
1 teaspoon salt
2 eggs
2 tablespoons onion, chopped fine
½ teaspoon pepper

Cook rice in top of double boiler, gently, for 40 minutes. While still hot, stir in all of above ingredients. Bake in greased square pan (9x9x2) 30 to 40 minutes in 350° oven, or until bubbling and brown. (May be cooked in casserole dish, but will probably need more time if dish is not as shallow as pan, and if it is glass, or other non-metal.) Of course, the longer it is baked the less moist it will be. It should be able to be taken up in flat slabs, not have to be spooned out.

A Variety
of Favorites
From Everywhere

ZUCCHINI PANCAKES

½ pound grated zucchini
2 tablespoons unbleached flour
1 tablespoon soy flour
1 tablespoon brewer's yeast
1 tablespoon wheat germ
½ cup parmesan cheese
2 eggs
½ teaspoon soda
dash pepper
dash marjoram

Mix all ingredients together and fry as pancakes. For variation, add fresh bean sprouts.

These pancakes may be served as a main course at breakfast or as a side dish at lunch or dinner.

SOYBEAN SOUP

1 cup dry soybeans
water
salt
3 tablespoons butter or oil
1 cup chopped onion
1 cup chopped celery
1 cup coarsely grated carrots
½ cup chopped ham
⅛ teaspoon tabasco sauce
1 clove garlic, chopped
1 bay leaf
3 teaspoons chicken broth
    concentrate
2 tablespoons chopped parsley,
    sour cream and chopped chives
    for garnish, if desired

Wash soybeans; cover with water and soak overnight in refrigerator. Drain. Place in 3-quart saucepan;

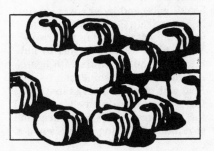

add 3 cups water. Bring to boil, covered, then turn to simmer and cook for about 2½ to 3 hours, or until tender. The last 10 minutes, add 1 teaspoon salt. To make soup; puree soybeans with cooking liquid in blender; set aside. Melt butter or oil in the 3-quart saucepan; add onion, celery and carrots and sauté until limp. Add 3 cups water, the pureed soybeans, ham, tabasco, garlic, bay leaf, chicken concentrate, and parsley. Cover and simmer for about 1 hour, or until desired consistency. Adjust seasoning. If desired, garnish with sour cream and chives. For a complete meal, serve with a tossed salad or coleslaw, bread and dessert.

Makes 6 servings.

HONEY GRANOLA

Mix together in large bowl:
7 cups oats (old fashioned rolled)
1 cup sesame seed (ground)
1 cup sunflower seed (ground)
1 cup wheat germ
1 cup bran
1 teaspoon salt
1 cup sliced almonds or cashews

In blender put:
1 cup oil (safflower or soy)
1 cup water or apple juice
1 teaspoon vanilla
1 cup fresh coconut, cut up
1 cup honey (less if apple juice is used)

Blend until coconut is coarsely chopped.

Mix well with dry ingredients in bowl.

Spread thin on baking sheets and bake in 200° oven for 2½ hours. Chopped dates may be added ½ hour before removing from oven. Stir occasionally. Cool. Store in containers.

PEP-UP DRINK

Mix in blender:
¾ cup cottage cheese
1 quart buttermilk
¼ cup dry skim (non-instant) milk
    powder
2 tablespoons wheat germ (optional)
1 raw egg
2 tablespoons cold-pressed oil
½ cup brewer's yeast

You can vary the flavors with different fruit juice concentrates. ☼

RECIPES FOR SHARING

YOPEACO ICE

2 cups plain yogurt
1/4 cup honey
1 cup fresh coconut, shredded
2 peaches

Mix yogurt and honey and add coconut. Cut up and mash peaches, leaving the skin on. Add to the yogurt mixture, stirring thoroughly. Freeze in refrigerator. To serve, add a slice of peach on top and a dribble of honey. Serves 6.

HIGH-FIBER "GO-NUTTY" MACAROONS

1 cup almonds
2 cups coconut, freshly grated
2 teaspoons almond extract
2 teaspoons vanilla extract
1/4 cup walnuts, chopped
1/4 cup dates, chopped
6 tablespoons honey
1 teaspoon sea salt
4 egg whites

Preheat oven to 350°.
Place almonds in blender for 1 minute or until they are about the consistency of flour, but not long enough to become a paste. Place coconut in medium bowl and sprinkle almond and vanilla extracts over it. Add the almonds and chopped walnuts. Mix well. Add dates, honey and salt. Mix again. Beat egg whites until stiff but not dry. Fold into coconut mixture. Drop by heaping tablespoonfuls onto lightly greased baking sheet. Bake for 10 minutes or until golden brown. These cookies will freeze well. Makes 25 large macaroons.

OATMEAL HEALTH BARS

1 cup oatmeal
1/4 cup sesame seeds, ground
1 cup nuts, broken
1/2 cup honey
1/4 cup carob powder (optional)

Mix all ingredients thoroughly. Shape into roll. Sprinkle carob powder over the whole roll. Then wrap in wax paper and refrigerate to harden. Slice as needed and use as after-school snack or while traveling or camping.

Extraordinary
cuisine for
Extraordinary
health

CAROB BROWNIES

1 cup raw sugar
2/3 cup peanut oil
2 eggs
1/2 teaspoon vanilla
1/2 cup unsifted, unbleached flour
1/2 cup soy flour
1 teaspoon baking powder
1/2 teaspoon sea salt
3 tablespoons carob powder

Preheat oven to 350°.
Mix together the raw sugar and oil. Beat in eggs and vanilla. Sift together unbleached flour, soy flour, baking powder, salt and carob powder. Combine the egg mixture with sifted dry ingredients. Mix well. Pour into well-buttered 9-inch square baking pan. Bake about 30 minutes or until done. Cut into squares or bars while still warm. Makes 16 to 20 squares.

KEN'S CRESCENTS

1/2 cup milk
1/2 to 1 cup butter (depending on richness desired) or safflower margarine
1/3 cup honey
3/4 teaspoon sea salt
1 package active dry yeast
1/2 cup warm water (110-115 degrees)
1 egg, beaten
2 cups unbleached flour
1-1/2 cups whole wheat flour
1/2 cup soy flour

Preheat oven to 400° F.
Scald milk and pour over butter, honey and salt. Cool to 110°. Sprinkle yeast on water, stirring to dissolve. When yeast mixture begins to bubble, add to milk mixture with beaten egg and 2 cups unbleached flour. Beat with electric mixer at low speed for 1 minute and at medium speed for 2 minutes. Add whole wheat and soy flours, stirring with wooden

spoon until dough leaves sides of the bowl. (Dough will be soft and somewhat sticky.) Shape dough into ball and place in greased bowl. Cover and let rise until double in bulk. (1 to 1-1/2 hours). Turn dough onto board and divide into two pieces. Cover and let rest for 10 minutes. Roll each half to make a 12-inch circle. Cut each circle into 12 wedges. Roll up each wedge from the wide end and place on two greased baking sheets. Curve ends to make crescents. Cover with towel and let rise until double in bulk, or about 45 minutes.
Bake for 15 minutes, changing position of pans after 7 minutes—move from middle to lower and upper racks. Remove from baking sheets and cool on wire racks.
Makes 24 crescents.

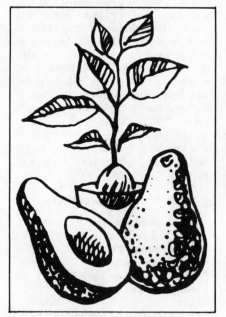

AVOCADO DIP OR GUACAMOLE

1 large ripe avocado
1/2 cup plain yogurt
1 green chili pepper, chopped or
2 teaspoons chili powder
juice of 1/2 lemon
1 teaspoon sea salt

Put all ingredients in blender and blend until smooth. Chill and serve as vegetable dip, dressing for tuna or chicken salad, or on crisp crackers or tortillas.

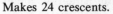

BLACK BEAN CASSEROLE

1 cup black beans
chicken broth or vegetable yeast
    extract to cover
1 large clove garlic, crushed
1 onion, finely chopped
1 stalk celery, chopped
1/2 cup parsley, chopped
juice of 1/2 lemon
sea salt and pepper to taste
2 tablespoons yogurt or sour cream

Soak beans overnight in enough water to cover. Drain and cover again with chicken broth or vegetable yeast extract such as Marmite. Add garlic, onion, celery, parsley, lemon and seasonings. Cook gently until tender, about 1 to 1-1/2 hours. Before serving, add yogurt or sour cream and reheat..

APPLE MUFFINS

Mix:
½ cup non-instant dry milk
3 teaspoons baking powder
½ teaspoon sea salt
½ teaspoon allspice
½ teaspoon nutmeg
1 teaspoon cinnamon
2½ cups whole wheat flour
Combine:
1 cup honey
1 cup oil
4 eggs
1 teaspoon vanilla
and add to dry ingredients.
Fold in:
1 cup grated apple
1 cup grated carrot

Pour into greased muffin tins and bake 15 minutes at 400°. Yields about 20 large muffins.

FISH AND ONION PIE

1 pound flat fish, filleted
2 tablespoons parsley, chopped
½ cup onion, chopped
4 potatoes, steamed
½ cup milk
salt and pepper to taste
2 tablespoons butter

Cut fish into small serving pieces. Cover bottom of buttered baking dish with a few pieces of fish. Sprinkle with parsley and onion and season lightly. Layer fish, parsley and onion until all

Eat well
if you want to
Live it up

are used. Mash potatoes, add butter and seasoning with milk, and spread over the fish, covering whole top of baking dish. Dot with butter and bake for half an hour at 350° F. Serves 4.

BEAN SPROUT EGG-DROP SOUP

3 cups clear vegetable, chicken or
    meat stock
2 cups soybean sprouts
2 beaten eggs
soy sauce

Heat stock to boiling and drop in soybean sprouts. Turn heat down and simmer for 10 minutes. Remove from the stove and slowly drip the beaten eggs from the end of a spoon into the hot broth. If this is done slowly enough, the eggs form soft, fine threads. Season

to taste and serve with a sprig of parsley. Serves 4.

CHICKEN AND BEAN SPROUTS

1 small chicken or 3 boned and
    skinned chicken breasts
2 tablespoons soy sauce (Tamari)
2 tablespoons peanut oil
1 clove garlic, crushed
1 tablespoon freshly grated ginger
    root
2 cups mung bean sprouts
1 tablespoon honey
½ cup mushrooms, chopped
1 cup chicken stock
1 tablespoon cornstarch

Cut chicken into very small pieces and season with salt and soy sauce. Heat the oil in a heavy pan or wok and stir-fry the chicken with the garlic and ginger until the chicken becomes white. Remove from pan and keep hot. Then fry the bean sprouts with honey and mushrooms for 1 minute. Add the stock which has been mixed with the cornstarch, and cook 1 minute more. Reheat the chicken. Serve with rice. If cooked chicken is used, omit the first cooking. Serves 4.

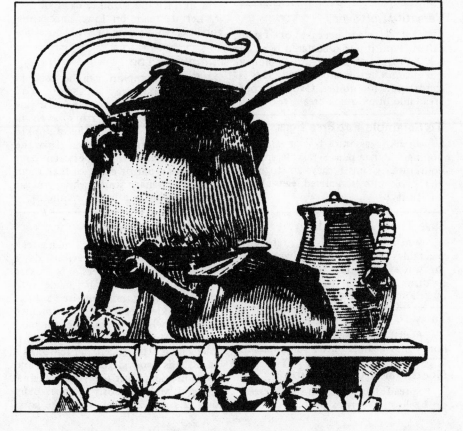

TREATS FROM YOUR BLENDER

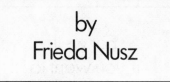

by
Frieda Nusz

My kitchen challenges me every minute of the time I'm in it—and I get the greatest pleasure out of figuring ways to save time (and money) while making every recipe easier and more tasteful. My kitchen is the place for imagination—and with me, anything and everything goes as long as what results is good for my family.

Here are a few ways to put your imagination to work—try them when you can. The results may stimulate you to figure out twice as many on your own!

Cook While You Sleep

A large roaster full of chicken can bake during the night. If you bake only one, add a little water. If you bake more than one, they form their own liquid. If you go to bed late, start the oven when you put them in, anywhere from 200 to 300 degrees. Or start them with the oven timer set about 3 or 4 in the morning. When it's time to get up or when you smell them, check on them to see if they are done. The meat can be removed from the bones and added to hot gravy made from the broth any time you want to use it.

Versatile Leftover

Got leftover pancake or waffle batter? Pour it into a buttered pan and bake. Frost with a mixture of honey and peanut butter mixed well. This is good bread for dinner. Good on corn bread and other quick breads too!

To Scramble Fat-Free Eggs

Break eggs into 1/4 or 1/2 cup boiling water in pan. Scramble and stir continuously until they go together and cook into scrambled eggs. Light and fluffy!

Save That Nutrition!

When using water to grate any vegetables in the blender always save the water for a place in a soup, gravy or drink, etc., that way you save the nutrition from the vegetables.

Tasty .. Tasty

A little molasses is tasty added to honey and peanut butter for a spread.

Good Flavor Combination

Spread thawed frozen strawberries or fresh strawberries on banana cake and let the juice soak in, either on the whole cake or on individual servings. This is a good flavor combination—and attractive.

Brown Rice That Looks White

Brown rice can be cooked either by starting it in cold water, or by having the water boiling first. Brown rice cooked with three parts of water to one part of rice, started on a high heat and then turned down to low heat until the rice has absorbed all the water, will be white and fluffy like white rice.

Making A Meal In A Hurry

Have to make a meal in a hurry, and no meat defrosted? Put frozen hamburger in the kettle with a little water. Let it cook, covered, and once in a while scrape off the defrosted meat. When it's all pretty well defrosted and crumbled, add onion (if you like it) and sprinkle basil all over it. Let it steam on low. This is real good served on rice or with potatoes.

Pumpkins, Too

Peeled pumpkin can be used in much the same way as carrots. You can grate it into salads and use it raw anywhere you use carrots, even in some blender drinks. The pumpkin seeds can be dried and eaten. Take the seed out of the shells between your teeth, like a parrot does, or take them out with a sharp knife while you sit watching television in the evening.

Multiple-Meal Dinners

School or other box lunches can be planned into the previous day's evening dinner or supper. A few extra potatoes cooked can be made into salad by adding mayonnaise, a little onion, pickle pieces, celery, pimento, parsley or whatever you like, the next morning. Most meats are good cold if dolled up a little, sliced and seasoned a bit. Rice is good mixed with fruit and sweet dressing. Just use your imagination and cook for both at once! Baby food jars and any small jars are good for packing good leftovers for box lunches.

Handed-Down Recipe for Bruises

From *Let's Live* magazine an article about one family's handed-down remedy for wounds or bad bruises: Grate a fresh carrot (preferably a home grown organic one) and apply as a poultice to the wound. There's no scientific basis for this, only the experience of one female correspondent that it works. She writes that she learned this from her husband's family. She also stated that it hurts more for a short while and then the pain lets up. We tried it once and it seemed to work. Tie the grated carrots on with a clean cloth and change, using fresh grated carrots, if needed. Our own Lane Alton got his finger smashed in something after I read this so I tied some grated carrots on and he was pleased with the relief.

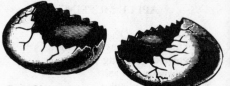

Egg Shortcut

To add cooked, chopped egg to a recipe like a sandwich spread or potato salad, you don't have to go through the work of cooking eggs in the shell. Break them into a hot skillet in a little water, butter or oil, and scramble them while they cook and add to the salad.

Easy-on Mashed Potatoes

Mashed potatoes are easily made from potatoes that were cooked with skins, if you own a ricer. When they are cooked soft, throw them into the ricer and rice away. The peelings are held back and you need only stir the riced potatoes with a spoon and add what you normally add: butter, milk, etc. and it's done!

Versatile Papaya

Have you tried papaya juice? This is a delicious drink and good for digestion. It seems to be highly recommended everywhere as a tasty addition to punch, milk shakes and drinks. I like to use it to make a drink out of water which was used to chop vegetables in the blender. Also makes good gelatin.

SOUPS, BEAUTIFUL SOUPS

FISH CHOWDER

2 tablespoons butter
1/2 cup onion, chopped
1/2 cup celery, chopped
1/2 bay leaf, finely crumbled
1/4 teaspoon fresh or dried dill
 weed (optional)
1 teaspoon sea salt or dulse
1-1/2 cups water
2 cups potatoes, diced
1 pound fish, cut in small pieces
2 cups rich milk (or 1/2 milk, 1/2
 cream)
1/4 cup parsley, chopped
paprika

Melt butter in heavy kettle; add onion and sauté until tender. Add celery, bay leaf and seasonings; mix well with onions and cook 1 minute. Add water, potatoes and fish. Cover and simmer very gently until potatoes are tender, 15 to 20 minutes. Add cream and milk; heat to serving temperature and serve in warm bowls. Garnish with parsley and dust with paprika. Fish may be cod, halibut, haddock, bass, snapper, bonita or other local varieties; or try this with scallops.
Serves 4 to 6.

From the book
Better Food for Better Babies
by Gena Larson.

MUSHROOM SOUP

1 ounce butter
1 small onion, chopped
1 medium-sized carrot, sliced
1 stalk celery, sliced
1/2 pound large mushrooms, sliced
1 heaping teaspoon yeast and
 vegetable extract
2-1/2 cups water
pinch of grated nutmeg
sea-salt and freshly ground pepper
 to taste
4 tablespoons heavy cream
1 tablespoon sherry (optional)

Melt the butter in a saucepan, add the chopped onion and cook gently until pale golden brown. Then add the vegetables, mushrooms, yeast extract and water. Bring to a boil, then turn heat to simmering point and cook for approximately 15 minutes, until the vegetables are tender. Place in electric blender for 30 seconds until smooth, then return to saucepan. Re-heat, add a miserly pinch of finely grated nutmeg (this gives a subtle flavor and also makes the mushroom flavor sing out), and seasonings to taste. Just before serving add the heavy cream. For special occasions add a tablespoon of sherry. Serves 4.

From the book
Recipe for Survival
by Doris Grant.

CHEESE SOUP

2 tablespoons onion, chopped
1 tablespoon green pepper, chopped
2 tablespoons carrot, chopped
4 tablespoons butter
3 tablespoons unbleached flour
1 quart chicken broth or stock
2 cups sharp cheese, grated
1 cup milk
sea salt and pepper to taste

In a large pot brown the vegetables in butter until tender (about 10 minutes), stirring constantly. Mix the flour with a little of the chicken broth, then blend in with the rest of the broth. Pour over the vegetables. Mix the grated cheese with the milk and seasonings and add, stirring, until the cheese is melted and piping hot. Serve with additional grated cheese on top.
Serves 4 to 6.

From the book
Three Worlds Cookbook
by Gayle and
Robert Fletcher Allen.

BEAN SPROUT EGG-DROP SOUP

2 cups clear soup, vegetable broth
 or stock
2 cups soybean sprouts
2 beaten eggs
salt or soy sauce

Heat the soup to boiling and add the sprouts. Simmer until tender, 8 to 10 minutes. Remove from the fire and drizzle into it the beaten eggs off the end of a spoon, slowly so that the eggs cook into soft, fine threads. Season to taste with salt or soy sauce.
Serves 4.

From the book
Add a Few Sprouts
by Martha Oliver.

LENTIL-CARROT SOUP

1 cup lentils
1 tablespoon butter
2 tablespoons onion, chopped
2 quarts soup stock (use concentrate
 if necessary)
1/2 teaspoon marjoram
1/2 teaspoon basil
1 tablespoon parsley, chopped
1 cup carrots, diced
1 cup lettuce, shredded
salt, cayenne
lemon

Soak lentils in 2 cups of water overnight. Melt butter in saucepan; add onions and brown. Add soup stock and herbs. Add drained lentils and cook slowly for 1 hour. Then add the carrots and lettuce and cook 1/2 hour longer. Rub through a food mill or sieve, reheat and add salt to taste and a dash of cayenne. Shave a washed lemon in very thin slices, put in a tureen and pour the hot soup over. Serve at once.
Serves 6.

From the book
Natural Foods Meals
and Menus for All Seasons
by Agnes Toms.

GREAT SOYBEAN SOUP

6 cups cooked soybeans
3 tablespoons vegetable oil
3 onions, chopped
2 carrots, chopped
1 green pepper, chopped
2 cloves garlic, minced
3 large tomatoes, peeled, seeded
 and chopped
2 tablespoons molasses
sea salt and pepper to taste

Heat the vegetable oil in a large kettle. Gently sauté the onions, carrots, pepper and garlic until the onion is translucent. Add the tomatoes, molasses and the cooked beans. Stir in enough water to make a thick soup. Cook 30 minutes to blend flavors. Add salt and pepper to taste and cook 10 minutes more. Serve hot. The soup may be as thick or thin as you please; add water to thin.
Serves 6, generously.

From the book
Super Soy!
by Barbara Farr.

SALADS, SALADS, SALADS!

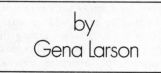

by
Gena Larson

GREEN BEAN SALAD

1/2 pound freshly cooked green
beans
2-1/2 red sweet peppers, diced
1 medium onion, diced

Marinate in dressing for one hour,
or overnight.
Serves 6.

MIXED BEAN SALAD

1 cup each green beans, kidney
beans and garbanzos— marinate as
above. If desired, 1 onion, diced,
may be added.
Serves 6.

DRESSING FOR GREEN BEAN
OR MIXED BEAN SALAD

3 tablespoons cider vinegar
3 tablespoons salad oil
1/2 cup chicken stock (see note)
1 teaspoon sea salt
1 teaspoon fresh dill weed, chopped,
   or
1 tablespoon fresh parsley, or
1/2 teaspoon dried parsley
1/2 teaspoon herbed seasoning

Beat with a whisk the vinegar, oil,
chicken stock, salt and seasonings.
Stir in the parsley and dill. Set aside
to blend. Chill. Can be made in a
blender.

Note: Poach chicken breasts or
thighs for salad. Save stock.

MOLDED FRUIT SALAD

1 envelope unflavored gelatin
1/4 cup apple juice
2 tablespoons raw honey
1 tablespoon fresh lemon juice
1 teaspoon vanilla extract
1-1/4 cups raw buttermilk (or 3/4
   cup nut milk blended with 1/2 cup
   yogurt)
1-1/2 cups fresh fruit, cut up
   (mixed apples, grapes, peaches,
   cherries, bananas)
1/2 cup chopped nuts

Soak gelatin in the apple juice—
place over low heat and stir until
melted. Add honey, lemon juice,
vanilla and buttermilk or yogurt
and nut milk. Chill until mixture
begins to thicken. Fold in the fruit
mixture and nuts. Chill until firm,
at least 4 hours, unmold on chilled

platter and decorate with pieces of
fruit and parsley.
Serves 6.

SAUERKRAUT SALAD

2 cups raw sauerkraut
1 cup pineapple juice, unsweetened
1/2 cup salad oil
1/4 cup cider vinegar
2 tablespoons honey
1 cup apple, diced, unpared
1/2 cup celery, sliced
1 large red or green sweet pepper,
   diced

Wash sauerkraut; drain well and
marinate in the pineapple juice overnight. At serving time, drain the
pineapple juice, reserving 1/4 cup
for the dressing. In serving bowl
place the reserved juice, oil, vinegar and honey; mix well. Add sauerkraut, apple, celery and peppers.
Toss and serve chilled.
Serves 6.

CHEESE AND
MUSHROOM SALAD

2 cups salad greens— washed,
   crisped and torn into bite-sized
   pieces
1/2 cup sprouts (any kind) chopped
1/4 cup marinated mushrooms
2 medium tomatoes, sliced
1/4 lb. Swiss cheese grated
1/2 lemon peel, grated

Mix greens, sprouts and mushrooms.
Toss with just enough dressing to
moisten well. Add sliced tomatoes
and top generously with grated lemon and shredded cheese.
Serves 6.

MARINATED MUSHROOMS

1/4 lb. tiny raw button mushrooms
   or large mushrooms, sliced

Cover with tangy salad dressing and
keep chilled in jar until needed.
When ready to serve, drain dressing
off in sieve and return dressing to
bottle. Toss mushrooms with green
salad.

SPROUT SALAD

1 cup sprouts, any kind
1/4 cup sugar peas—in the pod
1/2 cup carrot, shredded
1/4 cup celery, shredded

Chop sprouts and break peas in small
pieces. Mix with other vegetables
and serve.
Serves 4.

RAW-VEGETABLE SALAD

1 cucumber, sliced
1/2 cup cabbage, chopped
1 carrot, thinly sliced
1 green onion in 1 inch slices
1 zucchini, cut in half, then sliced
   in 1/2 inch pieces
1/4 cup parsley, chopped
1/4 cup celery, sliced
1/4 cup grated cheddar cheese
2 young beets, shredded

Mix all but beets very lightly with
an oil-vinegar dressing. Garnish each
serving with the shredded beet.
Serves 4.

WALDORF SALAD
WITH TURKEY

½ cup mayonnaise
¼ cup pineapple juice
¼ cup yogurt
1 tablespoon lemon juice
2 teaspoons sea salt
2 red apples, unpeeled
1 golden delicious apple, unpeeled
½ cup celery, sliced
½ cup pineapple, crushed,
   unsweetened
½ cup walnuts or pecans, broken
1½ cups diced cooked turkey or
   chicken
chopped parsley

Mix mayonnaise, pineapple juice,
yogurt, lemon juice and salt. Core and
dice apples into the dressing, turning to
cover thoroughly and prevent darken-
ing. Add celery, pineapple, nuts and
turkey; toss lightly. Trim with chopped
parsley. Serves 6. ☼

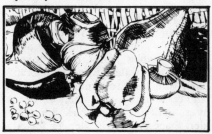

SANDWICHES TO LOVE

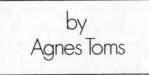

by
Agnes Toms

Make sandwiches ahead of time and freeze them. Place the wrapped frozen sandwiches in the lunch box. They will thaw out by noon.

To prepare sandwiches for freezing, butter bread, muffins or rolls to the edge. Place a thin layer of salad dressing over the butter. Place slices of ham, turkey, beef, tuna mixture or nut butter between the slices. Wrap sandwiches individually in plastic wrap, then wrap in foil and freeze. When preparing the lunch, wrap lettuce separately in plastic wrap, to be added later.

EGG SALAD FILLING FOR 8 SANDWICHES

Combine:
6 hard-boiled eggs, chopped
2/3 cup finely chopped celery
1/4 cup salad dressing
1 tablespoon prepared mustard
1/2 teaspoon salt

TUNA SALAD FILLING FOR 6 SANDWICHES

Combine:
1 can (6-1/2 ounces) chunk style tuna, drain and rinse in hot water then flake
2 hard-boiled eggs, chopped
3/4 cup finely chopped celery
1/4 cup chopped pickle (optional)
1/2 cup mayonnaise

PEANUT BUTTER CARROT FILLING

3/4 cup (not homogenized) peanut butter
2 tablespoons mayonnaise
1-1/2 cups finely grated carrots or alfalfa sprouts

Blend above ingredients. Makes about 2-1/2 cups.

CHEESE AND CABBAGE FILLING

1/2 cup finely shredded cabbage
2 tablespoons shredded cheddar cheese
1 tablespoon minced green pepper
1 tablespoon chili sauce

Mix ingredients well. Makes 1/2 cup.

SPROUT SANDWICHES

Spread thin slices of wholegrain bread with a butter-oil mixture. (Blend 1/2 cup butter with 1/3 cup salad oil.) Cover spread with cream cheese and a generous amount of alfalfa sprouts. Cover with buttered top slice.
Serves 8 to 10.

GOURMET CHICKEN SANDWICHES

1 cup chopped cooked chicken (or tuna)
1/2 cup finely chopped crisp celery
1/2 cup finely chopped cucumber
1/4 cup chopped walnuts
1/8 teaspoon salt
1/3 cup salad dressing
wholegrain bread

Combine chicken with celery, cucumber, nuts and salt. Add only enough salad dressing to moisten. Spread bread slices with softened butter. Use about 3 teaspoons of sandwich filling for each sandwich. Serves 10 to 12.

TURKEY AND CRESS SANDWICHES

Combine 2 cups chopped cooked turkey meat with 2 cups watercress leaves (no stems) and 3/4 cup mayonnaise. Season with salt to taste and 1/4 cup minced celery. Spread on buttered wholewheat bread. Makes 6 to 8 sandwiches.

CURRIED EGG SALAD SANDWICHES

Another tasty way to use up hard-boiled eggs. Combine 1/2 cup chopped pimiento-stuffed olives, 1/2 cup mayonnaise, 6 chopped hard-boiled eggs, 1/2 teaspoon curry powder, salt and pepper to taste. Mix well and spread on buttered wholegrain bread slices. Top with fresh lettuce leaves and remaining bread slice. Makes 2 cups spread.

PICKLED EGGS

6 hard-boiled eggs

3/4 cup liquid drained from cooked beets
3/4 cup vinegar
1 bay leaf
3/4 teaspoon salt
dash of pepper
1 clove garlic, crushed

Shell eggs and place in a quart jar. Combine beet liquid, vinegar, bay leaf, salt, pepper and garlic. Heat but do not boil. Pour over eggs. Cool, then cover and refrigerate overnight or longer.
Serves 6.

SANDWICHES YOU CAN FREEZE

1. Ground roast beef, lamb or chicken, moistened with mayonnaise and seasoned with grated onion.
2. Chopped cooked chicken livers or calf liver mixed with mashed hard-boiled egg yolk, minced onion and homemade ketchup.
3. Cream cheese, chopped olives and salted peanuts moistened with salad dressing.
4. Sliced roast lamb, on wholewheat bread spread with mint-seasoned butter. (Cream 1/4 pound butter with 1 tablespoon fresh mint.)
5. Peanut butter and applesauce or peanut butter and sliced pickle.
6. Chopped cooked chicken, chopped salted almonds and cream cheese.

OTHER SANDWICH SUGGESTIONS

1. Rye bread—liver sausage, ham or tongue.
2. Wholewheat breads—tuna, egg salad or meatloaf.
3. Boston brown bread—baked beans and finely chopped onion.
4. Oatmeal bread—chicken and chopped celery.
5. Cracked wheat bread—cottage cheese with grated raw carrot.
6. Soya bread—peanut butter with bananas or apple, never jelly or honey.
7. Onion bread—cheddar cheese and sliced tomatoes.
8. Pumpernickel bread—corned beef.
9. Meat and cheese stacks—no bread used.
10. Sweet breads—cream cheese with nuts.

WHAT TO DO WITH YOGURT AND KEFIR

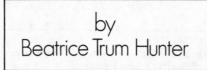

by
Beatrice Trum Hunter

How to Use Yogurt

Yogurt is best used fresh, before it is more than a week old. It should not be subjected to further heating. The bactericidal value is lost when yogurt is heated above 115° F. It is best to plan to use yogurt, whenever possible, in its natural state, or with fruit, in salad dressings, dips, cold soups and sherbets. It can be added to the top of baked potatoes in lieu of sour cream, or spooned over other cooked vegetables. It can be used as a garnish on top of hot soups, casseroles and baked apples.

If you do not like plain yogurt, try some of the following flavorings: cinnamon, nutmeg, unsulfured molasses, honey, carob, pure vanilla extract or pure almond extract. Or, top yogurt with ground nuts, sesame seeds or wheat germ. Yogurt combines very well with all fruits, berries and melons. Soaked, dried fruits such as prunes, dates, figs, apricots, peaches, apples or raisins are particularly good with yogurt, if you object to its normal tartness.

Yogurt salad dressing: Blend together in an electric blender a cup of homemade yogurt, 2/3 cup safflower oil, 1/3 cup apple cider vinegar, an onion quartered, 1/2 garlic clove, 1/4 cup celery leaves and 1/4 cup parsley leaves. Yields 2-1/2 cups of salad dressing.

Yogurt dip: Blend together in an electric blender a cup of homemade yogurt, two avocados, a garlic clove, and three tablespoons of minced chives. Yields a pint of dip. Serve on thin rounds of raw white turnips.

Yogurt-tomato soup: Blend together in an electric blender a quart of tomato juice, a pint of homemade yogurt, and a sprig of fresh tarragon. Chill. Serves 6.

Yogurt-cucumber soup: Blend together in an electric blender a pint of homemade yogurt, three peeled and coarsely chopped cucumbers, the juice of one lemon, a sprig of fresh dill, a garlic clove, three tablespoons of safflower oil and a tablespoon of fresh mint. If you wish to make a smooth-textured soup, remove the seeds from the cucumbers before putting them into the blender. Chill. Serves 6.

Yogurt sherbet: Blend together in an electric blender 1-1/2 cups of soaked and drained dried apricots or peaches with 1-1/2 cups of homemade yogurt. Turn this puree into six sherbet glasses. Chill. Serve garnished with ground sesame seeds. Serves 6.

These recipes are among many which are readily accepted and enjoyed by people who *think* that they loathe yogurt.

On the occasions when you wish to use yogurt in cooking, remember the following:

Yogurt, substituted for sour cream is less rich, but more tart.

Yogurt, substituted for buttermilk, in biscuits or pancakes, can be satisfactory. For each cup of buttermilk called for in the recipe, use one and one-half cups of yogurt. If baking powder is called for in the recipe, substitute one-half teaspoon of arrowroot flour to each cup of yogurt.

Cook yogurt at low temperatures, for a brief duration, and stir constantly. This will help to prevent separation. Cooking in a double boiler is advisable.

Yogurt may lose its flavor when cooked, but it still has the ability to intensify and blend the flavors of other foods. Yogurt is often used to blend herb flavors into sauces and gravies, or to marinate meat.

The Care and Feeding of Kefir

Preserving kefir grains for future use: If you plan to be on vacation and have no "kefir sitter" to nurture the grains in your absence, preserve them for future use. Store them wet, dry or frozen.

To store them wet, wash the grains thoroughly in a sieve with a stream of cold, running water. Place them in a clean jar, and cover them with cold *unchlorinated* water. Store in a refrigerator at 40° F. They will keep their viability for about a week, but lose potency if held much longer.

To dry the kefir grains, rinse and drain as above. Place them on two layers of clean cheesecloth. Air-dry them at room temperature for thirty-six to forty-eight hours. The room should have good air circulation, or use a fan. Place the dry grains in a paper envelope or wrap them in aluminum foil. Keep them in a cool dry place. Such dried grains are usually still active after twelve to eighteen months of proper storage.

To freeze kefir grains, rinse and drain as above. Place them in a small non-actinic bottle (light-excluding). Seal the bottle tightly and place it in a similar but larger bottle. Seal the edges of the lid of the larger bottle with masking tape to prevent any air from entering. Freeze, and thaw out to begin culturing again at a future date.

Reactivating stored kefir grains: You may find that kefir grains stored wet may be slightly slower in their culturing action. If so, leave them in the fresh milk somewhat longer than usual, or culture them at a slightly higher temperature than usual. In time, they should be restored to their full activity.

To reactivate the dried or frozen grains, first soak the grains overnight, or approximately twelve hours in *unchlorinated* water to cover, at room temperature. Drain, and transfer the grains to only *one cup* of milk. Allow this to stand, approximately twenty-four hours, at room temperature, or until the milk thickens. During this period, stir the mixture occasionally. Drain the grains from the milk, rinse, and transfer them to a fresh cup of milk. By then, the grains should be fairly active. They can be rinsed, drained, and transferred to *two cups* of milk. Continue, gradually increasing the number of cups of milk used, until ultimately the usual one quart of milk can be cultured with the grains. Continue to culture under the conditions that you have found produce the flavor and thickness which suit your taste.

Homemade kefir from freeze-dried grains: Sterilize all equipment. Heat a quart of fresh, clean milk to a near boil. Remove the pot from the heat, and cool the milk to 110° F. Stir in a teaspoonful of freeze-dried kefir grains, and blend thoroughly. Pour this mixture to fill a sterilized, warm container, cover, and place in a warm place, such as an oven at 100° F. Allow the container to remain undisturbed for twelve hours, while the kefir is incubating. Test the kefir with a toothpick to learn whether it has solidified. The toothpick, when inserted, should stand upright without support. If the test fails, incubate the kefir one to three hours longer. When the incubation is complete, refrigerate the kefir.

Homemade kefir buttermilk: Kefir grains can be used to prepare kefir buttermilk as well as to prepare the usual type of kefir fermented milk. Kefir buttermilk closely resembles churned or real buttermilk in flavor and consistency and has proved to be a popular item when it has been sold along with cultured buttermilk. Use either raw or pasteurized partially-skimmed milk (two to three percent butterfat content), or pasteurized sweet buttermilk, which is sometimes available from creameries where butter is made from sweet cream. Of course, it would also be available on a farm where butter is churned from sweet cream.

If raw milk is used, heat it to 165° F. Cool it to between 68° and 72° F. It is then ready for making the kefir buttermilk. Or, it may be kept in the refrigerator for later use. If sweet buttermilk is used, pasteurize it by heating at 180° F. for twenty minutes to expel all the air.

To prepare a small batch of kefir buttermilk, put the kefir grains in a cheesecloth bag. A half pound of grains will be enough to coagulate two gallons of milk in thirty-six to forty-eight hours at 68° to 72° F.

Place the milk in a porcelain, glass-lined or granite-iron container. Suspend the bag of grains near the surface of the milk. Incubate the milk at 68° to 72° F. until it is well set up, or until it shows an acidity of about 1 percent lactic acid. Then lift out the bag of grains, scrape off the adhering cream, and wash the bag thoroughly in cold, running water to remove all the sliminess from the outside of the bag, and the fermented milk from within. After squeezing the bag to remove the excess water, place it in a new supply of milk, and continue as before.

After the grains have been removed, stir the fermented milk slightly to incorporate all of the surface cream. Then cool it to 60° F. or lower. Then, using an eggbeater or other slow-speed type device, whip the mixture to break the curd. After the curd is broken, store the milk in bottles or in its original container at a low temperature until it is used.

Homemade kefir cheese: Pour cultured kefir (without the grains) into a pot, and heat very gently until the entire surface is covered with foam, just below the boiling point. Turn off the heat, and allow the heat to permeate the entire mixture for a few seconds. Then pour into another container for cooling. Cover, and allow to rest overnight. In the morning, strain through a cheesecloth bag. Kefir cheese is thick, and has large curds. To modify its bland flavor, a little grated Roquefort or blue cheese, or other strong-flavored cheese, can be blended with it.

Kefir summer cooler: Blend together in an electric blender a quart of homemade kefir, the juice of two oranges and two tablespoons of honey. Pour into glasses, chill, and top with a light dusting of nutmeg. Serves 4 to 6.

Kefir shake: Blend together in an electric blender a quart of homemade kefir, a half cup of wheat germ, and two tablespoons of honey. Pour into glasses. Serves 4 to 6.

Kefir summer soup: Blend together in an electric blender a quart of homemade kefir, one cup of raw, diced cucumber, one cup of watercress, and a sprig of fresh parsley. Chill and serve. Serves 6.

Kefir sherbet: Blend together in an electric blender 1-1/2 cups of homemade kefir, 3/4 cup unsweetened, pureed fruit, 4 tablespoons honey, and 1 teaspoon of pure vanilla extract. Pour into sherbet glasses, and refrigerate. Serve, garnished with unsweetened coconut shreds. Serves 4 to 6.

Quickie kefir dessert: Fold one cup of kefir into one cup of applesauce, and add 1/4 teaspoon of pure almond extract. Pour into sherbet glasses, and refrigerate. Serve, garnished with ground walnuts. Serves 4 to 6.

Baked apples with kefir: Wash and core raw apples. Arrange them in a baking dish with a small amount of water in the bottom. Fill the core cavities with raisins and almonds. Bake in a moderate oven for a half hour, and serve hot, with cold kefir drizzled over the apples.

Kefir fruit salad dressing: Blend together in an electric blender one cup of homemade kefir, one tablespoon of honey, two tablespoons of unsweetened orange juice and two tablespoons of unsweetened pineapple juice. This dressing is good over fruit salad, and also over cole slaw. Makes 1-1/2 cups.

Kefir dip: Mince a clove of garlic, and mix it with a teaspoon of safflower oil. Add a half cup finely chopped walnuts, a teaspoon of apple cider vinegar, and one cup of kefir. Mix well and chill. Serve with thin slices of raw white turnips. ☼

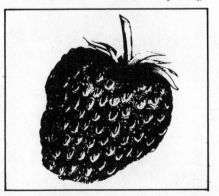

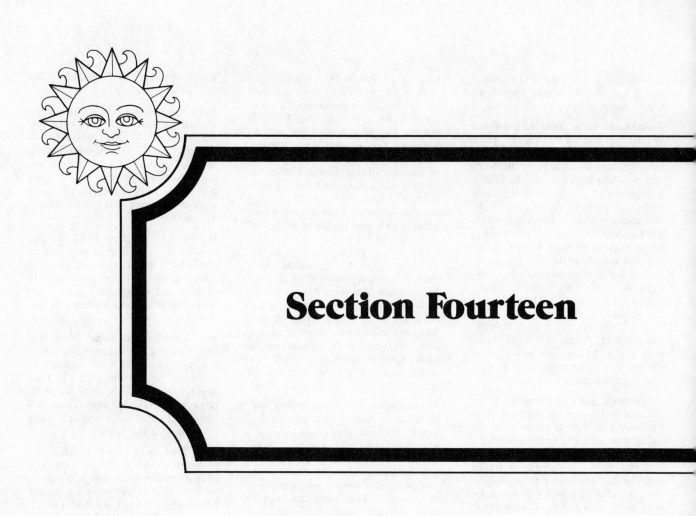

Section Fourteen

Prophets–
In and Before Their Time

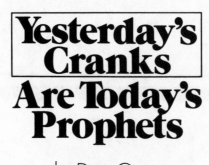

Yesterday's Cranks Are Today's Prophets

by Doris Grant

Since the early part of this century, a number of eminent medical experts have been stressing the close connection between wrong nutrition and disease and, in particular, the dangers to health of refined carbohydrates — white bread and refined white sugar. They were regarded by their fellow medics as cranks, however, and their warnings ignored.

That these experts are now being regarded as prophets way ahead of their time is due in large part to the research and writings, since about 1962, of a retired surgeon-captain of the British Navy, T.L. Cleave. His brilliant conception of a single "saccharine disease" linking many of the diseases of civilization to the same basic cause, the *consumption of refined carbohydrates,* has provoked great interest in the medical profession in Great Britain, and now in Germany and America. "Saccharine," incidentally, pronounced like the river Rhine, has nothing to do with the chemical sweetener, sacchar*in*, but means "related to sugar," and the term "saccharine disease" refers to all those conditions now linked to the taking of sugar, whether primarily as such, or secondarily via the digestion of starch in white flour, white bread or other carbohydrates. Captain Cleave's newest work on the subject, *The Saccharine Disease* was recently published in America by Keats Publishing. A growing number of surgeons and doctors enthusiastically support Cleave's concept.

Getting the message

Friends and correspondents frequently affirm that whereas a short time ago their doctors would have told them that whole wheat bread was no better than white, they are now recommending that they eat the whole wheat loaf and, moreover, that they take unrefined bran instead of laxatives!

That this conversion has now reached the British Government Health Service level would appear from a remarkable leaflet which the Medical Research Council is circulating at the present time. Entitled "Medical Research Council Diet and Health Enquiry," it appeals for "your help" in showing the value of natural foods, and states that "it has been suspected that certain diseases which have recently become common may be due to lack of vegetable fiber in the modern diet." Recipients of this leaflet are asked to answer the questions and return it to the MRC.

Taking the lid off bread

The new thinking regarding the role of nutrition and the vital importance of real bread is also reaching the national press. "Taking the Lid Off Bread", a special report in the *Sunday Mirror,* declared that "Give us this day our daily unadulterated bread" was the frequent cry from many doctors and nutrition experts, and quoted warnings from three well-known surgeons that the white loaf and white sugar, can predispose people to certain diseases.

The Sunday Times has been running a series of articles investigating the staples of the nation's diet, and has published revealing information debunking the popular conception of the safety and nutritional values of a number of these so-called staples.

In this series the white loaf came under particularly heavy fire. Disturbing revelations concerning the surprising ingredients which are put into it artificially after the natural nutrients have been knocked out must have alarmed many readers, especially with regard to one of these ingredients — *chlorine dioxide.* This "improver" has been in constant use since agene was banned, but it seems that *protective tests have never been done on it although these were recommended by the Government over twelve years ago!*

It has been reported that the baking industry now proposes spending $240,000 on a program to test the safety of chlorine dioxide, and that technologists and scientists are busily looking for an alternative to chlorine dioxide *in case it is needed!* The increasing medical acceptance of Cleave's "saccharine disease" concept has no doubt also contributed to the initiation of this new program.

British housewives are also "getting the message"

Women are becoming increasingly disenchanted with the British loaf, its cotton-wool texture, bland taste, and inferior nutritional value. There is now a widespread return to home-baking. Ironmongers claim that their sales of bread tins are remarkable, and health food shop owners tell me that their sales of yeast and 100 percent whole wheat flour have virtually trebled during the past few months. The whole wheat loaf is coming into its own.

Alas, habit dies hard; white bread will continue to be "a passport to disease" for many, many people. On the other hand, *the idea* of the vital role of diet in the causation and prevention of disease is being accepted at long last. How true it is, as Victor Hugo's dictum puts it, that *"All the armies in the world are not as powerful as an idea whose time has come."*

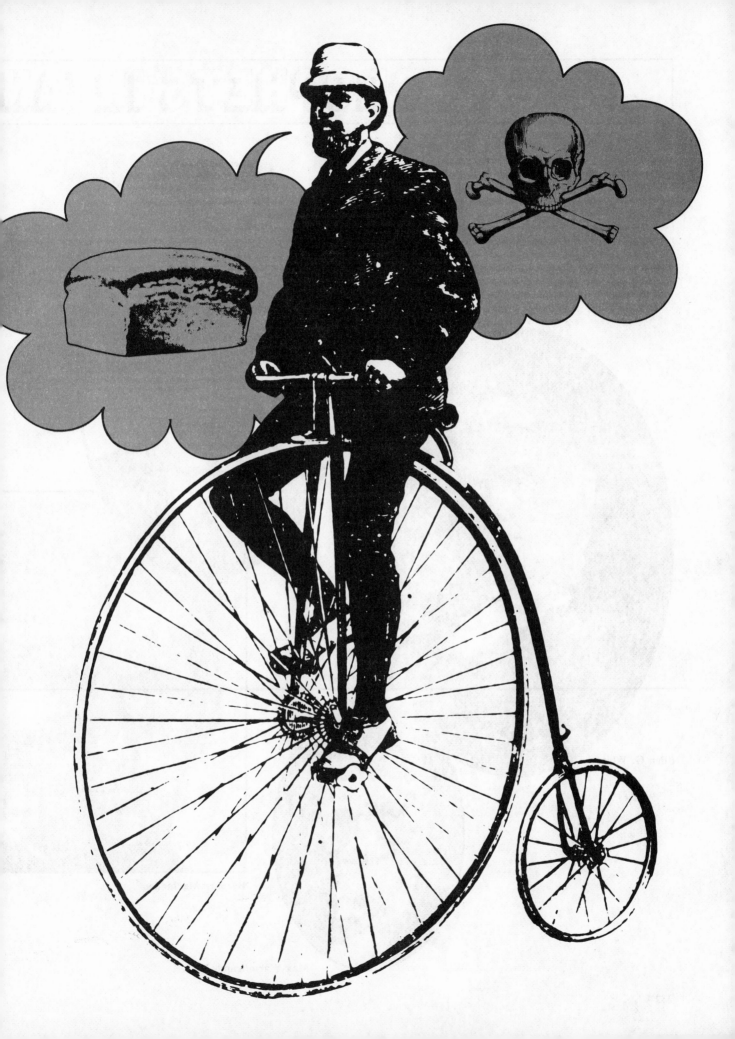

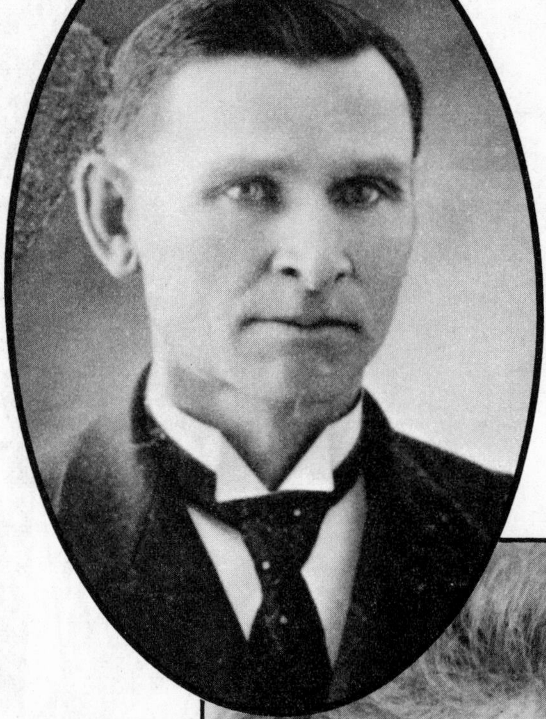

Jethro Kloss

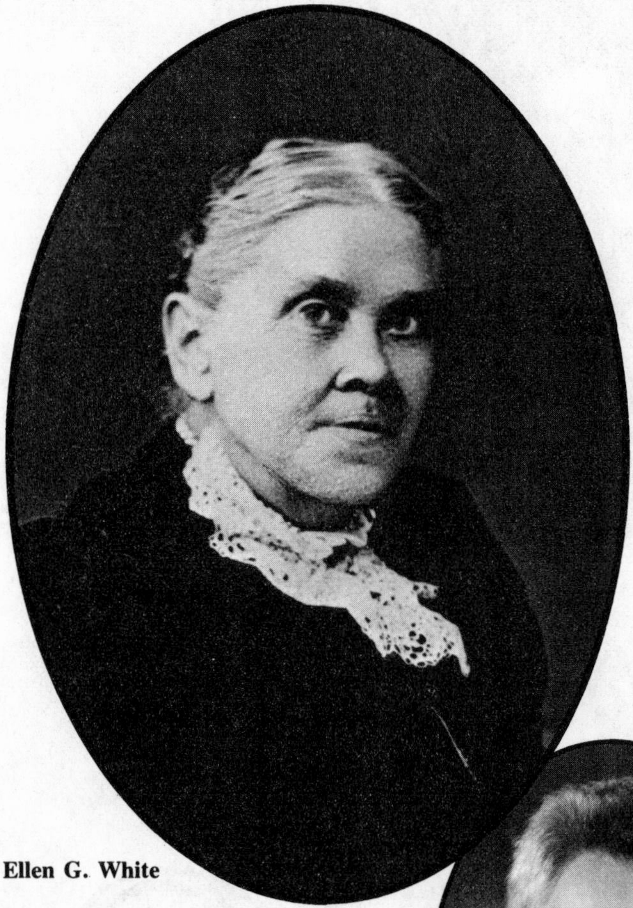

Ellen G. White

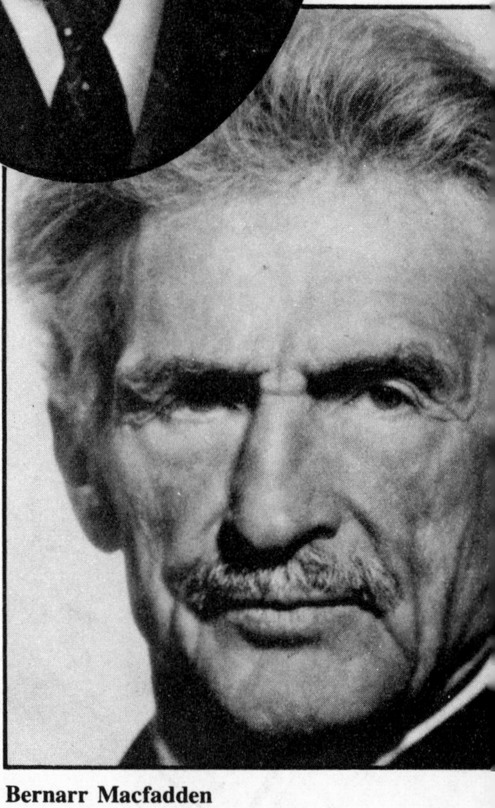

Bernarr Macfadden

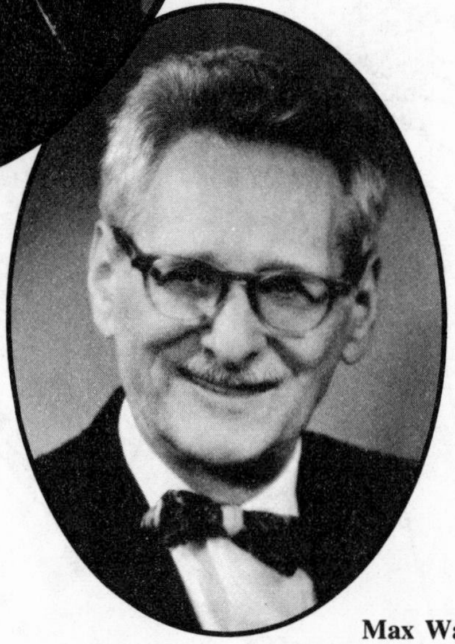

Max Warmbrand, N.D.

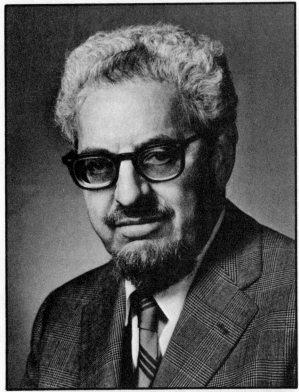

Jerome I. Rodale

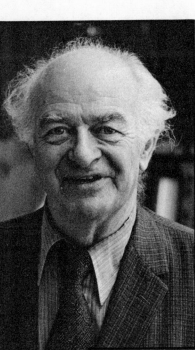

Linus Pauling

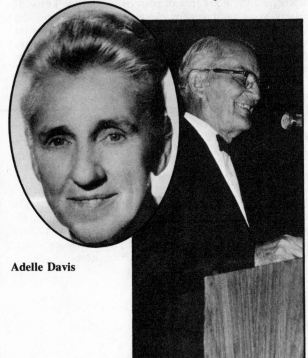

Adelle Davis

Roger J. Williams, Ph.D.

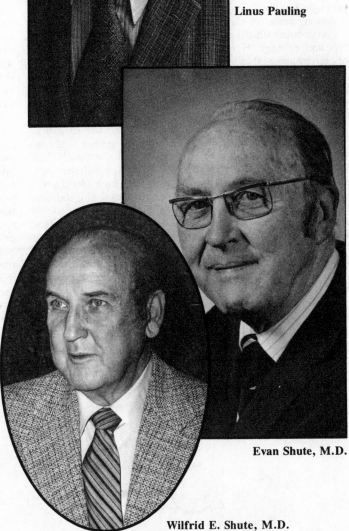

Evan Shute, M.D.

Wilfrid E. Shute, M.D.

Ellen G. White

Here was a visionary who warned others about the catastrophes she foresaw—with fervent urgency. Her insight ranges from advance, intuitive information on the destruction of San Francisco during the 1906 earthquake, to foreseeing the health dangers of tobacco and X rays. She also spoke out against the overuse of fats and refined sugar long before medical authorities came up with the now-familiar statistics on cholesterol and hypoglycemia. She was not a passive visionary, but an able and active organizer and teacher, and perhaps her most monumental achievement is her contribution, with her husband, to the founding of the Seventh-day Adventist Church which grew out of the Millerite sect. As an inspiration and leader of this church, it was she who counselled, and her directives were by no means confined to spiritual matters only. Nor was the continuance of her counsels left to the memory of her charges, but she committed them to posterity in voluminous writings. (Speaking of writing, she rose at three A.M. each day to answer the letters sent to her.) Her own energy, and the range of her activity, suggests the truth of her views on health.

Among some of the subjects Ellen G. White dealt with are vegetarian and unrefined-food diets, nutrition and healing, and ecology. Her academic training in the nutritional or environmental sciences was almost nil, nevertheless *she was always right,* and thus passed the strictest test of prophecy. She was right in 1905, when she condemned tobacco as a "slow, insidious, but malignant poison." She had it, right down to the word "malignant." She was also right in 1865, when she linked birth defects with the use of drugs. As early as 1884 Ellen G. White spoke out against the consumption of large amounts of salt. She did not totally ban its use, but cautioned that it should be added but sparingly to food. We now link salt consumption with high blood pressure, which is in turn linked with heart attacks. She did ban alcoholic beverages, contending that they had a permanent deleterious effect on the brain. Today it is explained that alcohol interferes with oxygen getting to the brain, liver and other vital organs, under which condition brain cells may actually die. In 1867 she, radically, counselled that the sick not be confined to bed, but that moderate exercise was an important aspect of curing illness.

During her lifetime she was accused of faddism and fanaticism. Reading, today, her book *Counsels on Diet and Foods,* the urgent pleas to cut out the use of sugar, refined foods and large quantities of fatty meats, or to give up cigarettes and alcohol seem almost trite, so familiar are we with the clinical evidence of their destruction of health. Ellen G. White was, in fact, conservative and sober in her directives on health, and in her life.

(1827-1915)

J.H. Tilden, M.D.

Dr. Tilden practiced medicine for sixty-eight years, and after the first eighteen years of his practice he used no "medicine." For the last fifty years of his practice he also ran a school and sanatorium in Denver, Colorado, devoted to teaching people how to have energy-filled and disease-free lives.

At the turn of the century, private physicians who demanded that their patients abstain from stimulants, drugs, fad diets, and surgery—and that they refrain from eating unless they have a keen appetite—who banned refined foods from the diet—and who also prescribed fasting to cleanse the body—were rare. They still are rare. His pioneering attitude brought censure, not praise, from the rest of the medical profession.

What he became convinced of was that illness and general debilitation were due to the buildup of poisons (toxins) and waste material in the body: in other words, toxemia. His medical practice was oriented toward guiding patients away from toxic substances such as coffee, alcohol, tobacco and sugar, and toward purer foods such as fruits, vegetables and whole grains which insure regular and efficient elimination of wastes from the body. His work foreshadows the present appreciation of dietary fiber, with its ability to rid the intestinal tract of a buildup of decayed food, and in the process to avoid a whole host of mechanical and chemical problems. His concept of toxemia as a cause of illness also anticipates our renewed interest in the value of fasting, and our discovery of the ability of the body to heal itself.

Diet was not the sole object of Dr. Tilden's concern when it came to detoxifying. He also recognized the value of exercise in keeping the body free of poisons. Today we know of the eastern yoga exercises for cleansing the lungs and the body. Another insightful element of Dr. Tilden's program was his urging that his patients eliminate stress, as much as possible, from their lives, giving us a new, medical-slant on the word "poise." How exciting to read, recently, clinical reports on studies of emotions and their effect on the levels of our brain waves, or of the connection between stress and heart failure. Dr. Tilden knew by close and open-minded observation what it is taking us years to validate. He realized that stress has a deadly effect on a healthy body, and inhibits the natural healing ability of a sick body. We know now that stress can cause a surge of hormones in the body, and that it can also deplete vitamin C, the B vitamins and calcium.

Dr. Tilden's ideas are handed down through his books: *Toxemia Explained* and *Food: Its Influence on Health.* During his lifetime he rose at three A.M. each day to work on the publication of his monthly, non-profit magazine, to further circulate his observations. Finally, his concepts are mirrored in the changes that are occurring now.

(1851-1940)

Jethro Kloss

M.O. Bircher-Benner, M.D.

Jethro Kloss is the prophet crying in the wilderness that if we would follow such simple laws of health as "proper diet, use of pure water, fresh air, sunshine, rest, and nature's remedies, herbs, etc., nature would restore the body to its original health." Daniel, an Old Testament prophet, "purported in his heart that he would not defile himself with the portion of the king's meat, nor with the wine which he drank." Instead, Daniel requested vegetables and water, and at the end of ten days Daniel and his band "appeared fatter and fairer in flesh than all the children which did eat the portion of the king's meat."

Brought up by pioneering parents in Wisconsin, Jethro Kloss learned the use and value of wild and cultivated herbs, grains, nuts, fruits and vegetables. He also began to realize that our Creator had indeed supplied life-giving properties to these foods in their natural state, and that overcooking them and dressing them up with sugar and other poisons was perhaps making them "fit for a king," but robbing man of physical well-being.

In his work at the Battle Creek Sanatorium (then revolutionary in its precepts) Jethro Kloss also quickly learned the dangers of the use of drugs (including alcohol, coffee and tobacco) not only to physically well people, but especially to the sick. He learned instead to treat illness with such natural and pure remedies as water, fruit and vegetable juices, and herbs (on which subject Jethro Kloss became authoritative). The extent of his use of herbs has hardly been equalled. Other unorthodox techniques were common at the Sanatorium, such as massage, hydrotherapy, fasting and exercise as remedial to health.

His classic book, *Back To Eden,* is an encyclopedia of natural treatments for illness, listing alphabetically a wide variety of diseases and emphasizing common disorders such as boils and insomnia which especially lend themselves to self-remedy. Particularly useful are his directions for such techniques as were used at the sanatorium, and for his guidance on the general care of those who are ill or convalescing. Part of the book is a complete herbal, whose main concern is with the medicinal application of plants. This section has been faithfully followed by millions of people

Back to Eden is also a basic guide to "unspoiled living," with discussions on soil, numerous recipes, and hints on food preparation, as well as personal anecdotes from Jethro Kloss's experiences on the farm and at the sanatorium.

Finally, the book is a hopeful testament to the fact that it was, after all, on Earth that Eden once existed, despite how impossibly incongruous that may seem now; and that at least several of the elements making up Eden—its variety of life-giving plants, sunshine and fresh air—are with us still.

(1863-1946)

It is easy to imagine this man peacefully gazing out of a window of his clinic on a hill overlooking Zurich. One guesses that he must have been a gentle healer, since his approach to health is so simple and sensible: healing through the regulation of a pure diet and pure and calm living habits. His "medicine" would include raw fruits and vegetables, soups, unrefined grains (especially the famous cereal mix, Muesli). One special aspect of food which Dr. Bircher-Benner also stressed was the importance of preparation. Foods were not to be mauled and then cooked until the life had left them. We now add to this that the vitamins are destroyed by oxidation and heat, and the minerals are leached into and discarded with the cooking water. In the case of many fruits and vegetables, Dr. Bircher-Benner preferred to use them raw—coining the delightful term "sunlight foods." He even claimed that, optimally, these foods should be eaten whole, rather than chopped or shredded.

This all sounds so easy and uncomplicated, but of course, there is more at work behind the scenes than we first notice. To be able to effect health cures by applying the right quantity, quality and combination of foods, water and rules for living, requires an intense knowledge of nutrition and of other aspects of human health. Max Bircher-Benner had that knowledge and he had the courage and insight to use it. Incidentally, he was also especially concerned with children and their diets. He felt that not only nutrition but correct habits must begin with the first foods that baby puts into its mouth. Now we realize the insidiousness of addiction to sugar and chemical additives that is formed early in a child's life, and also the difficulty of re-learning an appreciation for the taste and texture of unrefined foods.

There was and still is a revolutionary character to Dr. Bircher-Benner's teachings. The clinic was founded in 1897, and aroused a contempt which resulted in Dr. Bircher-Benner's ostracism from many of his colleagues. So, if we try to picture the man, let us put a light of conviction and strength in his eyes.

He did, determinedly, continue to treat patients with such "simple" methods as diet and nutrition, and his success brought people flocking from all over the world. They still flock to his clinic, a mecca for the sick as well as for dieticians and nutritionists seeking better training and answers to their questions. His books can answer our nutrition and diet questions, for he left us, among others: *Health-Giving Dishes, The Bircher-Benner Children's Diet Book* and *The Bircher-Benner Fruits and Raw Vegetables Book. Eating Your Way to Health,* by his daughter Ruth Kunz Bircher-Benner, is a further guide to Dr. Bircher-Benner's methods of healing and to his ideas about human well-being.

(1867-1939)

Sir Robert McCarrison

Max Warmbrand, N.D.

The initials of honors and degrees which follow Sir Robert McCarrison's name are impressive: C.I.E., M.A., M.D., D.Sc., LL.D., F.R.C.P. The most important things to remember are that McCarrison was a learned scholar, a doctor, and he was also a Major-General I.M.S. and was formerly Director of Research on Nutrition in India, for the British government. He spent much of his life in India, and had occasion to closely study some of man's most decimating diseases. His first work on the cause of sand-fly fever was closely followed by a study of goiter in the foothills of the Himalayas. This latter rigorous research is itself a classic. Now his mind began to ponder the problems of beri-beri in particular, and nutritional deficiencies in general. We are grateful for his subsequent pursuit of this last train of thought.

The finance and government officials trying to support a variety of concerns and services in a very needy country were not so grateful. McCarrison was stationed there to provide medical service, not to feed rats with oatmeal. Such originality did not contribute to the job at hand, according to a short-sighted view of things. So, with an empty room in which to set up his own apparatus, with assistants whom he paid from his own funds, his wife's cook to cut sections, and a clerk "lent" by the post office, this dedicated doctor carried on the research that would help wake our world to the truth of this statement: *Salus populi suprema lex;* or, "the destiny of peoples depends upon the food they eat."

In 1929 his work began to gain approval, and under the helpful insistence of Lord Linlithgow the Nutrition Research Laboratories were eventually established at Coonoor, and McCarrison was made Director at the age of fifty-one. But he was also well on his way to documenting the seriousness of a two-fold problem facing his world, and even more urgently, our world. The problem is this: first of all, how to provide adequate food for the rapidly increasing populations of the world; and secondly, how to avert the physical and mental disasters caused by the processing and altering of food.

The stamp and character of McCarrison's work is a fine blend of observation and experiment, the mark of a scientist. But his sensitivity and compassion gave him a broader, political outlook. "The greatest single factor in the acquisition and maintenance of good health is perfectly constituted food." These words became almost a motto for various organizations, and a guiding light to the United Nations Conference on Food and Agriculture held in Hot Springs, Virginia, in 1943, where they took it as a standard. Sir Robert McCarrison's thesis becomes more politically relevant as each day goes by, and food becomes an issue of power, along with armaments and oil. (1878-1960)

This sprightly, gentle man had an exceptionally active career as a successful nutritional doctor, lecturer, author and guest on radio and television. He had an endearing character, but was nonetheless firm for his amiability. Max Warmbrand was himself a testament to the benefits and feasibility of living, according to high standards, on unrefined natural foods. As a young man he determined to become a vegetarian, and he never shirked from applying to his own life the principles of nutrition that his interest and subsequent study revealed. He was aghast at the practice of polluting a sick body with drugs. He was saddened that most people failed to understand the diagnoses that their own bodies gave them, and the ability of their bodies to effect a cure.

Those fortunate patients who came under his care remained grateful to him throughout their lives—and they span three generations. Dr. Warmbrand's theories, based upon ridding the body of toxins, and proceeding with a fruit and vegetable diet (much in the same way as Dr. Tilden did), were always applied differently to individual patients. Each person had a tailor-made program for achieving maximum health. One of his principal concerns was with the suffering that arthritis caused so many people. He was particularly sought after for his success in alleviating this misery through remedial diet.

Abundant energy seems to be a trademark of our prophets. Some of them rose at the wee hours of the dawn to answer the voluminous correspondence of their followers, or to carry out further experiments and complete special projects before beginning their other employments as doctor, government official, or whatever else. Dr. Warmbrand used some of his abundant energy to establish a health spa in Florida where both body and spirit might be refreshed. (Again, it seems that his martial strictness about diet and living habits never interfered with his congeniality and enjoyment of life.) Energetically he continued to shuttle back and forth, until his death, from Connecticut to Florida.

During all this time he also kept up a vigorous writing career, giving us a legacy of such valuable books as *The Encyclopedia of Health* and *Living Without Pain.* His last book, *Overcoming Arthritis and Other Rheumatic Diseases,* was just being released at the time of his death at eighty-three.

Finally, we want to remind the reader that Max Warmbrand was not the only natural healer with a purely private practice. There are others who, at this moment, are healing without drugs and prescribing foods rather than penicillin. Dr. Warmbrand is presented here for his own merits, but also as a Type of Prophet. In recognizing him we recognize those others too, who are professionally shunned for their beliefs, but who are determined to heal and help. (1896-1976)

Jerome I. Rodale

Adelle Davis

J.I. Rodale might well be remembered for such achievements as the compilation of two, fine, standard reference works in the English language: the *Synonym Finder* and the *Word Finder* (of which over 200,000 copies are in use). He might also be remembered for his encouragement of the dramatic arts, and for his own numerous plays and skits. He might be remembered as the successful businessman who (with his brother) organized and administrated the Rodale Manufacturing Company, which has worldwide sales of almost 4 million dollars a year. J.I. Rodale is also, of course, a hero of the natural nutrition and organic gardening causes. For twenty-five years he braved severe criticism from the Establishment until, compelled by the witness of a consistently growing number of people all over the world, chemical companies and medical doctors began to realize that he was no wisp-in-the-wind popular leader, but a serious and correct teacher of health principles and agricultural reform. Rodale's intense concern that people learn the truth about health and about the incomparable benefits of organic gardening motivated him to begin the publication of two important magazines. That is, after he tested organic gardening for himself, having bought a farm in Connecticut and subjected the precepts to a rigorous examination, and having experienced and decided for himself the truth about "natural, whole foods." Perhaps it is because J.I. Rodale's convictions were based on real life experiences that they have such impact. He never was tied to conventions or to an unquestioned use of the ideas of others. An extremely active man, he became personally involved in the things that he viewed as valuable. And furthermore, he was eager to share any of the knowledge which he had gained.

His magazines, *Prevention* and *Organic Gardening and Farming,* were able to distribute high quality information and instruction to hundreds of thousands of people, in a language and style they could understand and use. Rodale kept people abreast of medical and agricultural news, he introduced them to the precepts of natural foods and non-chemical farming, he encouraged those who were carrying on the continual battle against refined foods, pesticides, and the other "enemies" widely recognized today. Rodale's books reinforced the work that his magazines were doing month by month. Such books include the *Encyclopedia of Organic Gardening* (1958), the *Health Finder* (1954), and the *Complete Book of Food and Nutrition.* The list goes on. These documents were written well before experts in the fields of nutrition and agriculture would accept them. Now they are finally, and fondly, regarded as reliable and intelligent works of scientific literature. (1898-1971)

Adelle Davis became a legend during her lifetime, acquiring a widespread following and fame that frequently elicited, instead of the honors she deserved, contempt from the medical establishment and from those who were opposed to placing an emphasis on nutrition and health problems. Her academic training would certainly pass the most orthodox muster, having received an education in such reputable schools as Purdue University, the University of California at Berkeley and at Los Angeles, Columbia University; and her Master of Science degree in biochemistry was received from the University of Southern California Medical School. Her subsequent jobs included work at Bellevue and Fordham hospitals in New York, consulting as a nutritionist to clinics in California, and eventually counselling patients referred to her by numerous specialists. She also planned individual diets for over 20,000 people suffering from almost every known disease.

But her major, priceless contribution to our society is the collection of four classic books on food preparation and nutrition: *Let's Cook It Right; Let's Eat Right to Keep Fit; Let's Get Well;* and *Let's Have Healthy Children.* It seems safe to say that no personal library would be complete without these basic guides to quality survival in relation to food.

Important leaders of nations, and persons in high positions of authority have confessed to being intimately familiar with her discerning guidelines for buying foods and food supplements. But it is always a confession. Even while sales of her books were hitting the 10-million mark, vehement attacks were mounted by the scientific community.

We can be thankful that her lucid discussions on the relation of vitamins to health did reach and will continue to reach a vast group of laymen and nonprofessionals, making it possible for the individual to determine intelligently a vitamin supplement program to suit his needs. We are thankful for other practices or concerns that Adelle Davis made well-known: the nutritional advantage of "undercooking" foods, especially vegetables, and of steaming food instead of boiling it; the concern for using cooking utensils and vessels that are not going to further contaminate our food; calling attention to the physical benefits to be derived from certain, usually overlooked foods such as brewer's yeast, sunflower seeds, and wheat germ; using nutrition to avoid the health problems often attendant on pregnancy, and to protect a child from all too common disorders.

Actually, in retrospect, it seems strange that Adelle Davis's work did arouse controversy. It is, above all, sensible; not radical but conservative as far as nutritional teaching today is concerned. (1904-1974)

Bernarr Macfadden

Weston A. Price, D.D.S.

In the beginning of his career, Bernarr Macfadden's ideas about physical well-being were scoffed at. The abandoned lifestyle of romantics, and then flappers, could admit no truth to his call for total abstinence of alcohol, tobacco and other drugs. Like so many prophets, the wisdom of his words was ignored because people abhorred the changes that the truth would demand of their own habits. Yet, in many ways, even during his lifetime, Bernarr Macfadden scoffed back. As an astute businessman he amassed a personal fortune of over $30 million, and in the 1930s he was head of a multi-million dollar publishing venture which included reputable newspapers and specialized trade papers, as well as lighter tabloids such as *True Love, True Romances* and *Ghost Stories.* But Bernarr Macfadden was well aware that money would not bring him any pleasure without health, that in fact health must be a prominent concern for everyone.

Some of the "crackpot" ideas that Bernarr Macfadden dared to voice were: as was mentioned, the abstinence from alcohol and tobacco; ending the use of drugs and patent medicines in restoring health; and the inclusion of raw vegetables as a major part of diet. Two ideas of his seem particularly visionary. He believed that occasional but regular fasting was important to keep the body cleansed and healthy. Not since the medieval European lenten practices, and not until the "spiritual" revolution of the 1960s was fasting practiced by more than a handful of mystics or clergy. Imported by aspiring, young, Eastern religion adepts, fasting began to be generally accepted for its benefits to health. Eventually science caught on, and today scientific reports are being prepared on the physiology and health value of fasting.

Another astounding insight concerned the importance of physical culture to promote and maintain health. Doctors *prescribe* exercise now. Health spas and resorts which stress sports, dance, yoga and exercise classes are booming. This was Bernarr Macfadden's most beloved weapon against disease. During the late twenties and early thirties he presided over a daily exercise program which was broadcast over radio to a large and faithful following. He also ran his own health studio, published the magazine *Physical Culture,* and wrote the book *Vitality Supreme.*

He believed in one more idea that still stands outside the gates of general acceptance: the value of nudity and exposure of the human body to fresh air and sunlight. John Ott has published a book on the subject of the relation of sunlight to health. A scientist at Massachusetts Institute of Technology is presently researching the effects of light on the pineal gland and its resultant controls on human sexuality. Bernarr Macfadden's suggestion may yet turn out to be wise fact. (1868-1955)

Weston Price was a giant in the early nutritional research field. He went to the root of our modern-day health problems by exhaustively studying the diets of primitive peoples. His scholarship is impressive and his discoveries profoundly significant. Most people who were aware of the difference between the excellent teeth of primitive peoples and the decay-ridden teeth of "civilized" cultures, focused their attention on what, by comparison, were those elements of civilization which were the culprits of dental problems. Weston Price had the insight to look instead at what made primitive teeth so good. He came to believe that we have lost track of the fundamental principles of living physically sound lives. The job ahead, as he saw it, was not to waste time clipping away at our present weakened wings, but to recover that basic health wisdom. This job was important enough to Weston Price that he left a successful dental practice in Chicago, and using his own funds as well as grants from generous patients and friends, delved into the study of fourteen different primitive tribes throughout the world.

In Dr. Price's search for the keys to healthy living, his study was directed to diet and nutrition, and this study is done with depth and attention to detail. But the study of nutrition led him to further considerations of agricultural customs and soil fertility. For instance, today the protein content of our wheat and other grains is declining; this is an indication of soil fertility, or rather the lack of it, and becomes an important factor in measuring nutrition.

Another aspect of Dr. Price's work is the realization that the crisis of poor nutrition snowballs from generation to generation, even if the nutritional conditions remain generally the same, simply because the nutritionally deficient children of a badly nourished mother produce offspring with even more health defects, and so on. This is a disturbing progression, and a clue to our present disease-ridden society: physical and mental *degeneration.* What enormous political impact this has—yet the book *Nutrition and Physical Degeneration* (1938) is not even available in many libraries.

Weston Price had other astonishingly revolutionary ideas. Here is a statement we are just beginning to fathom in relation to health: "Nature uses a written language which, without the keys, is made up of meaningless hieroglyphics, but which, with the proper keys, becomes a clear story of racial and individual history." Today we know that insufficient protein in a pregnant woman's diet may cause poor quality saliva in her child. Saliva normally has a detergent effect on the teeth, and its lack or improper consistency can lead to plaque formation and, ultimately, decay. This is an example of one small key, but it is enough to give us a notion of the impact that Price's ideas could have. (1870-1948)

Rachel Carson

When she was young, Rachel Carson had aspirations of becoming a writer. She would indeed be a writer, but she would first go on to become an outstanding marine biologist, serving on the staff of the United States Fish and Wildlife Service for fifteen years as a scientist, and for part of that time as editor-in-chief for the organization's publications. She received her education from Chatham College and John Hopkins University, and was an assistant in zoology at the University of Maryland.

In 1937 her career began as we are apt to remember it today: combining the two aspects of her skill, she became the first writer on natural history and environment to be widely read. Her first piece in this field was an article titled "Undersea" which appeared in *Atlantic.* Three best-selling books followed: *Under the Sea Wind; The Sea Around Us;* and *The Edge of the Sea.* These won her awards and recognition, but were minor victories compared to the book which shocked society in the early 1960s, and which awakened the world to the reality of ecological destruction: *Silent Spring.*

Having gathered information for four and a half years specifically on the topic of pesticides, she wrote with detail, yet in terms understandable to laymen, about the link between cancer and widespread use of certain chemicals. She warned of the genetic effects that certain chemicals have on the human body. And above all, Rachel Carson set down an outline of the environmental situation which would become the groundwork for many researchers after her. From the confusing jumble of misinformation and chaotic practices she extracted the essence of the infant science: ecology. She set the scene, giving our world a sense of the vast power that we exercise over nature, and our subsequent responsibility. In *Silent Spring* she also speaks of the natural enemies of insects and all the other checks and balances built into nature, and the consequences of our tampering with that natural order.

Rachel Carson's visionary intellect became the lens through which we could focus our attention on the physical world in a new and crucially important way. But it was her writing ability which made her message so outstanding and urgent. A lucid and dramatic style galvanizes the reader from the first paragraph, moving him with each flutter of the insect's wing, showing him the beauty of a grain of sand.

After her challenge of the chemical industry and her indictment of wrong-doing and irresponsibility, thousands of "concerned citizens" dared to fight industry and government. As part of her contribution to the cause of environmental protection and study, Rachel Carson was able to entrust to us a special legacy, the banning of DDT. (1870-1964)

Sir Albert Howard

Sir Albert Howard is another exemplary Englishman who made full use of a post in India to pursue his studies. His particular interest was the maintenance or restoration of soil fertility. Starting in 1940 he began to examine systematically both soil and agricultural practices, mainly in the West Indies, India (where he was Director of the Institute of Plant Industry in Indore, and Agricultural Advisor to States in Central India and Rajputana) and Great Britain. He discovered that nature, if untampered with, has its own built-in methods of soil management ("the forest manures itself"), and that cultures which used natural manures rather than chemical fertilizers had healthier crops. And he went on to test and document these discoveries.

Sir Albert Howard left us two specific legacies along these lines of study. As for agricultural reform, he established what he referred to as the Indore method of replenishing soil richness by adding humus from decayed vegetable and animal wastes. Today we call it composting, and take it for granted. However, when *An Agricultural Testament* was first published in 1940, Sir Albert Howard said in his Preface that he "hoped that they [his ideas on the importance of humus] will be discussed with . . . freedom and that they will open up new lines of thought and eventually lead to effective action." He had reason to be defensive on this point, since in 1931 he had already published *The Waste Products of Agriculture,* and the world still did not take his method seriously.

The second great contribution that Sir Albert Howard made to soil science was in emphasizing the little-appreciated factor called mycorrhizal association, or the living fungus bridge between "raw" nutrients in the soil and the ability of the plant to absorb these nutrients through its root system. Without the mycorrhizae the transition could not be made, and unless the soil itself was "healthy" and was treated correctly by the farmer, then the mycorrhizae would not be present. This is a crucial step in the food chain; information which we tend to take for granted.

Actually, the "we" who take these things for granted may not be the large-scale commercial farmer who is more concerned with soil productivity in terms of quantity than he is in quality. The average gardener is aware of the importance of humus, and most likely does use compost or green manure, but it is the rare, organic farmer who takes into account "the sacred duty of handing over unimpaired" and fertile soil to the next generation.

In our present age, Sir Albert Howard's work is the keystone of the organic gardening and farming movement (due largely to the championing of J.I. Rodale). Under growing pressure of world hunger and malnutrition, his work will be the genesis of agricultural reform. (1873-1947)

Roger J. Williams, Ph.D.

Evan Shute, M.D. and Wilfrid E. Shute, M.D.

Roger Williams received a Ph.D. degree in biochemistry from the University of Chicago in 1919. Since that time he has been an outstanding pioneer in biochemical research and is considered to be one of the most important living contributors to the field. He is a Founding Fellow and Honorary President of the International Academy of Preventive Medicine, a recently formed society of growing importance and prestige. He is also co-founder of the Clayton Foundation Biochemical Institute in Texas, and served as director from 1940 to 1963. This organization is responsible for the discovery of more vitamins and their variants than any other laboratory in the world. Roger Williams must take credit for the discovery and isolation of pantothenic acid, and for some of the first work on folic acid, which he named. He had the keen insight to foresee the importance of the B vitamins in treating illnesses, and is especially noted for his nutritional approach to combating alcoholism. A further crucial scientific contribution of Roger Williams is his concept of biochemical individuality, and the need for taking this individuality into account when diagnosing and treating disease (*You Are Extraordinary*).

He refuses to be confined to a specific field, and advocates a wholesome, broad nutritional approach to man's health. His emphasis is always on prevention of disease and maintenance of health. Much like the owner's manual that comes with each new car, Roger Williams's books are manuals for keeping the human body in good condition, and are written for the owner of the body. Here is the key to the motivation behind the writing of his bestselling books, some of which include *Nutrition in a Nutshell* and *Nutrition Against Disease*—so popular because they are easily understandable to laymen. His newest work, *Wonderful World Within You: Our Inner Nutritional Environment* is a mini-course in human life science, and a landmark in public education on nutrition. At the request of the medical profession he also has written the *Physician's Handbook of Nutritional Science*. One of the scientific premises on which all of these works are based is that "the microenvironment of our body cells is crucially important to our health."

As one of the leading authorities on nutrition he has received many honors and awards. Recognition of his expertise includes his election, as the first biochemist, to the presidency (1957) of the American Chemical Society. He is also a member of the National Academy of Sciences, and in 1972 served on the President's Advisory Panel on Heart Disease. He received the Mead Johnson Award of the American Institute of Nutrition, and the Chandler Medal. He is a member of the Association for Cancer Research, and the Biochemical Society.

These two far-sighted brothers are responsible for the astounding advances that have been made in the treatment of certain diseases, and the prevention of many ailments with the use of vitamin E. They are best known for their treatment of heart failures of all kinds, and related circulatory diseases—chronicled in such books as *The Heart and Vitamin E* by Dr. Evan Shute (1956) and *Vitamin E for Ailing and Healthy Hearts* by Dr. Wilfrid E. Shute and Harald Taub (1969) and Dr. Wilfrid E. Shute's *Complete . . . Updated Vitamin E Book* (1975). Their experience with actual clinical results goes back to 1937, when the two began treatment of angina pectoris with vitamin E.

Wilfrid Shute, especially, went on to lead a determined battle against heart disease, America's number one killer. He administered megadoses to cardiovascular disease victims—35,000 of them—saving over 10,000 lives. Through his efforts in books, articles, lectures and talks, he has made it clear that benefits can also be obtained by healthy persons taking vitamin E regularly. Yet despite the overwhelming clinical proof and well-documented case studies, drugs and other equally ineffective remedies are still being used on heart disease patients. No alternative to vitamin E therapy has been proven.

Evan Shute, a highly distinguished research scientist, is still involved in revealing the multitude of ways that vitamin E can help us to good health at the Shute Foundation in London, Ontario. He began his academic career exceptionally early, entering the University of Toronto at the unprecedented age of fourteen years. In 1933 he began to study a Danish veterinarian's suggestion that a "fertility vitamin" might be used to prevent habitual abortion in pregnant women. By 1937 Evan Shute was using vitamin E to treat various female disorders, and had realized that this new vitamin might have other applications. From this point on his research was a relentless hunt throughout human physiology to find out all that vitamin E was capable of. Some of his finds are: the use of vitamin E to heal burns and radiation reaction, with application in kidney disease, diabetic vulvitis, poliomyelitis, and also to prevent the formation of scars, or to diminish scars. His dedication helped make possible an understanding of the role of vitamin E in controlling the oxygen content of blood. And the list goes on.

We marvel at how some visionary pioneers were able to uncover essential, general principles of health and nutrition. We also marvel at the life-work of two men devoted to studying one substance, around which circles of understanding flow outward, like waves from the stone thrown into a pond.

Abram Hoffer, M.D. and Humphry Osmond, M.D.

Linus Pauling

Schizophrenia is a forbidding shadow hanging over the civilized world. For many years it has been the most prevalent mental illness and, of course, more schizophrenia exists than has been diagnosed. As a matter of fact, current research has uncovered a "family" of schizophrenias; many do not exhibit classical symptoms, and therefore remain untreated.

Not that treatment up until now has been so successful. Drs. Hoffer and Osmond despaired of the efforts of psychoanalysis or the administration of drugs to cure schizophrenia, or even to begin to alleviate its misery. They were searching for actual biological keys to the problems. In the process of studying mescaline psychosis they noticed a similarity of symptoms to both schizophrenia and pellagra psychosis. They knew that pellagra responded to niacin, and made a connection of that effect with schizophrenia. They discovered the use of megavitamin therapy, specifically prescribing massive doses of certain vitamins (especially niacin) and monitoring diet in order to remedy schizophrenia. With encouraging success these two doctors helped to usher in a new era in the treatment of mental illness.

Abram Hoffer and Humphry Osmond are two of the pioneers of this fledgling science—called fledgling not because its foundations are still shaky, but because it has only begun to grow. Perhaps recognition of orthomolecular medicine will cause the break between the new concepts of medicine and the orthodox drug-oriented approach to healing. Meanwhile, thousands of innocent patients are falling victim to addictive tranquilizers and other mind-altering drugs which do not always alleviate, and sometimes barely mask their health problems.

Dr. Osmond is currently director of the Bureau of Research in Neurology and Psychiatry at New Jersey Neuropsychiatric Institute. He has done much background work in the use and effects of drugs, having coined the term "psychedelic." He has also written the book *Models of Madness, Models of Medicine* with Miriam Siegler.

Dr. Hoffer currently continues a private practice in Saskatoon, Saskatchewan, in Canada. He is president of the Canadian Schizophrenia Foundation and also of its American counterpart, The Huxley Institute for Biosocial Research. His most recent book, written with Dr. Morton Walker, is titled *Orthomolecular Medicine,* an important introduction to the public of the principles and use of this new field of medicine.

Together Drs. Hoffer and Osmond are responsible for the writing of *How to Live with Schizophrenia,* which has been a valuable guide not only to those who suffer with this mental disorder, but especially for the families of those who have schizophrenia.

This man was awarded the Nobel Prize for Chemistry in 1954. He is famous for his "application of quantum mechanics to chemistry, his study of the effective sizes of atoms in molecules and crystals, his work in establishing the existence of helical structures in proteins, his development of a theory of metallic bonding, and his study of molecular abnormality in relation to disease." This overwhelming list may seem to suggest an unapproachable genius who confines himself to laboratory solitude. Linus Pauling has at least one other side to his nature—a warm compassion and concern for all humanity. In recognition of the excellence and devotion of his social awareness he was also awarded the Nobel Peace Prize in 1962, for his attempts to promote an international agreement to stop testing nuclear weapons.

His book *The Nature of the Chemical Bond* was a classic as soon as it was published in 1939. His textbooks on *College Chemistry* are professional bibles in that field. Besides the Nobel Prizes, he is honored by seventeen medals and awards, thirty honorary degrees, honorary memberships in twenty scientific societies. He has published over four hundred papers, and among his bestselling books is *Vitamin C and the Common Cold,* which caused a veritable revolution in public knowledge and use of this vitamin.

Linus Pauling's honors and degrees have not protected him from opposition and criticism. His work on vitamin C aroused disclaimers and defamers, while in his battles for social sanity he pits himself against the whole history of human aggression. He is no stranger to the battle against popular opinion, for the cause of right. The need for backbone and personal strength must have made demands on him early in his life. His father died when Linus Pauling was nine years old, yet he went on, by his own efforts, to put himself through school, eventually receiving his Ph.D. from the California Institute of Technology in 1925. The more than usual responsibility and financial obligations seem only to have strengthened his character.

Throughout his career Linus Pauling's constant concern has been the alleviation of human suffering. His scientific ability was focused on, among other things already mentioned, such topics as: the causes of genetic mutation and the transmission of aberrant genes. Paralleling these academic pursuits, just as his Peace Prize parallels his scientific honors, Linus Pauling has also turned his attention and efforts to advocating social attitudes and personal habits that would benefit mankind and the individual—speaking out against smoking, and other practices harmful to health. Presently he is researching the molecular basis of disease, contrary to the traditional germ and viral theories in use today.

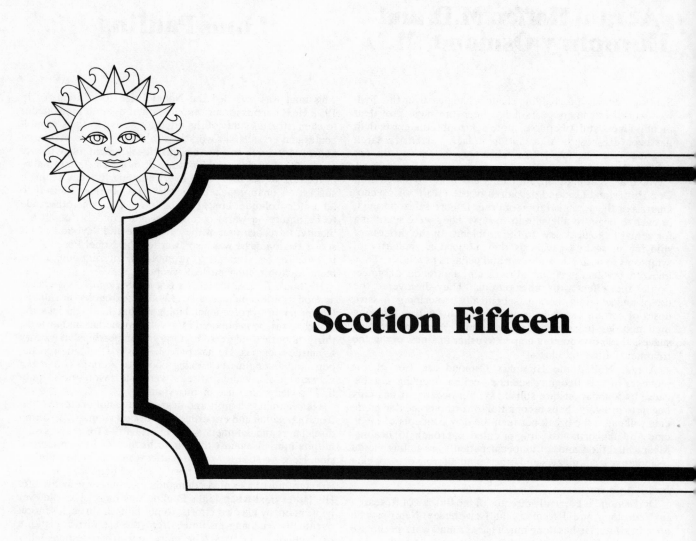

Section Fifteen

Nature's Big, Beautiful, Bountiful "Backyard"*

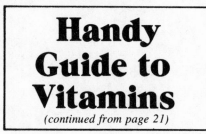

Handy Guide to Vitamins

(continued from page 21)

in water, but is readily destroyed by acid, light and extremely high temperatures.

BIOTIN aids in the metabolism of fatty acids and carbohydrates and is important to the normal utilization of amino acids, folic acid, pantothenic acid and vitamin B-12. It is necessary to the manufacture of glycogen, which is the form in which carbohydrate is stored in the liver. It can be manufactured in the intestine, unless the intestinal flora have been destroyed by antibiotics. Deficiencies can be produced by the ingestion of an enormous amount of raw egg white. Natural deficiencies are rare. Symptoms of deficiency may include dermatitis, pallor, muscle pain and depression.

Sources of biotin are organ meats, egg yolk, wheat germ, brewer's yeast and soy products. Biotin is water-soluble but heat-stable; it can be destroyed by very strong acids or alkalis.

CHOLINE is present in all body cells. Produced from methionine in the body, it is a constituent of lecithin which aids in the movement of fats from liver to cells. It emulsifies fat and cholesterol and is essential to the transmission of nerve impulses. It has been used in the treatment of alcoholism, kwashiorkor, hepatitis and cirrhosis of the liver. Deficiency may result in fatty deposits in the liver.

Choline is found in organ meats, wheat germ, legumes, lecithin and egg yolks.

INOSITOL is a component of brain, skeletal, heart and gland tissues and even human hair. It participates in nucleic acid formation, acts indirectly in stimulating synthesis of biotin in the intestine, and nourishes brain cells. Inositol appears to have a calming effect on the nerves. Deficiencies are uncommon.

Sources of inositol are whole grains and seeds (especially sprouted), lecithin, organ meats and nuts.

PANTOTHENIC ACID occurs in all living cells. It is essential for energy metabolism, fat and cholesterol synthesis and antibody formation. It is a necessity for proper functioning of the ad-

renal gland which affects growth. It aids in withstanding stress and is required in the utilization of riboflavin. It can be produced by intestinal bacteria. Deficiencies are rare, but would be characterized by adrenal malfunction, digestive disorders, fatigue and depression.

Pantothenic acid occurs in meat, poultry, fish, whole grains, legumes and brewer's yeast. It is destroyed by strong acids or alkalis.

PARA-AMINOBENZOIC ACID (PABA) aids in intestinal production of folic acid and pantothenic acid. As a coenzyme, it is important to protein metabolism and the formation of red blood cells. PABA also has the property of being able to block the sun's ultraviolet rays and is used in many sunscreen preparations. It is produced in the intestines. Induced deficiencies have caused fatigue, irritability, depression, nervousness, headache and digestive problems.

Natural sources of PABA are liver, brewer's yeast, milk, yogurt, eggs, whole grains and wheat germ.

B-15 (PANGAMIC ACID) is required to prevent the accumulation of fat in the liver. It also acts as a detoxicant. Although the U.S. government considers it useless, it has been used in Russia for many problems, especially circulatory and heart ailments.

B-15 occurs naturally in brewer's yeast, seeds and whole grains.

B-17 (LAETRILE) is even more controversial than B-15. It forms the basis of a cancer treatment which is not generally considered legal in the U.S. Since some cancer cases have reportedly responded to laetrile in Mexico, there is a growing movement to have it declared legal here. One judge recently allowed a cancer patient to bring laetrile into the country and use it for treatment. Though many researchers consider it harmless, it is found in seeds, such as apple seeds, which contain cyanide.

Natural sources of B-17 are sprouted seeds and the pits of fruits such as apricots and peaches.

THE VITAMIN C COMPLEX

THE VITAMIN C COMPLEX includes both vitamin C (ascorbic acid) and the bioflavonoids, also known as vitamin P. Ascorbic acid is a synthetic version of vitamin C and it is probably the only synthetic vitamin that is of great value. Natural vitamin C occurs in conjunction with the bioflavonoids in many substances, and can be used to supplement vitamin C obtained from ascorbic acid.

VITAMIN C (ASCORBIC ACID) is a water-soluble vitamin. It is necessary to the maintenance of collagen, a protein vital to the formation of skin, bones and ligaments. It aids in healing and strengthens blood vessels, thus aiding in the prevention of hemorrhaging. Vitamin C promotes resistance to virus, bacterial infections and allergens. It also seems to have an anti-anxiety effect. Vitamin C is essential to the production of adrenal steroids and aids in the detoxification of many substances such as pesticides and heavy metals. It is necessary to the absorption of iron and folic acid and helps intestinal regulation. It is also a natural diuretic. Vitamin C has been cited as an agent in cholesterol regulation, and is thought to retard the aging process. It has been used in megavitamin therapy to treat schizophrenia. Excessive smoking and the contraceptive pill increase the need for vitamin C. Stress also reduces the body's supply of C. Since excesses are excreted, vitamin C may be taken freely. The body cannot manufacture its own vitamin C.

Severe vitamin C deficiency results in scurvy, but lesser deficiencies produce such symptoms as bleeding gums, painful joints, retarded healing, a tendency to bleed or bruise easily and lowered resistance to infection.

Vitamin C is very fragile and can be destroyed by light, heat, air, copper and iron utensils, long storage, baking soda, loss in cooking water, and use of aluminum cookware. Sources of vitamin C include fresh fruits and vegetables, especially peppers, tomatoes, leafy greens, acerola cherries and rose hips.

VITAMIN P (BIOFLAVONOIDS) may help to prevent capillary fragility, as well as to protect vitamin C and adrenalin. It aids against bruising, and together with zinc, fights the effects of excess copper. Rutin, from buckwheat, is a bioflavonoid, as are citrin, hesperidin and quercetin.

Sources of bioflavonoids include buckwheat, citrus pulp, red peppers, black currants, apricots, cherries, blackberries, acerola cherries and rose hips.

II. THE MINERALS

Minerals in great variety are needed for the proper functioning of the human body. Some are needed in very small amounts, and these are called trace minerals. Most minerals are synergistic, that is, they need each other to produce maximum results. They also act together with vitamins. Trace minerals may be toxic in higher amounts, therefore, they are best supplied from natural sources.

CALCIUM is the most abundant mineral in the body and 99 percent of it is found in bones and teeth with the remainder in soft tissues. It aids in controlling blood clotting, and is important to normal muscle contraction, heartbeat regulation, and nerve transmission. Calcium absorption depends on the presence of vitamin D, parathyroid hormone, phosphorus, and vitamins A and C. The body's utilization of iron depends on calcium, as does the activation of several enzymes. A lack of magnesium can cause calcium deposits in the muscles, heart, and as kidney stones. Extra calcium intake requires extra zinc. Deficiencies can lead to soft bones (osteoporosis and osteomalacia), muscle cramps and insomnia. Calcium is abundant in dairy products and bone meal.

CHLORINE occurs in such compounds as sodium chloride and potassium chloride. It aids in the regulation of the body's acid-alkaline balance and aids in the digestive manufacture of hydrochloric acid. Excesses of chlorine are excreted. Chlorine is found in sea salt and kelp.

CHROMIUM is essential to the effectiveness of the insulin hormone which regulates the body's glucose level. Glucose is required for the function of every living cell. Chromium works in conjunction with zinc, calcium, magnesium and manganese. Chromium may be found in brewer's yeast, corn oil, liver and bone meal.

COBALT is a part of vitamin B-12 and is necessary to its production. Cobalt activates a number of enzymes and is vital to the normal function of red blood cells. The requirement for cobalt is very low, and it can be found in meats and animal products. (*See also* vitamin B-12.)

COPPER aids in iron absorption and formation of red blood cells. It is concentrated in the human liver, brain, kidneys and heart. Copper is present in enzymes and works with vitamin C to keep muscle fiber elastic. Deficiencies are rare: excesses can be dangerous. Smoking and the use of contraceptive pills can increase serum copper, and copper toxicity can result from water carried in copper pipes. A zinc deficiency can activate copper excesses. Copper may be found in organ meats, shellfish, nuts and dried legumes.

FLUORIDE is found in all body tissues and aids in the maintenance of normal bone and tooth structure. While sodium fluoride is added to drinking water to prevent dental caries, it is a by-product of industry, while calcium fluoride is the form found in nature. Natural sources of fluoride include tea and seafoods.

IODINE is an essential part of the hormones produced by the thyroid gland. Although excess iodine may cause nervousness, deficiency is more common and can produce hypothyroidism, goiter and cretinism. Sources of iodine are seafoods, kelp and sea salt.

IRON is vital as it combines with protein and copper to form hemoglobin. Iron losses through hemorrhage or menstruation must be replaced, or anemia may result. Iron is essential to the transport of oxygen in the tissues. Vitamin C aids in iron absorption, but sufficient hydrochloric acid must also be present in the stomach. Iron deficiencies may result in anemia, fatigue, headache and ridged, brittle nails. Iron is abundant, occurring in liver, organ meats, lean meats, dark green leafy vegetables, whole grains, dried fruits, legumes and molasses.

MAGNESIUM is needed for production and transfer of energy, normal muscle and heart contractions, protein synthesis and nerve health. Magnesium is combined with calcium and phosphorus in bones. A diet high in calcium increases the need for magnesium. Magnesium deficiencies occur in alcoholism and other diseases and may appear as depression, irritability and muscle tremors. Magnesium is found in milk, nuts, whole grains, green leafy vegetables and seafoods.

MANGANESE acts in conjunction with zinc to prevent excess copper. It is necessary for bone growth and development, normal reproductive function, fat metabolism, and nerve health. It is important in protein and nucleic acid synthesis, activation of enzymes, and proper thyroid function. Manganese is also necessary to the utilization of vitamin C and several of the B vitamins. An excess may cause a decrease in the storage and utilization of iron. Deficiencies are rare, but may be implicated in atherosclerosis and diabetes. Sources of manganese include nuts, seeds, whole grains, leafy vegetables, wheat germ, liver, buckwheat and bone meal.

PHOSPHORUS is the second most abundant mineral in the body. It functions in conjunction with calcium and is present in every cell. It is necessary to the metabolism of fats, carbohydrates and protein, and the synthesis of nucleo-proteins. Phosphorus also aids in acid-alkaline balance and the transport of fatty acids. It promotes hormone secretions, and normal nerve impulses and muscle contraction. Phosphorus absorption requires the presence of calcium and vitamin D. Excesses of phosphorus can result in loss of calcium. Phosphorus is found in organ meats, fish, legumes and dairy products.

POTASSIUM is important in maintaining the balance of cell fluids and the body's normal acid-alkaline balance. It helps to regulate nerve and muscle impulses, assists in the conversion of glucose, and aids in the formation of muscle protein. A diet high in fats, refined foods and salt can increase the need for potassium, as can stress, diuretics, prednisone, ACTH and digitalis. Symptoms of deficiency include muscle weakness, fatigue, constipation, apathy and slow heartbeat. As potassium is water-soluble, cooking water should be utilized. Potassium is found in green leafy vegetables, wheat germ, sunflower seeds, citrus juices, legumes and fruit.

SELENIUM can be dangerously toxic, but is an essential trace mineral. It protects against cadmium and mercury toxicity. It also increases the effectiveness of vitamin E and helps prevent chromosome breakage. Selenium is necessary for protein synthesis. The refining of grains destroys selenium. Abundant in human milk, though not in cow's milk, selenium is also found in brewer's yeast, garlic, liver and eggs.

SODIUM helps regulate the body fluids and maintain normal acid-alkaline balance. Kidney malfunction can cause sodium retention resulting in excess body fluid or edema. Excess sodium may aggravate high blood pressure. Sodium is abundant in almost all foods.

SULFUR is present in all body cells, especially skin, hair and nails. It aids in tissue respiration and detoxification. Sulfur is found in some B vitamins, and occurs naturally in eggs, garlic, onions, meat, fish, legumes and nuts.

ZINC is concentrated in the liver, pancreas, kidneys and spermatozoa. It is essential to proper tissue respiration, metabolism of alcohol and phosphorus. It also aids in protein synthesis and formulation of nucleic acid. Zinc is necessary for the health of brain and nerve tissues. Deficiencies of zinc can be caused by depleted soils, food processing and refining, over-consumption of refined foods, and discarding cooking

(continued on page 246)

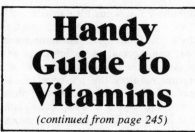

Handy Guide to Vitamins

(continued from page 245)

water, as zinc is water-soluble. Zinc deficiencies may result in dwarfism, reduced mental alertness, retarded healing, sexual abnormalities, stretch marks, painful joints and loss of taste. Excess zinc can cause losses of iron and copper. Zinc is found in shellfish, brewer's yeast, nuts and seeds.

III. THE FOOD SUPPLEMENTS

BONE MEAL is powdered, dried bone from young beef cattle. It is a good natural source of calcium, phosphorus, iron, magnesium and other trace minerals. It is a useful source of calcium for persons with an allergy to milk. Bone meal is available in tablets and powder form.

BRAN is the outer covering of the wheat kernel and contains B vitamins, iron and other trace minerals. It is also high in phosphorus, and should be supplemented with calcium when added to the diet. Bran has been highly publicized for its ability to aid fiber and bulk to the diet. Whole bran can be powdered in a blender, or soaked in liquid to make it more digestible.

BREWER'S YEAST is a marvelous source of protein, B vitamins and trace minerals. It is a non-leavening yeast originally produced as a by-product of the brewing industry, but now grown especially for human consumption. It is available in tablets, flakes and powders. Brands of brewer's yeast vary in strength, composition and flavor, so shop for a brand you like. Brewer's yeast may be added to baked goods, soups, stews, meatloaves and beverages as a nutritional supplement.

DESSICATED LIVER is made by drying beef liver at very low temperatures. It contains generous amounts of vitamin A, the B complex, iron and trace minerals. It is available as a powder which may be added to foods or in tablets.

KEFIR is a delicious milk product made by fermenting milk with kefir grains. It is useful in promoting healthy intestinal flora. More liquid than yogurt, it may be made at home quite easily using kefir grains.

KELP is seaweed, and is abundant in trace minerals. As a nutritional supplement it is available in granular, powder and tablet form. The powder and granular forms may be used in cooking, salads and as a seasoning. When using kelp, table salt should be eliminated or reduced drastically, as kelp has a high sodium content.

LECITHIN is a natural component of nonhydrogenated oils, egg yolks, soybeans and corn. As a nutritional supplement, it is derived from soybean oil and is available in capsule, granular and liquid forms. It is a natural emulsifier and is said to aid in control of cholesterol, dry skin, and many other ailments. It also contains choline and inositol, and aids in the body's utilization of vitamins A, D, E and calcium. Lecithin is a component of nerve tissue and comprises 17 percent of the human brain. Granular and liquid lecithin may be added to foods and beverages. In addition, liquid lecithin mixed with vegetable oil makes a terrific non-stick coating for baking.

ROSE HIPS are the roundish seed containers that remain when a rose has finished blooming. When they are bright red, they are harvested for their high vitamin C content. Fresh or dried, they are used to make soups, jams, syrups and teas. As nutritional supplements, rose hips are available in powders, syrups, tablets, capsules and combined with acerola cherries and vitamin C.

WHEAT GERM is the heart of the wheat kernel. It is an excellent source of protein, B-complex vitamins, vitamin E and minerals. It can be purchased raw or toasted. The raw germ is, of course, more nutritious. Wheat germ can be used in baking and cooking, and sprinkled over cereals, desserts and soups. Wheat germ is subject to rancidity and must be refrigerated in a tightly closed container.

YOGURT is milk that has been cultured with a special bacteria. It has a custardy consistency and a tangy flavor. It is rich in B vitamins and calcium and aids in maintaining healthy intestinal flora. More digestible than milk, it can be used in countless recipes. Some commercial yogurts contain undesirable ingredients, but excellent natural yogurts are widely available, and yogurt can be made easily and inexpensively at home. ☼

Vitamins: Should You Take Them and How Much?

(continued from page 25)

Pittsburgh, whose doctor prescribed 50,000 I.U. daily, was also apparently healthy. Many nutritionists usually settle for 25,000 international units per day, but that may or may not be the right amount for you.

Vitamin D in large doses, again for *some people*, has caused some minor disturbances. The beautiful thing is that if you should acquire any unexplained symptoms from too much A or D, all you have to do is stop taking the vitamin and the symptoms promptly subside. You have not been permanently damaged, merely temporarily inconvenienced. If you take vitamins correctly, this rarely, if ever, happens.

Synthetic vitamins in *large continued doses* can also cause trouble. This applies particularly to the B vitamins. But if you take a single B vitamin, such as B^1, B^2, B^3 (niacin), B^6, B^{12}, pantothenic acid, PABA, inositol, folic acid (all these and more are members of the vitamin B family or complex) then it is always wise to take natural foods *at the same time* which are rich in the entire B factors, such as brewer's yeast or lecithin or sprouts.

How Do You Know How Many Vitamins You Need?

I am asked again and again, "What vitamins should I take, and how many?" The answer is: nobody knows. Except you. Why? There are several reasons.

Roger J. Williams, the discoverer of the B vitamin, pantothenic acid, states that because there is such a great variety of individual difference, no single rule applies to everyone. No one has the same fingerprints. But the differences do not stop here. Anatomy books show pictures of hearts and other organs of many people. None are alike in size, shape, often in location! Obviously, if these organs are different in appearance, they may also work differently. So you cannot generalize on a *physical* basis that you need the same kind and amount of nutrients as your friends, your neighbors or even the members of your family.

Besides physical differences, each person possesses different genes. If your forefathers were Scandinavian, or

Italian, or Oriental, your *inherited needs* differ as previously described. So look to your ancestors and their many centuries of eating certain foods which may have conditioned your genes, thus your preference for those foods.

What about your *temperament?* Are you the emotional type or calm as a cucumber? If you are highly nervous, and/or an insomniac, it stands to reason that you are going to need more of the soothing foods such as B complex and calcium. These natural nutrients are far safer than tranquilizing drugs.

What is your *occupation*, or way of life? Is it sedentary or physically active? Do you walk to work or ride? Dr. Jean Mayer, nutritionist of Harvard University, is convinced that the amount of exercise you take determines the amount of food you should eat. Less active people, he believes, need less food, otherwise they store the excess as fat. More active people expend more physical energy and use up their fuel faster; they are rarely fat. They may need more food than their sedentary friends. Even the stress of a sedentary executive determines the amount of fuel he burns, whereas a relaxed secretary, also sedentary, may need far less than her high-strung boss. Actually, the amount of stress influences *everyone's* needs for more or less nutrients.

Your size and frame is another clue. Usually a large framed, active man or woman may need more food than a smaller, less active person, but not always.

What kind of food do you eat? A farmer who is raising his own organic food, natural dairy products and other goodies, certainly doesn't need the extra vitamins needed by city people who eat refined, processed foods. Our great grandparents ate whole natural food, got plenty of exercise and had never heard of vitamins. Today, people deprived of these whole foods need vitamin supplements as insurance to fill in the gaps of the missing nutrients.

Whole foods are extremely important. They are much more complete than partial foods. Partial foods include white bread, tampered-with cereals, white sugar, white rice, instant mixes, in fact all convenience foods. Whole foods include whole grains for cereals and breads, and whole brown rice instead of white. White rice has had B vitamins removed from its surface. Once you start using whole brown rice, which looks like and tastes like white rice, but is richer and nuttier in flavor, you will never go back to the white. It is a bit more expensive, yes, but a bargain in the long run,

because you get free B vitamins, too.

One nutritional physician uses the analogy of what would happen to you if you were marooned on a desert isle. Assuming the island is in the tropics, there would be a large supply of natural (unsprayed) fruit. If you ate only the fruit itself, our doctor tells us, you would receive some minerals and a few vitamins. But if you ate the kernels as well, you would get more vitamins, more minerals. And since the skin is unsprayed, if you added the skin of soft fruits, or the underlying skin if it is a citrus fruit, he says you have a sufficiently complete diet to remain well as long as you are a castaway. You would have been subsisting on a whole food which includes, not merely a single vitamin or mineral, but a large combination of them!

So, begin your new way of life by improving your over-all eating of whole, natural foods. Wait to give it a fair trial and see how you feel. Then very slowly, begin on natural supplements. They come, grouped together, available in health stores. One capsule will not hold all you need. There is no capsule large enough! Also, there is not enough of at least one of the most expensive, but necessary vitamins: vitamin E. Otherwise, it would make the all-in-one product too expensive. So you will have to add this separately to your vitamin intake. Vitamins (and minerals) are your friends and helpers. Don't ignore them.

Also, don't deny yourself foods which rebuild your body, for fear they may make you fat. You can eat less of those which are higher in carbohydrates, but you can reserve space for them by ignoring the partial carbohydrate foods which don't do a thing for you! And don't be misled by that myth that our foods today provide all the vitamins and minerals we need. *They do not!* This is why we have to take added vitamins and minerals and why millions are doing it because they feel better when they do. Remember, too, that *natural* food supplements save eating tons of food, including calories and carbohydrates!

You will have to use the trial-and-error method in choosing the best foods and vitamin products for you. You need not become a hypochondriac; just be intelligent until you learn what is the best program for *you.* Watch out for allergies. Almost everyone has at least one. Wheat and wheat products, and chocolate are considered by one large respected medical institution, as being the most common. But there are others, too.

How Should You Take Your Vitamins?

Vitamins, if from natural foods, as they should be, are food, and should be taken with food. Taking vitamins on an empty stomach may cause discomfort because they are so concentrated that, if taken alone, they may irritate the stomach lining. Also, read your labels. Since not everything can be put in one tablet or capsule, the label may read: "The following amounts are found in *six* tablets daily." This means, that to get everything in the necessary amounts, you do not take one tablet or capsule only, but six, usually dividing them throughout the day, probably two with each meal. People who do not read labels these days are missing a great deal of free education. Unfortunately, in some products, the government does not require the labels to state the ingredients. This applies to ice cream and other food products as well as cosmetics. This should not be. For the protection of the consumer, everyone should know what he is using in or on his body.

If you can find a nutritional doctor to help you, grab him! He is rare. If you can't find one, don't despair. Read the fascinating books in your health store and learn for yourself, as most of us have had to do. And remember, no one in the world has a right to dictate to you what you can and cannot eat. You know yourself and your reactions far better than anyone else who does not know you. Through self-discovery, you can work out a successful program of eating correctly, and taking the right supplements, so that you can control your weight and stay well too. ✿

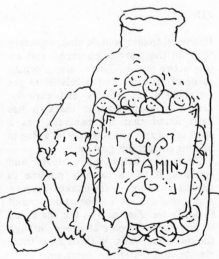

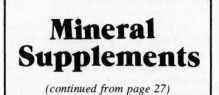

Mineral Supplements

(continued from page 27)

Copper aids in the oxidation of tyrosine, an amino acid, and works in the utilization of vitamin C. *Note:* Your bloodstream *must* have copper before iron can be properly assimilated. A deficiency may lead to Bang's disease, infections, weakened digestive powers, and forms of anemia. It should not be taken separately, but in natural organic mineral combination. Copper poisoning is not an uncommon disturbance.

SULFUR

We are gradually discovering this "beauty" mineral. Sulfur is able to give a natural gloss to your hair and to improve your skin health and texture. Sulfur has the power to invigorate your bloodstream to combat bacterial infections.

Sulfur also assists your liver in absorbing other vital minerals. A deficiency is seen in skin lesions, dandruff, and brittle fingernails. Sulfur is also a vital part of protein metabolism and body oxidative processes. Wounds have been found to heal more rapidly when the body has adequate sulfur.

SILICON

Silicon, another beauty mineral, is found in muscles, hair, nails, connective tissues, teeth, skin, and cellular walls. It joins with body fluorine to build strong bones and tooth enamel. A deficiency may cause skin flabbiness, eyes that are dull and without color, and a feeling of chronic tiredness.

ZINC

Nearly all tissues contain zinc, especially those in the thyroid, pancreas, and reproductive organs. Zinc is also a constituent of enzymes and is related to the metabolism of proteins and carbohydrates. In some diabetes cases, it has been found that the pancreas has a shortage of zinc and this may be a clue to helping correct this problem.

Zinc also helps store sugars and starches. It has a valuable purpose in tissue respiration — the intake of oxygen and expulsion of carbon dioxide and toxic wastes. Zinc acts as the sparkplug to help foods become absorbed through the intestinal walls. Without zinc, there may be constipation disorders.

Zinc further helps in the manufacture of various male hormones. It is needed to create energy because of its involvement in carbohydrate utilization. If someone feels tired or lazy and has a habit of malingering, this may be traced to a zinc as well as a basic mineral deficiency.

CHLORINE

Meet Nature's Broomstick. This mineral actually sweeps away toxic wastes from your body. How? Chlorine stimulates your liver to filter out many waste substances. *Note:* Chlorine is valuable for boosting the manufacture of hydrochloric acid needed in your digestive system for assimilation of food nutrients.

Chlorine is also found in the bloodstream where it helps to sweep out the nitrogenous end-products of metabolism. Deficiency symptoms may be hair and teeth loss, weak muscular powers, as well as impaired digestive abilities. It, too, should be taken in natural form; too much chlorine such as is found in some water supplies, has been found to affect the heart adversely.

SUMMING UP

You must have minerals! Daniel T. Quigley, M.D., in *The National Malnutrition,* declares, "We do know that the person who has a sufficient intake of calcium, iron and iodine . . . (plus vitamins) will have a resistance against disease in excess of the average person.

"Such persons will have more freedom from fatigue and greater ability to work; will live with the retention of all physical faculties to a greater age, and will have a better mind than the person who suffers from some single or multiple vitamin or mineral deficiency.

"The various vitamins and minerals are ALL necessary. *"Not one can be omitted if an individual would retain good health."*

Drs. Pottenger, Allison and Albrecht (*Report,* Merck & Co.), describe how minerals can promote miracle healing and restore vibrant health:

"Such varied symptoms (in human patients) were initially present as to be too baffling for accurate diagnoses. Yet they disappeared after consumption of trace element salts [medical terminology for minerals] and carefully regulated, high-protein, low-sugar diets during some 12 weeks or more.

"Relief occurred from this vast array of symptoms, which included aches of the back, shoulders and joints, allergies, arthritis, anorexia, hyperidroses, fever, constipation, enlarged spleen, mental depression and others amounting to a list reportedly as large as 200."

William H. Hay, M.D., author of

What Price Health? points to the values of minerals in improving health:

"Nature provides all her chemicals for restoration of the body in the form of colloids, organic forms, and Man has for a long time sought to imitate her in this, but he has not been so very successful that we are now able to insure the recouping of the mineral losses of the body by any artificial means, and must still depend on Nature's minerals as found in plant and fruit and food."

A valuable comment is offered by H. Curtis Wood, Jr., M.D., in *Overfed But Undernourished:*

"The skeptic will think that all this 'undernourished' business does not apply to him because he eats 'well-balanced' meals and may even take a pill with a few vitamins in it every day. This is not enough, for it has been estimated that one-third of our diets lack some of the essential nutritive factors, and some experts have even stated that vitamins alone — *in the absence of minerals* — are functionless. *We need them both.*

"Minerals may be thought of as the bricks, and vitamins as the mortar in the wall of health. Of the two, minerals may be the more essential, for it is possible to build a 'dry' wall without any cement at all."

Trace minerals are so described because they exist in foods in such minute amounts or traces. We may well agree with Dr. Michael Rabben, in *Modern Nutrition,* who says:

"While inorganic trace minerals are satisfactory for the treatment of acute conditions where they are employed as drugs, and as a temporary measure, the intake of natural trace minerals to maintain health is best. If they are to be taken as supplements, they should be in the form of an organic plant because Nature has balanced the constituents in a manner that is still beyond comprehension."

To help make up for any shortages, an all-purpose mineral supplement is your passport to better health and vitality — through Nature. ☼

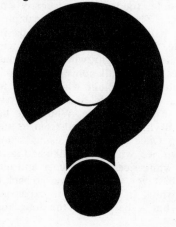

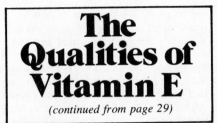

The Qualities of Vitamin E

(continued from page 29)

is especially useful after radical mastectomy, particularly where there is superficial irritation due to radiation. It not only reduces the toxic reactions but soothes and heals the irritated areas.

Vitamin E ointment is also useful on acne scars and on scars about the face due to laceration from windshield glass in automobile accidents. Not long ago my two-year-old grandson, standing up on the front seat of the car, was precipitated onto the rear view mirror. An elliptical piece of skin approximately 1 by 2 cm from his forehead was left on the mirror.

My grandson was seen very soon afterward by his local general practitioner. The doctor told my daughter to bring him the piece of skin. He washed it in saline and sewed it into the defect—an amazingly dextrous job on a two-year-old since he had, of course, to tease the contracted piece of skin back into approximately normal size and shape.

I chanced to arrive on the scene on the day the stitches were removed, and there was certainly grave doubt then that the patch would survive. It was raised in the center and quite inflamed around about half its periphery. As soon as the stitch holes sealed over, Vitamin E ointment was liberally applied with the result that although there was a very small area of superficial necrosis in the center, the cosmetic results six months later were excellent. The patch continues to improve and is now scarcely noticeable. The child's physician does not know the ointment is being used, and my daughter happily relates this excellent physician's surprise at the steady and unexpected improvement.

Vitamin E ointment has another specific use—namely, in the treatment of nerve root pain. Intercostal neuritis or neuralgia, sciatica and various cases of myositis (muscle inflammation) respond to Vitamin E inunction. Drs. Burgess and Pritchard of the Montreal General Hospital long ago reported that Vitamin E could be recovered at the periosteum of bones and joints shortly after the ointment was rubbed into the overlying skin. The ointment, rubbed in gently for ten minutes and followed by the application of heat for ten minutes over the nerve roots of the sensory nerves involved in a

neuritis, will relieve the condition in a majority of cases. If it does not do so within one to three nights of application, however, it is unlikely to help.

A great many doctors, especially in Canada, have long scoffed at manipulation. They have given excellent reasons why manipulation cannot help and I expect that this has been taught in every medical school, as it was in mine. However, there is now an association of trained physicians manipulating patients with the various neuritic lesions. Many surgeons attempt manipulation under anesthesia as do many in the new specialty of physical medicine.

About 50 percent of patients who have had myocardial infarcts or angina often also have pains in the chest unrelated to coronary artery disease. The cervical root syndrome closely mimics heart pain. Many of these cases respond to manipulation. Dr. Paul Goodley described such a case at the fifth International Congress of Physical Medicine in 1968. His patient, a fifty-two-year-old longshoreman, had suffered serious neck injuries in a car accident. His severe pain of fifteen months duration was completely relieved by manipulation under anesthesia. Incidentally, this doctor of medicine was refused permission to do this manipulation in his hospital.

At the same meeting Dr. Janet Travell, Associate Clinical Professor of Medicine at George Washington University, and Dr. John Mennell, Associate Professor of Medicine and Rehabilitation at the University of Pennsylvania, reported on the virtues of manipulation. Manipulation can give instant relief from pain and from restriction of movement in some cases.

Vitamin E ointment somehow does the same in most cases of sciatica, intercostal neuralgia, frozen shoulder and others of that type. Many cases of months or years duration respond. When they do not, we have for years sent patients for manipulation with excellent results, again in most cases.

An interesting instance of Vitamin E—but not, apparently, E ointment—helping in a muscular condition, occurred in Chicago. Some years ago, a Chicago newspaper contained an account of an unusual case involving a ten-year-old boy whose leg muscles had become so hard, owing to calcium deposits, that they were described as "turning to stone." The newspapers said that the boy's doctors believed that "highly concentrated doses of Vitamin E" had helped him so that he could walk a few steps. They were, they said, expecting considerably more improvement. In 1965 Drs. R.H. Brodkin and J. Blei-

berg reported that there can be allergic reactions to Vitamin E applied locally. We have noted this from the very beginning of its use and have warned all patients, for years, that about 10 percent of people cannot tolerate the full-strength ointment on open wounds or ulcers. Before it is applied to the whole area, Vitamin E should always be used on one corner of the ulcer or sore until it is evident that it does not cause a local reaction. We first published this caution in 1950.

The ointment is a 30 IU per gm of alpha tocopherol in a petroleum jelly base, and those who cannot tolerate a full-strength ointment can often derive benefit without reaction from a half-strength dilution. If there is still reaction to the local application of the ointment, opening a capsule of the succinate preparation and scattering the powder over the ulcer can often be tolerated and can be very effective.

We decry the use of Vitamin E for any nonmedical reason. We were horrified at its use as a deodorant. Had the companies concerned bothered to consult us, we could have told them that many users would show allergic reactions. However, our main objection arises from the fact that this substance is often in short supply as the result of its rapid acceptance for prophylactic and therapeutic use in medicine. It is a shame to see it wasted.

The mechanism by which the Vitamin E ointment functions is quite unknown and very puzzling. New uses for it, however, keep cropping up constantly. Often we hear about them only by letter. In this connection, let me quote three paragraphs from a letter:

"I was born with a hemangioma (birthmark) on my face. It covers my left eye, forehead, cheek, nose and upper part of my left lip.

"As my sister, who is a medical doctor, read your book on Vitamin E, she thought it would be advisable that I take Vitamin E. I started with 400 units for a period of 6 months, then increased to 600, and since August 1973, to date I am taking 800 units per day.

"During the first six months I was taking Vitamin E I did not notice any change on my hemangioma but suddenly I started noting that it was fading out little by little and right now it has faded out almost one centimeter all around the birthmark. At the same time that I was taking Vitamin E, my sister ordered from Canada Vitamin E ointment and I applied it on my face with a lamp (200 watts). I think the birthmark started disappearing since I started applying the ointment and taking the Vitamin E. I have applied 3 jars of ointment."

☼

BREWER'S YEAST

Brewer's yeast is one of the biggest food finds of the century. This is not a calculated guess; it is a fact as proved with thousands upon thousands of cases of health improvement resulting from its use. A list of its contents explains why it is such a high-powered food. It contains all of the major B vitamins (except B-12, which can be especially bred into it), nineteen amino acids (making it a complete protein), and eighteen or more minerals. Except for vitamins A, E and C, which it lacks, it can be considered a whole food.

A more detailed list of its contents follows:

Vitamins: B-1 or thiamin, B-2 or riboflavin, B-3 or niacin, B-6 or pyridoxine, choline, inositol, pantothenic acid, PABA and biotin. B-12 does not occur unless especially "bred" into nutritional yeast. Ask for it at health stores.

Protein (amino acids): lysine, tryptophane, histidine, phenylalanine, leucine, methionine, valine, glycine, alanine, aspartic acid, glutamic acid, proline, hydroxyproline, tryosine, cystine and arginine.

Minerals: calcium, phosphorus, potassium, magnesium, silicon, copper, manganese, zinc, aluminum, sodium, iron, tin, boron, gold, silver, nickel cobalt and iodine.

Brewer's yeast, originally a by-product of beer, is a powdered, dried residue. It has been "killed" by heat; it will not cause bread to rise, or, by the same token, feed upon your intestinal vitamins and multiply in your body, creating gas. It may cause gas for some people, as any high protein food can, but the addition of hydrochloric acid can prevent this problem.

Brewer's yeast is becoming so popular as a food that it is now being made specifically for that purpose. It is often called nutritional yeast. Instead of being available in powder only, it is now made in large and small flake form. Both Adelle Davis and I have listed examples galore of the improvement of health through the use of brewer's yeast or nutritional yeast. I will mention here only one benefit, in addition to the value of being a good reducing food. It increases energy.

I have tried yeast for energy myself and I have watched my children and grandchildren use it as a pickup. My elder daughter, particularly, when she feels slightly fatigued, will automatically go to the yeast cannister, kept beside the flour, raw sugar and other staples, stir a tablespoon or so into liquid and drink it down. Within about ten minutes a pickup is noted, which, unlike the temporary lift of coffee or tea, lasts for several hours. Most people begin with a teaspoon in fruit juice or tomato juice or hot bouillon, which blends with the slightly savory flavor of the yeast. Later, people work up gradually to one-fourth cup daily, and they no longer bother about putting it in juice, but add it to plain water and gulp it down.

Yeast flakes are somewhat milder in flavor, but it takes more of them to provide the equivalent of the powder. Yeast tablets are also available but it takes twenty-four tablets to equal one tablespoon of yeast powder or flakes. Health stores, of course, provide all forms. If you take separate B vitamins, which are almost always synthetic, it is very important to take brewer's yeast the same day. The yeast is a source of natural B vitamins, which prevents vitamin B imbalance.

Because brewer's yeast, like other protein foods, is high in phosphorus, it is advisable when taking it, to add extra calcium. (Phosphorus, a co-worker of calcium, can take the calcium out of the body with it, leaving a calcium deficiency.) The remedy for this is easy. Mix up your pound of yeast with one-fourth cup of calcium lactate powder (available at health or drug stores). Mix well and keep in any container. It need not be refrigerated. The calcium corrects the calcium-phosphorus imbalance so that leg or other cramps can be prevented. By having the mixture premixed, it is convenient when you want to use it quickly.

WHEAT GERM

Wheat germ is a superior food. The United States Department of Agriculture considers it an excellent food for the following reasons: "A grain of wheat, like all seeds, contains the nutriment needed for germination and growth of the seedling. Protein, minerals, B vitamins, fat and carbohydrates are present in the right proportion . . . the germ or embryo contains a large proportion of the vitamins and protein of superior quality. White flour, as it is milled today . . . has removed the germ, also the greater part of the minerals and vitamins and much of the protein."

In a later yearbook it adds: "Losses in milling are even higher for some less familiar nutrients. For example, vitamin E is present in high concentrations in the oil of the wheat germ. Nearly all of this vitamin is removed with the germ." This tells the story of wheat germ in a nutshell. As we have said again and again: Because the wheat germ is removed from bread and cereals to protect the shelf life, our bread and cereals are lacking vitamin E, which comes from wheat germ. Cattle, deprived of wheat germ and vitamin E have dropped dead of heart disease. Many Americans are following suit. When the wheat-germ vitamin E was restored to the cattle feed, the deaths from heart disease ceased. This valuable nutrient is not restored to the food for people. They must take it on their own. Meanwhile, the Drs. Wilfrid E. and Evan V. Shute have rehabilitated the hearts of thousands of people with vitamin E.

Wheat-germ oil has been tested by various laboratories on animals and humans, especially athletes. It has been found invaluable in building energy and outwitting fatigue. Both wheat-germ and wheat-germ oil, once opened, should be kept refrigerated to prevent rancidity. The raw wheat germ is less tasty but valuable for adding to baked products. The toasted type, usually vacuum-packed to prevent rancidity until opened, is tasty and children love it when it is floated on top of milk as a cereal. It can also be used instead of bread crumbs for breading meat and vegetables, or added to meat loaf, breads, biscuits, muffins, waffles and hot cakes.

There is a newer type of wheat germ now available in most health stores. It is called a high potency embryo chunk-style wheat germ. This does not mean that it comes in chunks, but that it is not rolled flat. (The chunks are noticeable only under a magnifying glass.) This type is less subject to rancidity, due to underprocessing.

ANALYSIS OF WHEAT GERM

	(per ounce)
Vitamin B-1	.45 mg.
Vitamin B-2	.14 mg.
Vitamin B-3 Niacin	.5 mg.
Vitamin B-6	.45 mg.
Vitamin E	7.00 mg.
Oil	8.4%
Protein	23%
Copper	.4 mg.
Iron	2.5 mg.
Manganese	4.0 mg.

SUNFLOWER SEEDS

Most seeds are an excellent source of many nutrients, but sunflower seeds take the prize. Whenever your children, or you, feel the need for a snack to hold you together until mealtime, sunflower seeds are a natural. They are good for that four o'clock slump and save a low blood sugar reaction if taken with coffee. They are also said to be good for the eyes.

Sunflower seeds should be eaten hulled and raw. Cooking them causes a loss of some valuable nutrients. They should be refrigerated after opening. Otherwise they can become rancid. If a jar or other container of sunflower seeds should smell rancid, return it, explaining the reason to the health store operator. (He knows that rancid foods can be disturbing to health, even dangerous.)

If you are traveling and want something to nibble while you wait for a bus, train or plane, a few sunflower seeds will give you a lift within minutes. I always carry them with me. For victims of hypoglycemia (low blood sugar) they are invaluable. They raise the blood sugar naturally through the protein content and are much wiser to take than something sweet. Here is the analysis:

ANALYSIS OF SUNFLOWER SEEDS PER 100 GRAMS OR ¼ POUND

Minerals

Phosphorus	860.0 mg.
Iron	6.0 mg.
Calcium	57.0 mg.
Iodine	0.07
Magnesium	347.0 mg.
Potassium	630.0 mg.
Manganese	25 ppm
Copper	20 ppm
Zinc	66.5
Sodium	.4
Vitamin A	68 I.U.

B Vitamins

B-1 (Thiamin)	2.2 mg.
B-2 (Riboflavin)	0.28 mg.
B-3 (Niacin)	5.6 mg.
B-6 (Pyridoxine)	1.1 mg.
B-12	.04 mcg. per gm.
PABA	62. mg.
Biotin	0.067 mg.
Choline	216. mg.
Inositol	147. mg.
Folic acid	0.1 mg.
Pantothenic acid	2.2 mg.
Pantothenol	3.5 mg.
Vitamin D	92 USP units
Vitamin E	31 I.U.
Protein	25%
Sunflower oil	48.44%
(over 90% unsaturated)	

ALFALFA

Alfalfa is one of the most complete and nutritionally rich of all foods tested. In addition to a fabulously high potency of vitamins as well as minerals, it is high in protein and contains every essential amino acid. Its antitoxin or detoxification properties surpass those of every food tested: liver, brewer's yeast and wheat germ. Although these foods, too, have antitoxin properties, alfalfa is superior in this respect. It has been found to provide resistance to disease and seems to help those ailments that end in "itis" such as arthritis. It also helps to prevent exhaustion and provides an excellent calcium-phosphorus ratio (2:1).

Alfalfa seems to be most effective when it has had the fiber removed before being pressed into tablets. (The fiber upsets some people's digestion.) Alfalfa is an outstanding natural product as the following analysis shows.

ANALYSIS OF DEHYDRATED ALFALFA

Vitamins	*Per 100 Grams*
A	up to 44,000 I.U.
D	1,040 I.U.
E	50 I.U.
K	15 I.U.
U	unknown
C	176 mg.
B-1	0.8 mg.
B-2	1.8 mg.
B-6	1.0 mg.
B-12	0.3 mcg.
Niacin	5 mg.
Pantothenic acid	3.3 mg.
Inositol	210 mg.
Biotin	033 mg.
Folic acid	0.8 mg.

Other Content

Fiber	25%
Protein	20%
Fat solubles	3%

Minerals

Phosphorus	250 mg.
Calcium	1,750 mg.
Potassium	2,000 mg.
Sodium	150 mg.
Chlorine	280 mg.
Sulfur	290 mg.
Magnesium	310 mg.
Copper	2 mg.
Manganese	5 mg.
Iron	35 mg.
Cobalt	2.4 mg.
Boron	4.7 mg.
Molybdenum	2.6 ppm

Trace Minerals
Nickel
Strontium 90
Lead
Paladium

RICE POLISHINGS

Rice polish (or rice bran) is loaded with B vitamins. It is the outer covering removed from whole, brown, natural rice.

Rice polish has a mild flavor and its use is an excellent method of fortifying foods. Usually, after it is taken off the white rice, it is sold back to the public in vitamin preparations. It is less expensive, in the long run, to buy it in powder form at health stores and add it to breads, biscuits, muffins, pie crust, meat loaf and cereals. It can be used cooked or uncooked. Cooking does not destroy its value.

CULTURED MILKS

The cultured milks are of great value for health. They help to stabilize the intestinal flora so that digestion is improved and many B vitamins can be synthesized in the intestines. After taking antibiotics, it is imperative to take acidophilus or one of the cultured milks, for the antibiotics kill the friendly intestinal flora that must be reestablished to encourage the return of health. In Italy, doctors routinely prescribe a cultured milk product when prescribing antibiotics.

The cultured milks include kefir, cultured buttermilk and yogurt. These can be purchased, but it is also possible to allow your own milk to clabber at room temperature; or with the aid of a starter which can be purchased from health stores, make your own. Kefir is liquid. Yogurt is more custard-like. Directions are supplied when you purchase the starter.

There is some indication that, whereas powdered skim milk has been used to make yogurt more solid, it is better to use a minimum because it is rich in galactose, an antagonist to vitamin B-2 (riboflavin). Animals made deficient in riboflavin have developed cataracts. Yogurt starter may be perverted by artificial additives (colorings and flavorings). Countries that have used it for generations for health use it plain.

BLACKSTRAP MOLASSES

Blackstrap molasses is a food that you may hear belittled. Those who do not understand nutrition may consider blackstrap a fad. As we have said, no single food is a panacea; but blackstrap, as you will note in the accompanying analysis supplied to me by the medical profession, is a truly rich source of minerals and vitamins.

(continued on page 252)

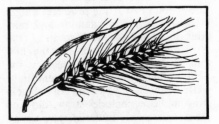

ANALYSIS

Five tablespoons of blackstrap molasses contain:

Calcium	258 mg.
Phosphorus	30 mg.
Iron	7.97 mg.
Copper	1.93 mg.
Potassium	1500 mg.
Inositol	150 mg.
Thiamin (B-1)	245 mcg.
Riboflavin (B-2)	240 mcg.
Niacin (B-3)	4 mcg.
Pyridoxine (B-6)	270 mcg.
Pantothenic acid	260 mcg.
Biotin	16 mcg.

What about other sweeteners? White sugar contains no nutrients and is pure carbohydrate. The best form of sugar, if you must use it, is Yellow D sugar. It is a rich brown sugar made from cane molasses and it contains natural vitamins and minerals. It is called a raw sugar. Turbinado sugar is also acceptable. Fructose—fruit sugar—is now also available.

Better than raw sugar as a sweetening, however, is natural, unrefined, unclarified and unheated honey. If it is unprocessed and unrefined, it contains vitamins and minerals. Honey labeled as "pure, deluxe" and so clear that you read the label through it is robbed of its nutrients, so that it will look pretty. Reject it in favor of the cloudier, natural honey. That found in the comb is probably even richer, nutritionally, because it has not been tampered with in any way.

To produce molasses, sap from the sugar cane is collected. The first extraction, after boiling, is crystallized raw sugar (such as Yellow D). Usually it is later refined into pure white sugar thus being robbed of all nutrients. It encourages tooth decay, low blood sugar and a host of other ailments because it robs the body of B vitamins.

The second extraction produces a light molasses, richer in vitamins and minerals than raw sugar. Blackstrap, the third and last extraction, at the bottom of the barrel, so to speak, is the richest of all. Most of the nutrients have settled there. If you hear that blackstrap molasses includes straw, dirt and other extraneous material, pay no at-

tention. It has served people well for centuries, and has improved health. It contains more calcium than milk, more iron than many eggs, more potassium than any food and is an excellent source of B vitamins. It contains no sugar at all. It can be added to yogurt, used for cooking. If it is taken straight, the mouth should be rinsed immediately, because any sticky substance encourages tooth decay. Blackstrap has been found to recolor hair in some cases, has prevented anemia (because of its high iron content) and has even been credited with stopping falling hair.

LIVER

Liver has been considered one of the best "health foods" for many years. It contains vitamin B-12, and doctors and nutritionists advise eating it once or twice weekly. It provides protein, vitamins, minerals and energy, as proved by experiments with laboratory animals. Many doctors consider it a necessity for regaining or maintaining health. One physician says: "Adding liver to your diet invariably has resulted in a lasting improvement, often evident within a few days."

The reason liver is so effective is that it is a depot of all vitamins and minerals taken into the body. This is a plus factor, but there is also a minus factor in our present-day polluted civilization. The liver is a depot for poisons and pesticides which can lodge there in the fatty tissues. (Pesticides are always stored in fat.) For this reason many people are afraid to eat liver these days. Fortunately, there are several solutions to the problem. Organically raised meat does not come in contact with pesticide sprays or other chemical poisons. Therefore organic liver is safer. But some people do not like liver. In this case, desiccated liver, dried at low temperature to retain the nutrients, can be taken in powder or tablet form. One company derives its liver from animals raised in Argentina, where sprays are not used. Other companies now de-fat their desiccated liver which removes not only the fatty tissue but the pesticides and other poisons stored there.

Liver has been given (in desiccated form) to athletes to provide stamina. It, too, has recolored some cases of prematurely gray hair. It is a powerhouse of nutrients and, in its safer forms, should be high on your list of high-power foods.

ANALYSIS OF LIVER

(in 100 grams or about 4 ounces fresh liver—an average slice)

Calcium	8 mg.
Phosphorus	486 mg.
Iron	7.8 mg. (hamburger contains only 2.8)
Vitamins:	
A	53,500 I.U. (hamburger contains none)
B-1	.26 mg. (hamburger contains .08)
B-2	3.96 mg. (hamburger contains 1.19)
B-3 (niacin)	14.8 mg. (hamburger contains 4.8)
C	31 mg. (hamburger contains none)
B-12	35-50 mcg. (hamburger contains 2-5 mcg.)

From *Heinz Nutritional Data*, Fifth edition, published by Heinz Research Center.

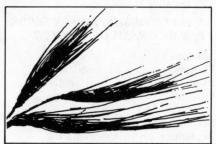

SPROUTS

Many seeds and nuts are nutritionally rich. They contain vitamin E (the germ for regrowth upon planting) as well as protein, other vitamins and minerals. They are most nutritious when eaten raw, since cooking destroys much of their value. However, there is a way of using seeds that really hits the jackpot, nutritionally—sprouts from seeds. You can sprout them at home, or buy them already sprouted at the health store and some supermarkets. They can be germinated from any whole unhulled seeds or beans. The most popular are mung, soy, alfalfa and wheat. If you grow them yourself, do not buy those seeds coated with fungicides, mercury or other poisons. These are usually found at seed stores. Those at the health stores are safe.

The Chinese, of course, have used bean sprouts for centuries. Sprouts can be added to salads, sandwiches, or dropped at the last minute into soups, casseroles or omelets, so that they will remain crisp and not be damaged by cooking at high heat.

Each person who sprouts seeds has his favorite method. I like mine because it is so simple and easy. Soak the seeds overnight. In the morning drain them. Place a white paper towel in a colander. Spread the seeds, one layer thick, on the towel. Cover with another paper towel. Hold the whole thing under the water spigot and gently allow cold water to run over the towels, soaking them and the seeds. Drain again. Put the colander away in the corner of the kitchen counter and forget about it until the next morning. At this time, re-irrigate in the same way.

Dampen the seeds every morning. Within a few days they will develop little "tails" or sprouts. When these are about an inch long, remove the towels, wash the sprouts and refrigerate them.

A friend of mine lived next door to a physician. Both had children, and my friend always kept a bowl of sprouts on the table for the children and their friends to eat as snacks after school. They loved them. Later, the physician and his family moved away. After some time had passed he wrote: "As long as we lived next door to you, our children remained healthy. Since we have moved, they have been less healthy. The only way I can account for this change is that the sprouts must have contributed to their health.

"We are going to make them a habit in this family from now on."

There is no doubt that sprouts are nutritious; they contain a fantastic amount of vitamins B, C and E. When seeds sprout, the vitamin content increases, depending upon the vitamin, 10, 50, 100, 500 and 1,000 percent. They are one of the cheapest sources of natural (not synthetic) vitamins you can find.

Catharyn Elwood tells the full story of the increase of the vitamin content of sprouts. I am going to quote one analysis to give you an idea of how sprouting seeds increases their value.

ANALYSIS OF B VITAMINS IN SPROUTED OATS

Niacin	500% increase
Biotin	50% increase
Pantothenic acid	200% increase
Pyridoxine	500% increase
Folic acid	600% increase
Inositol	100% increase
Thiamin	10% increase
Riboflavin	1350% increase

We come to the end of this discussion of high-power foods. Don't let anyone kid you into thinking there are no such things as wonder foods. ☼

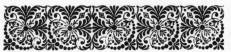

Soybeans

(continued from page 45)

☐ "For a number of years I had been troubled with chronic constipation and while temporary relief was afforded by the use of ordinary cathartics, I found no permanent cure could be made by their use and that it was likely to become habit forming. I then tried the various mineral oils which I found to be much more satisfactory than the cathartics but which were objectionable because of leakage.

☐ "In June, 1942, I visited the U.S. Regional Soybean Laboratory at Urbana, Illinois, in company with Mr. Morse and brought up the question of using soybean oil for constipation, found that some use had been made of it, but the results were not generally known. I then obtained a quart of soybean oil and for the past year have been taking a tablespoonful each night before retiring. Let me say here and now that the decision to try soybean oil was a happy one for I am no longer troubled with constipation, there is no leakage and I have been able to reduce the dosage to thrice weekly instead of daily. In addition I have recommended it to several of my friends who were suffering with constipation and a check showed they had the same results that I did."

☐ Soybeans have proved to be an excellent food for those with food allergy. They clear up pimples, rashes, eczema, and other skin troubles. They are valuable in arthritis, rheumatism, and allergy-caused asthma. The reason that soybeans are recommended for use in cases of eczema and other skin diseases is that they render unnecessary the use of animal proteins—meat, eggs and milk—and thus lessen the inflammatory activities in the skin. The soybean user is therefore free from any sensitivity-producing tendencies or allergic reactions which so frequently attend the use of all animal proteins.

☐ Consequently soy milk is of great value to persons who are allergic to cow's milk. It is estimated that there are 2 percent of such people in this country.

☐ Dr. Wolfgang Tiling, by the use of soy milk and soy flour, has successfully treated during the last eleven years hundreds of children and infants who were allergic to cow's milk and were suffering from eczema, asthma, diarrhea and sprue. He found that soy milk and soy flour promoted growth, improved appetite, revived the destroyed intestinal motility and digestive function, and restored the general disposition, psychic behavior, and mental alertness that were altered by the sickness. Some cases of recovery have been almost unbelievable. In one such case a sick child was admitted to the clinic with a most seri-

ous case of marasmus (progressive emaciation), the result of sprue due to allergy to cow's milk. She was restored to perfect health in six months when cow's milk was replaced by soy milk.

☐ At Columbia University, Drs. Charles A. Slanetz and Albert Scharf once conducted some interesting and effective experiments which were aimed toward the solution of the problem of recurrent summer itch. The experiments dealt with the effects of soybean phosphatides on the utilization of vitamin A and carotene. Two percent soy lecithin was fed to dogs infested with summer itch or whelping eczema, with excellent results. The scientists explain that the introduction of the new factor, while helping the utilization of vitamin A, has in turn its effect on skin condition.

☐ Professor Mader of the University of Frankfurt, Germany, showed that infants can be cured of pyurea on a diet containing soy flour. The beneficial results of his experiment may be explained by the fact that the alkalinity of a soybean diet increases the resistance of tissues to infection.

☐ A newly developed oil emulsion is aiding patients who are unable to utilize fats taken into the stomach, but who can use fat injected into the bloodstream as a water emulsion. Of the many commercial emulsifiers tested for making oil-in-water emulsions, only a few hold promise. The naturally-occurring phosphatides, principally soybean lecithin, are currently being used for this purpose because of the absence of hemolytic activity.

☐ It is thus evident that whether persons are in a state of health or disease, soybeans occupy a prominent place in their diet. ☼

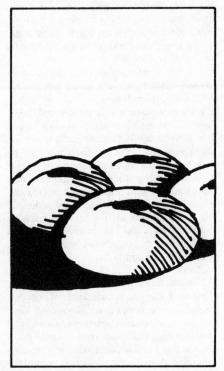

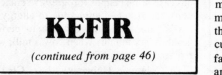

KEFIR

(continued from page 46)

be removed. You can give them to a friend, neighbor or relative who is anxious to begin culturing kefir. (Such extra grains are excellent fund-raising items for worthy causes.) Or, you may decide to preserve the grains for future use (see below). Or, you can culture more kefir than you can use as a beverage, and turn the surplus into kefir cheese (see below).

In culturing kefir, you can control the flavor as well as the consistency. If you enjoy it tart, culture for a longer period of time; if you like it mild, culture more briefly. If you enjoy thick kefir, allow a large quantity of grains to remain in the culture; if you like thin kefir, remove the excessive grains as they multiply.

Preserving kefir grains for future use: If you plan to be on vacation and have no ''kefir sitter'' to nurture the grains in your absence, preserve them for future use. Store them wet, dry or frozen.

To store them wet, wash the grains thoroughly in a sieve with a stream of cold, running water. Place them in a clean jar, and cover them with cold *unchlorinated* water. Store in a refrigerator at 40° F. They will keep their viability for about a week, but lose potency if held much longer.

To dry the kefir grains, rinse and drain as above. Place them on two layers of clean cheesecloth. Air-dry them at room temperature for thirty-six to forty-eight hours. The room should have good air circulation, or use a fan. Place the dry grains in a paper envelope or wrap them in aluminum foil. Keep them in a cool dry place. Such dried grains are usually still active after twelve to eighteen months of proper storage.

To freeze kefir grains, rinse and drain as above. Place them in a small non-actinic bottle (light-excluding). Seal the bottle tightly and place it in a similar but larger bottle. Seal the edges of the lid of the larger bottle with masking tape to prevent any air from entering. Freeze, and thaw out to begin culturing again at a future date.

Reactivating stored kefir grains: You may find that kefir grains stored wet may be slightly slower in their culturing action. If so, leave them in the fresh milk somewhat longer than usual, or culture them at a slightly higher temperature than usual. In time, they should be restored to their full activity.

To reactivate the dried or frozen grains, first soak the grains overnight, or approximately twelve hours in *unchlorinated* water to cover, at room temperature. Drain, and transfer the grains to only *one cup* of milk. Allow this to stand, approximately twenty-four hours, at room temperature, or until the

milk thickens. During this period, stir the mixture occasionally. Drain the grains from the milk, rinse, and transfer them to a fresh cup of milk. By then, the grains should be fairly active. They can be rinsed, drained, and transferred to *two cups* of milk. Continue, gradually increasing the number of cups of milk used, until ultimately the usual one quart of milk can be cultured with the grains. Continue to culture under the conditions that you have found produce the flavor and thickness which suit your taste.

Homemade kefir buttermilk: Kefir grains can be used to prepare kefir buttermilk as well as to prepare the usual type of kefir fermented milk. Kefir buttermilk closely resembles churned or real buttermilk in flavor and consistency and has proved to be a popular item when it has been sold along with cultured buttermilk. Use either raw or pasteurized partially-skimmed milk (two to three percent butterfat content), or pasteurized sweet buttermilk, which is sometimes available from creameries where butter is made from sweet cream. Of course, it would also be available on a farm where butter is churned from sweet cream.

If raw milk is used, heat it to 165° F. Cool it to between 68° and 72° F. It is then ready for making the kefir buttermilk. Or, it may be kept in the refrigerator for later use. If sweet buttermilk is used, pasteurize it by heating at 180° F. for twenty minutes to expel all the air.

To prepare a small batch of kefir buttermilk, put the kefir grains in a cheesecloth bag. A half pound of grains will be enough to coagulate two gallons of milk in thirty-six to forty-eight hours at 68° to 72° F.

Place the milk in a porcelain, glass-lined or granite-iron container. Suspend the bag of grains near the surface of the milk. Incubate the milk at 68° to 72° F. until it is well set up, or until it shows an acidity of about 1 percent lactic acid. Then lift out the bag of grains, scrape off the adhering cream, and wash the bag thoroughly in cold, running water to remove all the sliminess from the outside of the bag, and the fermented milk from within. After squeezing the bag to remove the excess water, place it in a new supply of milk, and continue as before.

After the grains have been removed, stir the fermented milk slightly to incorporate all of the surface cream. Then cool it to 60° F. or lower. Then, using an eggbeater or other slow-speed type device, whip the mixture to break the curd. After the curd is broken, store the milk in bottles or in its original container at a low temperature until it is used.

Homemade kefir cheese: Pour cultured kefir (without the grains) into a pot, and heat very gently until the entire surface is covered with foam, just below the boiling point. Turn off the heat, and allow the heat to permeate the entire mixture for a few seconds. Then pour into another container

for cooling. Cover, and allow to rest overnight. In the morning, strain through a cheesecloth bag. Kefir cheese is thick, and has large curds. To modify its bland flavor, a little grated roquefort or blue cheese, or other strong-flavored cheese, can be blended with it.

Homemade kefir from freeze-dried grains: Sterilize all equipment. Heat a quart of fresh, clean milk to a near boil. Remove the pot from the heat, and cool the milk to 110°F. Stir in a teaspoonful of freeze-dried kefir grains, and blend thoroughly. Pour this mixture to fill a sterilized, warm container, cover, and place in a warm place, such as an oven at 100° F. Allow the container to remain undisturbed for twelve hours, while the kefir is incubating. Test the kefir with a toothpick to learn whether it has solidified. The toothpick, when inserted, should stand upright without support. If the test fails, incubate the kefir one to three hours longer. When the incubation is complete, refrigerate the kefir.

Kefir summer cooler: Blend together in an electric blender a quart of homemade kefir, the juice of two oranges and two tablespoons of honey. Pour into glasses, chill, and top with a light dusting of nutmeg. Serves four to six.

Kefir shake: Blend together in an electric blender a quart of homemade kefir, a half cup of wheat germ, and two tablespoons of honey. Pour into glasses. Serves four to six.

Kefir summer soup: Blend together in an electric blender a quart of homemade kefir, one cup of raw, diced cucumber, one cup of watercress, and a sprig of fresh parsley. Chill and serve. Serves six.

Kefir sherbet: Blend together in an electric blender 1½ cups of homemade kefir, ¾ cup unsweetened, pureed fruit, 4 tablespoons honey, and 1 teaspoon of pure vanilla extract. Pour into sherbet glasses, and refrigerate. Serve, garnished with unsweetened coconut shreds. Serves four to six.

Quickie kefir dessert: Fold one cup of kefir into one cup of applesauce, and add ¼ teaspoon of pure almond extract. Pour into sherbet glasses, and refrigerate. Serve, garnished with ground walnuts. Serves four to six.

Baked apples with kefir: Wash and core raw apples. Arrange them in a baking dish with a small amount of water in the bottom. Fill the core cavities with raisins and almonds. Bake in a moderate oven for a half hour, and serve hot, with cold kefir drizzled over the apples.

Kefir fruit salad dressing: Blend together in an electric blender one cup of homemade kefir, one tablespoon of honey, two tablespoons of unsweetened orange juice and two tablespoons of unsweetened pineapple juice. This dressing is good over fruit salad, and also over cole slaw. Makes 1½ cups.

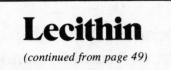

Lecithin

(continued from page 49)

the American Lecithin Company, as follows:

"Cholesterol in the bloodstream does not in itself cause atherosclerosis. It is not until it has been precipitated out of the bloodstream upon the arterial surface, whether from chylemicrons or from giant molecules, that it can act to produce characteristic atheromatic lesions. This precipitation is due to disturbance of the delicate balance necessary for the maintenance of colloidal stability. Fat and cholesterol *per se* are insoluble in water and equally in blood plasma. A lipid particle containing fat or cholesterol is maintained in colloidal dispersion in the plasma by means of stabilizing, solubilizing, or emulsifying agents.

"In order to be an effective stabilizing or solubilizing agent, a compound must have both fat-soluble and water-soluble groups. The simple explanation usually given for this type of emulsification is that the fat-soluble groups are anchored in the fatty substrate of the particle with the water-soluble polar groups extending out into the aqueous medium. Soy lecithin has been well known for many years to be a very effective emulsifying and solubilizing agent for lipids.

"In the bloodstream, also, it has been believed for many years that lecithin and other phospholipids act in a similar manner, along with other emulsifying or hydrotropic agents. These include the proteins, and to a lesser extent, cholesterol esters.

"It is not difficult to believe that the concentration of lecithin and other phospholipids or, more appropriately, the ratio of phospholipid: cholesterol or phospholipid: total lipid (cholesterol plus fat) may be significant in maintaining stable colloidal dispersion.

"Thus, for example, with a given physical stress, such as vibration, an unstable lipid dispersion may be precipitated, while a relatively more highly solubilized or stable dispersion will not be precipitated.

"In coronary thrombosis both phospholipids and cholesterol increase in the patient but cholesterol rises at a more rapid rate than the phospholipids. As the phospholipids (in lecithin) are believed to be the controlling factor in keeping the cholesterol dissolved in the blood, the importance of influencing the disturbed balance is stressed. It can be achieved by either reducing cholesterol without lowering the phospholipid content of the blood or, in reverse, elevation of phospholipids and maintenance of the cholesterol at a constant level."

Note: As stated earlier, egg yolks have high levels of cholesterol and also lecithin. But the ratio is such that the liberation of cholesterol is favored. Egg lecithin is also high in *saturated* fatty acids. This makes egg lecithin a less desirable source of helping to wash away body cholesterol.

The phosphatides of soybeans contain lecithin which is a prime source of *unsaturated* fatty acids, making this lecithin source much more desirable.

Soybeans as well as soybean oil and soybean foods are regarded as the best source of lecithin. Soybean oil is reportedly highest in the essential fatty acids and lecithin, all of which are helpful in maintaining better heart health. In various reported tests, soy lecithin (whether in the form of oil or granules) was more effective than other forms of lecithin in helping to lower the blood cholesterol levels.

Soy lecithin is a prime source of phosphatides as well as *sitosterols,* substances which have been found to lower the blood cholesterol levels. (From sitosterol is prepared the male sex hormone, testosterone, which has the action of promoting growth and normal functioning of the accessory male sex organs and the development of secondary male sex characteristics.)

Soybean sterols are also used for preparing cortisone, an adrenal cortex hormone that helps control and heal problems of arthritis distress. In brief, soy lecithin contains three heart-helping substances: (1) essential fatty acids, (2) lecithin, (3) sitosterol, along with other needed sterols. Most important, health stores sell soy lecithin as a *natural* heart and health saver!

The noted Lester M. Morrison, M.D., author of *The Low Fat Way to Health and Longer Life,* cites many medical reports telling of the use of this all-natural lecithin as a means of helping to combat problems of cholesterol. Dr. Morrison feels that with a doctor-supervised program, lecithin is able to dissolve and remove atherosclerotic plaques from the bloodstream.

"In the course of our research," says Dr. Morrison, "we have found that lecithin apparently has the ability to increase the cholesterol esterases in the human bloodstream. These esterases are enzymes, or activators, that aid in the metabolizing of fats."

Furthermore, Dr. Morrison tells us that patients who followed the oil-free, soybean lecithin program experienced a sense of well-being. "They said they had more vitality, did not grow tired so quickly as they had formerly, and were in better health than before." He emphasizes that "lecithin is one of our most powerful weapons against disease. It is an especially valuable bulwark against development of 'hardening of the arteries' and all the complications of heart, brain and kidney that follow."

Dr. Lester M. Morrison also suggests the use of doctor-supervised vitamin and food supplementation. He offers a five-step program for his patients:

1. Include daily, as a food supplement at breakfast, two to four tablespoonfuls of lecithin extracted from soy beans.
2. Add to your diet each day B-complex vitamins in the most potent form. Avoid the cheaper preparations which provide only small and ineffectual quantities of the vitamins, and have little or no effect on your body. Your doctor or druggist can advise you which brands provide potent quantities of the vitamins.
3. Also add to your daily diet at least 25,000 units of vitamin A and 150 milligrams of vitamin C.
4. Take two tablespoonfuls of soybean oil, corn oil or safflower oil daily to provide the essential fatty acids necessary to proper nutrition. The oil may be used as a salad dressing, taken with tomato or fruit juice, or in any way you prefer.
5. Include in your diet two to four tablespoons of whole wheat germ each day. This may be eaten as a breakfast cereal with fruit, or sprinkled in your salad.

Dr. Morrison tells of a forty-five year old housewife who had fat plaques of yellowish hue on her skin because of fatty deposits. After she took lecithin as the doctor prescribed, the patches disappeared and soon vanished entirely. It is known that the same "washing" of fat occurred within her arteries.

Dr. Morrison also tells of a forty-five year old baker who was troubled by chest pain (known as angina, caused by an interference with the blood supply to the heart muscle). The man could not work. When examined, the doctor noted he had yellowish-brown plaques under his eyes. He also had a cholesterol level that was "high in the abnormal range." The doctor prescribed a low-cholesterol and low-fat diet for the man. Then he gave him prescribed amounts of lecithin and high-potency vitamins. Within a few months, his chest pains were gone. His cholesterol level was lowered appreciably. His fatty plaques (xanthalasma)

(continued on page 256)

Lecithin

(continued from page 255)

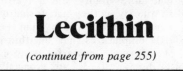

vanished from his face. Thanks to the doctor-prescribed low-cholesterol and low-fat diet, and the taking of lecithin and vitamins, this forty-five year old baker enjoyed better heart health . . . the natural way!

Writing in *Let's Eat Right to Keep Fit*, nutritionist-author Adelle Davis gives us a hopeful picture of the healing power of lecithin:

"Another cousin of the fat family, lecithin is supplied by all natural oils . . . Lecithin is an excellent source of the two B vitamins choline and inositol; if health is to be maintained, the more fat eaten, the larger must be the intake of these two vitamins. This substance can be made in the intestinal wall provided choline, inositol and essential fatty acids are supplied.

"Lecithin appears to be a homogenizing agent, capable of breaking fat and probably cholesterol into tiny particles which can pass readily into the tissues. There is evidence that coronary occlusion is associated with deficiences of linoleic acid and the two B vitamins, choline and inositol, and perhaps with a lack of lecithin itself.

"Huge particles of cholesterol get stuck in the walls of the arteries; they might be homogenized into tiny particles if sufficient nutrients were available for the normal production of lecithin. When oils are refined or hydrogenated, lecithin is discarded."

Note: Again we see the importance of pure and unrefined and non-hydrogenated or pure oils, such as sold in many health food stores. These pure oils contain lecithin, the heart saving nutrient.

Adelle Davis further lauds lecithin in *Let's Get Well* by explaining how it aids in the transportation of fats; helps the cells to remove fats and cholesterol from the blood and to utilize them. This action further boosts the production of bile acids made from cholesterol, thereby reducing the amount in the blood.

"Lecithin is a powerful emulsifying agent and for this very reason is particularly important in preventing and correcting atherosclerosis. *Although blood is essentially water into which fats cannot dissolve, lecithin, if present in normal amounts, causes cholesterol and neutral fats to be broken into microscopic particles which can be held in suspension, pass*

readily through arterial walls, and be utilized by the tissues."

Soy lecithin reportedly is able to flow into the arteries of people troubled with atherosclerosis and is able to change blood fat particles from large to small size so that they may pass through the arterial walls.

Your physician will advise you how much to take for your individual case. In one situation (Dr. E. R. Diller in the *Journal of Nutrition,* Vol. 73, No. 14), four to six tablespoons of soy lecithin were given daily to people with heart trouble. No other dietary change was made. After three months of daily lecithin intake, their blood cholesterol readings dropped. In one case, a patient who had a 1012 count was able to have the reading dropped to a more healthful 186 milligrams of cholesterol in the bloodstream—thanks to lecithin!

Generally speaking, doctors administer about two tablespoons of soy lecithin daily and have reported it is helpful in controlling cholesterol and boosting better heart health.

If you want to include lecithin in your diet, the key word here is "natural." Select natural seeds and nuts, whole grain cereals, millet, natural brown rice, cold-pressed oils and unbleached soy flour. These products (sold at most health food stores) contain lecithin as placed there by Nature. But . . . hydrogenation, processing, heating, refining, bleaching, all tend to destroy lecithin. Therefore, you should use *natural* food sources of lecithin as listed above.

Health stores also sell cold-pressed soy oil as well as lecithin in the form of granules or tablets which may be taken as regularly as prescribed by your doctor for your individual case.

So go ahead and do your heart a favor—take lecithin! ☼

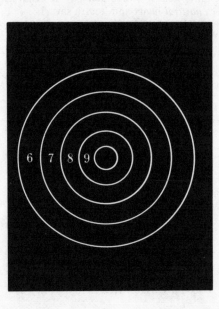

Piimä — Remarkable Culture from Nomad's Land

(continued from page 51)

acidophilus. Both are given by the nursing mother to her baby. The bifidus can now be purchased from your health food store, usually in a malted milk base (Eugalan Forte), sometimes in a liquid concentrate. The bifidus can be added to your piimä and cultured right along with it. This is an easy way to supply this vital substance and also be sure that it goes along its way in friendly and supportive company.

Bifidus Piimä

Place 1/2 teaspoon piimä in a pint, wide-mouth jar. Add 1/2 cup milk and mix well. Now add 2 tablespoons bifidus powder and gently stir and mix. Fill jar with milk and proceed as usual. Serve within a day or two and always use plain piimä for a starter.

Use no other substance or additions in making your piimä except the bifidus in the previous recipe.

Piimä Eggnog

1 cup piima yogurt
2 fertile eggs
1 teaspoon or more, food yeast
1 teaspoon vanilla
1 tablespoon honey, sorghum or molasses

Buzz in blender just long enough to mix.

Variations: Add one or more of the following:

1 tablespoon carob powder and
1/2 to 1 medium banana
1/2 cup raw fruit
1/2 cup thick fruit juice
1/3 cup of very sweet fruits such as dates

Berry Shake

2 cups piimä yogurt
1 cup frozen berries (unsweetened)
1 teaspoon honey (or to taste)

Place in blender and buzz until thick and creamy. Serve topped with a sprinkle of nutmeg.

Party Bavarian

2 tablespoons gelatin
1/2 cup cold water or juice
4 eggs, separated
2 cups strawberries or fresh fruit
2 to 4 tablespoons honey (depending upon sweetness of the fruit)
2 tablespoons grated lemon peel
2 tablespoons lemon juice
2 cups piimä cream

Dissolve gelatin in water. Melt over hot water or low heat, stirring constantly. Place egg yolks in blender bowl and whites in a bowl to be beaten stiff. Add to the blender bowl the strawberries, honey, lemon peel and juice. Add melted gelatin with blender on low. Place in refrigerator while beating egg whites until stiff. Stir gelatin mixture into the piimä cream and fold in beaten egg whites. Turn into large mold or individual serving dishes and chill. Garnish with fresh berries and mint leaves.

To make a pie of the above desserts, make a crust of
1/3 cup freshly ground almonds (or Malted Almonds)
1/3 cup freshly ground sesame seeds
1/3 cup freshly ground sunflower seeds
1/3 cup soft butter
1/2 teaspoon cinnamon
1/2 teaspoon nutmeg

Mix in bowl until crumbly, then pat into pie pan. If your filling has gelatin in it you may, if you wish, omit the butter as the gelatin will firm the crust.

Cheese Cake

Line a spring form pan with one half the pie crust mix above, without butter if desired. Reserve the other half for topping.
2 teaspoons gelatin (if you use yogurt you will need 1 tablespoon)
1/4 cup water or pineapple or apple juice
2 cups cottage cheese (or piimä yogurt)
2 cups piimä cream
4 eggs (fertile, if possible)
1/4 teaspoon sea salt
1-1/2 tablespoon vanilla
Grated rind of 1 lemon
1 tablespoon lemon juice

Dissolve gelatin in water or juice and melt over low heat or hot water, stirring constantly.

Place in blender cottage cheese (or yogurt), piimä cream, eggs, salt, vanilla, and lemon juice and rind. Blend until smooth and turn to low. Slowly add melted gelatin (this will fill a 5 cup blender). If your blender is smaller, make in two parts.

Pour this mix into spring form pan and crumble remainder of the pie crust mixture on top. Chill until firm. This makes a nice birthday cake decorated with strawberries or use the berries as birthday candle holders on the cake. Serves 8-12.

Vegetable Sprout Salad Mold
1 tablespoon gelatin
1/2 cup cold water
1-1/4 cups broth or water

juice of 1 lemon
1/2 teaspoon grated lemon rind
1/2 teaspoon herbed seasoning salt

Dissolve the gelatin in the cold water in a small saucepan, then heat over low heat, stirring constantly until gelatin is melted. In a 3 quart bowl mix the broth, lemon juice and rind and the seasoning salt. Add the melted gelatin and stir gently. Chill while preparing vegetables.
1/2 cup mung bean sprouts, chopped
1/2 cup wheat sprouts
1/2 cup celery, chopped
1/2 cup cabbage, chopped
1/2 cup carrots, shredded
1 tablespoon chives, finely snipped
1 tablespoon parsley, chopped

Stir into the gelatin mixture. Pour into individual molds or tea cups. Chill until firm. Serve on mounds of alfalfa sprouts and top with piimä yogurt, seasoned with a dash of curry powder and food yeast.

To use piimä in your own favorite ice cream recipe use piimä milk or piima cream as a direct substitution for the plain milk or cream called for in your recipe. You will find you can make this change in almost any recipe you now cherish.

Rosy Coconut Slaw
1 cup cabbage, shredded
1/2 medium raw beet, shredded
1/4 cup coconut, freshly shredded
Frozen pineapple juice to moisten
Piimä cream or milk
Toss gently until just moistened. Top with a spoonful of cream or yogurt.

Yogurt Sundae

Place a large scoop of yogurt in a dessert dish. Top with honey, molasses or thick fruit puree. Or mix crushed juice-packed pineapple with berries, peaches, pears, apples, or any fruit in season. Top with chopped nuts or seeds.

Other uses for piimä

Use cream or yogurt to top a zesty enchilada or baked potato.

Add to mashed avocado to make a creamy dressing.

Try just plain cooked beans with a spoonful of thick piimä cream or yogurt on top.

Add, at the last moment, to any Stroganoff dish.

Serve over any lightly steamed vegetable as a luscious natural sauce.

Add to mayonnaise or French dressing for a creamy variation.

Moisten a variety of chopped fresh fruit with a little frozen pineapple juice, then top with a dollop of yogurt or piimä cream. ☼

Garlic:
(continued from page 53)

In the *Review of Gastroenterology* for January-February, 1944, H. Barowsky and L.J. Boyd, both doctors, tell of using garlic on fifty patients who suffered various gastro-intestinal disorders. Flatulence was relieved in a vast majority of the cases, and relief from nausea, vomiting, gas, abdominal distention and after-meal discomfort was "sufficiently regular and marked." In the same review for May, 1949, F. Damran and E. Ferguson, report that cases of gas and nervous dyspepsia were improved by garlic, and that the garlic had a sedative action on the stomach and in the intestines: belching, nausea, and after-meal discomfort were all relieved.

From the German *Pharmaceutical Magazine* (February 1, 1950), we are told that patients having garlic treatments speak of a feeling of well-being and increased vitality after a short time:

This possibly may result from the ability of garlic to reduce blood pressure as well as to effect dilation of the blood vessels and detoxification of the entire organism. Patients also reported themselves freed from apprehensions and neuroses . . . It tends to detoxify the entire organism with special influence upon the heart, blood vessels and blood pressure, especially in the aged. This attribute may be responsible for its successful use on excessive tobacco users in chronic nicotine poisoning.

In 1965 two Germans, Dorfler and Roselt, had this to say about garlic and its general effect on indigestion and other disorders:

The use and healing properties of garlic are manifold. The volatile oil exercises a fine influence on the digestive system; smaller doses activate the peristalsis, larger ones, however, have a calming effect on it. Through the activation of the secretion in the alimentary canal appetite is increased. Since the volatile oil effectively eliminates intestinal parasites, boiled garlic water or freshly squeezed garlic juice are used in the fight against maggots. Boiled garlic water or fresh juice are taken internally as an enema, and garlic is further used in cases of arteriosclerosis.

Arteriosclerosis

Recent medical studies support the claim that garlic actually affects the factors responsible for arteriosclerosis or hardening of the arteries: Hyperlipemia (excess blood cholesterol levels) and hyperglycemia (high blood-sugar levels associated with diabetes). In a December 29, 1973 issue of the prestigious British medical journal, *The Lancet*, letters from two cardiologists, Drs. Bordi and Bansal, of the Department of Medicine, R.N.T. Med-

(continued on page 258)

Garlic

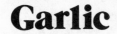

(continued from page 257)

ical College, Udaipur, India, stated that the addition of garlic to the diets of test subjects actually controlled the amount of cholesterol in the blood. These tests were conducted on five subjects with garlic juice, and on another five subjects using the oil extract of the juice. All subjects were in good health, and the garlic juice and oil extract produced similar results.

THE TESTS

The doctors added to the regular meals of their subjects 100 grams or 1/4 pound of butter. Three hours later, the subjects averaged a blood cholesterol of 237.4 milligrams percent, which was up from a fasting level before the meal of 221.4. When the juice or oil from 50 grams of garlic was added to an identical meal with the same amount of butter, the blood cholesterol level three hours later was only 212.7 milligrams percent, which was *down* from a fasting level of 228.7 before the meal.

The addition of butter without garlic also brought the level of plasmafibrinogen (the precursor of fibrin which is involved in the blood clotting mechanism) to 320.9 up from a fasting level of 249.8. When garlic was added the level was 256.4 which, again, was down from a fasting level of 281.3. These are both significant drops especially in view of the fact that the garlic brought the cholesterol and fibrinogen levels down below the normal levels before the addition of the fat. Bordi and Bansal concluded that:

> It is obvious that garlic has a very significant protective action against hyperlipemia and blood coagulation changes, which are normal after fat ingestion.

In discussing the other drugs on the market which control these blood factors — drugs which are either very expensive or transient in effect — these researchers added finally that:

> Clinically, garlic could avoid most of these drawbacks and could be recommended for long-term use without danger of toxicity. It would be particularly useful in preventing alimentary hyperlipemia *in persons who do not have manifest signs of arteriosclerosis but are predisposed on account of diabetes, hypertension, family history of stroke and heart-disease.* (Italics mine.) *(The Lancet,* Dec. 29, 1973, pp. 1491-2)

Well, that means *me,* and millions of other Americans. If there was ever a doubt in my mind about why I am taking a lot of garlic in my diet, this statement by Bordi and Bansal erases it.

Another letter in the same *Lancet* came from three doctors; Jain, Vyas, and Mahatma, also from the R.N.T. Medical College. They showed that garlic is effective in controlling blood-sugar levels. Garlic's hypoglycemic action, although a little slower than tolbutamide, an oral drug for diabetics, was equally effective (and more effective than onion). Their tests were conducted with four groups of rabbits: each group was given glucose plus either garlic, onion, tolbutamide, and in the case of the control group, distilled water.

Heart Disease in Garlic-Eating Cultures

Harald J. Taub, in his article "Garlic Oil for Healthier Arteries" (*Prevention,* April, 1974), reviews these statistics and concludes that garlic in the diet is indeed a contributing factor in the lower incidence of arteriosclerosis and heart attack among the garlic consuming people of Italy, and especially Spain. Taub cites the fact that in the U.S., one in three deaths is caused by heart disease. In Spain only one in seventeen are due to heart disease. If one looks at the rate of heart disease deaths per 100,000 population, the variation between garlic-eating and garlic-avoiding nations is phenomenal:

U.S.A.	319.5 (per 100,000)
Italy	208.9
Spain	71.3

These statistics were acquired by Taub from the United Nations Demographic Yearbook for 1966.

These kinds of statistics have been pointed to before in making claims for garlic. Other garlic eating cultures are also said to have low incidence of heart disease — Korea, Slavic countries, certain areas of Russia, the south of France. But these statistics alone do not prove that garlic is the sole factor responsible for the low incidence of heart disease in these countries. If one examined Spain, Italy and the U.S. from the point of view of "stress," or the level of technological development, one could conclude that the lower incidence in heart disease is due to a lower level of stress and competition within the culture. Stress is being recognized as an important contributor to degenerative disease in highly developed countries. America must rank as the number one stress culture.

But with the evidence supplied by Bordi and Bansal, and others, for the direct effect of garlic on blood cholesterol and glucose levels, it becomes more likely that garlic in the diet *is* a significant factor in the control of heart disease and heart attack. ☼

What Makes People Sick?

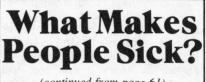

(continued from page 61)

While the germ theory contributed handsomely to our understanding of disease, the science of diet and nutrition, as well as hormones, suffered considerable neglect. Even in the nineteenth century, much information was available which showed that cretinism and goiter (reflections of low thyroid state) were in some manner related to iodine intake. Regrettably, because of the fashionableness of the germ theory, most scientific authorities at that time attributed hypothyroidism to exogenous toxins (poisons produced by germs). It was this same philosophy that slowed down progress with beri-beri.

This history of nutrition may be grouped into three significant eras. The first, the *naturalistic* age blossomed from about 400 B.C. to 1750 A.D. Its major contribution is essential to life. The *chemicoanalytic era* (from 1750 to 1900) dissected the prevailing unity into four parts and put into perspective the biologic importance of fat, protein, carbohydrates and minerals. Thus, the major foodstuffs were recognized. Finally, the *biological period,* extending from 1900 to the present, brought attention to the minute fractions, the vitamins and the trace minerals. Perhaps even more important, the emphasis had shifted from the relationship of *specific* nutrients to *specific* disease entities (e.g., scurvy, pellagra, beri-beri) to the *nonspecific* role of the interplay of nutrients in diseases heretofore regarded as nonnutritional in origin.

Today, much data, indeed, is appearing in scientific literature regarding the role of diet and nutrition in infertility, obstetrical complications, congenital defects, mental retardation, psychologic imbalance, oral disease, heart ailments and cancer.

The evidence is in, and has been for a long time, that numerous factors enter into the cause of a particular disease, even in the case of an acute infectious problem. Increasing interest is being generated in the soil (body) versus the seed (germ). The *science* of medicine, if not the *practice* of medicine, now knows some of the ingredients of the host state. Included in this group is diet. Precisely the role played by diet depends upon recognition of the fact that *undernutrition* and *malnutrition* are distinct but interdependent entities. In other words, the *importance* of diet is clear. ☼

cults from practicing less harmful palliations. How many reputable physicians have the honesty of Sir James Mackenzie?

In spite of Mackenzie's high and worthy ambitions, he could not get away from the profession's stereotype thinking. The early symptoms of disease he declared held the secret of their cause, and he believed an intense study of them would give the facts. But functional derangements are of the same nature and from the same universal cause that ends in all organic so-called diseases. All so-called diseases are, from beginning to end, the same evolutionary process.

The study of pathology — the study of disease — has engaged the best minds in the profession always, and it surely appears that the last word must have been spoken on the subject; but the great Englishman believed, as all research workers believe, that a more intense and minute study of the early symptoms of disease will reveal the cause. There is, however, one great reason why it cannot, and that is that all symptom-complexes — diseases — from their initiation to their ending, are effects, and the most intense study of any phase or stage of their progress will not throw any light on the cause.

Cause is constant, ever present, and always the same. Only effects, and the object on which cause acts, change, and the change is most inconstant. To illustrate: A catarrh of the stomach presents first irritation, then inflammation, then ulceration, and finally induration and cancer. Not all cases run true to form; only a small percentage evolve to ulcer, and fewer still reach the cancer stage. More exit by way of acute food-poisoning or acute indigestion than by chronic diseases.

In the early stages of this evolution there are all kinds of discomforts: more or less attacks of indigestion, frequent attacks of gastritis — sick stomach and vomiting. No two cases are alike. Nervous people s[...] and some present all kinds [...] symptoms — insomnia, head[...] Women have painful menstr[...] hysterical symptoms — [...] morose and others have ep[...] the more chronic symptom[...] those of the lymphatic tempe[...] not suffer so much. As th[...] progresses, a few become p[...]

develop pernicious anemia, due to gastric or intestinal ulceration and putrid protein infection; in others the first appearance of ulcer is manifested by a severe hemorrhage; others have a cachexia and a retention of food in the stomach, which is vomited every two or three days, caused by a partial closing of the pylorus. These are usually malignant cases.

To look upon any of these symptom-complexes as a distinct disease, requiring a distinct treatment, is to fall into the diagnostic maze that now bewilders the profession and renders treatment chaotic.

It should be known to all discerning physicians that the earliest stage of organic disease is purely functional, evanescent, and never autogenerated so far as the affected organ is concerned, but is invariably due to an extraneous irritation (stimulation, if you please), augmented by Toxemia. When the irritation is not continuous, a toxin is eliminated as fast as developed, to the toleration point, normal functioning is resumed between the intervals of irritation and toxin excess.

For example: a simple coryza (running at the nose — cold in the head), gastritis or colonitis. At first these colds, catarrhs, or inflammations are periodic and functional; but, as the exciting cause or causes — local irritation and Toxemia — become more intense and continuous, the mucous membranes of these organs take on organic changes, which are given various names, such as irritation, inflammation, ulceration, and cancer. The pathology (organic change) may be studied until doomsday without throwing any light on the cause; for from the first irritation to the extreme ending — cachexia — which may be given the blanket term of tuberculosis, syphilis, or cancer, the whole pathologic panorama is one continuous evolution of intensifying effects.

Germs and other so-called causes may be discovered in the course of pathological development, but they are accidental, coincidental, or at most auxiliary — or, to use the vernacular of law, *obiter dicta*.

The proper way to study disease is to study health and every influence favorable or not to its continuance. Disease is perverted health. Any influence that lowers nerve-energy becomes disease-producing. Disease cannot be its own cause; neither can it be its own cure, and certainly not its own prevention.

After years of wandering in the jungle of medical diagnosis — the usual guesswork of cause and effect, and the worse-than-guesswork of treat-

ment, and becoming more confounded all the time — I resolved either to quit the profession or to find the cause of disease. To do this, it was necessary to exile myself from doctors and medical conventions; for I could not think for myself while listening to the babblings of babeldom. I took the advice found in Matt. 6:6. According to prevailing opinion, unless a doctor spends much time in medical societies and in the society of other doctors, takes postgraduate work, travels, etc., he cannot keep abreast of advancement.

This opinion would be true if the sciences of medicine were fitted to a truthful etiology (efficient cause) of disease. But, since they are founded on no cause, or at most speculative and spectacular causes, as unstable as the sands of the sea, the doctor who cannot brook the bewilderment of vacillation is compelled to hide away from the voices of mistaken pedants and knowing blatherskites until stabilized. By that time ostracism will have overtaken him, and his fate, metaphorically speaking, will be that of the son of Zacharias.

An honest search after truth too often, if not always, leads to the rack, stake, cross, or the blessed privilege of recanting; but the victim, by this time, decides as did Jesus: "Not My will, but Thine, be done;" or, as Patrick Henry declared: "Give me liberty or give me death!" The dying words of another great Irishman is the wish, no doubt, of every lover of freedom and truth:

That no man write my epitaph; for, as no man who knows my motives dares now vindicate them, let not prejudice or ignorance asperse them. Let them and me rest in peace, and my tomb remain uninscribed, and my memory in oblivion, until other times and other men can do justice to my character. When my country takes her place among the nations of the earth, then, and not until then, let my epitaph be written. (Emmet.)

The truth is larger than any man, and until it is established, the memory of its advocate is not important. In the last analysis, is not the truth the only immortality? Man is an incident. If he discovers a truth, it benefits all who accept it. Truth too often must pray to be delivered from its friends.

I must acknowledge that I have not been very courteous to indifferent convention; and the truth I have discovered has suffered thereby. It has always appeared to me that the attention of fallacy-mongers cannot be attracted except by the use of a club or shillalah; and possibly my style of presenting my facts has caused too great a shock, and the desired effect has been lost in the reaction.

(continued on page 260)

Toxemia, the One Disease Everyone Has

(continued from page 259)

That I have discovered the true cause of disease cannot be successfully disputed. This being true, my earnestness in presenting this great truth is justifiable.

When I think back over my life, and remember the struggle I had with myself in supplanting my old beliefs with the new — the thousands of times I have suspected my own sanity — I then cannot be surprised at the opposition I have met and am meeting.

My discovery of the truth that Toxemia is the cause of all so-called diseases came about slowly, step by step, with many dangerous skids.

At first I believed that enervation must be the general cause of disease; then I decided that simple enervation is not disease, that disease must be due to poison, and that poison, to be the general cause of disease, must be autogenerated; and if disease is due to autogenerated poison, what is the cause of that autogeneration? I dallied long in endeavoring to trace disease back to poison taken into the system, such as food eaten after putrescence had begun, or from poisoning due to the development of putrescence after ingestion. In time I decided that poisoning per se is not disease. I observed where poisoning did not kill; some cases reacted and were soon in full health, while others remained in a state of semi-invalidism. I found the same thing true of injuries and mental shock. It took a long time to develop the thought that a poisoned or injured body, when not overwhelmed by Toxemia, would speedily return to the normal; and when it did not, there was a sick habit — a derangement of some kind — that required some such contingency to bring it within sense-perception.

To illustrate: An injury to a joint is often complicated with rheumatism; the rheumatism previous to the injury was potentially in the blood.

Just what change had taken place in the organism which, under stress of injury or shock of any kind, would cause a reaction with fever, I could not understand until the Toxemic Theory suggested itself to my mind, after which the cause of disease unfolded before me in an easy and natural man-ner. And now the theory is a proved fact.

After years of perplexing thought and "watchful waiting," I learned that all disease, of whatever nature, was of slow development; that without systemic preparation even so-called acute systemic disease could not manifest.

In a few words: Without Toxemia there can be no disease. I knew that the waste-product of metabolism was toxic, and that the only reason why we were not poisoned by it was because it was removed from the organism as fast as produced. Then I decided that the toxin was retained in the blood, when there was a checking of elimination. Then the cause of the checking had to be determined. In time I thought out the cause. I knew that, when we had a normal nerve-energy, organic functioning was normal. Then came the thought that enervation caused a checking of elimination. Eureka! The cause of all so-called disease is found! Enervation checks elimination of the waste-products of metabolism. Retention of metabolic toxin — the first and only cause of disease!

Those who would be freed from the bondage of medical superstition should consider this theory of Toxemia. ☼

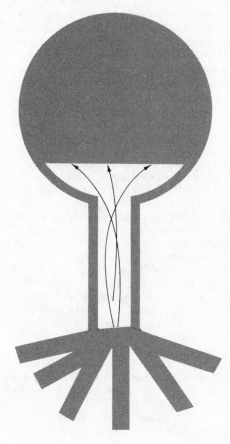

Baby's First Years

(continued from page 65)

If pasteurized milk is all that is available, try to get the product "Eugalan," a cultured powder made from mothers' milk. This contains millions of the friendly *lacto-bacillus bifidus* which aid in digesting and assimilating pasteurized milk. Look for it in your health food store. The powder is easily mixed by pouring 4 oz. of lukewarm water into a jar. Add 3 measuring spoons of the powder, cap the jar and shake. The resulting liquid can be kept in the refrigerator. Add 1 teaspoonful or more to each bottle of milk you prepare for your baby. Your doctor will help you decide how much water, molasses, brewer's yeast and other supplements if any, to add to the bottle also.

If baby must be fed from a bottle, hold him in your arms while he is eating. Yes, I know you are busy; but you need a moment to rest and relax, and your baby needs most urgently the contact of your warm and loving arms to let him know he is safe with you and that you love him.

La Leche League, a nursing mothers organization whose whole sole purpose is to aid nursing mothers and all mothers everywhere, will be happy to offer helpful advice and suggestions. To learn more of La Leche League, write to 9616 Minneapolis Ave., Franklin Park, Illinois 60131, for brochures and information on the group nearest you. Or call your local childbirth education society. Mothercraft classes are sometimes taught at the YWCA, and the teachers will know of local La Leche Leagues. Look for their very fine book —*The Womanly Art of Breastfeeding* — at your local library or bookstore. It can also be ordered by mail from La Leche League, address above.

How Long to Nurse: One week is better than none. One month is better than one week. Three months is still better. Ideally, the infant thrives best if nursed from one year to eighteen months, or even two years if possible.

If the little one is completely breastfed, with no solids or supplements before the age of six months, the well nourished mother will have an ample milk supply.

One wise doctor in our town tells anxious young mothers who are asking about supplementary foods for their babies, "Fine, fine — whatever you think he needs, *you* take it and he will get it."

Adequate sleep as well as good nutrition is necessary for the manufacture of vitamin B in your body. This controls milk production. Do not be too quick to supplement if your milk supply lessens temporarily. Listening to your hungry baby cry is the most effective milk production stimulant known.

The child who is *not* nursed may need a natural vitamin-mineral supplement. Try to find one prepared from organically grown cereal grass juices or other plants.

When mother is ill (unless the illness has directly involved the mammary glands), do not deprive your baby of the antibodies in your milk at a time when he needs them most. He will be exposed to air-borne bacteria and virus in the air, not from your milk. You can wear a mask while you are nursing if you wish.

When to Nurse: Nurse the young infant when he cries to be fed and *only* when he cries to be fed. Between meals he should sleep or play as long as he wishes. Let him take as much milk as he wants but do not urge him to take one more swallow than he wants. If the mother's supply of milk is ample, the baby should be able to drink his fill in ten to twenty minutes. This type of demand feeding is based upon the belief that a normal healthy child will take enough food to supply his own nutritional needs. Life for both the mother and baby is more comfortable than with a rigid schedule. Mother is able to provide comfort whenever the child cries and he soon learns that he is in the hands of someone who loves him.

One young woman, wise in the art of "mothering," told me that when she takes her baby up for his feeding at night or in the early morning hours, she places in the baby's bed a heating pad turned on medium heat. After the leisurely feeding, she removes the pad and places him back in a warm and cosy bed.

Take It Easy: When you feed the baby, put your feet up and relax. Some mothers, especially for the first few weeks, will enjoy lying down to nurse the little one.

Take a nap each afternoon when the baby naps. Try to rest *before* you get tired.

If possible, hire a helper. If you can't, get your relatives to help. They will be anxious to get acquainted with the new baby anyway. Try to drink lots of liquids and eat many good fresh foods each day.

Don't try to reduce at this time, for if you have gained a few pounds they will gradually slip away as the months go by.

Cuddle your baby. Love and enjoy him. Housework will wait but babies grow up faster than you would ever believe.

So many young mothers have told me that the use of brewer's yeast in their diet has helped them to produce an ample quantity of high quality milk, that I must mention it here. Adelle Davis gives detailed instructions for the use of this and other supplements in her fine book, "Let's Have Healthy Children" now off the press in a revised form. Many libraries have a copy that you may borrow.

Minor Illnesses

Any new food in the mother's diet should be taken in moderation at first. If some food eaten by the mother gives the baby a loose bowel, one teaspoon scraped raw apple may be fed him. Carob powder is helpful also. One teaspoonful may be mixed with ¼ cup warm water and ¼ teaspoon raw honey and fed in a bottle, or from a spoon. Acidophilus concentrate (1 teaspoonful) added to water or juice, is often of benefit. This concentrate may be found in your health food store. If the diarrhea is severe, stop all food but the acidophilus and water and call your doctor at once.

If a mild sore throat develops in mother or baby, raw pineapple juice, (1 to 3 tablespoonful) taken every hour during waking hours will often digest the troublesome virus and eliminate the need for harmful drugs or antibiotics.

It is important to know that the chief cause of infant indigestion is toxic bile from the liver of the child. During the first three years of life, this green-colored bile is thrown into the baby's bowel for elimination. Even mother's milk may form rubbery curds at such times. When this occurs limit the baby's food to mineral-rich water or to fruit and vegetable juices greatly diluted with the mineral water. Continue for as long as necessary for the baby's comfort. If using cow's or goat's milk, dilute with half mineral water for a day or two. Of course, if the parents are in radiant health at the time of conception, the child will not be born with a load of toxins in the liver and gas and indigestion in the baby — and worry and loss of sleep for the mother — will be avoided.

Colic: New findings indicate that most colic may be avoided if the feet of the tiny baby are kept warm and comfortable. The many nerve endings in the bottom of the infant's feet are very sensitive to changes in temperature. Warm booties, soft warm socks, or an extra little blanket will keep the child's feet warm and colic at a minimum.

Constipation: Babies who are nursed will rarely be troubled with constipation but if this should occur (or if the child is not being nursed), Dr. Kurt Donsbach has this suggestion: "Equal parts butter and raw honey or safflower oil and honey is a fine natural laxative for the infant. One half to one teaspoonful as needed. This tastes good, has no irritants and causes no griping."

Baby's First Food

Minimum equipment: A stainless steel food grater, cheesecloth or nylon net and a food grinder. A blender and a juicer will be very helpful also.

From two to four months, your nursing infant will need little, if any, other food. If you wish, you may offer him mineral-rich water in a bottle from time to time, but don't expect him to be very excited about anything in a bottle. If you can obtain organically grown oranges, you may offer him the strained juice (about ¼ teaspoon) from the tip of a teaspoon or mixed with water in a bottle, at about four months. If safe oranges are not available, sweet red peppers may be chopped and soaked, and the baby fed a tiny bit of the soaking water, strained.

Sometime between four and six months, you may wish to add codliver oil to your baby's diet: ¼ teaspoon to begin, gradually increasing the amount to ½ teaspoonful by the time the infant is about eight months old.

If your child indicates that he is beginning to need additional food (by a suddenly increased demand for nursing that continues for several days) it is time to introduce him to solid food. Usually this occurs between five and six months of age.

For the first few weeks, offer the new food midway between nursings, or after nursing, before he gets too hungry to be in the mood for something new. When a new food has been introduced, do not start another in less than five days. In this way, if the baby develops a sore bottom or other indications that he is not handling that particular food well, you can feed less or eliminate it for two or three days. Once a food has been started, however, it should not be omitted from the diet for any length of time, but a small portion fed at least once or twice a week; otherwise, it is possible for him to have an allergic reaction to his food when it is offered later.

The first feedings of solid food are usually easier if you hold your little one on your lap, in much the same familiar nursing position. If you let his head tilt back a little as you introduce each new spoonful, the food will go in with little difficulty. Start with ¼ to ½ teaspoon of any new food, increasing gradually as he becomes used to it.

Juices from organically grown fruits and vegetables are good first foods. Grate them fine and squeeze the juice through cheesecloth or nylon net. If you have a juicer or can obtain organically grown juices from your health food store, that is fine, too. Start with one to three teaspoons daily, of any one kind. Apple or carrot are good starters Dilute with safe water or the mineral-rich water. Feed at room temperature from the tip of a teaspoon or from a bottle.

Mashed ripe banana may be offered at this time. Please *do not* purchase canned banana for your little one. Why should you buy an inferior food for over a dollar a pound when you can prepare in an instant quality food for a few cents? *All* commercial baby foods should be avoided. Most contain harmful chemicals and far too much salt and sugar to be considered good foods. Thin the mashed fruit with mineral-rich water or certified raw goat or cow's milk.

As the weeks pass by and baby's appetite increases and his digestive system develops and is ready for increased solid foods, give him the good natural foods that nature intended children to have. Ripe papaya and peaches, pears, and nectarines are spoon

(continued on page 262)

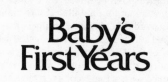

Baby's First Years

(continued from page 261)

ready. Just mash, dilute with mineral-rich water and serve. As your infant grows, use less and less water to dilute his food. Avocados are usually relished at the first taste, and your good homemade yogurt can be offered now. Try scraped raw apple or beets; sieved cottage cheese will be enjoyed. Mashed ripe persimmons in season, or mashed dates are good foods that require a minimum of preparation. Potatoes and sweet potatoes may be grated and the juice pressed through cheesecloth or nylon net; add to carrot or apple juice for a better flavor. Berries may be blended and strained or mashed with water and pressed through a sieve for a delicious juice. Raw peas or green beans may be blended or chopped, soaked in a small amount of water, then strained. Raw almond butter may be offered at about ten months; dilute at first with mineral-rich water. Acidophilus concentrate may be added to this or any seed or nut milk made for baby.

After the little one is eating a variety of solid foods, one or two of them can be spoon fed each day, but some of the others — such as mashed avocado or steamed, pureed vegetables — may well be thinned with mineral-rich water and fed from a bottle with a crosscut nipple. Various supplementary foods can also be added to these feedings such as a bit of brewer's yeast, bone meal, or molasses.

Sometime after nine months, you may wish to offer your baby milk to drink from a cup once or twice a day. Try to find a safe raw certified milk or goat milk for him. If that is not possible, get the best milk you can and add to each cup 2 teaspoonsful of "Eugalan," cultured from mother's milk, and available at health food stores.

Dissolve the day's supply of the powder, 6 to 8 teaspoons, in 4 ounces of lukewarm water in a jar with a tight cap. Shake to mix and keep chilled. Add 2 teaspoons of the prepared liquid to each cup of milk.

At ten or eleven months, baby will begin to show some interest in feeding himself. Encourage him by giving him a chicken bone to hold and crunch on, or a spoon of his very own to use at the beginning of a meal when he is eager to eat. You can finish up the feeding but he will slowly learn to handle a spoon and how to use it. Smile to show him your pleasure in his accomplishment. He will quickly learn also to eat carrot sticks or apple wedges or raw peas with his fingers.

If the family meals are well planned and nourishing, very soon the little one will be eating some of the good things from the family table.

Sometime after about one year, you may wish to introduce raw fertile egg yolk. Start with 1/16 of a teaspoon, and increase it just a tiny bit daily. You can add it to a bit of mashed avocado, or banana for variety. Baked potato may be served once a week now if you wish to add cooked foods. Mash with a little yogurt. Raw vegetables may be pureed in the blender, or very finely grated and added to mashed avocado, or thinned with a little carrot juice. Finely grated apple and carrot or apple and beet are good combinations.

Fresh, lightly steamed vegetables, pureed in the blender or pushed through a sieve and thinned with a little milk make very fine soups for little ones. Organically grown brown rice, baked sweet potato, or other complex starch foods may be served to the child over one year of age. Until that time the enzyme ptyalin, essential for the digestion of starch, is not present in the baby's saliva. A good hard crust of whole-grain bread is a help with teething. Raw kelp or lightly broiled fish, from a known source, may be chopped and soaked and the resulting liquid fed to the child for iodine and other sea minerals.

If you wish your child to have meat, and can find a safe source, it may be added to his diet after fourteen months (or before, if your doctor suggests it). It can be lightly broiled, then blended with a little water. When the child is older, he can eat a patty of broiled ground meat with his fingers. Organ meats, such as heart and sweetbreads, may be steamed, then finely chopped or ground. Fish, from a known safe source, is a good food for baby; steamed or broiled, and mashed or cut up to suit his age, it will add many essential minerals to his diet.

Homemade soups made from organically grown vegetables and safe chicken or meat, cooked at a very low temperature, may be pureed in your blender and frozen in ice-cube trays. Remove and store in a plastic bag tightly sealed in the freezer until needed.

Many vegetables may be finely grated and fed raw to the child eight months or older. (Before that time, grate raw vegetables and squeeze juice through a square of nylon net; feed only the juice to the baby.) Grated carrot, sweet potato, zucchini, parsnips, turnip, potato or rutabaga will be relished by almost every baby. Beets are good too, but very concentrated. Start with only a half teaspoon of beet, added to a food already established in the diet, such as banana or avocado.

Remember the little one's taste buds have not been perverted by sugar foods, spices and seasonings. Natural foods taste *good* all by themselves.

Be persistent about offering raw romaine and other salad greens so your child will grow up with a fondness for health-giving green salads. At first you can blend the greens in a bit of mineral water in the blender. Later they can be squashed through your grater before feeding and finally, when the baby's teeth are here, he can do his own chewing.

Any vegetable or fruit that you prepare for your family can be pureed or blended for the baby. Cook with very little water at the lowest possible temperature and use every drop of the cooking water. If the food is too thin, thicken with a little wheat germ. To prepare in advance, proceed as above then freeze in small cups or ice-cube trays. Store in a plastic bag in the freezer until needed. Remove from freezer and place in a small custard cup or other heat-proof dish to thaw. At meal time simply set the cup or dish in a pan of warm water until it is the proper temperature.

Fresh raw blender applesauce or dried apricot sauce may be served to the infant plain or blended into mashed banana.

Dried prunes should be soaked two days in the refrigerator — use apple juice to soak if you have it — then pit and puree in your blender (or put through a food grinder or mill if you have no blender). The prune sauce is luscious spooned over a scoop of yogurt or mixed with a tablespoon or so of wheat germ. If sweetening is desired, use a bit of honey. *Sugar* is at the top of the "No No" list for both baby and mother.

Don't have any "junk" foods in the house, then they simply will not be available to the child, or to his parents.

Weaning

Every child sets his own timetable for weaning. Some babies nurse or drink from a bottle longer than others because they feel need for this security. Others, more adventurous and secure, look forward to drinking from a cup.

Withdrawing just one feeding from the daily schedule and offering milk from a cup at that meal only, is a gentle way to begin the weaning. A little extra attention and a loving cuddle or two during the day will make this time easier for the little one. The following week, if all goes well, another feeding can be withdrawn. As the child becomes more and more interested in the wonderful world around him and is enjoying at each meal a tummy full of hearty natural foods, he needs less nursing and usually tapers off to just a pre-bedtime snack. There is no harm in continuing this token feeding as long as the baby wants it. Even after the mother has considered the baby completely weaned, he may decide he wants to nurse a little "just for old times' sake." Usually he will be satisfied in a moment or two and this may well be his final nursing.

Most important to remember is that babies can actually *die* without a constant supply of love and loving — as well as milk.

☼

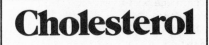

Cholesterol

(continued from page 67)

Sea salt is 1.9 percent chlorine, 1.0 percent sodium, 0.135 percent magnesium, 0.08 percent sulfur, 0.04 percent calcium and 0.038 percent potassium, with much less phosphorus. Most of the sulfur is as the sulfate, which is easily used by ruminants but not by man. The main extra mineral to be obtained from the use of sea salt on your egg is magnesium.

It is true that the egg is high in cholesterol, averaging 275 mg. Since the average daily consumption of cholesterol is about 800 mg, you can see that eggs are a major contribution. The individual who eats no eggs or organ meats probably takes in about 200 mg of cholesterol a day. If he or she uses skim milk and vegetable margarine, the intake may be as low as 100 to 150 mg per day.

Our recommendation may exceed the generally advised upper limit; however, this amount of balanced egg cholesterol has not been proven to be harmful. Furthermore, it is substantially less than the 1 to 2 gm the body manufactures every day. Dr. Roger Williams says that it is a fundamental nutritional error to exclude eggs from the diet. He believes that the cholesterol will be utilized if the other foods eaten contain the needed trace metals. Doctors and others worried about heart disease have unduly placed the blame on the egg.

Egg eating does not explain or cause heart disease. Instead of blaming eggs, it would seem wiser to concentrate on correcting an otherwise poor diet. As we have seen, nutrients such as vitamin C, niacin, magnesium, zinc and chromium, possibly lecithin, and other factors such as natural carbohydrates and regular exercise produce and maintain lowered cholesterol levels, which are negatively associated with atherosclerosis. High cholesterol levels are promoted when the diet is mainly refined junk foods without trace elements.

The high-risk cholesterol patient should be tested for adequate zinc, excess copper levels and his spectrum of serum lipids. He can then be advised as to whether his total nutritional status will allow the addition of eggs to his diet. The person who eliminates eggs will still have the basic problem which allowed the initial build-up of cholesterol in the arteries in the first place! So, by all means, unless you are a high-risk coronary patient, have your one or two eggs a day for good economical nutrition.

The cholesterol war between the American Heart Association (AHA) and the egg industry continues, with the public trying to guess how it will all turn out. Both sides appear to be short on science and long on hot air. Perhaps some quotes will illustrate.

Dr. Jean Mayer: "Both sides are fighting over your heart." He advocates only two eggs per week and calls the egg industry "the heart-disease Mafia."

The egg industry: " . . . absolutely no scientific evidence that eating eggs, even in quantity, will increase the risk of a heart attack . . . Eggs do not contain food additives."

Dr. Roger Williams: "I think the egg advertising tends to counteract the anti-egg promotion of the AHA which is not justified. They're such good food. I believe the cholesterol in eggs will take care of itself if the other foods you eat are good."

Dr. Ray Reiser, Professor of Biochemistry at Texas A & M: "First recognize individual differences. There's no increase in risk at cholesterol levels below 240, and such people are in no danger from eating eggs. The advice is: See your doctor, find out your cholesterol level and be treated as an individual."

A Standard Brands subsidiary has a cholesterol-free egg substitute called Egg Beaters which is sold in the frozen state. When thawed, this product has the appearance of beaten eggs but is mostly egg whites with selected vitamins, minerals, fat and even protein added. The 1-pound package is said to be the equivalent of eight large eggs and without detectable cholesterol. A prominent label says, "Cholesterol-free Egg Substitute." In fine print, we find "egg white, corn oil, non-fat dry milk, emulsifiers (vegetable lecithin, mono- and diglycerides and propylene glycol monostearate) cellulose and Xanthan gums, trisodium and triethyl citrate, artificial flavor, aluminum sulfate, iron phosphate, artificial color, thiamin, riboflavin and vitamin D." The tinkered product has lost almost all zinc, all usable sulfur, all B-6, all vitamin A and all niacin, not to mention the trace metals and nutrients which allow a whole baby chick to develop from the yolk.

What happens to all those yolks from the tinkered eggs? A company public relations man says that various things such as cosmetics, bakery products and pet food absorb the yolks. Dr. Roger Williams says, "The dogs are again better fed than man." We say, "Let them eat their tinkered eggs. Whole fresh eggs or fight is our motto!" ☼

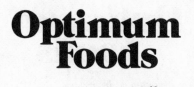

Optimum Foods

(continued from page 69)

consumer, can be highly injurious to his health when consumed over a long period of time. Often salt is included in foodstuffs without being listed.

When the hearings on chemical additives in foods were held back in the 1950s, it was admitted that some 700 chemicals were being added to American foodstuffs. Grave doubt existed as to the safety of at least 150 of them. Since then, the total number of chemical additives in food has soared. Official estimates today reach up to 10,000. To list and describe fully all food and color additives that have received government sanction now requires a directory of five volumes, and there is no exact knowledge of the number in present use.

What harm can chemical food additives do? Some additives produce chemical changes in the food itself by altering its biological structure. Others produce disorders in the human system so insidious that they do not become apparent until long after the original exposure to the chemicals. Because of this, the additives may not even be suspected as the original instigators of trouble. The earliest signs of damage to vital organs may be indicated by microscopic changes that can be detected only by a trained pathologist.

Many chemical food additives interfere with the normal function of vitamins and enzymes, which work closely together in the body. Vitamins play an important role in releasing energy for all physiological processes, including cell repair. Closely associated with them are the enzymes, which are the effective agents of the whole life process. As long as each cell lives, it is continually being broken down and rebuilt. Energy is needed for this repair process. In a vitamin deficiency, where energy liberation is interfered with by the introduction of chemical food additives or other substances, the rebuilding process slows down or ceases; the cells die. When enough cells sicken and die, the body dies.

Injury or deterioration of the cells is recognized by physicians who are aware of vitamin and enzyme deficiency symptoms. Patients are easily fatigued, show such symptoms as weakness, constipation, loss of appetite, headache, dis-

(continued on page 264)

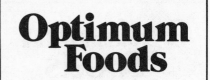

Optimum Foods

(continued from page 263)

turbance of sleep, excessive irritability, depression, inability to concentrate, odd feelings in the fingers and toes, burning tongue, gas, and many other strange bodily sensations. These symptoms all too often may be classified vaguely as nervousness, neurasthenia, or imagination, when in reality they may stem from impairment of the vitamin-enzyme system of the body.

Commonly used chemical food additives, such as sulfur dioxide, sodium nitrate, food dyes, certain hormones used to stimulate plant and animal growth, antibiotics used in food production, fluorides used in processing water, and pesticides are all acknowledged enzyme destroyers.

According to medical researchers, adverse effects can occur even when the chemicals are present in exceedingly small amounts. For example, as little as 0.4 parts per million of DDT can inhibit a vital enzyme in human blood.

Catalase is one important enzyme found almost universally in living cells, not only in human beings but also in animals, plants, and even in bacteria. This particular enzyme plays many vital roles. It is intimately related to cell respiration and buffers the cell from toxic substances, infection, virus, radiation, and cancer. The normal cell maintains a specific balance of catalase and hydrogen peroxide. Catalase controls the hydrogen peroxide at a very low level, converting it into oxygen and water. However, many substances, including some chemical food additives, destroy catalase. When this happens the level of peroxide rises. In turn, there results in the electron-transport system of the cell a slowing down or stoppage. Cellular abnormalities may then develop and the cell becomes predisposed to tumor formation.

It is evident that if this fundamental biological mechanism is interfered with for a long enough time by physical and chemical agents present in our environment, whether in food, drink, or the air we breathe, then we shall see in peoples so exposed a progressive increase in the incidence of tumors. To help arrest this condition it is important to abolish some of the chemicals currently added to food and drink for preservation or coloring.

The ultimate would be to eliminate major toxins—such as salt, coffee, cigarettes, drugs (legal and illegal), alcohol—out of the human diet. However, to be realistic, this would cause a collapse in a way of life for a great many people, both figuratively and literally. This would certainly happen if they were asked to stop smoking suddenly, or to not have their morning coffee, or sleeping pills, or their pep pills and tranquilizers—the latter in some instances being used to produce a quieting effect from the extra pep derived from the pep pills.

However, there are people, young and old, who today want to live a life free of disease, and bear healthy children. How do I know this? It is a sign of the times. On my recent annual vacation tour from California to Colorado, up through Montana then back home, I noticed many hot dog and taco stands had closed. At the same time, I found health food businesses booming, with more and more people being attracted to this new way of life. More people are planting organic gardens, wherever they can find the space to do so. Increasingly, more women are baking their own bread and feeding their families simply, buying good, wholesome foods.

Now, with emphasis on wholesome foods that will, in my opinion, help you toward a healthy life I offer my Optimum Food List:

Proteins:
Rare beef and lamb
Raw egg yolks
Raw milk
Pecans, almonds
Fish, sea food (boiled)
Chicken (boiled or broiled)

Starches:
Whole grain bread (preferably make your own with no salt, little sweet, or shortening)
Boiled potatoes, brown rice
Cereal and grains
Bananas

Sugars:
Raw sugar
Dark brown sugar
Maple sugar
Raw honey, molasses

Fats:
Raw cream
Unsalted butter
Avocado
Apricot kernel oil
Olive oil

Vegetables:
Cooked:
Soft squashes
String beans (yellow and green)
Chinese peas
Potatoes.
Chard and beet-tops
Fresh corn
Chinese cabbage
Raw:
Lettuce, celery, cucumbers
Alfalfa sprouts, water cress
Fruit:
Apples, bananas
Babcock peaches, pears
Blueberries, orange, grapefruit
Raspberries, watermelons
Cantaloupes
Papaya, grapes
Pineapple, cherries

Some of the foods I consider most helpful to normalize activity of the endocrine glands are included in the following list.

For the Adrenal Glands:
Raw egg yolks, fish, meat, raw milk
For the Gonads—Sex Glands:
Meat, eggs, fish, oatmeal, whole wheat bread and wheat germ, lentils, whole barley, liver, kidney beans, black molasses
For the Pituitary Gland:
Potatoes, lettuce, wheat germ, almonds, liver, agar-agar (a sea moss), raw egg yolks, parsley, meat, fish, raw milk
For the Parathyroid Glands:
Oranges, apples, cabbage, cucumber, lettuce, radishes, watercress, whole wheat, honey
For the Pancreas:
Eggs, milk, meat, fish, cabbage, lettuce
For the Thyroid Gland:
All sea food, particularly oysters, shrimps, and fresh salmon

Foods that I consider to be in the "twilight zone" are those that should be eaten in small amounts, if at all, and only when the person is in good health. The protein group of this category consists of cottage cheese and yogurt. Commercial cottage cheese has too much salt. Most commercial yogurt has synthetic lactic acid. Processed cheddar cheese and Swiss cheese—in fact almost all processed cheeses—are loaded with salt and preservatives. It always should be remembered that cheese is a decayed food, and should be eaten in small amounts if at all.

The third food category—the "don't touch" list—contains the toxic food poisoners: white sugar, white-sugar products, white-flour products, soft drinks (dietetic as well as regular); in fact, any and all dead food that has been devitaminized and demineralized. What many people do not realize when shopping is that they sometimes buy a foodless food that contains potentially harmful hidden ingredients, not advertised on the product's label. ☼

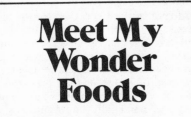

Meet My Wonder Foods

(continued from page 73)

30 percent.

Yogurt and the acidophilus cultured milks have undergone many ups and downs in popularity. They have been advocated for everything from "that tired feeling" to typhoid fever. My interest in yogurt is wholly concerned with *nutrition,* and from a nutritional point of view it is tops.

Bulgarians are credited with retaining vigor, vitality, and the characteristics of youth to an extremely advanced age; their longevity is traditional. Yogurt and certain cultured milks constitute a major item of diet for the Bulgarian peasant. To state that all of these virtues stem solely from the consumption of yogurt is to treat the subject most superficially; climate, heredity, and other factors must be considered. But clearly the Bulgarians have established the nutritional excellency of yogurt. That, and that alone, first attracted me to yogurt and caused me to investigate and study it. Its superior nutritive qualities caused me to recommend it to my students, and my faith in it has been justified in every respect. The extent to which the bacteria present in yogurt may reach the colon is to me of incidental interest only. They are "friendly" and helpful bacteria, active in the synthesis of certain B vitamins, and the acid they produce from milk sugar tends to suppress the activities of pathogenic and putrefactive types of organisms. If yogurt eaters receive these benefits in any measure at all, they are just that much ahead.

While excellent yogurt can be purchased in dairy and food stores, the homemade variety is far less expensive and can be made with inexpensive skim milk. With the growing popularity of the home yogurt-maker, there has been a growing sophistication about the taste of good, fresh yogurt.

Yogurt can be eaten plain, seasoned with chives or other herbs, served with fresh or canned fruits, or made into a sundae with maple syrup, honey, or molasses. Real yogurt connoisseurs prefer it plain! I'm indeed sorry that many dairies now sell "jazzed-up" yogurt, loaded with white sugar and glucose preserves. Buy it plain or—better still—make your own.

The World's Best Cereal—Fresh Wheat Germ

Fresh wheat germ is worth its weight in gold. It takes its place on my list of wonder foods as an outstanding source of vitamin B1. One-half cup provides about three and a half times my generous daily allowance of this important vitamin.

Fresh wheat germ should be sprinkled over hot or cold cereals. Excellent hot cakes, waffles, muffins, and breads can be prepared by substituting from one-half to one cup of wheat germ for an equivalent quantity of flour. If you own an electric blender, you can make delicious drinks with a pint of any fruit juice, a small section of banana, and half a cup of wheat germ.

Wheat germ also contains vitamin E. Man, over centuries of time, became adapted to the consumption of whole cereal grains, including the germ. He cannot now lightly drop the germ from his diet. Many modern processes of refining natural foods have led to a number of dietary deficiencies, some of them dramatically clear-cut, others more subtle and difficult to identify.

If at all possible, do get the fresh wheat germ. If you live near a mill that produces it, by all means buy it directly. If not, you will find it on sale at your local health food shop. Not only is the fresh wheat germ better for you but it will cost about half as much as the processed toasted wheat germ. Stored in a tight can or jar in a cool place, it will keep its freshness for a month. And above all, avoid the "processed" wheat germ that has other ingredients added—especially foodless white sugar. The best wheat germ is made in France. There the Moulin de Paris exposes the freshly milled wheat germ to the rays of a powerful ultraviolet lamp, which adds sweetness and brings out the natural flavor of the "heart of the wheat."

Unsulphured Molasses

For many years I have advocated the use of blackstrap molasses because it is an unusually rich source of iron and the B vitamins. The late Dr. Tom Spies, of Hillman Hospital in Birmingham, Alabama, first told me of the wonders he performed with it. It has long been an important staple in the diets of many Southerners in the United States. However, because of its unusual taste, it invokes in most people a strong *yes* or *no*—and, unfortunately, more often *no* than *yes*. So, if you are one of those who say *no* to blackstrap molasses, use instead the darkest molasses you can find, or mix a little blackstrap in with your regular molasses, which should be the unsulfured kind. Molasses is made from the residue left from making sugar out of sugar cane. "Sulphured" molasses is bleached with potassium to make it more attractive. This process, of course, destroys important nutrients.

Molasses is an excellent source of nutritionally available iron. Moreover, it is the best source of natural sugar, and it also provides significant quantities of thiamine and riboflavin.

I list it as a wonder food primarily for its rich iron content. It lends itself in dozens of ways to the preparation of foods; added to muffins, waffles, spiced cookies, and the like, it enriches them significantly with much-needed iron. Milk is poor in iron, yet the growing youngster requires three or four glasses a day; a tablespoonful of molasses stirred into each glass turns an iron-poor food into an iron-rich one, providing from 50 to 75 percent of the daily iron allowance. Used in place of table syrups, which for the most part are nascent sugar solutions, its nutritional superiority is undoubted.

Six-Course Dinner Growing on One Tree

Mother Nature put many of her best ingredients into a fruit-vegetable that grows on a tree—the avocado. In each avocado (or alligator pear) are combined the proteins of meat, the fat of butter (unsaturated, as an extra bonus), the vitamins and minerals of vegetables, and the flavor of nuts. You might say that the avocado is a complete meal from soup to nuts.

The protein content of the avocado is the equal of many kinds of meat; when fully ripe, the fruit contains little starch and practically no sugar. It offers generous quantities of calcium, magnesium, potassium, sodium, copper, phosphates, manganese, and iron. It is loaded with vitamins A, B1, B2, and C and has some vitamins D and E.

About one fourth of the avocado consists of fat or oil. What makes avocado oil so valuable is its high percentage of polunsaturated fatty acids. This oil gives the avocado its mellow texture and nutlike flavor. The Mexicans call the soft green pulp "butter growing on trees"; and they spread it generously on their tortillas. A very ripe, soft avocado, mashed with a few drops of lemon juice and spiked with herbs, makes an utterly delicious dressing over fruit and vegetable salads. Because the vegetable oils are easily burned by the body, even overweighters can enjoy this "green butter."　☼

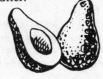

the sea. It was even suggested that iodine vapor was carried inland by sea breezes and fertilized coastal land with iodine. This notion has now been wholly discounted. Countries like Holland, close to the sea, and where there is no lack of iodine, nonetheless, has a high incidence of goiter in some regions. (H. O. Hettche, *Aetiologie, Pathogenese und Prophylaxie der Struma*, Munich, 1954) We now know that there are a number of other factors which, in an area where iodine intake is low, makes goiter more apt to occur. Cabbage leaves, turnips, kale, cabbage seeds, mustard seeds and grape seeds all contain certain sulfurous substances which block the utilization of iodine. When eaten in great quantities, over a period of time, they act as goitrogens. Water that is high in calcium and magnesium is also another factor.

Medical Problems of the Program

As with other well-intentioned programs of food supplementation, iodized salt raised a new set of unanticipated problems. Many dermatologists warned that certain individuals could not safely tolerate the added iodine. Certain skin diseases such as acne are aggravated by iodide.

Other professionals pointed out that it is wrong to think that iodide's only biologic effect is on the thyroid. Iodine also has an ability to increase an inflammatory response, which may be harmful as well as beneficial. (*Nutrition Today*, Summer 1969)

After iodized salt usage reached its peak during World War II, it began to decline. By 1947, U. S. Public Health Service reported that newer surveys showed a rise in the incidence of goiter in certain geographic areas. Public health officials lost faith in the voluntary iodization program. They began to push for mandatory legislation to have *all* table salt iodized.

At this point, professional objections were raised. The New York Society of Dermatology opposed such mandatory legislation. The group went on record as stating that such legislation "would mean a tremendous increase in iodic eruptions of the skin."

The Cleveland Dermatology Society, while approving the use of iodized salt for persons who could benefit from its use, nevertheless disapproved of mandatory iodization of *all* table salt. The Society stated its objection: "A serious result of the universal use of iodized salt would be a great increase of severe iododermas, at times causing hospitalization for several months, and even death—from induced sensitivity caused by iodine-contained salts and suddenly manifested by submedicinal doses of iodine." Other dermatology groups followed suit.

Despite these warnings, proponents of mandatory legislation were so convinced that iodized salt was the panacea for eradication of goiter that they even suggested having iodized salt extended for uses in food processing as well as in the home. Fortunately, the food processors resisted this measure. Their rejection was based on practical considerations. Any shift from untreated to iodized salts would have created complex technical problems in food processing. If they had agreed to use iodized salt, the total dietary iodine in today's food would have been pushed to an even higher level.

Both untreated and iodized salt are presently available. Persons who do not need medication with an iodide may be using iodized salt anyway. And to the unenlightened, the idea that "a little is good, more is better" is fraught with danger, if it results in iodine being ingested at a high level.

Too Much Dietary Iodine?

According to Dr. Robert L. Vought, Chief of the Metabolic Diseases Epidemiology Unit of the National Institute of Arthritis and Metabolic Diseases, proof is lacking that iodized salt is essential for the diet of most Americans. Iodine intake from food alone is entirely adequate for most of our population. Vought reported that recent data suggest that we may be suffering from *"an iodine surfeit"* from too much dietary iodine.

Food Processing, Food Contamination, Food Choices and Iodine

Surprisingly high, and increasing amounts of iodine in the present American diet were found by M. Z. Nichaman and his associates, from the Preventable Disease and Nutritional Biochemistry Section of the Center of Disease Control (HEW), Atlanta, Georgia, thus confirming Vought's findings. Data were gathered by means of analyzing the iodine excreted in human urine, as well as the iodine composition of specific foods. Nichaman *et al* admitted that the dietary sources responsible for the high iodine content are not well defined. The traditional sources have been from seafood and

from iodized salt. But these two sources do not appear to account for the high levels of iodine excretion that they observed in human urine. They suggested that possible changes in food processing have introduced new sources. The use of iodine in food preparation and processing introduces unquantified and potentially large amounts of iodine into foods. The specific health hazards are not well defined. From a public health standpoint, they suggested, it would seem wise to avoid adding large amounts of iodine to foods during production and processing, particularly when alternative techniques are available.

Baked goods are sources of iodine, from the potassium or calcium iodate permitted in these products as dough conditioners. In the decade from 1955 to 1965, the American consumption of baked goods jumped a whopping *65 percent*. This greatly increased consumption inevitably leads to higher levels of dietary iodine.

Salts blocks, used in animal feeding, may contain an assimilable source of iodine for supplementing the animals' diet. At a later stage, iodine from this source may turn up in products such as milk and other dairy foods, consumed by humans.

Among the most surprising, and heretofore unrecognized, sources of iodine in food is from a widely used food dye. Erythrosine (FD&C Red No. 3) is tetraiodofluorescein, a compound that contains a form of iodine. Rat experiments with this dye suggest that significant deiodination can occur, and as much as one-fourth to one-third of the total iodine can be converted to iodide and be metabolized in the rat. This was demonstrated in three separate feeding experiments, in which an erythrosine-containing commercial breakfast cereal was fed to rats for three to five weeks. At the end of each study the animals were examined. It was found that the dye in the cereal exerted an effect on the uptake of iodine in the following: (1) in the thyroid gland, (2) in the protein- and non-protein bound iodine in the serum. and (3) in the urine.

At present, it is not known whether this dye is metabolized to an equivalent extent in humans. If this deiodination of erythrosine is quantitatively similar in the human to that in the rat, it is estimated that a single serving of a breakfast cereal containing this dye would increase the daily intake of available dietary iodine sufficiently to cause problems if the cereal is eaten regularly over a period of time. The researchers suggested that "Whether or not this amount of iodide, especially when added to that derived from bread, iodized salt, and various other colored foods and drugs, *will enhance the incidence of iodide goiter* cannot be readily predicted from information presently available." (Emphasis mine.) *(Journal of Clinical Endocrinology and Metabolism*, Vol. 34, No. 4, 1972)

Erythrosine is found in many other processed foods in addition to breakfast cereals. It is also used extensively in candies, confections, bakery goods, dessert powders, maraschino cherries, beverages, pet foods, and to a lesser extent, in ice cream, sherbet, dairy products, snack foods and meat inks. The dye is also a popular one for pharmaceutical products, and to a lesser extent, it is used in cosmetics. Erythrosine was originally approved in 1907, so it has been around for a long time. It can be readily seen that the extensive use of this dye, with a wide variety of consumer goods, may expose a large percentage of the population to another source of dietary iodine.

Our foods may also inadvertently be contaminated by iodine from various sources. Recently, milk contamination by iodine was traced to the practice of dipping cows' teats in a solution containing approximately 5,000 parts per million of activated iodine, used as a sanitizing agent. (*Dairy Research Digest*, October 1975) FDA agents seized over 700 pounds of breaded onion rings which had been sprayed illegally with an iodine-based sanitizer, directly onto the sliced onions before they were breaded. (*FDA Consumer*, November 1975)

Official Pronouncements and Consumer Options

Many indications, abstracted from reliable sources, attest to the surfeit of dietary iodine in the present American diet. But the data are at loggerheads with present FDA policy. Although this agency generally rejects the idea of negative labeling (it would look askance, for example, at a label stating that produce has been grown without pesticides, or that eggs were produced without antibiotics in the feed), in this instance, the agency insists that *non*-iodized salt be labeled with the warning "This salt does not supply iodide, a necessary nutrient."

As one consumer advocate wrote, "in these days of class action suits, those who overseason their food because of a plug for iodized salt may well have a legal case against the federal government on the basis of HEW's labeling requirements. ☼

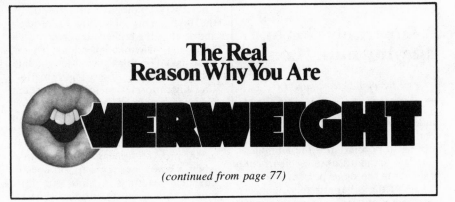

The Real Reason Why You Are OVERWEIGHT

(continued from page 77)

I know of one couple in this metabolic category. The man has been greatly overweight until recently (a doctor spotted his problem and helped him trim down). His wife, who actually eats more than he does, remains a svelte size eight. In such physical disturbances, the doctor can help to establish the cause.

Glands, Exercise and Zig-Zag Dieting
Grant Gwinup, M.D., says, "Many fat persons console themselves with the idea that their glands are at fault. They are only kidding themselves; I believe glands rarely cause obesity. That rumor has persisted for more than 60 years, but it is usually untrue. Neither the pituitary nor the thyroid gland is guilty. About five million men and women today are taking thyroid pills unnecessarily. The pills do nothing for them except cause nervousness and weakness if the doses are large."

But there is another opinion. Dr. Mayer believes that the greatest cause of overweight is inactivity. Research proves this to be true with animals, as every farmer knows. He believes that self-indulgence or a combination of the above factors can cause overweight.

He — and others — deplore the on-again, off-again dieting, which Dr. Mayer terms "the rhythm method of girth control." It has been found to throw glandular machinery out of kilter in regulating the body machinery. The glands become so confused by the constant changes that they finally break down in their efficiency. Avoid see-saw dieting, he warns.

It is true that if you did not eat at all, you would lose weight sooner or later. It is also true that if you eat more food than you need, you will store that food and become overweight. It is a simple case of body mechanics. All foods are a source of energy (some more, some less), and energy is used up by the body either in movement or by producing heat. If less is eaten, any existing fat is taken out of storage. If more is eaten than is used, it is put into storage. Therefore, for a fat person to lose weight, he has two choices: he must either eat less, or exercise more to keep his weight in balance. Once a desired weight is attained, the food intake and output must

be balanced by checking scales regularly and adjusting eating or exercise accordingly. This will no doubt help you to maintain the weight you wish but it will not insure good health! So now we are finally coming to the secret of accomplishing this goal.

Grant Gwinup, M.D., has apparently stumbled upon part of the secret: He says, "Practically every reducing diet — no matter how well it works at the start — is doomed to fail. The proof is apparent. The average person stays on a particular diet for a couple of weeks and then he or she is looking around for a new one. All diets fail after a few weeks. And for a good reason. All diets have a common basic fault."

Now comes the clincher: Dr. Gwinup says, "The fault of the reducing diets is that they are physiologically unsound and therefore unacceptable to your body."

I would like to put it more bluntly: the reason that the average reducing diet does not work, does make you nervous and irritable, does play havoc with your skin and hair, as well as your nerves and makes you feel worse rather than better, as well as ravenously hungry, is that *it induces malnutrition* and actually starves you to death. No wonder you cannot stay on it for long! Malnutriton is now beginning to be considered a *disease* and reducing diets induce this disease. It is possible to feed your body *what it needs,* prevent that gnawing hunger, and at the same time make you *healthy as well as slim.* ☼

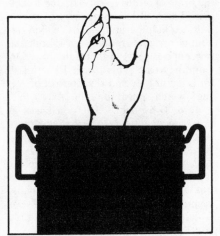

under resting conditions show the same tendencies. The rate of blood pH returning to normal after the administration of a standard dose of bicarbonate is slower in the older person. The same is true of the other variables, concerning their recovery to normality, when challenged. Thus, an obvious and fundamental conclusion is that one of the characteristics of physiological aging is this reduction in reserve capacities. Besides the decline in production of numerous body components such as hormones and enzymes, it has been established that a number of enzymes also increase in concentration as the body ages.

Many view aging as occurring when cells die out. As Dr. Comfort, in a January 1970 issue of *Gerontologia* puts it: ". . . like so many lights on a theater marquee [the cells die], eventually shutting off the entire network." Others prefer to view aging as the biological mechanism that occurs prior to, and is responsible for, the cells dying out. *Cellular aging underlies aging of the whole person.* The body consists of some sixty trillion cells of various types. These cell types age at different rates and by different mechanisms.

Dr. Charles Barrows of the Gerontology Center, a section of the National Institute of Health, wrote in *Parade* in 1970: "We know, from animal studies, that death of cells in certain organs and tissues accompanies age." We can count the cells and note the reduction. It is as great as 55 percent in the skeletal muscles of extremely old rats. We know also that the weight of a seventy-five-year-old man's brain is less than that of the brain of a thirty-year-old, due to cell loss. This cell loss is greatest in nerve, muscle, kidney, and glands, which accounts for the gradual loss (about 0.6 percent per year) of their functions. Dr. Comfort wrote in his article "Experimental Gerontology and the Control of Aging," which appeared in the March 1970 issue of *Geriatrics,* "The consensus at the moment appears to be that aging represents the loss of biological information. This is only another way of saying that, with aging, the stability of the living system is progressively impaired, but by putting it in this way, we may become more alert to the kind of loss which is taking place and to its possible site."

The loss of biological information by the body components that reproduce and control the body is then responsible for aging. Obvious questions begging to be asked by this explanation include: What causes this loss of information? Can this information loss be restored, or at least stopped? What is the mechanism causing the information loss? In order to answer the first two, the last question has to be answered first. The aging process appears very complex when viewed as a group of specific chemical reactions, but one simplified view is to concentrate primarily on the loss of information in the molecules responsible for reproducing the body's proteins.

The Underlying Cause of Aging

Fundamentally, the free-radical theory first conceived by Dr. Denham Harman of the University of Nebraska states that in the body, the random and irreversible reactions initiated by free-radicals (highly reactive chemical groups) produce a multiplicity of harmful reactions. The damage occurs from the primary reactions of free-radicals with DNA (the body's genetic material and protein synthesizer) and other enzymes or cell membrances, as well as by secondary damage.

The Importance of Undamaged DNA

Proteins are the indispensable constituents of life. The chief reason they hold this key position is that all enzymes are proteins and cause physiological reactions to proceed at rates compatible with life. The job a particular protein is delegated to do in a cell depends upon its structure and seemingly small differences produce major consequences.

If the DNA molecule loses information, for example, by alteration of one or more of its nucleotides, life is impaired and an important body function is destroyed. The alteration results in either no protein or a wrong protein ("clinker") being built. A "clinker" inflicts damage by causing an immunological reaction, by using up required nutrients, and by strangling cells with waste material.

Retarding the Aging Process

My approach to aging research is aimed, first, at finding ways to slow the aging process. This approach is simpler, safer, and has a higher probability of producing relatively rapid results than direct rejuvenation attempts. After slowing the aging process, we can then seek to reverse them. Gerontologists such as Bjorksten are presently seeking to reverse the aging process.

A simple solution to the aging process is to destroy the free-radicals before they can do harm to DNA, enzymes, or other macromolecules in the body. Antioxidants are scavengers (inactivators) for free-radicals. Since collagen, which makes up 30 percent of the body's protein, is very subject to cross-linking initiated by free-radical attack, it is easy to see that neutralizing the free radicals with vitamin E and promoting the growth and health of collagen with vitamin C will help slow the aging process. Several researchers (including Drs. Denhan Harman and Alex Comfort and myself) have increased the mean life spans of rats and mice significantly by feeding them antioxidants.

A combination of radiation absorbers and antioxidants would do more to slow the aging process. Chemicals in the body that can absorb radiation before it reaches critical body components will protect them and prevent free-radicals from being initiated. In addition, the presence of antioxidants will back up the radiation protectors by squelching the reaction in the oxidation stages. Of course, these solutions do not help the body components already destroyed by free-radical attack or radiation. They only prevent or minimize further deterioration.

The aging process cannot be significantly altered without controlling either the missynthesized material or repairing the damaged body components. The latter hasn't been accomplished yet and shows little promise that it will be, but several scientists are pursuing this research as part of science's continuing routine and thorough investigation.

Antioxidant therapy alone should add five to ten years to the human life span; radiation protection alone should add two to five years; and success with protein missynthesis re-sorting alone should add five to ten years. The three protection mechanisms together will act synergistically, potentially producing a life span increase of thirty to forty years of youthful life.

Ingredients can be selected so that each chemical performs at least two of the above functions and each enhances the action or lowers the toxicity of another ingredient.

A companion antioxidant, vitamin C, can work in the water-based fluids as vitamin E works in the fat-based membranes. Both vitamins C and E help circulation, so that cells are nourished and remain vital. Vitamin C also helps regenerate used vitamin E. In addition, vitamin C is needed for healthy collagen, the protein substance that makes up more than 30 percent of our body. A deficiency in vitamin E results in abnormal collagen which constricts blood vessels and chokes off adequate blood supply to the tissues. The diminished blood supply reduces the nutrients reaching the tissues, resulting in cell death and loss of reserve. *The loss of cells from any cause results in aging. Environmental poisons, including air pollution, some food additives, smoking, and alcohol can all cause cell loss. Vitamins C and E both help secondarily to protect against these environmental poisons.* There are other factors affecting aging, including mental attitude, exercise, and genetics, but they should be discussed more fully as separate topics.

Sulfur compounds that are excellent radiation protectors are also free-radical scavengers, peroxide decomposers, and catalysts of sulfhydryl-disulfide exchange; possibly they can implement repair of damaged sites. Sulfhydryl compounds and vitamin E also increase the body's tolerance to selenium, so that quantities normally toxic can be used to protect against free-radicals.

Selenium Compounds Protect Against Radiation

Selenium and certain organic-selenium complexes help the body assimilate vitamin E (a natural antioxidant), are free-radical scavengers themselves, and may play a key role in protein missynthesis re-sorting.

An analogy often used by gerontologist Dr. Alex Comfort in his 1970 *Gerontologica* paper is that the taking of chemicals such as antioxidants and radiation protectors guard the cellular-synthesis program "like protecting a phonograph record by lubricating the needle to reduce scratching with use that would make it unplayable."

The Effect of Vitamin E on Aging

In gerontology there are many theories and not enough gerontologists. However, it is easy to prove the effect of antioxidant vitamins such as vitamin E on animal health and life span. Thirty to forty (control group) mice may be raised on a normal and nutritionally adequate diet, another thirty to forty mice on a vitamin E fortified diet, and a third thirty to forty mice on a vitamin E deficient diet. I have undertaken this experiment and so have other scientists; most experiments have yielded the following observations:

1. Vitamin E deficient diets lead to premature death.
2. Vitamin E supplemented diets lead to longer actual mean life spans (the age at which 50 percent of the original group has died), but so far, yield no significant increase in *natural* maximum life spans (the length of time the animal should live, if in an optimum environment).

I think an analogy with humans is valid,

but of course, the correlation may never be proved. With a balanced diet, people should live closer to the natural mean life span of eighty-five years. With a balanced diet and vitamin E supplementation, people should live closer to the potential natural maximum life span of 120 years. In essence, vitamin E, in addition to a balanced diet, overcomes many problems that arise because we do *not* live under perfect conditions. Research with animals and other laboratory models indicates that vitamin E is related to the aging process in two primary and several secondary ways. The two primary ways are through protection of cell membranes and through the deactivation of free-radicals. Protection of cell membranes is essentially a nutrition function, wherein a deficiency of vitamin E causes membrane damage, while an excess of vitamin E offers little additional membrane protection. The deactivation of free-radicals, on the other hand, is related to total vitamin E concentration and appears to offer additional benefits above the level of vitamin E required for nutritional purposes. Few scientists would question the role of vitamin E in membrane protection, but its role as a free-radical scavenger is not as widely known.

Vitamin E Extends Cell Life Span

Recently scientists have learned to grow living tissues in laboratory containers. The tissues grown in this manner are known as cell cultures, and they allow scientists directly to study interactions between chemicals and cells, without the complicating interactions that may occur within a host animal.

In normal cell cultures, cells have a definite life span. Human embryonic lung cells will divide and reproduce about fifty times before they die. However, in a vitamin E enriched medium cell lives are dramatically extended; physiologists Drs. Lester Packer and James R. Smith of the Lawrence Berkeley Laboratory have found that cells have divided 120 times and are still dividing at this writing (October 1974); moreover, the cells are young and healthy. Thus, vitamin E has unquestionably retarded the normal aging process in laboratory-cultured human cells. The researchers reported their full findings in the December 1974 *Proceedings of the National Academy of Sciences*. Dr. Packer has been quoted by reporter Robert Joffee in the September 29, 1974, issue of *The Washington Post* as saying, "Cells might not necessarily have a finite life span, but their death might be influenced by compounds called free-radicals that combine to form such large, insoluble molecules that cells

become clogged." Dr. Packer went on to say, "We don't know how vitamin E works, but it seems that damage which accumulates in the cells is reduced [by it], thus enhancing their chances to live."

I have reached several conclusions about aging based on laboratory experiments and human observations.

1. A deficiency in vitamin E (or any nutrient) will cause premature aging. Vitamin E is more critical than others because it is involved in membrane protection; it is lacking in most diets. Vitamin E's possible role in slowing the aging process is not accepted as fact by all scientists, even though they are aware of such experiments as described above.

2. Vitamin E will protect the body against many pollutants and poisons. This too is not accepted as fact by all scientists, although it can be demonstrated by animal experiments and "uncontrolled" clinical studies.

3. Vitamin E will protect cell membranes, aid circulation, and reduce cell loss; a deficiency will cause greater cell loss, and a slight excess over the suggested RDA will add greater protection because of better replacement efficiency. A larger excess will not give greater membrane protection, but may play other roles. Some scientists argue against this strenuously, although the work of Dr. Lester Packer has confirmed it.

4. In my opinion, if everyone received adequate amounts of vitamin E, the *actual* mean life span of seventy years would increase. In summarizing the above three points, I conclude that the role of vitamin E in aging is twofold: a deficiency causes accelerated aging; a nutritional excess may inactivate free-radicals. Although vitamin E supplements may shift the *actual* mean life span, they will not significantly shift the *natural* mean life span, the life span of those individuals living under perfect conditions. ☼

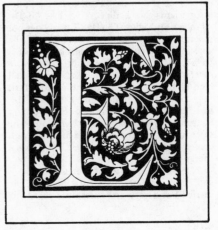

Hypoglycemia

(continued from page 83)

Every 2 hours until bedtime—4 ounces of milk or a small handful of nuts.

Allowable vegetables: Asparagus, avocado, beets, broccoli, Brussels sprouts, cabbage, cauliflower, carrots, celery, cucumbers, corn, eggplant, lima beans, onions, peas, radishes, sauerkraut, squash, string beans, tomatoes, turnips.

Allowable fruits: Apples, apricots, berries, grapefruit, pears, melons, oranges, peaches, pineapples. May be cooked or raw, with or without cream. *Note:* Do not use sugar! Canned fruits should be packed in water, not syrup. Read the label.

Eat all you want: Lettuce, mushrooms, nuts.

Drink all you want: Any *unsweetened* fruit or vegetable juice *except* grape juice or prune juice.

Beverages: Weak tea (tea ball, not brewed); decaffeinated coffee and coffee substitutes.

Desserts: Fruits, unsweetened gelatin, junket (made from tablets, not mix).

Alcoholic and soft drinks: Club soda, dry ginger ale, whiskey and other liquors.

AVOID ABSOLUTELY

Sugar, candy and other sweets, such as cake, pie, pastries, sweet custards, puddings and ice cream.

Caffeine: Avoid ordinary coffee, strong brewed tea, beverages containing caffeine. Consult with your physician about these taboo beverages for your individual case.

Avoid potatoes, rice, grapes, raisins, plums, figs, dates and bananas.

Avoid spaghetti, macaroni and noodles. *(Editor's suggestion)*: Other high sugar and/or carbohydrate foods to avoid are pretzels, biscuits, crackers, etc.)

Avoid wines, cordials, cocktails and beer.

(Editor's note: We have included bacon, ham, soft drinks and distilled liquors in this diet, as Dr. Abrahamson does, but it would be wise to eliminate them, too. And be sure to remember that you must obtain a complete examination by your physician and then request his personally-prescribed food program for your specific condition.)

Seale Harris, M.D., the pioneer-discoverer of the hypoglycemic problem, puts his patients on a diet very close to Dr. Abrahamson's diet. The Harris plan does not recommend avocado or beets, and the amount of nuts eaten for snacks is limited to a handful. The amount of in-between-meal milk is reduced to four ounces and ham or bacon is not suggested for breakfast.

Psychiatrist Juan Carlos DeTata, M.D., in a medical paper entitled *Research on Relative Hypoglycemic Syndrome,* tells of treating neurotic patients at a mental health center by using prescribed nutritional therapy.

Dr. DeTata writes of the results:

"We have at this mental health clinic carried out a very simple research consisting of 23 patients who came for outpatient pschiatric treatment in which we suspected the presence of relative hypoglycemic syndrome.

"We utilized a very similar diet to the so-called Harris Diet and we were able to bring about a tremendous (mental) improvement in those patients who cooperated with the diet.

"It is also interesting to note that the local people's diet is mostly starchy, consisting of rice and some vegetable products and they have tremendous difficulty in following a high-protein diet. Also, they are reluctant to abandon coffee. However, in the few cases that did follow our diet, they improved wonderfully.

"Increased ingestion of *calcium* to improve their concomitant hypoglycemia was also recommended ... We certainly insist that every patient with emotional upset try to discover if he is not suffering concomitantly from relative hypoglycemia."

The well-known John W. Tintera, M.D., writing in the *New York State Journal of Medicine* (Vol. 55, No. 13, page 1875) states clearly that *eight out of ten patients in mental hospitals may be victims of hypoglycemia.*

This is quite startling and should alert the medical profession and lay populace to the need for testing for hypoglycemia as part of the routine examination.

Dr. Tintera's hypoglycemic diet agrees with the basic diets listed above except that he recommends acidophilus milk, peanut butter, soybeans and soybean products. Also, he adds hot and cold cereals to the foods to *avoid.*

Dr. Harry Salzer in his article, "Frontiers of Hospital Psychiatry" in *Roche Reports,* emphasizes the strong relationship between emotional disorders and how they may be corrected by strict adherence to a diet regimen which would consist of:

1. High protein
2. Low carbohydrate
3. Frequent feedings
4. No caffeine

In the *Journal of the National Medical Association* Dr. Salzer tells of treating some 300 mental patients. All had previously been treated with sedatives, tranquilizers and even electro-shock therapy. No improvement was noted. Dr. Salzer then tried this special and all-natural hypoglycemia diet:

1. Vegetables included fresh broccoli, Brussels sprouts, cabbage, cauliflower, carrots and others low in carbohydrates.

2. Non-sweetened all-natural fruits such as apples, berries and grapefruit.

3. *Taboo* were sugar-rich soft drinks, caffeine-containing coffee which would affect and disturb sugar metabolism. (Editor's note: high protein was also recommended such as lean meat, fish, and cheese.)

Dr. Salzer reports that more than eight out of ten of the institutionalized inmates were either greatly improved or entirely recovered. A wholesome, natural and low-sugar, low-starch, high-protein diet had turned the tide and restored mental-emotional health.

Dr. Abrahamson tells of treating a middle-aged woman. She was emotionally ill and had a long history of mental depression. For seventeen years, she had been out socially only four times. She had been treated by more than sixty doctors. She had gone to more than twenty sanatoriums. Doctors advised shock treatments but these were never given.

Instead, she was put on the special low blood sugar diet. She began on Tuesday. By the following Saturday, she was so improved that she asked her husband to take her to a movie for the first time in years. This corrective diet therapy helped her improve her emotional disorder within one short week!

WHY A SUGAR-FREE DIET HELPS EMOTIONAL HEALTH

It has often been suggested that a good way to raise the sugar in the blood is by eating sugar or sugar foods. But the problem here is that foods containing refined sugar or starch (which is quickly changed into sugar) create internal upheaval. The body's mechanism for handling sugar is either triggered too rapidly or is first delayed and then set into action very speedily.

If triggered too rapidly, the blood sugar shows little or no rise following the eating of sugar.

If the body first delays and then sets speedy action, the blood sugar rises abnormally high and then drops abnormally low.

It is this see-saw and up-and-down insulin yank that leads to erratic and disturbed emotional temperament. A sugar-free diet is beneficial in that it permits the body's sugar-handling mechanism to be more stabilized by slow-metabolizing protein and healthful fats.

What about strong coffee or commercial tea?

Again, these substances, like alcohol and tobacco, act as a stimulant because they contain caffeine or tannic acid. Drug-like, they whip up the adrenals and trigger a reaction similar to that of eating sugar. That is, there are quick spurts of energy followed by quick let-downs. Again, it becomes a vicious up-and-down emotional cycle.

Nearly all cola drinks, chocolate and cocoa contain caffeine and create the same effect upon the body and the mind. Therefore, it is best to eliminate these non-foods from your corrective eating program.

HOW A "MENTAL CASE" USED THE ABRAHAMSON DIET TO COME BACK TO THE LIVING

A woman told her tragic story to columnist Mary Haworth in the *Washington Post.* This woman suffered emotional depression because of hyperinsulinism (another name for hypoglycemia). Unaware about corrective diet treatment, she underwent suffering and costly medication. In her own words:

"I began drinking much coffee, heavily sweetened, to clear my head and spur myself to longer, harder hours of work. Result: more depression, worsening symptoms. Suicide beckoned, but I made a desperate search for help. I had simple surgery, blood transfusions, hormone

270

therapy, sedatives, tonics. No improvement. A certain tranquilizer put me in lower spirits than ever. Finally psychiatry!"

She tells of having one brief interview with a psychiatrist (no physical or laboratory tests) and her husband was informed that she should have electro-shock treatments. She was sent to the hospital, underwent the treatment. She resolved to escape. She pretended optimism "even while wanting to scream out against this excursion into Hell."

After ten treatments in two weeks, she was taken home, supposedly "well" but worse than ever. She felt totally lost, completely disoriented. She had forgotten how to cook. She could not add. Her clothing was strange. She forgot the names or identities of neighbours and friends. She suffered from dizzy spells, blackouts and was obsessed with wanting to die.

Someone sent her a copy of the Abrahamson book and its diet. She tried it. She went to a physician who gave her special blood sugar tests. Now, the reason for her mental disorder was identified as low blood sugar. She went on the above described corrective diet. "Three months later, I have a wonderful sense of well-being and look thirty years younger than I did eight months ago."

It was natural nutrition that restored her sanity!

PROPER DIET HELPS RESTORE MARRIAGE

Many marriage counselors have reported that family strife can be healed with dietary improvement. For example, Cecilia Rosenfeld, M.D., wrote in *New Medical Horizons* (Humanist Council of Southern California), "In my own practice, I found that a surprising number of 'broken marriage' spouses suffered from a blood-sugar imbalance. Many of these husbands and wives showed symptoms of irritability, violent temper, abnormal sensitivity and extreme fatigue."

Dr. Rosenfeld finds that hypoglycemia is a prime cause of marital discord. She offers this case as an example:

T.E., a fifty-three year old business executive, suffered for ten years from such symptoms as intense migraine headaches, constant depression and irritability.

He was so difficult to live with that his wife finally gave up in despair and started divorce proceedings. Fortunately, the family physician noted that T.E. had a serious low blood sugar problem. The doctor put him on the special diet with emphasis on high-protein and low-sugar and low-carbohydrates. Within two months, the symptoms disappeared. Dr. Rosenfeld reports that he and his wife became happily reunited. Now he was a joy to live with.

Just as in T.E.'s case, others who suffer from hypoglycemia with its related emotional disorders, are put on a program that forbids these foods: candy, cake, chewing gum, pastries, pie, puddings, jelly, ice cream and other sugar-laden foods. The benefit here is to help reduce the excessive sugar-starch intake and normalize the hormonal balance. Since starches are broken down into sugar by the body, there has to be a restriction of these starch-rich foods: beans, noodles, potatoes, rice, spaghetti, etc.

Hypoglycemic sufferers feel many emotional disturbances in early mid-morning and mid-afternoon. For this reason, a hearty breakfast and between-meal feedings of milk and fruit are advised to prevent any slackening off of blood sugar levels which are prone to occur two to three hours after eating. Those who note emotional symptoms occurring in mid-morning and/or mid-afternoon would do well to obtain doctor-prescribed dietary suggestions to help maintain a tranquil blood sugar level.

CORRECTIVE NUTRITION EASES INBORN ERRORS

A specialist in internal medicine, Nicholas R. Occhino, M.D., writing in *Nutritional Reviews* describes persons suffering from symptoms of mental illness who were restored to emotional health by following a corrective food program to help normalize the blood sugar level.

Dr. Occhino says that *inborn errors of metabolism resulting in mental disorders may often be corrected by properly prescribed natural nutrition.*

This offers much hope for those who claim they were "born" with a mental illness.

Please note: The various food programs presented have some contrasting items, because health is as personal as your fingertips, and so there are differences in programs. It is essential to seek your own doctor-prescribed personal diet. The preceding is presented solely as an informative guideline.

But in any diet, always select natural, whole grain, unbleached and chemical-free foods. These are brimming with Nature-bestowed vitamins-minerals-proteins-enzymes that help build body-mind health.

We now have enough evidence to show that emotional illnesses ranging from daily tensions to institutionalized confinement can respond to proper, doctor-prescribed nutrition. It offers hope for the future of emotional health—the natural way. ☼

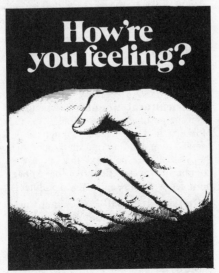

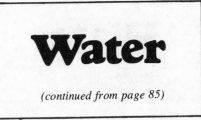

Water

(continued from page 85)

million. This means there are 50 million people dependent upon individual home supplies of water which is anything but drinkable.

☐ Our country's most navigable rivers are also the most heavily populated in terms of shipping and cities. They are to all intents and purposes open sewers. The Ohio, the Mississippi, the Hudson, the Missouri and the Colorado are polluted. Water is everywhere, true, but it is unfit to use. Here are more reported facts:

☐ **New York:** A Long Island housewife draws a glass of "fresh" tap water and discovers it has a two-inch head of foam. No, it is not beer. It is polluted water with an oily, fishy taste.

☐ **Mid-West:** A community in Kansas, faced with recurring problems of drought, tries to recycle water from its sewage treatment plant directly into its purification plant. Yes, the water meets "health standards" but the "foam" rises in every glass, piles up in fifteen foot billows at the water works and blows like snow!

☐ **West:** Along the Animas River in Colorado and New Mexico, where a uranium mill dumps its waste, drinking water contains 40 to 160 percent more than maximum safety levels of radioactivity.

☐ **Eastern Seaboard:** An outbreak of hepatitis along the Eastern Seaboard is traced to oysters raked from the Gulf of Mexico and to clams taken from New Jersey's Raritan Bay and along the Connecticut coast. These waters filter into tap water.

☐ **Missouri:** Gas bubbles rise from the sludge in the Missouri River below Sioux City, where a packing house unloads tons of animal entrails. Downstream, Omaha uses the river for drinking water.

☐ **New England:** Typhoid fever breaks out in New Hampshire. Hepatitis cases set a new record. Leptospirosis, known as "sewer worker's fever," suddenly crops up in the area. Health departments in a number of cities note an upsurge in diarrhea, intestinal disorders and stomach sickness. In each case, water is the obvious virus carrier.

☐ In the publication, *Community Water Supply Study,* issued by the Environmental Protection Agency, Dr. Charles C. Johnson, Jr., has written this warning:

(continued on page 272)

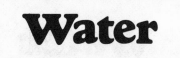

Water

(continued from page 271)

☐ "Our water resources, more perhaps than any other, illustrate the interaction of all parts of the environment, and also the recycling process that characterizes every resource of the biosphere. Everything that man injects into his environment —chemical, biological or physical—can ultimately find its way into the earth's water. These contaminants must be removed by nature or man before the water is potable.

☐ "Concern for our water quality until quite recently has centered principally on the danger of bacteriological contamination from inadequately treated sewage discharged from our rivers and streams. Today we are confronted with the fact that chemical pollution of source waters poses additional and possibly even more difficult problems. Moreover, we deceive ourselves if we assume that even the most complete and effective treatment of municipal and industrial wastes can ever remove all threats of water contamination. Actually, several million people drink water containing potentially hazardous amounts of chemical or bacteriological contamination."

☐ Dr. Johnson's study points out that most of our municipal water supply systems were constructed over twenty years ago; and that since they were built, the populations that they serve have increased rapidly, thus placing a greater and greater strain on plant and sand distribution system capacity. Moreover, he writes, when these systems were built, not enough was known to design a facility for the removal of toxic chemical or virus contaminates. They were designed solely to treat raw water of high quality for the removal of coliform bacteria. Such facilities, he shows, rapidly become obsolete as demands rise for water.

☐ Chemical contaminates in our environment have been on the increase for about twenty-five years, the report goes on, due to the dramatic expansion in the use of chemical compounds for agricultural, industrial, institutional and domestic purposes. There are 12,000 different toxic chemical compounds in industrial use today, and more than 500 new chemicals are developed each year. Wastes from these chemicals—synthetics, adhesives, surface coatings, solvents and pesticides—are already entering our ground and surface waters, and this trend can only increase.

☐ The extreme danger in all this, the Johnson report demonstrates, is that we know very little about the environmental and health impacts of these chemicals. We know very little about their genetic effects. We have difficulty in sampling and analyzing them—and finally, therefore, we cannot determine their contribution "to the total permissible body burden from all environmental insults."

☐ Are we drinking reasonably decent water today? Listen to Dr. Johnson's conclusion: "Consideration of these findings leaves no doubt that many systems are delivering drinking water of marginal or sub-marginal quality on the average, and many are delivering poor quality in one or more areas of their water distribution systems today."

Consider the water we drink

☐ Perhaps we might begin with some kind of definition of the ideal, or almost ideal, safe water. What is it? To begin with, it is free from harmful bacteria, free from viruses and unnecessary man-introduced chemicals. It should look clear, and should be free from objectionable odors or tastes. While some off-odor or off-taste does not necessarily suggest danger, it might suggest an unusual condition leading to unhealthy water or water to be avoided. For example: **1.** An off-color may be the result of the presence of inorganic materials or metals; **2.** An off-taste may suggest the presence of many inorganic materials that cannot be properly handled by the body; **3.** Turbidity (cloudiness) should alert the user to the fact that the water has been improperly treated and that it contains insoluble material.

☐ Actually, however, the ideal in water for most people is a figment of the imagination—for if most of the tap water of today was analyzed, this is what we could expect to find:

☐ **Silt**—soil suspended in water because the chemicalized soil was washed out by rain from land devoid of cover.

☐ **Municipal sewage**—because of the increased dumping of untreated or insufficiently treated sewage into the nation's waterways.

☐ **Industrial waste**—because the increase in industrial effluent and inadequate sewage means that such pollutants as detergents, pesticides, bleaches and soap suds are increasingly infesting our waterways.

☐ **Agricultural pollutants**—resulting from the pesticides and billions of pounds of insecticides and weed and fungus killers sprayed over and dug into the ground over the years. It is believed that almost all community water supplies have been poisoned with these agricultural pollutants.

☐ **Detergents**—daily so much non-biodegradable (hard soap) detergents have been dumped into our waterways that control, local ordinances notwithstanding, become empty gestures. Decomposing or so-called "clean" detergents are also in our water but these, too, are unsuitable in pure drinking water which should contain no additives.

☐ **Radioactive wastes and fall-out** —radioactive raindrops disturb man and his water supply, as well as milk and growing crops. This waste and fall-out finds its way into our drinking water—carried on clouds and in the air. We inhale them every time we leave the house, thereby increasing the hazard to our health.

☐ **Thermal pollutants**—the result of the presence of hydroelectric plants, steam/electric factories and other industry complexes, and the resulting high heat and water temperature have adverse effects on the growth of oxidating bacteria and plants. Not to mention the damage and ecological upset they cause through mass milling of fish and wild life.

☐ **Transportation pollutants**—resulting from the heavy shipping along our inland waterways and in our oceans. The *Torrey Canyon* disaster was the most dramatic recent example of this. And there have been many other instances of oil waste discharge from ships killing sea birds and fouling beaches. Actually, few tankers and other ships afloat have suitable facilities for waste treatment. Garbage and effluent are usually dumped over the side, and the same cavalier treatment is usually given our waters from the oil and smoke discharged by outboard motors and other boat engines. All contaminate and contribute to the toxicity of our aquatic life.

Our Ever-Widening Water Crisis

☐ The urgency of our water problem today increases with the demand for ever more water. Very soon, the daily per capita consumption of water is expected to rise to 165 gallons. Five gallons of water, for example, are needed daily to wash our hands and face, shave and brush our teeth. Every time a toilet is flushed, seven gallons of water are used. Washing machines, air conditioners, garbage disposals and dishwashers generate heavy demands on our water supply. Domestic irrigation, watering of lawns and gardens can become critical factors in the increased use of water in the average residential community.

☐ To add to the crisis, our population has been constantly exploding in the direction of the suburbs, leading to almost overwhelming demands on our water supply from hundreds of new industries, countless new shopping centers and thousands of new homes.

☐ And while this is happening, salt water continues to intrude into our inland waterways and wells from our oceans and gulfs; the wasteful stripping of land goes on with its replacement of trees and undergrowth by paved streets and parking lots, causing quick, unexpected run-offs of rain into swiftly overflowing streams and rivers. The pollution expands—with billions and billions of gallons of potable water being contaminated in all ways, and for all the reasons we have already mentioned.

□ A victim of mighty pollution is the lower Colorado River, which in one way or another serves about fifteen million people. All rivers have natural salts, but the Colorado is not only unusually salty, it is also used for agricultural irrigation for some farms as far away as 150 miles. As the water travels over the irrigation ditches, it leaches salt from the soil and is returned to the river bed saltier than ever. Environmentalists warn that with the added pollution from industry, and expanding residential developments and resort complexes crowding its banks, the great Colorado River is overdrawn and on its way to bankruptcy. Nor can the leaching of salt and minerals from the soil benefit the food grown on the farms that use the river's waters.

□ Nature's systems are being distorted —the self-renewing cycles that rhythmically rejuvenate the land, air and water. While the land is being leached of nutrients and chemically exhausted and the water is becoming unfit to drink, we continuously pump millions of tons of solid matter and noxious gases into the atmosphere. This protective covering shields us from otherwise deadly radiation and admits the sun's lifegiving light and heat. It releases water as rain or snow to nourish plants and animals. It restores rivers and lakes. Solar energy gives water vapor back into the atmosphere from nearly three-quarters of the earth's surface covered by water. This vast amount of vapor is drawn up, chilled and distilled, then released in order to sustain all of life below—only to be corrupted by pollutants in the air and in the soil.

□ Nature's superb distilling system is designed to save our planet from extinction. About half of today's known chemical elements (in abundance and in traces) have been found dissolved in natural waters that you eventually drink. Lakes, streams and oceans contain quite concentrated solutions of literally thousands of substances in ionic form, metals as well as non-metals, with an average of up to 35,000 parts per million in sea water, somewhat less in fresh water. But when the vapor rises, it leaves chemicals and minerals behind. Only the purest of all water in the form of vapor is carried into the atmosphere.

□ As this vapor cools, it collects into little droplets which join others and fall to earth. It is the first drop beneath the clouds that contains the purest of all water. This is the drop Nature intended us to drink. It is pure H_2O, or distilled water. As soon as these drops descend, they begin to perform a twofold function: to purify the atmosphere and to pick up minerals for the plants below.

□ But our air has now become poisoned, our soils contaminated with chemicals such as pesticides that travel through the food chain to contaminate our bodies in turn. We have accumulated dangerous amounts of such poisons as mercury, lead, DDT, strontium 90 and nitrates in our bodies.

□ Nitrates are particularly hazardous to health. It is believed that nitrates in drinking water have caused "blue babies"; and they are at such a dangerous point of saturation that wells need to be dug deeper. This would be but a temporary measure, since as the water gets harder, the nitrates settle into the deeper wells. Furthermore, the faster that pumps are run, the more nitrates are leached into the water. Nitrates are considered as toxic as cadmium, nickel, lead or mercury. They belong in the chemist's laboratory and not in your drinking water.

□ What other problems are involved with drinking polluted water with its inorganic minerals? Since your body cannot assimilate inorganic minerals, they settle themselves into your joints in the form of arthritis, or in your kidneys and liver as "stones" or in the artery walls; they pave the way to a score of illnesses.

□ These are just a few of the hazards that cause trouble in the water that pours from your tap to be used by your body processes as a lifeline of health. Environmental deterioration has accelerated until it has reached the point of crisis. We must understand the problems we face if we are to solve them. It seems evident that as an important step, you should find the way to safe, healthy and nourishing water as close to the distilled water of nature as it is possible to get. ☼

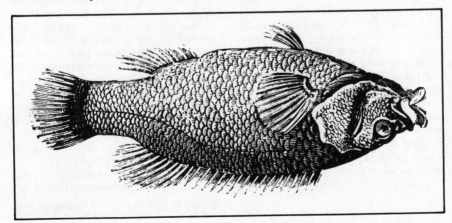

New, and Natural, Hope for the Arthritic

(continued from page 87)

and/or the unsalted, dehydrated vegetable powders to enhance the flavor of vegetables—this makes them more pleasurable, especially for those who previously have eaten little of these foods.

For those who feel the need for more substantial fare, the following menu is an example of how a wholesome, natural diet can be planned.

Breakfast

Any fresh fruit or berries in season, such as peaches, melons, grapes, apples, pears, raspberries, etc. Those who find this insufficient may add a very ripe banana.

If the above breakfast is inadequate, the following meal should prove more satisfactory:

1. Any fresh fruit or berries in season (from those mentioned above).

2. A small serving of natural brown rice or some natural whole-grain cereal, served with stewed fruit such as stewed peaches, apple sauce, baked apples, or baked or stewed pears. These should be eaten slowly and chewed thoroughly. (Various wholegrain cereals, and natural brown rice, are obtainable at health food stores.)

3. A cup of alfalfa tea or any of the other bland herb teas such as camomile, sassafras, linden blossom, etc., slightly sweetened with honey, or one glass of raw, skimmed milk. No sugar should be added to the stewed fruit and when milk is used, it should be sipped slowly or taken with a spoon.

Lunch

1. A large, raw vegetable salad.

2. Corn on the cob, baked or boiled unpeeled potato, or yams, or sweet potato, or wholewheat toast, with—or without—two steamed vegetables.

3. Baked apple, or stewed or soaked prunes, or any other unsulphured and unpreserved stewed fruit may be used for dessert, if still hungry.

Remember that fruits must be prepared without sweetening, and no salt or butter should be added to vegetables.

A large fruit salad composed of fresh fruits and berries in season with 4 to 5 oz. of either cottage, pot, farmer, or ricotta (Italian cottage) cheese,

(continued on page 274)

also provides a very satisfactory and wholesome lunch. (The British equivalent is curd or St. Ivel cheese.) We must be careful not to use cream cheese as it is too rich in fat.

Dinner

1. A large, raw vegetable salad.
2. A small portion of your favorite protein food.
3. One or two steamed vegetables.
4. Raw fruits or berries for dessert, if still hungry.

Those who choose the cheese meal mentioned above for lunch, would do well to use baked or boiled unpeeled potatoes or another wholesome starch food, in place of the protein, with their evening meal.

The soft, bland cheeses, lentils, the young, green (cooked) soy beans, or garbanzo beans, provide valuable protein but should be used in moderation. Almonds, sunflower seeds and pumpkin seeds, are other fine sources of protein, and may be used in small amounts in place of the protein foods suggested above. Those who cannot do without meat or fish may use small portions of lean fish or poultry or any lean meat, in place of the other protein foods, about two or three times a week. These foods may be served broiled or baked, but never fried.

The above illustrates the sort of diet that can be planned for those who suffer from these distressing ailments. The meals may be varied to suit individual taste, but should always be composed primarily of wholesome natural ingredients.

Make the Salad Your Main Dish

At this point we wish to reiterate that *uncooked natural foods provide the best and most valuable nourishment for the body.* Unless contraindicated because of certain digestive difficulties, raw vegetable salads should make up the major part of the meals, while the foods that are not eaten raw should be prepared only in the simplest way possible. Steaming or baking is best, to repeat once more.

Other Food Facts Worth Remembering

Bread, cereals and other grain foods should be used only very sparingly or not at all. Potatoes, carrots, beets and parsnips provide easily-digestible starches and are to be greatly preferred. Potatoes should be baked or boiled in their skins and eaten without any butter or salt.

The use of fats must be strictly controlled. Cold-pressed natural ôils such as soybean, safflower, wheat germ, or corn may be used in small amounts on the raw vegetable salad to enhance its flavor. *No fats should be used in cooking and again, no fried foods!*

Eggs contain valuable protein. However, they are rich in fat and contain a high amount of cholesterol. For these reasons they are best omitted from the diet. Other foods with a high cholesterol content are butter, cream, milk, fatty meats and the fatty cheeses. This includes practically all types of cheese, except Italian ricotta, cottage cheese (pot cheese), farmer cheese, or the unprocessed goat cheeses.

It should be obvious that the many refined sugars and sweets such as ice cream, candies, cakes, pastries, must be completely omitted. Even the highly concentrated natural sweet foods, e.g., figs, dates, raisins and honey, must be used very sparingly or not at all. Patients should obtain their sugar from fresh fruits: apples, pears, grapes, melons, as well as from the root vegetables: carrots, beets, parsnips, potatoes, yams, etc. Concentrated sugars, even those taken in natural form, lead to excessive fermentation and overstimulation and are not recommended.

Coffee and tea have to be eliminated. Alfalfa, alfa-mint, or any of the other herb teas may be substituted for coffee or regular tea and make fine beverages. A cup of hot vegetable broth made at home out of fresh vegetables, or prepared by adding one heaping teaspoonful of your favorite vegetable broth powder to a cup of boiling water, provides a desirable hot drink. Vegetable juice combinations—carrot and celery; carrot, celery and apple; carrot, cabbage and apple; carrot, celery and parsley—also provide excellent liquid vegetable nourishment. These juices should not be taken in too great quantities; not more than 6 to 8 oz. at any one time. Other beneficial mixtures of vegetables may be used.

A "juicer," or machine for extracting fresh, raw vegetable juices, and a blender are valuable additions to the home. These machines, together with a great variety of vegetable broth powders and tasty herb teas, are available at all good health food stores.

Steamed vegetables are delectable even when prepared without any seasonings, but those who have been accustomed to spices and condiments sometimes find these foods too bland at first. The addition of onion, garlic, dill, sage, assorted herb flavorings, or the vegetable broth powder will improve their flavor.

All irritating spices and condiments such as salt, pepper, mustard, vinegar, etc., and stimulants such as coffee and tea should be avoided. Alcohol is a depressant and must be eliminated. There are many ways of preparing enjoyable, tasty meals without resorting to irritating, health-damaging substances.

Under these circumstances, it seems to us that those who are in search of renewed health and well-being would derive infinitely more benefit if, instead of placing their faith in injections, potions, or medicines, they turned to natural food substances to obtain their required nutrients.

At this point it would be well to define the difference between the vitamins and other food supplements derived from natural sources and those produced synthetically from coal tar products or other chemicals. While chemically they may appear alike, nutritionally they are very different. The natural vitamins and food supplements derived from plants and other natural sources, especially when obtained in complete and unprocessed form, provide vital substances essential to life; those that are synthetically manufactured are mere chemical substances and can scarcely be regarded as foods.

We must realize that natural foods provide not only a wide variety of vitamins and minerals, but also many other vital constituents such as enzymes, co-enzymes, trace elements, protein and undoubtedly many more that have not yet been identified. All these are necessary for sound nutrition and have to complement each other if real and lasting benefits are to be achieved. Synthetic vitamins—even those in multiple formulae—are devoid of these associated nutrients and while, like drugs, they sometimes seemingly provide a temporary lift, they cannot be depended upon for permanent results. If used indiscriminately, they can even contribute to an upset in the body chemistry. *We have pointed out on many occasions that a deficiency of one vitamin or mineral presupposes a deficiency of other vitamins, minerals and associated nutritional factors.* ☼

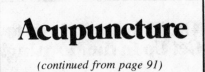

Acupuncture

(continued from page 91)

in the western world, and in Britain in particular, is that it defies any specific explanation. But who can explain how aspirin works? Digitalis, the heart drug made from fox-glove, slows the heart beat and increases its force, but nobody knows how it achieves this effect.

Adrenalin constricts the blood vessels in normal doses and acts as a dilator in minimal doses—for no explained reason.

They are all empirical; used as the result of observation and experiment, but with no irrefutable scientific explanation.

Acupuncture falls into exactly the same category. It has been used with great effect for thousands of years by a nation distinguished for its civilization, but there are no clinical test reports to say why.

But perhaps the greatest single proof of its effectiveness lies in the fact that for centuries it has been the practice of Chinese doctors only to charge fees as long as their patients remain healthy. If a patient is ill he pays no fees.

If is because of this that acupuncture has been developed with the emphasis on preventive therapy. The Chinese acupuncturist is skilled in recognizing an oncoming complaint and treating it before the symptoms have a chance to manifest themselves in pain and ill-health.

Certainly the training for acupuncturists is detailed and practical, and the graduate is permitted no margin of error if he wishes to qualify.

Exact copies of the human body in bronze, and perforated with the points of acupuncture, are kept in medical centres. For examinations, the holes are filled with wax, and the figure is covered in fine rice paper. The examinee is told to place the needles at certain points, and the needle must be inserted into the correct filled-in hole, or the student fails.

While it is easy to place the needles painlessly in a patient the practitioner must know what he is doing. There are certain points of acupuncture that should never be used by the unskilled.

Sceptics, of course, dismiss all this as some kind of primitive mumbo-jumbo, but fortunately there are a number of distinguished people who are more open-minded.

Aldous Huxley commented only a few years ago: "The fact remains that there are pathological symptoms on which Old Chinese methods work well."

For Dr. Moss the proof is contained in scores of letters from patients telling at length how his treatment by acupuncture has relieved and cured them of complaints which had defied the efforts of conventional medicine. And a patient's cure must surely be the most potent proof of the success of any medical treatment. He says: "They were told by the medical authorities to live with their pain or take aspirin, but what I have done to relieve them can soon be learnt by any medical practitioner who cares to study and follow my techniques.

"The suggestion that acupuncture achieves its results through some form of hypnotism is made nonsense of by the fact that it is employed in the treatment of sick animals."

The theory and practice of acupuncture is rooted in the Chinese concepts of life—the Tch'i—which, according to the old writings, is the beginning and the end, life and death.

In order to become a practising acupuncturist it is vital to study and understand the Chinese traditional medicine and philosophy, which is based on the interpretation and conception of Tch'i.

The belief, which has been handed down for thousands of years, is that all things animate and inanimate have a built-in factor of energy. This stabilizes the chemical composition of matter and when this matter is broken down, energy is released.

A simple illustration is contained in the fact that man is made of matter, and he also has life. These are his two sources of energy. The one is the electrical energy created by the biophysical and biochemical changes in his cells, and the life that is given to him at his birth.

But the Chinese in their medical teaching depart from the western view of life by believing that we are all one with the cosmos, obeying the rhythms of the natural order.

This oneness with the entire universe is represented by two forces contained within the Tch'i, known as the Yin and the Yang.

Yang is the positive force in man and nature—powerful elements such as heat, energy, virility, the lush, growing period of summer, the sun.

Yin, on the other hand, is the passive, almost negative force, seen at its most obvious during winter, when plant growth almost comes to a stand-

still, when certain animals hibernate. It happens daily in man when he sleeps.

A common example which we all experience is the low resistance we have to infection during the winter, and the surge of energy we experience in the spring, when nature is coming back to life.

Seasonal changes apart, it is a well known fact that the human body responds to barometric pressure. On a close, muggy day, the body feels heavy and listless, and everything we do is an effort. But on bright, sunny days, we literally bound with energy and enthusiasm.

People who suffer from rheumatic pains frequently claim they can forecast a change in the weather by the onset of pains, and many people respond emotionally to the flow of energy in their body. They can feel full of life, or deeply depressed for no apparent reason.

The condition of the energy flows can also be markedly influenced by the food we eat. Unsuitable food moving sluggishly in the digestive tract can create an unsatisfactory environment for the body, and the poisons produced by it will weaken certain digestive organs.

For really good health it is essential for the Tch'i to circulate in a balanced and unbroken manner. In the ancient Chinese treatises it is asserted: "The blood circulates following the energy. If the energy circulates, the blood circulates; if the energy is trapped, the blood stops."

According to the ancient Chinese system of medicine there are two categories of organs associated with the Tch'i. They are called the Tsang and the Fou.

The Fou is that group of organs which absorb food, digest it, and expel the waste products. They are all hollow organs such as the stomach, large and small intestines, bladder and gall-bladder, and are Yang by nature.

Tsang organs are all associated with the blood—the heart which circulates the blood around the body, the lungs which oxygenate the blood, the spleen in control of the red corpuscles, and the liver and kidneys. These are of the passive Yin force.

Both the Yin and the Yang have three grades of strength. In the case of Yang they are maximum, balanced and weak, and maximum, medium and weak for Yin.

It is vital in treatment to understand the flow of the energies. In the upper limb the three Yin meridians carry Yin energy which gradually

(continued on page 276)

Acupuncture:

(continued from page 275)

becomes Yang energy as it flows into the three Yang meridians of the upper limb. As the intermingling of energies takes place towards the end of the Yin meridians and the start of the Yang meridians, the energy is found to be unstable at the fingers, therefore it has been found that the best area for treating inbalance of energy is between the elbow and the fingers.

A similar mingling of the Yin and Yang meridians takes place in the lower limb, and the points for correcting inbalance are between the knee and toes.

The vital Tch'i, central to the whole balance of energy, flows through the meridians from the lungs to the large intestine, to the stomach, spleen, heart, small intestine and bladder on to the kidneys, circulation-sex, triple warmer, gall-bladder and liver, and then starts again.

For the flow of energy to remain steady it is dependent on the energy of one organ to another being unimpeded. If the organ is weak the resultant energy passed on to the next organ is weakened.

Acupuncture comes in as the stimulant to the meridian which corrects the fault.

Good health is dependent on the balanced flow of the Tch'i maintaining an unending cycle of energy. The fact that energy is not confined to the interior of the body is confirmed by western research over the last thirty years which has shown that there are great variations in the electrical potentials of the skin, and that certain areas show a much lessened resistance than the areas surrounding them. These areas follow certain well defined longitudinal lines and along them at certain points of the skin electrical resistance reaches zero.

Experiments by physiologists and electronic engineers using highly sensitive and sophisticated electronic apparatus discovered nearly 800 points of acupuncture.

It is an extraordinary coincidence that the Chinese over the centuries have identified nearly 800 points of acupuncture.

In other words, the human body is a highly complex electrical circuit, formed by biochemical processes in the body. Like any electrical circuit it must be kept in good working order if it is to function effectively. If you take a bulb out of a set of Christmas Tree lights the set will not work. If the human circuit breaks down the result is illness, or even death.

This basically is what acupuncture is all about—it keeps the human circuit in good order.

There can be no doubt in this day and age that the stress of modern life is an environmental condition which is reflected by the nervous system. A considerable body of opinion believes that the prime cause of illnesses, such as coronary thrombosis, high blood pressure, gastric and duodenal ulcers and rheumatic pains is not due so much to faulty feeding, bad teeth, draughts or dampness, as to the stress of modern living.

Our reactions to general environmental conditions are governed by the nerve endings. If it is cold, nerves cause the tiny blood vessels in the skin to contract, causing more blood to go into the deeper arteries and so prevent heat loss from the body. If the body is too warm, these nerves cause the skin blood vessels to relax and expose a larger amount of blood to be cooled.

These nerves are under the control of what is called the autonomic or "self-governing" nervous system. The autonomic nervous sytem is formed by two sets of nerves arising from the spinal cord, called the sympathetic and para-sympathetic. The impulses originating from these nerves must always be balanced to co-ordinate the functions of the various organs and to keep the body in good health, just as the Chinese affirm that the Tch'i must flow evenly through the whole extent of the network of the twelve meridians and the various linking channels.

Acupuncture is quite clear that there is a complete association between the brain and the various nervous systems controlling the movement of muscles and joints, therefore the stimulation of the nerves of one system that supplies an organ or structure will often influence other points served by different nerves. It is what is known as reflex action.

An illustration of this is the example of a painful neuritis down the arm being a frequent symptom in diseases of the heart. Pneumonia may refer pain to the region of the appendix, and pain in the region of the appendix may be referred to the chest. An infection of the gall-bladder or stomach may refer pain to the muscles of the lower shoulder girdle. These findings could be multiplied ten-fold showing that there is a two-way connection between the skin and all the organs in the body. ☼

Oh, How You'll Love to Get Up in the Morning!

(continued from page 105)

or trimming the vegetables; let everyone prepare their own. Just place a large bowl on the table to hold the egg shells, vegetable peelings, and the like.

Cheese Pudding

If you find it more convenient you can assemble the Cheese Pudding an evening in advance and refrigerate it until morning. You can then put it in the oven first thing and prepare the rest of breakfast while it bakes.

12 slices stale whole-grain bread
12 ounces cheese, sliced or grated
4 eggs
2 cups milk
1 teaspoon salt
1/2 teaspoon dry mustard powder
1 tablespoon butter

Arrange pieces of bread over the bottom of a greased, shallow 2-quart baking dish. Cover with cheese and repeat the layers, ending with bread. Beat eggs, add milk and seasonings. Pour over bread and cheese and dot top with butter. Bake in a 350° oven 20 minutes. Let set 5 minutes and serve.

Makes 6 servings; each furnishing 450 calories and 28 grams protein.

Cottage Cheese Fondue

A Cottage Cheese Fondue served with fresh fruits for dipping is a fine idea for company breakfasts and informal breakfast buffets in particular.

2 tablespoons butter
2 cups (1 pound) cottage cheese
3 tablespoons milk
2 tablespoons honey
1 teaspoon grated lemon rind
1/4 teaspoon cinnamon
1/8 teaspoon nutmeg

Melt butter in saucepan. Add cottage cheese, 1/2 cup at a time, and stir over moderate heat until cheese becomes liquidy and curd separates out. After all the cheese is added and the mixture is soft, but lumpy, transfer to a blender container and process at low speed until smooth and creamy. Pour into a fondue pot and set over the warmer. Add the milk, honey and grated lemon rind and stir until smooth and warmed through. Sprinkle with cinnamon and nutmeg. To serve, skewer tangerine sections, whole berries, pineapple chunks and other fruits of your choice on fondue forks and coat with the creamy cheese mixture.

Makes approximately 2-1/2 cups fondue; 1/2 cup furnishes 166 calories and 12.5 grams protein.

Fish Hash
When made with an inexpensive variety such as cod or haddock, Fish Hash is economical as well as good tasting. Only minutes to prepare.
1 pound white-fleshed fish, filleted
4 tablespoons fresh bread crumbs
2 tablespoons oil
1 tablespoon salt
1/2 teaspoon sugar
dash of pepper
1/4 cup yogurt

Cut fish fillets into bite-size pieces. Sauté fish and bread crumbs in oil, stirring until fish separates easily into flakes. This will take, at the most, 10 minutes. Add seasonings, remove from heat and stir in yogurt. Serve plain or on toast.

Makes 4 breakfast servings.

Sardine Spread
1 can (about 3-3/4 ounces) sardines
2 tablespoons cottage cheese
2 teaspoons lemon juice
1/4 teaspoon mustard

Mash together all ingredients and spread on crackers or toast. Serve cold, or better still, broil quickly, about 1 minute, to heat through.

Makes about 1/2 cup spread; enough for 8 crackers or 2 pieces of toast.

"Gothic" Brunch
Gets rave reviews served over hot biscuits, English muffins, or small baked potatoes.
2 cups canned salmon (1 pound)
skim milk
2 tablespoons chopped onion
2 tablespoons oil
2 tablespoons cornstarch
pepper
1-1/2 cups cottage cheese

Drain liquid from salmon and add enough milk to it to equal 1 cup. Sauté onion in oil until tender and transparent. Remove from heat and, using a wire whisk, stir in cornstarch to make a smooth paste. Add liquid and stir over moderate heat until thickened, 5 to 10 minutes. Season with pepper, stir in cottage cheese, and heat, stirring gently, until cheese melts. Add salmon, stir, warm, and serve immediately.

Makes 4 servings. ☼

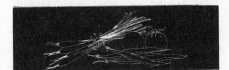

The Magic of Sprouting... How Does It Happen?

(continued from page 107)

folic acid in the germinating seeds of peas *(Pisum sativum)*, mung beans *(Phaseolus aureus)*, rice, wheat, Bengal gram *(Dilichos lablab)*, lentils, horse gram *(Dolichos biflorus)*, gram or chickpeas *(Cicer arietinum)*, Kalai *(Phaseolus mungo)*, barley, cow-gram or black-eyed peas *(Vigna catiang)*, and kidney or haricot beans *(Phaseolus vulgaris)*. In the early 1940s the United States Army had sponsored investigations in sprouted seeds, hoping to establish their suitability for military use; they found similar rises in the B-vitamin contents of peas, soybeans, navy beans, kidney beans, pinto beans and lima beans. These investigations were based on earlier work by Paul Burkholder and Ida McVeigh on wheat, barley, corn, oats, soybeans, mung beans, lima beans and peas. All of these investigators found significant increases in B vitamins and usually waxed enthusiastic over the prospect of incorporating sprouts into the diet. Dr. Burkholder concluded, "If the food value of germinated seeds is to be judged by their content of vitamins and readily available amino acids, then it appears that the common use of sprouts in the diets of Oriental peoples rests on a sound nutritional basis and should be introduced on a wide scale among Occidentals."

Peaks of the various B-vitamins seem to occur at different stages of the germinating process. Thiamine, vitamin B-1, which was originally known as the anti-beriberi vitamin, shows a maximum use at 120 hours in lentils and Kalai (an Indian pulse known as urd or black gram), but peaks at 48 hours in black-eyed peas and chick-peas. Increases are not nearly as spectacular as in some of the other B-vitamins, however, and agreement on them not nearly as universally held, with some investigators finding no appreciable change in the thiamine content during the first four days, the stage at which consumption is recommended, others recording small increases, especially in the grains; and others, apparently using a different method of bioassay, reporting increases from 400 to 2,000 percent in thiamine content after five days of germination. After the appearance of leaves and the changeover from stored energy to photosynthesis, thiamine increases greatly, and the last-mentioned figures could

possibly be explained in this way. Feeding experiments attempting to find a cure for beriberi or polyneuritis, as it was called at the time of these experiments, show that sprouts may be a good source of vitamin B-1; pigeons with severe beriberi were cured on a ration of one and one-half grams of sprouted mung 'beans daily. Another feeding experiment found that one-half gram of the dried sprout maintained the weight of experimental animals, but one gram of dried beans was ineffective in prevention.

Riboflavin, or vitamin B-2, which is considered the growth promoting factor of the B-vitamins, is universally reported as increasing markedly in all parts of the seedling, especially when grown in the dark. Riboflavin is the only B-vitamin destroyed by the presence of light, but it is continually synthesized in seedlings, and thus even seeds germinated in direct sunlight contain more B-2 than dormant seeds do. Under natural conditions, of course, seeds sprout in the ground or under some sort of cover; normally, they are not exposed to light until the cotyledon pushes the leaves above the surface of the earth, when photosynthesis begins. Most researchers report increases of at least 100 percent in B-2 during this stage; several find much greater increments. Methods of storing and handling of foodstuffs that can be a reliable source of this vitamin may ignore its light-sensitivity; milk that is bottled in clear glass may lose most of its B-2 with only a few hours' exposure to sunlight. The interdependency of the B-complex makes it important to have a good source of every one of them, and sprouted seeds are an excellent source of this especially elusive one.

Niacin, or nicotinic acid, the pellagra-preventing vitamin, also increases markedly during germination. Pulses (leguminous seeds) contain approximately three times the original amount of niacin in the seed after four days of germination. Whole wheat grains are rich in the entire B-complex group; their niacin content almost doubles with germination.

It is suspected that the entire B-complex has yet to be isolated and identified; nine factors in addition to the three well-studied ones above have been isolated and named, but experimental animals do not thrive on synthetic diets that contain only the identified vitamins. (Perhaps this is the strongest argument against depending entirely upon the use of synthetic vitamin pills, which may be incomplete in these unknown substances, and an equally compelling

(continued on page 278)

The Magic of Sprouting... How Does It Happen?

(continued from page 277)

reason for choosing a variety of natural food sources of vitamins. The unknown substances probably occur as part of the growth process, even though they are unknown, unnamed and unsung in the literature.) Pantothenic acid, para-aminobenzoic acid, pyridoxine (B-6), choline, inositol, biotin, orotic acid and vitamin B-12 are all found in germinating seeds, and although the increases are by no means equal, all show some rises as a result of germination. The reports on folic acid are mixed; one researcher reports an increase and another a decrease. Substantial increases in biotin, choline, inositol, and pantothenic acid are well-documented.

Vitamin B-12 of which milk is one of the few good sources, increases in germinating seeds; one serving of sprouts provides the amount needed daily. Leafy vegetables contain no B-12 unless grown on manured soil. Yeast, wheat germ and soybeans contain traces. Many vegetarians who eliminate eggs and milk from the diet may suffer from a dangerous-and-difficult-to-recognize deficiency of B-12,

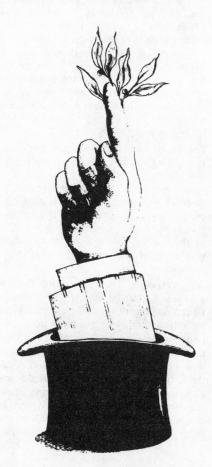

especially when masked by an abundance of folic acid, usually richly supplied in vegetarian diets. Studies now going on in Great Britain on multi-generation vegetarians may indicate an imbalance of the B-complex that could be irreversibly dangerous. In our country, the sale of folic acid tablets has recently been severely restricted by federal law. Work done so far on the folic-acid B-12 ratio of sprouts points to a much more favorable balance for vegetarians than most other foods contain. More research in this area is urgently needed.

The vitamin C content of sprouted seeds has been demonstrated by their historical context; long before vitamin C was identified and isolated, the anti-scorbutic qualities of malt and sprouted beans were being exploited in many parts of the world — in times of famine and on long ocean voyages. The recent controversy over the use of massive doses of vitamin C as a cure for the common cold has refocused attention on this vitamin, but it is not my intention to enter this fray, since the amount of vitamin C that one can consume in a single reasonable serving of sprouted seeds does not approach megavitamin treatment. However, this reasonable serving of sprouts provides approximately the recommended adult daily requirement of vitamin C — 70 milligrams (U.S. National Research Council). One-third of that amount has been shown to effectively prevent scurvy in man.

The initial vitamin increment during germination is so pronounced, however, that sprouted seeds have been used in studies of vitamin C formation pathways. The mechanism is enzymatic in nature and takes place at the expense of sugar. Legumes are generally better sources than grains. Whether the increment is measured by chemical methods or by feeding trials on guinea pigs, the vitamin C content of sprouted seeds is remarkable; 100 grams of mung beans (about 3½ ounces), when sprouted, contain 120 milligrams of vitamin C. The same weight of Bengal gram or chickpeas yields 75 milligrams. The vitamin content of these legume sprouts compares favorably with orange juice, tomatoes and lemon juice as a source of vitamin C.

Germination in any seed is always accompanied by an intense enzymatic hydrolysis of protein. This means that stored proteins are broken down into their component amino acids, just as they are when the body digests them. This explains why sprouts are more easily assimilated and less gas-forming than dried beans; they are already partly digested. On the average, digestibility doubles with sprouting.

Amino acids increase in number (on a dry weight basis) as germination continues at the expense of carbohydrates and fats as the plant synthesizes proteins appropriate to its new needs. The whole process takes

place because the protein needs of a seedling are different from those of a seed. Reserve proteins, stored by the seed for just this event in its life, are broken down. One might compare this situation with a complicated house of cards, which is demolished so the cards will be available to construct an entirely different but equally complex house. The blueprint for the new house is called DNA; the builder is called Messenger RNA. The plant is capable of making both blueprint and builder all by itself.

The biological value of sprouted seeds, which is measured by the weight gained as a proportion of the total weight of sprouts eaten, surpasses the biological value of seeds in every case. The reason for this may be that the composition (i.e., relative balance) of the amino acid pattern changes little, but essential amino acids increase in value at the expense of nonessential ones. All amino acid values go up, increasing both in number and in concentration. Total protein content of sprouted seeds, then rises significantly during germination. Mung beans contain 25.07 percent protein, but sprouted mung beans contain 37.30 percent (on a dry weight basis); yellow soybeans increase from 42.99 percent protein in dry seeds to 50.26 percent in sprouts.

For centuries it has been observed that heating improved the value of legume seeds, but only recently has the limiting factor been isolated. A heat-labile trypsin or proteolytic inhibitor, which interferes with the utilization of protein, is present in all raw beans and peas. Why beans and peas should manufacture this substance is not known; it may act as a natural preservative during the drying process. Cooking for as little as five minutes destroys 95 percent of the trypsin inhibitor, and this improves digestibility and biological values for legumes. The trypsin inhibitor retards the very hydrolysis (digestion of protein) that germination begins; thus, germinated raw beans have a higher biological value than ungerminated raw beans. This explains why the nutritive value of raw germinated soybeans is higher than that of raw meal, even though the trypsin factor is unchanged. Cooking germinated legumes additionally improves their values; the efficiency (i.e., percent of protein absorbed) of protein in cooked germinated legumes rates higher than that of raw seeds, raw sprouts or cooked seeds. The value of an amino acid pattern may be judged by comparing it with egg protein, the most useful for humans; if eggs rate 100 (gain in weight per gram of protein consumed), raw soybeans rate 39, cooked soybeans rate 68 and cooked sprouted soybeans rate 75. Heating also makes the limiting amino acid in legumes, methionine, more available. Grains do not contain the trypsin inhibitor; it is therefore not as important to cook them before eating.

The proteins of all grains and legumes are incomplete in some ways, although soybeans and whole wheat are nearly as good as meat; for a thorough discussion of protein completeness and supplementation, see Frances Moore Lappé's *Diet for a Small Planet,* published by Ballantine.

Germination is also characterized by a decrease in the dry weight of the seed. (The swelling of the seed due to imbibition makes it weigh a great deal more, of course; the dry weight is what is left after all the water is taken out. Dry weight is the only accurate way to measure real changes, since only then are we making a true comparison of seed with sprout. Even the driest, hardest seed does contain some, but not much, moisture.) The overall loss in dry weight is 20 to 25 percent; this is due to respiratory losses, leakage of soluble materials and the energy loss when the reserve protein and carbohydrate are metabolized. Loss in dry weight reflects a loss in caloric content. This is a real gain in any diet, for one exchanges high-calorie fats and carbohydrates for vitamins and protein that are more difficult to find. The carbohydrates are changed to sugars, the same ones found in the fresh fruits and recently picked vegetables that give them their superlative flavor. As the root emerges, the sugar content rises rapidly. By the sixth day, starch is reduced from 30 to 5.4 percent; total sugars rise from 1.5 to 8.3 percent. The enzyme responsible for this is alpha-amylase, which is found in the mouth of every human above the age of six months; immediately after the imbibition phase, this enzyme shows a great increase. Oils are also depleted, and play an important role in carbohydrate metabolism. The free fatty acid percentage of crude fat present in the seed rises, even though the total fat content changes very little; the saturated fatty acid content drops after four days. The tocopherol content increases during germination and the alpha-tocopherol especially; this last mentioned one is the elusive vitamin E. From the point of view of human nutrition, these last two metabolic patterns are extremely fortunate; vitamin E is highly unstable since it is quickly destroyed if exposed to air. Oils and whole grains, refined, hydrogenated and heated to high temperatures in processing, contain little. Saturated fats (butter and animal fats as well as hydrogenated oils and natural coconut and palm kernel oil) seem to be used more widely than unsaturated liquid vegetable oil in our diet; a good balance is half saturated, half unsaturated, but few average diets maintain this. Sprouts provide us with an excellent, yet inexpensive, way to obtain these difficult nutrients. ☼

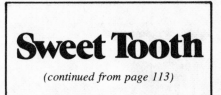

Sweet Tooth

(continued from page 113)

tion. He points out that the addition of sugar to all commercial and bottled baby foods, besides soft drinks and sweetened cereals and all the other treats children consume, has greatly increased the number of fat children.

Also, he states, "You may find it difficult to believe, but when you have really become used to taking very little sugar in your food and drinks, you will notice that all your foods have a wide range of interesting flavors that you had forgotten. Swamping everything with sugar tends to hide the flavors and blunts the sensitivity of your palate. You will especially notice how much you enjoy fruit — all the subtle difference between one sort of apple or pear or orange and another."

Natural ingredients should be used not only for health reasons, but also for their superior taste and flavor. Natural fruit sugar can be just as concentrated as refined sugar, but it hasn't been subjected to chemicals, and, in addition, it contains valuable minerals. Also, the type of sugar found in whole foods is more complex than the refined sugar you buy in a store. Natural fruit and grain sugars are absorbed differently by the body, and additionally they contain nutrients that aid in digestion and assimilation. They also take more time to be digested, since they must first be broken down into simpler forms.

What about brown and raw sugar? The amounts of vitamins and minerals in both of these products is very small — just a smidgen more than in white sugar.

Ecologically, natural foods are the most logical ingredients to use. Refined flour and sugar have not only lost most of the original nutrients (refined sugar is almost completely devoid of any food value except calories), but the refining process itself is costly in terms of manpower and energy and more expensive in the long run because of all the waste that is produced.

Fresh fruits are cheaper when used in season. Therefore, follow the availability of goods according to season. Frozen or canned foods should never be used. Dried fruit that has been sun-dried rather than treated with sulfur dioxide is another handy natural sweetener and rich in nutrients as well.

Honey and maple syrup should be omitted for similar reasons. Tastewise, many foods contain so much natural sweetness that adding extra sweetness in the form of cane sugar, honey, or even maple syrup is unnecessary. Also, many leading nutritionists, such as Adelle Davis, warn that, although honey is a naturally sweet food, it contains only small traces of nutrients and appears to cause tooth decay as quickly as does refined sugar. And many honey users often go overboard by eating large amounts that put on extra weight (honey is far more concentrated and higher in calories than table sugar). Besides, honey is not a food created for man — but for bees! Our greed for honey is quickly producing a worldwide honey shortage. DDT and other pesticides have drastically reduced the number of bees. Honey production has also been decreasing because many beekeepers are selling all the honey bees produce, rather than reserving some for the bees during the winter months. As a result, bees are fed sugar water, which weakens them, and their numbers continue to decrease. From just the ecological viewpoint, honey is not an ideal sweetening agent.

(continued on page 280)

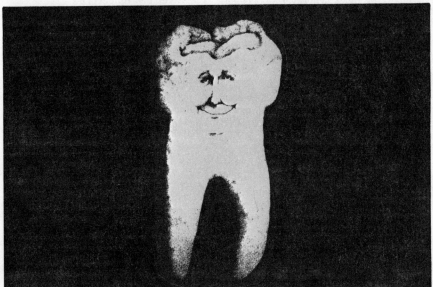

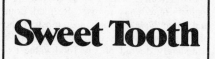

Sweet Tooth

(continued from page 279)

Maple syrup and forms of molasses are also refined products to some extent — ecologically, maple syrup is a poor food because many gallons of sap must be concentrated through high heat to form crystallized sugar or syrup. Real maple syrup is a much better food than cane sugar, but it is very expensive and often hard to find.

If you are just getting accustomed to breaking the refined sugar habit, you may want to use a little honey or maple syrup during your withdrawal phase. However, I suggest that you first try doing without these concentrated sweetening agents and experience the honest sweetness of natural foods.

Rather than honey, maple syrup, or brown sugar, use barley malt extract, both because of its nutritional properties as well as its refined nature.

Almost all fruits and grains become sweeter the longer they are cooked. As the excess liquids are cooked out and the natural sugars broken down, the sweetness becomes more concentrated. Cooking is a form of alchemy — the art of changing foods and flavors through the use of time, pressure, and fire.

Organic apple juice or other fruit juices are convenient to use as quick sweeteners in cooking, and so are many kinds of dried fruit. Other liquids, such as grain coffees (those that are made from whole roasted grains and are commercially available in health food stores), and herbal teas can also be used to flavor desserts.

Salt also helps to bring out the natural sweetness of foods. However, too much salt can sometimes make a dessert taste slightly sour.

Pan roasting grains or flour in a dry cast-iron skillet before mixing with other ingredients gives them a richer, almost nutty taste.

But starting from scratch with natural foods doesn't mean that you have to spend hours cooking. Nor do healthful desserts have to be dull!

I firmly believe that good food should not only be nutritionally satisfying but should captivate the senses and appeal to everyone. This approach to cooking can open an exciting field of exploration to the experienced cook as well as the novice anxious to learn. ☼

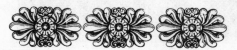

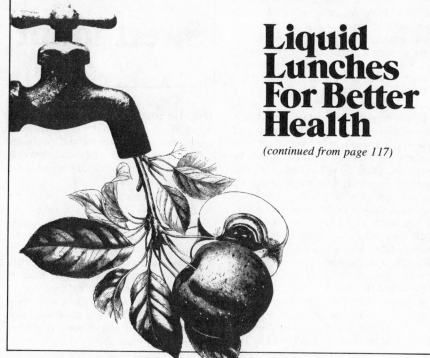

Liquid Lunches For Better Health

(continued from page 117)

The Coffee Break

1 cup Witches' Brew
1 cup whole skimmed milk
2 T. instant coffee*

Mix all ingredients in a blender.
**Nutritional values: Calories: 440
Grams of protein: 64**
Plus all vitamins, minerals, amino acids as contained in the basic Witches' Brew formula.

*Instant de-caffeinated coffee can be used.

The Blue Max

1 cup of Witches' Brew
1 half cup fresh, unsweetened blueberries
1 half cup unsweetened grape juice

Mix in blender.
**Nutritional values: Calories: 490
Grams of protein: 57**
Plus all vitamins, minerals, amino acids as contained in Witches' Brew and 15 mg. vitamin C from blueberries.

The Tart

1 cup of Witches' Brew
1 cup tomato juice
1 t. lemon juice
Worcestershire sauce to taste

Mix in blender.
**Nutritional values: Calories: 400
Grams of protein: 55**
Plus all vitamins, minerals, amino acids as contained in Witches' Brew and 39 mg. vitamin C from tomato juice.

The Berry Batch

1 cup of Witches' Brew
½ cup fresh or frozen (unsweetened) strawberries
½ cup orange juice

Mix in blender. Makes approximately 1 pint.
**Nutritional values: Calories: 415
Grams of protein: 55**
Plus all vitamins, minerals, amino acids as contained in Witches' Brew and approximately 100 mg. (more than the recommended minimum adult daily requirement) of vitamin C from the orange juice and strawberries.

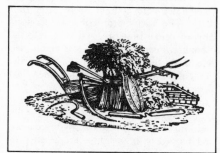

There you have five variations based on Witches' Brew . . . one for each workday of the week. There's actually no limit. Try cranberry juice in place of orange, add raspberries instead of strawberries . . . let your own imagination take over and you, too, can make a magic cauldron out of your blender. And there's one thing in your favor, you can't really ruin the brew. Anything you do to it is almost certain to improve the flavor and nothing you do is likely to detract from the nutritional value.

So bottom's up. Skoal. To your health! ☼

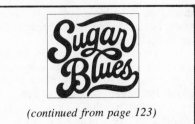

(continued from page 123)

The wise people who understood what sugar blues were all about had been driven underground. Their litany of signs and warnings that the human body and brain cannot handle sugar was driven underground with them. It would take centuries for these signs and warnings to be rediscovered. Eventually, those zealous missionaries of Christianity would take the cross and the flag and the sugar cube and the Coke machine around the world. The church blessed slavery abroad in the sugar business as salvation for the heathens' black souls. Physicians and priests condemned natural healers at home as witches and consigned them to damnation.

Much of that deep historical antagonism is buried in language and symbols. Christians called natural healers sorcerers, from the Latin word which meant someone who drew lots, or Tarot cards, or yarrow sticks to foretell the future. Christians began to call all unbelievers pagans. Pagans called their natural healer the good woman. The natural healer dealt with herbs and potions. These were mysteries to the priests, who felt it necessary to maintain a total monopoly on all·mysteries. Centuries of horror are buried in the saga of the transformation of the natural healer into the Halloween witch.

In the summer of 1973, I walked through a primeval forest in a remote area of southwestern France with a natural herbal healer and watched him perpetuate what his ancestors had done without interruption for more than four hundred years. It was like going back on the time track all the way. This remote forest resembles our images of the Garden of Eden. We walked gingerly, taking care not to trample or disturb the sacred order of the universe underfoot. He knelt to taste the early morning dew. He passed by dozens of growing things to pause before one, then picked it as carefully as one might lift a baby from its mother's lap. He pressed it to his face and his inhalation became a kind of prayer. We retreated to an ancient wooden shed where plants were arranged on racks to dry. Each had been picked at the proper time, according to the moon and the stars as well as to the time of maturity. They are stacked to dry for days, hours, weeks. Each has

its own timetable. Everything in its own season. The wood is preserved intact, inviolate, an inexhaustible source of natural healing remedies, some to be used singly, others in combination. Some are for infusions, to be drunk before meals. Others are for fomentations in which ailing people soak their hands and feet.

The healer learned all this from his father, who used to lie in the fields—studying the insects, the birds, the bees, and the animals, learning their secrets by observation—like Darwin and Goethe and Paracelsus—then checking his conclusions against ancestral documents maintained for centuries and verified constantly by trial and error, practice, and more practice...the *practice* of herbal healing. His father had taken him on herb-collecting trips all over the countryside, by the dawn's early light as well as by the dark of the moon. People came from miles around to consult with his father about their miseries. Sometimes they would be given potions to take home. Perhaps a hot tub might be prepared with a selection of dried branches; the patient would soak away his pain in the tub in the kitchen. No one with the miseries ever left the healer without being questioned on eating and drinking habits. One would be cautioned about the quality of the bread being eaten, the wine being drunk. Always a stern injunction was given against sugar.

In the remote corner of Gascony where I visited herbal healer Maurice Mességué, the Inquisition had passed them by. However, the disasters of World War II—the fall of France, the Nazi occupation—had finally reached the village. The young apprentice healer left his village and journeyed to the outside world. When the son repeated elsewhere the simply natural cures that his father, grandfather, and great-grandfather had accomplished every day, they were taken either as miracles or as quackery, according to which modern superstition viewed them. Mességué successfully treated personages such as Admiral Darlan, Mistinguette, and Jean Cocteau, as well as the then president of the French Republic, Edouard Herriot. Monsieur Mességué's simple cures were sometimes so spectacular that his famous patients talked too much. He came to represent a threat to orthodox medical authorities which they could not ignore. He was hauled into courts throughout the French Republic on more than forty occasions for practicing medicine without a medical degree —for daring, like the witches, to cure without having studied in official institutions.

The trials were spectacular advertisements for herbal medicine. The orthodox diseasestablishment in France made Maurice Mességué famous. Judge after judge duly found him guilty, sentenced him to a fine of one or two francs, then sought his professional services for the ailing wife or mistress waiting in the chambers. Eventually, the healer wrote three books—all bestsellers in Europe—about his adventures and his natural cures. In each he repeats the simple prescriptions learned from his forefathers: Whole natural food, naturally grown. What the avant garde of modern medicine has just now begun to tell us, his ancestors have been preaching for over four hundred years: stay away from all refined cane and beet sugar in all forms and guises. He returned in triumph to Gascony, where he was duly elected mayor of the beautiful city of Fleurance. He lives in a magnificent chateau where his mother had toiled as a maid. He became the owner of a huge primeval forest, where he walks in the morning. This vast tract of land is held in trust as an inexhaustible source of natural herbs and plants with which to minister to a polluted and chemicalized world outside.

In 1964, I prepared a translation of the first of some fifty books written by a Japanese natural healer. My introduction to Sakurazawa's *You Are All Sanpaku* detailed the experiences I had had healing myself according to his simple teachings.

The book contained a chapter on sugar which said, among other things:

"Western medicine and science has only just begun to sound alarm signals over the fantastic increase in its per capita sugar consumption, in the United States especially. Their researches and warnings are, I fear, many decades too late...I am confident that Western medicine will one day admit what has been known in the Orient for years: sugar is without question the number one murderer in the history of humanity—much more lethal than opium or radioactive fallout—especially those people who eat rice as their principal food. Sugar is the greatest evil that modern industrial civilization has visited upon countries of the Far East and Africa....Foolish people who give or sell candy to babies will one day discover, to their horror, that they have much to answer for."

Natural healers today may differ on many points, but on one thing they agree: The human body cannot handle man-refined sugar...sucrose. ☼

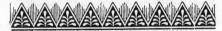

branes to an unnaturally fierce attack by the gastric acid which may result in an ulcer. In places like India and Japan the refining of the rice leads to even more ulceration than occurs in this country. Hence the importance of the second rule set out above.

Obesity (Overweight). — Obesity stems from the appetite being deceived by the unnatural concentration present in white flour and in sugar, so that a person eats too much. For example, the average consumption of sugar today is about 5 oz. per head per day (against less than 1 oz. about a century ago). This 5 oz. is contained in nearly 3 lb. of sugar-beet or in up to a score of ordinary apples. Who would consume this quantity of sugar in its natural, dilute form? The same argument applies to white bread, and other articles containing white flour, as compared with unrefined wholemeal bread.

By following Rule 2, above, the natural fiber (roughage) is restored to the diet, and the natural dilution is restored also. As a result the appetite can again be allowed to regulate the amount to be eaten, as it is designed to do, and we can ignore any question of calories, just as all creatures in the wild state ignore them (and they never suffer from overweight).

For the removal of overweight already present, a certain amount of starvation may be necessary, as in the omission of breakfast and afternoon tea — to be done under medical supervision.

No forced exercise is advised in obesity.

Diabetes and Coronary Disease. — The causation of these conditions is likewise connected with over-eating, through the appetite being deceived by concentration in the food, and the same unrefined diet is indicated. Any other treatment must be under medical supervision.

Simple Constipation, and Its Complications of Varicose Veins and Hemorrhoids (Piles). — Simple constipation is caused solely by the removal of fiber (roughage) in the manufacture of white flour and sugar. Varicose veins and hemorrhoids arise from the fact that in constipation the unnatural accumulations in the bowel press on the great veins in the abdomen which are bringing up blood from the legs (thus causing varicose veins), or on the veins bringing up blood from the back-passage (thus causing hemorrhoids). None of these conditions is seen, even in pregnancy, in native races who do not consume these refined foods. The basic treatment of all these conditions lies in the restoration of the natural fiber to the diet, as in Rule 2, above.

Primary *E. coli* Infections. — Appendicitis, cholecystitis (inflammation of the gall-bladder, with or without gall-stones), diverticulitis (inflammation of the bowel), and cystitis (inflammation of the bladder) all arise from the hordes of microbes subsisting on unnatural food surpluses in the gut, which result from people eating too much, for the reason given. If this over-consumption is prevented in the basic manner just described, the microbes are starved out. Hardly any of these conditions are seen in those races who do not eat white flour or sugar. In the fully developed acute attack, antibiotic treatment and surgical operation may be essential.

Certain Skin Conditions. — The bacterial decomposition just described leads to much offensiveness in the motions and in any wind that is passed. These offensive products when absorbed into the bloodstream may be responsible for certain skin conditions, such as acne, chronic boils, and many cases of eczema.

It may be noted at this point that the most delicate test of the correct application of the two rules given above lies in the disappearance of this offensiveness from the motions, etc.

Applying The Rules

In spite of the simplicity of the diet, it is essential to know the following points about its practical application.

1. Flour. — White flour in the kitchen has to be replaced by a true wholemeal flour. The latter flour can be bought or ordered from a good grocer, but it is far from easy to lay your hands on a true wholemeal bread. Many brown breads are by no means wholemeal. This matter will probably need consultation with your bakery, grocery or health store. There are also books on sale showing how you can bake a true wholemeal bread yourself, without any kneading.

Next, it is essential not to eat your bread too new. New bread forms pasty lumps in the mouth, which do not properly mix with the saliva and are exceedingly indigestible. Bread should therefore be exposed to the air for at least two days before it is eaten. This should be done by wrapping it up in a cloth, not enclosing it in a breadbox or tin (which fosters mildew).

In the eating of rice or a refined breakfast cereal, a tablespoonful of unprocessed bran, as described below, could be added to each plateful, to restore what has been removed. This would not be necessary with an unrefined cereal like Shredded Wheat or bran. The former may be rendered crisper by slight toasting in an oven. Sugar must only be used sparingly with all these (see below).

2. Sugar. — The chief problem in the present diet, however, concerns how to avoid eating ordinary sugar, and all the sweet things containing it. The ideal solution to this problem, undoubtedly, lies in substituting natural sugar, by eating raw fruit or dried fruit (but not canned fruit, as this contains added sugar). For example, instead of sweetening a rice pudding with sugar, eat a banana or two with it, or make the pudding with some raisins. The substitution of raw fruit involves little or no loss in pleasure, but it does involve some extra expense.

It should be added that although honey appears to be a natural food, it should be taken just as sparingly as ordinary sugar. Under natural conditions mankind would have great difficulty in getting honey away from the bees, and even Solomon advised using it in very small quantities. Similarly, the date, containing some ten times as much sugar as an English apple, is not a natural food for the white races, and should be taken sparingly, preferably with other things, such as a glass of

It must also be realized, especially in cases of obesity, that beer and similar drinks contain large quantities of malt sugar, and are immensely fattening.

Finally, the use of the chemical substance, saccharin, is not an obvious solution to the avoidance of sugar-consumption, since it is an unnatural material. For this reason, the suggestions set out above are considered unquestionably preferable.

3. Ready-mixed Foods. — Avoid eating these, the reason being as follows: If, to take a simple example, you eat boiled eggs, bread, butter, and even a little sweetened tea, in accordance with your personal tastes, you will consume the quantities of each of these foods you are best able to digest; but if the eggs, flour, butter, and sugar are all mixed up by someone else, like the cook when making a cake, the proportions of each may not be nearly so accurately attuned to your particular digestion. This is also the reason why fried foods are often difficult to digest. For with these, if you are a Jack Sprat, you will be forced to eat fat you do not want, in order to eat eggs, fish, meat or potato you do want.

4. Cooking. — The closer food is to the natural state, and the less it is cooked up, the better. Overcooked brown meat, for example, is less easily chewed and digested than underdone red meat. Boiled and steamed foods are still more easily digested. Pickled foods are even further from the natural state than overcooked foods. The lean parts of ham and bacon have been considerably altered from the natural state and should be approached with caution.

As regards potatoes, it is recommended that these be boiled, and eaten with the skins still left in position. They are not then more fattening than any other natural food. Boiled potatoes are clearly more easily digested than baked, roasted, or fried potatoes.

5. Acid Stimulants. — Certain foods strongly stimulate the flow of gastric acid, but neutralize none of it. Such foods include coffee, meat extracts, and especially alcohol. These foods are to be avoided, especially in those who suffer from indigestion and ulcer. They are at their most dangerous when taken by themselves.

6. Sandwiches. — These are also likely to cause trouble with anyone who suffers from indigestion, unless carefully planned. First of all the bread must be as described above, Next, the amount of butter must be the amount desired by you. Then, if you do not like bread and butter when eating meat, but do like it when eating cheese, sardines, or eggs, make your sandwiches with one of the latter. Lastly, any unwanted bread in the sandwiches should be left uneaten.

7. Canned Foods. — These are not actually harmful, unless they contain added sugar, as in canned fruit, but fresh foods are always much more appetizing, and are therefore much to be preferred.

8. The Teeth. — It is most difficult to digest raw fruit and other desirable natural foods if they cannot be properly masticated. Therefore, it is quite essential that the bite, if inadequate, should be rectified by proper dental treatment. Until this is completed, natural foods should be mashed up carefully before being eaten.

9. The Use of Bran. — The present diet will itself usually correct constipation. If it does not, do not resort to drugs but have resort instead to ordinary unprocessed bran, which can be obtained from corn and seed stores, health stores, and even pet shops. The cost is quite negligible. The bran should be taken at first in teaspoonful doses *before* meals (otherwise the stomach may become overfilled), and the dose gradually increased, if necessary, to suit individual needs. For example, some people may need several tablespoonfuls a day. Bran cannot be swallowed in the dry state and it is best taken in soup, or in unrefined breakfast cereals with milk, or just washed down in a glass of water. It is sure to cause some flatulence at first, but this slowly vanishes. If bread is made at home, a good thing to do is to incorporate extra bran into the flour — up to 10 per cent by weight of the wholemeal flour — thus making a "bran-plus" loaf.

10. Changes in Diet to Be Made Gradually. — Lastly, and perhaps most important of all, the transition to the present diet must be made slowly, *so as at all times to keep in step with the appetite — i.e., with the liking for the natural foods indicated.*

An effort has been made to set out the basis of a natural diet, which may be expressed as "follow the natural instinct of appetite, as long as it is allowed to play on natural foods." Both halves of this statement are essential. Eating natural foods that you do not desire will achieve very little; and eating unnatural foods that you do desire will achieve infinitely less.

Since we have become adapted to cooking over thousands of years, foods showing simple cooking count as natural, but refining by machinery is so recent a practice that we are not adapted to it at all. That is why foods containing white flour and white or brown sugar are exceedingly dangerous. If these two groups of foodstuff are avoided, and with due regard to the few items mentioned above, you can and should eat whatever you like, such as meat, fish, eggs, cheese, milk, butter, and any fruit or vegetable.

It must be noted, however, that though the alterations recommended in the diet are so few, they must be very carefully followed. These notes must be frequently consulted and the correct habits built up and maintained. Success will depend on realizing it is health, above all, that governs happiness, so that first things are put first and kept that way. People are prepared to take endless trouble over the maintenance of a motor car, but over the maintenance of that infinitely more delicate mechanism, the human body, they are seldom prepared to take any trouble at all. ☼

Hunza Food, Recipes for the Beautiful Life

(continued from page 129)

but to produce their apricot oil. The results prove worthwhile, as it tastes delicious, it enriches the flavor of the food, and is supposed to be rich in polyunsaturated fats. The freedom from circulatory disease, heart attacks, and strokes that the Hunzakuts enjoy makes one wonder .

Meat

The Hunza people are not vegetarians, but they eat very little meat and it is served only on special occasions. And when they cook it, it is prepared in a form of a stew, and small portions are dished out. Chickens until recently were not allowed to be brought in, for fear they would destroy the crops by pecking the seeds. Recently this has changed, and you can find a few chickens wandering around. Children play with them, since there are no dogs or cats, for lack of food to feed an extra animal. The chickens take the place of a family pet. Then, of course, the eggs have enriched the diet! An additional supply of proteins is a great luxury.

Occasionally, these people run out of food at the end of the winter season. Until the new crop is available, they have practically nothing to eat, and water has to suffice. Apparently it nourishes them well, and they easily survive the period of near-starvation. We would call it "fasting," a method which has been adopted by a number of sanatoriums and clinics all over Europe, especially in Switzerland and Germany.

Hippocrates, the father of medicine, suggested fasts up to seven days and stated: "Hunger reacts in the nature of man with great power and can be considered the means that leads to recovery from disease." He was a great believer in fasting and also in a natural way of eating, in exercising, and in morning walks. He said, "Your food should be your medicine."

The Hunza palace cuisine would please the most critical gourmet, and I enjoyed many exotic, delicious new dishes while I was there. Most of the meals were served formally, but the buffet dinners served from time to time, with their natural informality, were very pleasant.

The Hunzakuts work very hard from sunrise to sunset, six days a week, and

(continued on page 284)

Hunza Food, Recipes for the Beautiful Life

(continued from page 283)

use a tremendous amount of physical energy. Nevertheless, they eat little and do very well on their frugal diet, compared to the variety and quantity of foods the average American thinks he needs each day to survive. My housekeeper, a wonderful person, is quite argumentative when it comes to meat. She claims that without eating meat at least twice a day, she doesn't have physical strength to work. I don't intend to convince her, but I have seen and lived with the Hunza people. Excess weight is unusual among them. They enjoy good teeth, sturdy bone structure, good eyesight, normal digestion, and sound hearts. A general condition of perfect health is the rule rather than the exception in Hunza. So who can argue with them?

Above all the Hunzakuts demonstrate that a peaceful life can be enjoyed. People can shake off a heritage of greed, jealousy, and craving for power. The Hunzakuts have demonstrated that love and a spiritually inspired life brings happiness. When we truly learn to understand each other, to fulfill the precepts of brotherly love and live a simple life, then we, too, will be able to find peace within ourselves.

Captured by the spell of the whole valley, the friendly and joyous people, I saw everything in a new light. Why can't we learn that the readiness to enjoy life is no shallow childishness but the deep source of blessed living?

HUNZA RECIPES

The following recipes were given to me by the gracious Rani who taught me how to cook the Hunza way. Of course, I've more or less adapted certain recipes to include nutritional products and natural ingredients obtainable in our own country.

Kamali — Plain Chapatti

(Basic Recipe)
2 cups whole wheat flour (stone ground)
1/2 teaspoon vegetable salt or sea salt
3/4 to 1 cup water
Blend flour and salt together. Stir in just enough water to make a very stiff dough. Knead dough on a lightly floured surface until smooth and elastic. Cover with a wet cloth: set aside for 30 minutes. Break the dough into one inch balls, and roll out into very thin rounds, about 8 inches in diameter. Bake for 10 minutes on a hot, lightly greased griddle over low heat; turn often. It makes 20 chapattis.

Kalchar — Small Chapattis

2 cups of whole wheat flour (stone ground)
1/2 teaspoon mineral sea salt
1/8 pound of margarine (rich in unsaturated fatty acid)
1/2 cup buttermilk
Blend flour and salt together.
Mix margarine with flour, then blend milk in a little at a time.

Variations:

1. Chapattis on grill — thin and crisp. Roll dough paper thin and cook on pre-heated griddle. It is excellent with salads or soups. Can be kept in an airtight container and it will remain crisp for future use.
2. Roll dough about 3/4″ thick and cut out like small biscuits. Bake in oven in greased pan. Pre-heat oven to 350° then turn down to 250° and bake until done.

The Hunza stone-ground flour contains more bran than our usual flour. Therefore, the consistency might be different and it is advisable to add some bran flour to the mixture. Also they do not use salt, as their food is full of natural minerals. Our taste requires flavoring of food. We suggest using sea salt or vegetable salt.

Piti-Chapatti

(Basic Recipe)
2 cups whole wheat flour (stone ground)
3/4 cup milk and lukewarm water (half-and-half to equal the 3/4 measurement)
1/2 teaspoon vegetable salt
1/4 cup safflower oil
Mix flour with milk and water, add oil and salt. Make into a dough and roll out to a 1/2-inch thick loaf and bake in a 350° oven (pre-heated). Mix dough thoroughly, stirring mixture by hand. The longer you stir the dough, the more you develop the gluten in the flour and the more elastic it will become and the lighter the bread will be.

Cheese Chapatti

1/2 cup whole wheat flour
1-1/2 cups buckwheat flour
1/2 teaspoon baking powder
1/2 teaspoon vegetable salt
3-1/4 cups buttermilk
2 tablespoons sweet butter or preferably safflower oil
2 eggs
Sift flour and then add salt and baking powder. Pour into a bowl, add buttermilk and melted butter or safflower oil, beat egg yolks and add. Then blend dry ingredients and beat the batter until it is smooth and elastic. Add the stiffly beaten whites of the eggs. Bake chapattis on a medium hot griddle following customary rules. Makes 8 large chapattis.

Filling:
Blend 2 cups of cottage cheese with buttermilk until smooth, add vegetable salt to taste. Lay out one chapatti and spread cheese all over, cover with another and repeat till all are used. Let stand 2 hours then cut like a cake and serve.

Millet Bread

1 cup millet flour
1 cup grated golden carrots
1 tablespoon honey
1 tablespoon vegetable salt
2 tablespoons corn oil
2 eggs
Combine in bowl: Millet flour, carrots, oil, honey and salt. Mix well, then stir 3/4 cup of boiling hot water into the mixture. Beat the egg yolks well, adding 2 tablespoons of cold water, continue to beat and then add to the mixture. Fold in stiffly beaten whites of eggs and bake in hot, oiled pan at 350° for about 40 minutes.

Millet Casserole

2 tablespoons safflower oil
1 cup hulled millet
1/2 cup diced carrots
1/2 cup diced green fresh peppers
1 cup fresh mushrooms (cut)
1 teaspoon vegetable salt
1/4 teaspoon salad herbs
1/4 cup whole almonds
Heat the oil in a heavy skillet, stir the millet and brown slightly. Add the chopped vegetables and vegetable salt, and stir for three minutes. Put the mixture into a covered saucepan, adding enough water to cover about one inch above the millet. Add almonds and cook over low heat for 15 minutes, then continue for a while in a double boiler until tender (6 servings).

Millet — Hulled

1 cup water
1 cup milk
1/2 cup hulled millet
    dried apricots — (soaked in bottled water overnight, just enough to cover the fruit)
1/2 teaspoon vegetable salt
Heat water and milk in top part of double boiler and add millet and steam over boiling water for 30 minutes or until millet is tender. Add apricots and liquid and serve hot. (Sun-

flower seed meal and almond meal or ground nuts can be added). Millet is very nourishing and rich in proteins. For a quick breakfast, prepare in double boiler the night before. (4 to 6 servings).

The Hunzas use millet frequently, serving with dried apricots or fresh in season. They don't use any sweetening, but their fruit has an entirely different taste. If you prefer it sweet, honey is advisable.

Whole Buckwheat Groats

1 cup whole buckwheat groats
2 cups of water*
1 teaspoon vegetable salt
2 tablespoons of safflower oil
1 egg

Heat the oil in a heavy skillet, stir in the buckwheat mixed with the beaten whole egg. Add the vegetable salt and brown slightly, keeping it stirred with a spoon. Finally, add the water, bring to a boil, then reduce the heat. Cover tightly and let cook until all liquid is absorbed. It must never be mushy. Every grain should be separate. (6 servings.)

*Instead of the water you can use vegetable broth in the form of a powder. (The health food stores have a variety of vegetable broth brands.) Pour a cup of hot water over a teaspoon of the powder. It makes a delicious soup and can also be used instead of water in the buckwheat groats.

Hunza Mint Soup

To any broth such as lamb, beef or chicken, the addition of a tablespoon of chopped mint per serving will greatly improve the flavor. Also, blend in some buckwheat groats.

Hunza Golden Brown
Lamb Pillau

2 large onions (could be omitted)
1/2 cup of safflower oil
1 pound of carrots
2 pounds of meat (lamb)
1 pound of brown rice
   enough water to cover rice
2 teaspoons vegetable salt
Cut onions finely and brown in oil. Blend in carrots cut into squares. Keep stirring for about 10 minutes over low heat. Add meat cut up into fairly small pieces and cover with water. Let it cook until the meat is done. Keep it covered all the time. Take out meat only, strain soaked rice and add to the soup. After 1/2 hour, add the pre-cooked meat and cook a little longer, covered with a lid. ☼

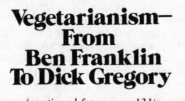

Vegetarianism— From Ben Franklin To Dick Gregory

(continued from page 131)

Oneida community primarily obtained their income by trapping animals for furs. By 1864, annual sales from furs amounted to about $100,000 with the manufacture of close to 300,000 furs. Noyes and members of the community took great pride in the superior efficiency of their traps.

Gradually the community died out, probably because the children of the original founders grew up and drifted away from the communal pattern of their parents, although their childhoods seemed happy and outwardly unaffected by the living arrangements and education.

John A. Collins, an abolitionist from Boston, founded a commune in 1843 at Skaneateles, New York, where vegetarianism was also practiced. Organized religion was forbidden and divorce was encouraged so that happiness within marriage was always obtainable. Eventually Skaneateles also disbanded because of the jealousies and petty arguments that developed among the colonists.

Another commune advocating vegetarianism was established in Benton County, Arkansas, where a small group of anarchists settled in 1860 and called themselves the Harmonial Vegetarian Society. However, it was their advocacy and practice of free love that caused a sensation in conservative Arkansas, rather than their meatless diet. What might have happened to the commune is conjecture since the imminent Civil War led to its disbandment. Confederate soldiers took possession of the various buildings and seized their official publication, *The Theocrat*.

One would think the author of *Walden* would have embraced a simple, meatless diet. Yet Henry David Thoreau, who chose solitude rather than communal living as a means of experimentation, advocated vegetarianism but practiced it for only a few years. "Like many of my contemporaries," he wrote, "I had rarely for many years used animal food, or tea, or coffee; not so much because of any ill effects which I had traced to them, as because they were not agreeable to my imagination." Thoreau recognized that one's repugnance to animal flesh is mental rather than a genuine repulsion; that most sensitive men have, at one time or another, thought of abstaining from animal food.

Needless to say, Thoreau's exaltation of civil disobedience and the abandonment of the complexities of society have been far more influential than his contradictory views on vegetarianism. Another nineteenth-century innovator, Ellen G. White, had a greater influence on the national spread of the meatless diet.

The Seventh Day

Ellen G. White, who was then Ellen Harmon, was in the original group of New Englanders who began the Adventist movement, an outgrowth of the Millerite movement. The importance of this Christian sect in a history of vegetarianism may be explained by their present number of followers: there are about 2 million Seventh-day Adventists around the world and approximately 500,000 in the United States. Fifty percent of all Adventists are lacto-ovo-vegetarians.

The success of the sect is due largely to a tight web of educational programs that involves separate schooling—from elementary school through college—a continual magazine, book publications, and international missionary work. Contributions are authorized by a strict interpretation of the Bible.

Vegetarianism in the Seventh-day Adventist movement is the direct result of Ellen White, who believed the body to be God's temple and that therefore any abuse of one's body is also a violation of Him. With that principle in mind, she denounced tobacco, alcohol, and meat.

Although not a nutritionist, Ellen G. White applied common sense to various health problems that afflicted America during the nineteenth century and of course many of the excesses she pointed to still apply today .

A Seventh-day Adventist whose name is as well known as the cornflakes that he invented was the vegetarian Dr. John Harvey Kellogg. His involvement with the Adventists began in 1864 when, at the age of twelve, he started as an apprentice at the Review and Herald Press, the Seventh-day Adventist publishing company still in existence today. Kellogg received his medical degree from Bellevue Hospital in 1875. In 1876 he returned to Michigan and took over the Adventist sanitorium, which soon became a non-profit and non-sectarian health institute that reflected the personal stamp of Dr. Kellogg.

For over sixty years, Kellogg edited *Good Health Magazine,* which promoted vegetarianism in almost every

(continued on page 286)

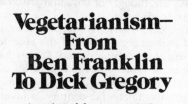

issue. His nutritional ideas were always undergoing modification, but his dedication to fruits, nuts, and grains as the natural and best diet for man remained consistent throughout his life.

A significant aspect of the endorsement of a meatless diet by the Seventh-day Adventists has been the development of meatless protein dishes, such as soyburgers, soy milk, and various canned plant protein foods flavored to resemble meats and poultry. Their dietary explorations have inspired researchers trying to find low-priced, high protein solutions to the problem of providing nutritious and economical meals for schoolchildren in this country and around the world.

Upton Sinclair

In Upton Sinclair's obituary in *The New York Times* in 1968, twelve reforms that he advocated are listed: vegetarianism is one of them. In fact, Sinclair practiced a meatless diet for only about three years when he experimented with nutritional benefits in 1911; yet the label stuck, even posthumously.

One obvious reason for this was his novel *The Jungle*, famous exposé of the fictitious "Packingtown." The meatpacking industry is the background Sinclair made use of to describe his central theme—the plight of the working class. Yet the nation was ready for Sinclair's explosive and visual words about the meat industry, although they occupy only 12 pages of a 340-page novel. It was this material that gained instant national fame for the struggling novelist. As Sinclair often commented, he aimed for the hearts of Americans but reached them through their stomachs.

One summer Sinclair decided to take his wife and young son, along with his friend Mike and his family, to the coral reefs of Bermuda. There his experiments with a meatless diet became an obsession and proved the inspiration for *Good Health and How We Won It,* published in 1919. Thirty years later, in *American Outposts,* Sinclair tells his readers that he is so ashamed of his dietetic treatise he will not reveal the title. In *Good Health,* Sinclair advanced numerous physiological reasons for giving up meat, basing many of his conclusions on the studies of Horace Fletcher at Yale University, and on the increased endurance of vegetarian, as opposed to meat-eating, groups. Sinclair described his regime: two meals a day, never eat before sleep, no drinking during meals, using only fresh foods, adequate ventilation, play as the best exercise, and careful chewing of food to allow enough nutrients, but in smaller quantities. He even provided daily menus and recipes.

Fasting—a purely hygienic procedure to Sinclair—was a practice he pursued all his life as a cure for any illness provoked by overwork or other causes. He broke the fast with orange juice and advised against any solid foods until the third day. The social reformer certainly proved an advocate for vegetarianism indirectly through *The Jungle,* even though he avoided the label.

Vegetarians for President

When five hundred delegates to a convention of the American Naturopathic Association met at The Hotel Commodore in New York on July 28, 1947, it proved to be the birth of the American Vegetarian Party. At eighty-five, Dr. John Maxwell, a naturopathic doctor and vegetarian restaurant operator from Chicago, was nominated for candidacy in the presidential election of 1948. Symon Gould, public relations director and associate editor of *The American Vegetarian,* was nominated for Vice-President. Gould remained the force behind the American Vegetarian Party, but it wasn't until 1960 that Gould himself finally ran for President. He continued to keep vegetarianism and pacifism in the forefront of the public mind through his 1962 campaign for state senator from New York. His opponent, Jacob Javits, had been his classmate at Public School 40 in New York.

Gould's political career was a joke to some, annoying to others, and appreciated by only a few fellow believers, since he alienated so many other American vegetarians who believed that a meatless diet should take place at the dinner table, not in discussion after the meal. Gould died of cancer in 1963, at the age of seventy: the American Vegetarian Party died with him.

Modern Times

What is the situation in America today regarding organized vegetarianism? There are some notable advocates, such as Will Durant, author of the multivolume *The Story of Civilization;* Dick Gregory, comedian and political activist: Scott and Helen Nearing, socialists and authors of *Living the Good Life;* and some actors and actresses, such as James Coburn and Susan St. James. Yet it is not a cause that is openly discussed and debated by the intellectual community. Many doctors, educators and celebrities are silent about their meatless diet and ethics.

One eclectic faction, located in New York City, is the Vegetarian Feminists, who are part of the Vegetarian Collective. A headline in the *Majority Report,* organ of the women's liberation movement, stated:

WOMEN, ARE YOU *STILL* HUMAN CHAUVINISTS? THE ALL COMPASSIONATE FEMINIST IS A VEGETARIAN!

Their point is well taken, but even more effective is a three-minute film they distribute, portraying the activities inside an actual slaughterhouse. Even thirty seconds of this grueling film is enough time to get the message.

Ottoman Zar-Adusht Ha'nish, raised in Tibet and Iran by monks, began the Mazdaznan movement in Chicago in 1890. This group, still active today, is a modern adaption of Zoroastrianism. The four basic principles are: vegetarianism, distilled water, no tea or coffee, and sun worship.

Also located in Chicago are the headquarters of the Natural Hygienists, who follow the principles of Herbert Sheldon. They are that man is constituted in perfect health and that any illness may be traced to a breach of naturalness. The best way to recover genuine health is by fasting.

The American Vegan Society, founded by Indian-born Jay Dinshah, follows similar views but enhances them with Jainist attitudes of *ahimsa* and the elimination of all animal products and clothing apparel. Both groups are the extremist vegetarian sects in America today.

That vegetarianism is a growing movement in contemporary America is undeniable, as evidenced by the appearance across the country's college campuses of vegetarian alternatives for meals in dormitories and cafeterias. Vegetarianism offers idealistic youth a way for each person to fight the unharnessed aggression and violence associated with earlier generations. It is also an expression of the growing affinity with Eastern philosophies. Furthermore, vegetarianism offers a way of returning to nature. In addition, the high cost of meat is forcing people to adopt a diet that consists of fewer animal products; starting under external impetuses, many persons choose to continue such a regimen when they discover that it is possible to eat both pleasantly and humanely. ☼

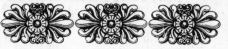

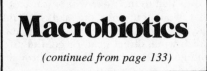
There is nothing more appropriate for a slice of halibut or swordfish than, before broiling, to pre-soak it in soya sauce flavored with ginger.

Daikon is a Japanese radish which looks like a gigantic white carrot. Heavy eaters find it helpful after an exaggerated intake of liquid and food. It is a great aid to digestion. Besides its medicinal values, it has a subtle taste akin to the radish, nevertheless retaining its own unique quality. It is excellent raw, pickled or cooked. Japanese stores also sell it shredded and dried.

Lotus Root is sold in Chinatown in New York City and San Francisco. It is available fresh or dried. Fritters can be made by soaking and deep-frying it. Kohren tea is the name given to its powdered form, used mostly to fortify weak lungs.

Jinenjo must be growing somewhere in the mountains of the U.S.A. However, if you live on the plains it can be obtained at Japanese stores. A long and heavy root the size of a policeman's club, it tastes like potato when sliced and deep-fried in oil. For the cerealian, jinenjo is a very strengthening food. When grated raw and mixed with soya sauce, it is excellent for anemia.

Condiments

Sesame Salt, or Gomasio, is a combination of toasted sesame seeds and genuine sea salt, ground together. It is a balanced table condiment, good for people who tend to drink too much. One uses it sprinkled on grains and vegetables.

Soya Sauce is also called Tamari or Shoyu in Japan. Good-quality Tamari is twice as expensive as the chemicalized, quickly-processed variety. Made from wheat, soya beans and water, it is fermented over a period of two years. It is used in sautéed vegetables, soups, sauces, fish, etc.

Miso is a soya-bean paste made from the same ingredients as soya sauce. It is used in the famous Miso Soup, enhances the taste of a pâté, and makes good spreads and sauces. Unique in value, its richness has no limit and plays a most important role in body metabolism. It is a great energy-source for those wishing to accomplish hard work.

Seitan: Your guests will almost certainly mistake this for meat. Teeth find it pleasant to chew. A combination of wheat gluten, wheat soya beans, water and salt, it comes in handy when mixed with vegetables, sauces and soups.

Salted Plums, or Umeboshi, are Japanese plums pickled in salt for three years. For centuries the Japanese have been using them to make the best-tasting and most harmless vinegar. They have hundreds of practical and successful medicinal uses.

Sesame Butter, in Arabic countries, is known as Tahini or Tahina. Its uses are unlimited — if your imagination is! It makes a delicious spread when mixed with miso, and is excellent in sauces, creams, cookies and custards.

Tofu is another name for soya-bean curd. In Chinatown, you'll see it in wooden barrels. It looks like Greek feta cheese and is excellent served with sautéed vegetables, sauces, fried or cooked in Miso Soup.

Kuzu can be bought in any natural-food store. It is a twin brother of arrow-root. While kuzu is most often used for colds and digestive troubles, arrow-root is used for thickening sauces and pie fillings.

Bonita (or Bonito) and *Chirimen Iriko* are sold in Japanese markets and in Chinatown. Chirimen Iriko is a tiny fish, the size and shape of a vermicelli noodle. Bonita comes in a hard stone-like form or shredded and packaged. Both are excellent for flavoring soup stocks.

Sea Salt is not the conditioned, sparkling salt usually sold in grocery stores. The true one comes from the ocean, while the other comes from laboratories. There is a gray, unwashed kind which we use in our home, and there is a lighter one which has been previously washed in sea-water. Both of these contain many natural mineral salts. Some cerealians roast their salt before using it to liberate excess chlorine gas.

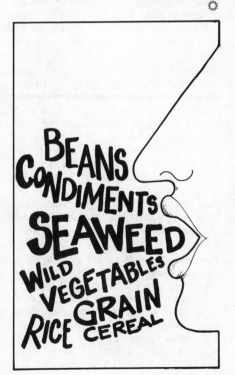

The Pleasures of Container Gardening

(continued from page 143)

If you do use my suggestion of soil and planter mix, sow the seeds directly in the planters to avoid damaging the seedlings in the process of transplanting. In areas where frosts linger you can buy individual seedling peat pots to be used to start the seeds. These pots are made from compressed peat moss and can be filled with soil or soil and planter mix, but plant no more than three seeds per pot. When the seedlings develop two sets of leaves or more, simply thin them to the strongest single plant and sink the plant, peat pot and all, into the soil of your permanent container. The roots grow right through the peat container, which disintegrates as the plants grow. Seedlings should not be fertilized as young plants cannot accept a concentration of nutrients and will shrivel up. Do not add any fertilizer until the plants have reached a height of 4 to 5 inches. Then select a fertilizer with your nursery clerk and follow the directions carefully for the amount and frequency. A good, mild, all-around fertilizer is fish emulsion, which can be purchased in any nursery. It works well on all vegetables, and if you buy young tomato plants it can be applied directly after you have transplanted them into the permanent containers.

Mixing the Soil

If you have an old tub, use it to mix your soil combination. Moisten as you mix to keep the dust down. The mixture settles as it becomes damp, so it is important to get it nicely damp before transferring it to the planters.

If you aren't using casters, first place your planters where you want them and make the drainage arrangements. Then move the soil to the planters (large, full planters can become very heavy). Mix several batches to fill the larger planter. To help with drainage, it is a good idea to put a layer of coarse sand on the bottom of the planter before putting in the soil mixture.

Choosing Your Crop

The selection of vegetables depends on the size and number of planters and on your own taste. Remember that leafy vegetables will give a higher yield per area, but you may want to try a few root vegetables too.

Seeds

Seed racks are found in nurseries, in

(continued on page 288)

The Pleasures of Container Gardening

(continued from page 287)

hardware stores and, very commonly, in markets.

Carrots: Home-grown carrots are so delicious you will certainly want to try growing some. I suggest either the midget variety, which matures most quickly, or the short, fat type, which is very tasty. The longer carrots may present a problem unless your planters are good and deep. Sow early in spring, and when the seedings get to be 1 to 1½ inches tall, thin them to about 1 inch apart. Then, after a month or so, thin them to about 3 inches apart. Incidentally, you can enjoy the sweet taste of these tiny thinnings in salads. Generally it will take eight to ten weeks for full maturity.

Radishes: Both carrots and radishes can take an early sowing. Radishes grow beautifully in these soil combinations and should be eaten as soon as they are mature because they quickly get dry and pithy. Thin them to an inch apart after they are about 2 inches tall, and they should be ready to eat in a month, or earlier. When you pull a radish, replace it with another seed and start a second crop.

Onions and shallots: Sow seeds very early in spring. Even better, start onions and shallots (the delicate little bulb that is a cross between onion and garlic and is used in French cooking) with "sets," very young plants that are available at nurseries. Separate the sets and plant an inch apart, and the bulbs will be ready to eat in a month to six weeks. When an onion top falls, it's time to pull the onion; then let it dry in the sun for several days to a week. Ask your nursery clerk for specific directions on the variety you choose.

Beets and turnips: These are very good for planters as you can eat both the root and the greens. Sow early in the spring and when the plants have grown to about 1½ to 2 inches, thin them to 1½ inches apart. Thin again when they have reached a height of 7 to 8 inches. They are best when young, so don't let them get larger than 2 inches in diameter.

Swiss chard and spinach: Swiss chard is usually much better as a summer crop than spinach, which does not flourish in hot weather. One exception is New Zealand spinach, an extraordinarily hearty variety that will grow and spread for months. Young tips can be picked throughout the summer months. Chop fine for salads and cook longer than ordinary spinach, for this plant is tougher. It is also considered to be more nutritious. A vinelike quality makes New Zealand spinach a good hanging plant.

Kale: This plant is new to most people, or known only as cattle food. It is well worth growing because it has the heartiness of a weed and grows all year in many areas. Treat it as you would any green, but pick it young and discard any tough stalks. It takes longer to cook than spinach or chard and is very high in nutritional value.

Lettuce: It is best to select leaf varieties rather than the heading type. They are easier to grow and quicker to produce for eating. You can eat the thinnings in a few weeks or, if you do as I did one year and accidentally overplant, you can eat the delicate seedlings in salad in ten days. Keep thinning as the lettuce grows, and pick the outer leaves. If it is hot when your lettuce is in the seedling stage, cover the planter with window screening to diffuse the heat and light. When the plants begin to toughen and go to seed, continue to keep them moist and wait until they produce new leaves again in the early fall. Remember, lettuce likes cool weather, so you may have to move it occasionally when the sun is very hot.

Beans: Both bush and pole beans will do well in a container garden with a good soil mixture and will give a good yield if watered well. Sow when the weather is warm and follow the directions for sowing on the package. Beans do well in pots. Tell your nursery clerk what you are doing and ask his advice on the best container. Pole beans will have to be staked.

Squash: All summer squashes are surefire crops for a beginning gardener. They grow rapidly and can be eaten when they are very young. In fact, they should be eaten young not only for taste, but because they will grow weighty and cumbersome for the container. Use a large, round, and deep container if you can, as squashes have a long root system, and sow according to the directions on the package. When they have grown into young plants, do not overwater or you will have more leaves than vegetables.

Tomatoes: Tomatoes are a joy to grow because they are so prolific, but they take longer to germinate, and must be sown when the weather is warm or indoors in peat pots for transplanting in warm weather. It is advisable to start with small plants until you are gardening with confidence. Most larger tomatoes will have to be staked and the plants tied to the stake with a soft cloth that won't cut into the stalks. Plant them securely, protect them from too much wind, direct heat, or cold nights, and give them plenty of water throughout their growth period.

Tomatoes generally produce later in the growing season because they have to be grown in warm weather. Do not be put off by the scraggly vines as they get older, especially if they give a good yield. For your first gardening experience, it would be best to try a cherry tomato which grows anywhere and produces a sizable crop, or the Pixie variety which yields a slightly larger tomato. Any tomato plant larger than a cherry variety needs room for roots—at least 1½ feet of soil. When transplanting, feed with fish emulsion (½ teaspoon to each ½ gallon of water). Repeat every five days for two weeks. Do not overwater, but keep moist.

Herbs: I think a container garden is complete only with herbs, and if your space is very limited, they may be the only crop possible. For the beginning gardener, small plants bought in the nursery are advisable, although parsley, dill, and savory germinate quickly and grow especially well from seeds. Herbs should be snipped frequently to insure proper growth and a bushing effect.

Snip the tiny top leaves with your nail or small scissors. If you do this continually, your herbs will grow very thick. When the plants are young, be very careful not to break or injure the main stem or stalks of the nonbushy herbs like tarragon, dill, or basil. Snip off the leaves, not the stems, until they grow larger and produce many shoots. Bushy herbs like thyme or oregano have many stalks and cannot be injured easily, but you must be gentle with all young herbs. When the weather gets too cold you can bring the pots into the house and put them in a well-lighted place for the winter. If you do this, continue to feed and fertilize. When they get beyond your ability to utilize or begin to lose life or go to seed, they should be picked for drying and storing.

Sowing, Watering, and Thinning

Sowing: It is important not to overseed your container, for an excess of seedlings makes the thinning process quite a chore. After you have sown according to the package directions, cover each container with plastic in which you have punched holes to allow air to circulate. I find it helpful to put a stake (a chopstick is good) in each planter to give a tentlike space for air circulation under the cover. The plastic cover acts as an incubator and greatly speeds up germinations, as well as protecting the seeds from browsing birds.

Watering: Remove the plastic to water lightly. Use a fine spray attachment on the hose, or a watering can. You must water carefully to avoid routing and floating the seeds or damaging the delicate seedlings. Watering depends on the amount of sun on your garden and how quickly the soil dries out. The soil should be kept moist, but not soggy. When plants are 1½ to 2 inches high, remove the plastic: at first, roll it back during the day but keep the plants covered at night, then gradually remove it altogether.

Thinning: If you have a good soil you can be assured that the majority of seeds will germinate. Follow the directions on the package for sowing and thinning. When you begin the thinning process, use a pair of tiny pointed scissors. Clip off the seedlings at the soil line for nonroot vegetables, and pull out the excess root-vegetable seedlings with tweezers. Keep the thinnings to use in your salad of the day.

Predators

It is unlikely that in a container garden you will have much trouble with insects, and a healthy plant, like a healthy body, has good resistance to disease. Keeping the soil moist helps ward off insects. All strong-smelling flowers, like marigolds, and herbs and onions will act as insect repellents, and are good companions for your vegetables.

A special dinner for mature plants can be made by placing a few days' vegetable parings, scraps, and egg shells in the blender and, with some water, blending into a liquid. Pour this into the soil around the plants every two weeks for extra nourishment.

Mulching for the Next Year

To prepare the soil for the next season when your crops have completed their yielding cycle, you can compost and mulch the soil for reuse. For a month or two after harvest, continue to pour the liquid dinner into the soil, turning under with a trowel, or in larger containers with a hand spade. Chop vegetable parings fine and turn these under too. If you have some fertilizer left over from the growing season, add it to the soil. Then cover all the containers with whatever mulch you have collected (oak leaves, lawn clippings from a park, or even hay), and let it decompose through the winter months. It will be fine to cultivate the following spring. Or, if you have had immense success with your summer crops, start investigating what you can grow throughout the winter. ☼

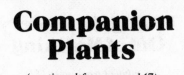

Companion Plants

(continued from page 147)

of produce and the health of consumers.

Teas are a good means to transfer neighborly impulses from one plant to another. When the leaves carry the active principle, the plant for tea must be gathered early in the morning, not later than ten o'clock and before blooming — while the blooming process is still found in the leaves before it has dissipated into the blossom. It has been proved in this case that older plants do not have the same strong effect. Dry in the shade and store in a dry place, preferably in tin boxes. For many herbs like Camomile, Yarrow, St. Johnswort, and others the blossoms are the part used.

To make an herb tea to be used as a spray: cover the medicinal plant with water in the pot, bring just to the boiling point and take off the fire. This infusion should be diluted with four parts water. It is recommended that the fluid be stirred for ten minutes. It should then be used immediately.

Stinging Nettle tea will combat plant lice or aphis.

Chives tea is useful to overcome apple scab. Use dried Chives. Do not boil Chives but instead pour boiling water over dried Chives and leave it to infuse 15 minutes. Dilute the infusion with 2 or 3 times as much water and stir. The best results have been obtained with a comparatively strong solution.

Chives tea is useful to combat gooseberry mildew.

Horse-radish tea fights monilia in fruit trees. Use young horse-radish leaves at the beginning of the attack. Make the tea as explained above and dilute with 4 times as much water.

Most vegetable plants have inconspicuous flowers, or in the case of root crops, no blossoms at all the first year. This makes for a one-sided atmosphere among the vegetable plants, lacking in the realm of blossoms formed by warmth and light. If the garden is surrounded by borders of summer flowering plants of mixed varieties, the latter will attract a wide and balanced variety of insects thus promoting pollination of all neighboring vegetation. Some of the summer flowering plants and shrubs which have a beneficial effect are: Wild Rose, Elderberry, Buddleia, Privet, Goldenrod and Bee Balm.

Some herbs may be scattered about the garden, for instance, one herb clump

at the end of each raised bed, to help overcome the monoculture and to create a lively aromatic atmosphere in the bed where it is growing. Small herb hedges may be grown, for instance of Hyssop or of Lemon Balm. When Hyssop is in bloom, it is bedecked with all manner of moths and butterflies, and wild honey bees and other flying insects, all of which benefit the whole garden. Parsley and Dill, Coriander and Bee Balm, allowed to blossom will provide welcome for honey bees and butterflies who bring their good influence to the heavier vegetables which are confined there.

INSECT PESTS

Insect pests, when they get out of hand, are one sign of upset balances in nature. Restore the right proportion in nature and pests gradually become less troublesome. This does not mean we shall ever be without insects. In a balanced scheme they are a necessity but because of man's interference their destructive powers occasionally become abnormal. Even more disturbing today is man's economic insistence that agricultural products must be large and unblemished by insects. One of the tasks of the Bio-Dynamic farmer and gardener today is to restore conditions which approximate those of nature without using unnatural substances. Making use of plant combinations which repel troublesome insects or which attract helpful insects is one part in this restoration of natural conditions.

INSECT PESTS AND PLANT CONTROLS

Insect	Plant Antagonist
Ants	Spearmint, Tansy, Pennyroyal
Aphis	Nasturtium, Spearmint, Stinging Nettle, Southernwood, Garlic
Bean Beetle, Mexican	Potatoes
Black Fly	Intercropping, Stinging Nettle
Cabbage Worm Butterfly	Sage, Rosemary, Hyssop, Thyme, Mint, Wormwood, Southernwood
Cucumber Beetle, Striped	Radish
Cutworm	Oak Leaf mulch, tanbark
Flea Beetle, Black	Wormwood, Mint
Flies	Nut trees, Rue, Tansy, spray of Wormwood and/or tomato
Grub, June Bug	Oak leaf mulch, tanbark
Japanese Beetle	White Geranium, Datura

(continued on page 290)

Companion Plants

(continued from page 289)

INSECT PESTS AND PLANT CONTROLS

Insect	Plant Antagonist
Lice, Plant	Castor bean, Sassafras, Pennyroyal
Mosquito	Legumes
Mosquito, Malaria	Wormwood, Southernwood, Rosemary, Sage,
Moths	Santolina, Lavender, Mint
	Stinging Nettle, herbs, (See also APHIS)
Potato Beetle, Colorado	Eggplant, Flax, Green beans
Potato Bugs	Flax, Eggplant
Slugs	Oak leaf mulch, tanbark
Squash Bugs	Nasturtium
Weevils	Garlic
Woolly Aphis	Nasturtium
Worms in Goats	Carrots
Worms in Horses	Tansy leaves, mulberry leaves

INTERCROPPING

When several crops are grown on the same space, they are intercropped, and harvesting takes place at different times. After the first crop is harvested, the second crop remains as a ground cover until it is ready for harvest. With a crop like broad beans it is a great help to grow an intercrop like spinach which shades the soil and prevents a cracked and crusted soil surface.

Here are some further examples of intercropping according to F. Caspari: Bush or dwarf peas, when planted with early potatoes grow poorly; the neighborhood of carrots enhances their growth. For a long time Dutch gardeners have grown leek and onions with carrots. Onions are also friendly to red beets, strawberries and tomatoes. In good soils some Camomile scattered between onions is said to be helpful to the onions. Growing bush beans adjacent to onions is not good practice. Celery does better when intercropped with members of the cabbage family, especially cauliflower. Cucumbers like to have other plants growing around the edges, such as beans or corn, which will protect them from the wind in a slightly enclosed space. Also cucumbers grow well between annual "hedgerows" of corn.

Taking the Mystery Out of Mulching

(continued from page 151)

floor. You can learn more about the health of your forest from the depth of the humus at your feet than from the height of the trees above your head.

If the layer of leaf mold and humus is thick, rejoice! Your forest is in natural, healthy condition and you do not need mulch — in fact, if your forest is in that good condition, you do not need this article.

On the other hand, if you are restoring a piece of abused land, you are probably not so fortunate. Fire may have burned the leaf mold away; people, vehicles, or cattle may have pulverized or compacted it; or you may have just planted a new forest where the trees have not yet begun to build up their mulch beds.

Any bare — or balding — piece of land can benefit from mulching. Placing mulch around a tree is both helpful and natural. Other places that can use mulch, urgently at that, are bare slopes or disused road beds and around trees suffering from compacted soil.

What kind of mulch? The longer you mulch, the more prejudices and stubborn attitudes you will probably develop, until you eventually become so crotchety, opinionated, and impossible that everyone will consider you an expert.

My own hang-up was rotten horse manure. I attributed all sorts of magical properties to The Stuff. I knew of several stockpiles from old stables, and I cherished these bits of knowledge as a prospector might cherish his mines of gold.

Yet, to be honest about it, any vegetable matter will do as a mulch. Some, of course, are better than others. Some are more acid, others more base. Some have more nitrogen than others. Some rot faster and others more slowly. If you are raising vegetables, delicate flowers, or exotic shrubs, you might worry about these fine points. But for general wild-land management, any organic matter is better than bare ground. What you use will probably depend on what you can get. One word of warning, though: do not use an inflammable mulch in a high-fire-hazard area. Dry sawdust in particular has been known to ignite by spontaneous combustion.

Here is a list of some of the more commonly available mulches, and a few comments.

HAY Look for "spoiled hay," that is, hay that has been ruined by rain and is no longer good for animal feed. The farmer's woe can be your delight. You can often get spoiled hay free for the hauling. It makes a fast-rotting, excellent mulch. It is easy and pleasant to handle, and it is the best mulch you can get for erosion control.

LEAVES Obviously the most natural mulch for trees. Before collecting them from city streets or parks, think about how to compress them in the back of your truck. Some sheets of plywood and a few stones might help.

Oak leaves and pine needles have a reputation for making the soil acid. I generally wouldn't be too concerned about this, but if you mulch often with these leaves, an application of lime won't hurt any.

LAWN CLIPPINGS This is perfectly good stuff, and city parks departments will often give it to you free. Don't lay it on much thicker than six inches, because bigger piles of green lawn clippings sometimes heat up ferociously as they decay.

SAWDUST Personally, I hate sawdust. I find it hard to handle and boring to shovel, it looks dull and sodden when wet, it tends to blow away when dry, and it makes me sneeze. Other people use it regularly, and some people even prefer it. Different strokes for different folks, as they say. If you live near a sawmill, you may get it free and help reduce air pollution at the same time.

One occasional problem with sawdust is that sometimes the first application creates a nitrogen deficiency in the soil. It seems that the organisms that digest cellulose use up lots of nitrogen, which they borrow from the soil. Once the sawdust starts to rot, however, the organisms die off and return the nitrogen to the soil, so the problem is short-term. If a recently mulched tree shows signs of nitrogen starvation (look for a yellowing of the leaves), add some sort of nitrogen-rich compost or fertilizer.

WOOD CHIPS Wood chips are another of my favorites. They don't decay as fast as sawdust and have none of sawdust's drawbacks. They are often available from utility companies or anyone else with a chipper.

OLD CHRISTMAS TREES Why not? Returning a Christmas tree to the soil would be an excellent Christmas present for your land. And soliciting Christmas trees from the community is a fine way of getting people involved. DRY WEED STALKS AND

HAY If you are planting trees in the middle of an old pasture, you might bring along a sickle or scythe and cut weeds and hay right from the site. Don't worry about weed seeds. They won't stand a chance if you make the mulch deep enough.

AGRICULTURAL AND FOOD PROCESSING WASTES Depending upon your local agriculture and industries, you might get buckwheat hulls, ground corncobs, rice or wheat stalks, crushed sugar cane, peanut hulls, spent brewery hops, cocoa bean hulls, or well-rotted manure. Look around, become mulch conscious, and remember: *any* organic material (no matter how weird it smells) is better than bare soil.

Applying the mulch: There's really not much to it. If the soil is hard and compacted, you might rototill the area first. Otherwise, just dump the stuff around the tree. Don't even dig up the weeds and grasses; unless the sod is exceptionally thick, bury them! If the mulch is deep enough, the weeds and grasses below will rot and add to the mulch.

After you've dumped the mulch and spread it around a bit, you must rake it away from the tree trunk. If you leave it piled around the trunk, the millions of little beasties will soon arrive to nibble away at the bark. Spread the mulch so that most of it is under the *drip line* — the area underneath the outermost branches of the tree. If the material is light you can throw some sticks, branches, or logs over it or wet it down so that it won't blow away.

Afterwards: After you've mulched, there is nothing else to do. Nothing. Please don't cultivate the ground with the idea of working some of the mulch into the soil. If the mulch has not yet decomposed, cultivating won't do any good and might even steal moisture and nutrients away from the roots. If the mulch has decomposed, then it is soil, organic soil, and the earthworms will have an absolutely ecstatic time mixing it with the mineral soil underneath. If you want your share of ecstasy, there is nothing better you can do than watch the earthworms. ☼

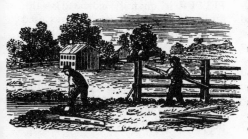

Whatever Happened to Tomatoes

(continued from page 153)

own. I had to do this so that I could experience the sublime flavor of corn, picked just before cooking, and cooked just before eating. There are those who will not eat corn that is more than a few hours picked. I have eaten such corn, and I found it to be a different vegetable altogether, in the same way that canned peas are different from fresh ones. Starting May 1, but taking a small gamble on it, I plant an extra early variety, like Early Sunglow, for corn on the Fourth of July. The same day, I put in a 78-day variety, like the scrumptious Honey and Cream (also known as Butter and Sugar), to take up when the early variety gives out, about two weeks later, and a main-crop yellow corn, like Iochief, if it should happen to be dry and hot, and a white corn, like Silver Queen, if it should be a good growing season. The flavor of Silver Queen is unbelievable, even in February when you take it from the freezer. The sweetness of this variety may be due to the long growing period, for these last two are both 90-day varieties. So they will be our mainstay in early and mid-August. Succession plantings of these last two varieties will keep us in corn until frost, in mid-October around here. Meanwhile, a little freezing will insure that the flavor of fresh corn will be a winter treat too. Don't try to freeze it all at once. When you pick the corn for dinner, about 6 P.M. when the sugar content is highest after a day of sun and photosynthesis, gather an extra dozen. Steam-blanch with the corn for dinner, and after your coffee, cut off the extra dozen and pack into freezer boxes, the work of but a few minutes. This way, corn gets into the freezer without an exhausting day of steaming and cutting in the heat of afternoon. You inspect the corn-patch each afternoon, to be sure that the gradually maturing ears don't slip by you and get too old, and when the first frost threatens, there's no panic to grab it before it's all gone. You can afford to leave a few for the pheasants.

We are now into a good-sized gardening plan, but there are more "flavorite" varieties in store for us. Cantaloupe is cantaloupe to most people, but that is because most commercial growers use only one variety, which is picked green and allowed to ripen in transit. The new, extra sweet varieties, when allowed to ripen on the vine until the stem falls off with a touch of the thumb, make the old ones seem insipid and blah. "Ambrosia" and "Luscious" are two variety names for the new sweet cantaloupes, and the names are not mis-

leading. These two are not more than three years old in the home gardening catalogs, but they may make you feel that you have never tasted cantaloupe before.

With an eye on superb flavor, we would next mark off a corner of the garden, or a bit of the perennial border, for a small herb garden. A sprinkling of fresh herbs can make the difference between a good soup and a marvelous one. A circle of parsley round the outside, and then six wedge-shaped plots of chives, thyme, sage, basil, mint and oregano will fill all of my herb needs. The oregano is one plant of great age, used in tomato juice, pizza sauce, spaghetti and bouquet garni. I planted it from seed, several years ago. It seems to benefit from the mild pruning of its tips when it is needed. The chives multiply so rapidly that I am constantly digging up little chive plants and giving them away. This was also from seed, and is used in cottage cheese, soup, and salads, and can be frozen, chopped, for use in the winter. The mint, likewise a perennial, I transplanted from the woods, and it makes dandy tea, mint jelly and garnishes. The sage needs to be pruned to keep it from being too leggy, since it grows bigger every year. It finds its way into dressings, tomato juice, and sachets, and is available all winter. The thyme, also perennial, is one plant that grows slowly, but makes up for what I use each year. Indispensable in pizza sauce, pot roast, spaghetti, and tomato juice. The basil, for tomatoes in any form and soup in general, must be replanted every year, as does the parsley, which I use in everything, including "pesto" sauce and salads. The herb garden takes very little work for the joys and flavors it provides.

A row of dill I usually save for the garden, because it grows four feet tall and destroys the symmetry of the herb patch. Imperative for dill pickles.

Those dill pickles bring up another vegetable where the consumer in the supermarket ends up with the less flavorful choice in favor of the seasoned traveler. Cucumbers come in a wide variety of types — Burpee lists sixteen, some of the subtle differences among which elude even me, and the top one in my opinion, for flavor and beauty, is never found in the store. "Burpless" is a long, smooth, slim cuke with a thin skin, and it is supposed to agree with people who have trouble with cucumbers. As to this quality I cannot testify, because I love all cucumbers, but this one is tops in my book because it is firm, never pithy, has small seeds, a fragile and delicate skin, never like the heavy plastic coats some cukes seem to get when older, does not seem to turn bitter in hot, dry weather, and makes exquisite dill pickles as tall as a quart mason jar. When packed full-length, in a wide-mouth quart, they look like a *(continued on page 292)*

Whatever Happened to Tomatoes

(continued from page 291)

How to Resist

(continued from page 159)

Herbs, Spices and Seasonings

(continued from page 165)

treat from an epicure shop at $5 per jar. They are fun to eat. What more do you want?

Another neglected variety is the lemon cuke, a charmer exactly the size and color of a ripe lemon, but sweet and tender and with practically no skin at all. My husband swears that, dilled whole when the size of golf balls, they are his favorite pickles.

Glancing through a seed catalog can be an enlightening experience for a city dweller. Most people aren't aware that carrots come in a huge variety of shapes, from short and fat to very long and thin, with nine gradations of these extremes between, and that cauliflower comes in green and purple besides basic white, and that cabbage comes in early, midseason, late, red, savoy and Chinese types. Within each of the above categories, there are three or four varieties from which to choose, for flavor, color, shape, size, weight, and resistance to disease.

In an age when we get more choices among laundry detergents than we really need, and a bewildering variety of cold prepared cereals, we must make do with one variety of vegetable of each kind, when there are usually dozens. Plant breeders generally do not look for what I want in food, and when I see the words, "good shipper," "huge size," "heavy yield," or "resistant to everything," I just keep reading until I see what I want in a vegetable: "wonderful flavor," "sweet and tender," and my favorite: "our most delicious variety." Why settle for less? ☼

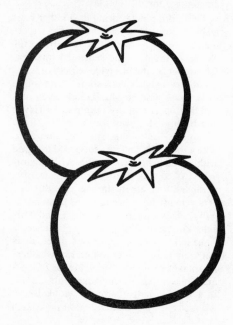

How to Resist the Resisters

Today, if you can become steward of a piece of land and have 35 cents for a packet of seeds, you can afford dozens of heads of lettuce, real and fresh, or a hundred pounds of winter squash, real and sturdy enough to last well into the next winter.

The best way to get the word around and convince resisters is to grow good vegetables. Ask people to visit and look at the organic gardens, and, in fact, turn your gardens into demonstration centers. Let the skeptics see for themselves how successful they can be. And how beautiful sometimes, when decorated here and there with bright nasturtiums, neat white feverfew, blooming mints, and clean, rugged, dark-green parsleys and other herbs.

Start Organic Gardening Clubs

Another good way to spread the word is to establish organic gardening clubs and encourage people to come and hear about others' experiences. And offer to go to talk to already founded garden clubs. Also join the work of ecology groups, pollution fighters, organizations working for recycling collections and detergent-abatement programs. Look up and join natural or organic food cooperatives.

How to Convert the Resisters

If you do not grow fruits and nuts yourself, send away for some. Bring out some of your best vegetables and other produce and get people to taste how good organically grown, untreated fruits, nuts and vegetables can be. Get them to taste utterly fresh foods. Explain how the nutritional values can be kept from dissipating by certain protections you can give them, and how you don't have to throw them away as Americans so often do—through carelessness, wastefulness, or ignorance.

Write articles for bulletins, papers, magazines and any others who are willing to publish what you have to say. And give talks to clubs and on the radio to tell the public what organic gardening is. There are still people who have never heard of it. Take photographs and show slides. Explain about organic sprays and companionate planting. Many are eager to learn what these mean as soon as they hear of them. ☼

MUSTARD, symbolizing indifference, is a widely used condiment. The whole seed is used in pickling and salad dressings. Powdered mustard adds tang to sauces and dressings, or can be mixed with liquid to make hot mustard paste. Fine mustards are prepared in Dijon and Dusseldorf, and a delicious, grainy, farmstyle mustard is occasionally available. Mustard seed sprouts are deliciously peppery. The young shoots of the mustard plant in the spring contribute zest to any green salad and provide a wealth of vitamins and minerals as well.

NUTMEG is the seed of an Indonesian tree. It is best used in whole seed, grated as needed. The subtle flavor lends magic to custards, pies, cheese dishes and cream sauces. Nutmeg should be used sparingly.

OREGANO may also be known as wild marjoram. Another member of the prolific mint family, oregano gives pizza its characteristic flavor. It is also widely used in Italian, Greek, Mexican, Spanish and Caribbean dishes. The flavor of oregano is strong and the herb should be used lightly.

PAPRIKA is an abused spice. The most commonly available variety is almost tasteless, lending color, but little flavor, to dishes in which it is used. Paprika is made from dried, ground peppers, and the best comes from Hungary. The flavor is pungent, ranging from mild to fiery. It is delicious in meat, fish and poultry dishes and is compulsory in Hungarian cooking.

PARSLEY symbolizes both revelry and victory. It is very rich in vitamins A and C, and trace minerals. Both the flat-leafed (Italian) variety, and the more common curly-leaf variety are easy to grow, and readily available in season. Dried parsley should be bright green. Parsley should be used liberally.

PEPPER in quantity indicated wealth during the Middle Ages, and was used as a method of payment as late as colonial times. The same fruit produces black, white and green pepper. Our common black peppercorns are unripe berries, sun-dried. White pepper simply has the black outer coating removed. For superior flavor, white and black pepper should always be freshly ground.

Green pepper is made from pickled, immature pepper berries and is used in meat and seafood dishes.

POPPY SEEDS come from the lovely poppy flower, though NOT the opium poppy. The delicious nut-like seeds are delightful in desserts, pastries and baked goods. They are a marvelous garnish for buttered noodles or vegetables.

ROSEMARY symbolizes remembrance. Hundreds of years ago in the British Isles, rosemary was said to flourish in gardens where "the mistress was master," and insecure husbands would covertly uproot it. Fresh rosemary is most flavorful but the dried form is also pungent. Rosemary is a natural complement to lamb, and delightful in marinades and salad dressings.

SAFFRON is extremely expensive because it takes the stigmas of 4,600 saffron flowers, handpicked, to make one ounce. Luckily, a little goes a long way in rice and fish dishes.

SAGE symbolizes domestic virtue. Easy to grow, fresh sage has a wonderfully pungent flavor, delightful in salads and stuffings.

SAVORY was used generously by the Romans. It has sometimes been called the "bean herb" because it is not only delicious with dried beans, but helps to reduce flatulence. Bees are fond of savory, too. Savory is good in soups, salads, sausage, fish and poultry dishes.

SESAME is used as a flavoring both as seeds and oil. Toasted sesame seeds are wonderful in baked goods, salads, sauces and French dressing. Sesame oil is an important ingredient in Chinese and Japanese cooking. Tahini, a paste made from ground sesame seeds is used in Near Eastern cooking.

TARRAGON symbolizes generosity. Native to southern Europe, tarragon is an essential ingredient in tartare and Bearnaise sauces, goes well in poultry, veal and egg dishes, and is the essence of tarragon vinegar.

THYME symbolizes courage. The wild thyme growing on the slopes of Greece's Mount Hymettus flavors a wonderful honey. Thyme is one of the most basic herbs in French cuisine. Dried thyme has a strong flavor and can be used sparingly in soups, stews, sauces and vegetable dishes.

TUMERIC is a relative of ginger, but has a vastly different flavor. Tumeric root is peeled, dried and powdered to produce a bright yellow powder which lends color and flavor to curries, pickles, rice, sauces and mayonnaise.

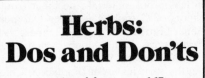

Herbs: Dos and Don'ts

(continued from page 167)

your herb infusions. They may impart a bitter *(better)* taste to a given remedy, and, with the roots, are most useful as a tonic in general debility, weakened gastro-intestinal conditions and rheumatic complaints. Do balance with aromatics. All Gentian parts are used in making wines.

16—Do be adventuresome and prepare your own coffee substitute. The vegetal ingredients include Chicory and Dandelion roots, sliced in long, thin strips, the shells of Nuts—Acorns, Groundnuts and Peanuts—and Soybeans, Chickpeas, Rye, Barley and Peas. These are roasted together for an hour to a deep brown in an oven, on the stove, or in the fireplace. (Years ago I'd roast them in an outdoor fireplace.) Try to achieve a uniform color.

17—Do prepare your own soil enricher. Find a well-humused wastefield in late fall and transport much of its composted material to your garden area. Mix it well into the soil. In the following late spring and early summer, after you have finished planting the *vegetable* seeds, stir a handful of fresh (or last summer's) plants of Dandelion, Mustard, Pigweed (Amaranth), Burdock and especially Nettle, a tablespoonful each of Chamomile and Sage, and two tablespoonfuls of *dried* horse or cow manure in a tub or barrel of five or more gallons of water. Place the container in warm sunshine for four or five days, stirring the contents daily. Dilute one or two cupfuls in four or five gallons of water and spray over the soil of the vegetable garden twice a week. Do *not* apply to the herb area.

Alone or in combination, weeded plants, grass and shrub cuttings, and vegetable discards (e.g. Pea pods, Corn husks) make good mulches.

18—Do include more of these ever-present wildlings in your herb teas and simple remedies: Birch, Yarrow, Linden, Goldenrod, Mints, Catnip, Alfalfa, Clovers, Dandelion, Pine (leaves), Sassafras, berry leaves, Sweet fern, Bayberry, and Meadowsweet.

19—Do make greater use of your pretty Nasturtiums. They are a tangy adjunct to a salad, soup, or omelet, and are a most acceptable replacement for a close

relative, Watercress. And whether you are an organic gardener or not (better if you are), protect your cultivated vegetables with frequent plantings of this delightful herb. Have it reside among Tomatoes, Potatoes, Squash and Radishes, to protect them against harmdoers.

20—Do make various herb vinegars via conventional recipes. Use aromatics of your choice or any of these: Wild Allspice, early Tansy leaves, Mints, Catnip, Wild Onion and Garlic, Horseradish roots, Masterwort, Wild Ginger, Penny grass, Sassafras twigs and bark, Wormwood, Bayberry leaves, *and* citrus peels. Always use cider, wine or malt vinegar. The finished product not only serves in salad dressings, sauces, bastings and marinating liquids; it is often employed as a gargle, liniment, poultice and hair rinse.

21—Do prepare a herb pillow with (1) kitchen food-seasoners—Marjoram, Thyme, Lavender, Lemon Verbena, et al. (2) wildlings such as Sweet Fern, Sassafras, Pine, Bayberry, Mints, Sweet Clovers, et al. (3) garden favorites—Lilac, Sweet Violets, Lily of the Valley, Rose buds, Heliotrope and (4) pillow-stuffers like Hops, Milkweed silk and Life Everlasting. (The latter three alone make separate products.) These pillows will aromatize a room, may be slept on, are suitable Christmas and birthday gifts, and excel as conversational pieces.

The same herbs plus the rinds of the citrus cousins are also ingredients of sachets and potpourris. The two-by-two-inch sachets (or sweet bags, as they were called in my youth) are usually kept in closets and drawers, and with stored clothing to disperse their delightful scent. Some say they deter moths.

22—Do include "bitter" herbs in your herb teas (tisanes): Horehound, Blue Verbena, Yarrow, Boneset, Sage, Barberry, Mugwort, Gentian, Wormwood and Goldenrod. They're better for you and will sweeten and invigorate the entire system. The strong taste is gone far sooner than imagined.

23—Do make better use of the common Smooth and Staghorn Sumacs: A tea of the early fruits becomes a delightfully refreshing "Indian Lemonade." A simmered infusion of the mid-summer fruits helps to remove catarrhal deposits from the alimentary and bronchial passages and to reduce temperature in feverish colds; a decoction of the fall-collected fruits, an effective mouthwash or gargle for all mouth and throat irritations, sores and cankers.

(continued on page 294)

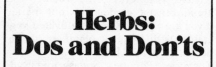

Herbs: Dos and Don'ts

(continued from page 293)

The hardened excrescences (warts) and late fall bark yield a high content of tannic and gallic acids which renders a fast healing effect to sores, cuts, and minor skin problems.

24—Do prize Sassafras for its many virtues. Its leaves may be cooked in a gumbo-like soup, in stews, casseroles, and with other vegetables; powdered and incorporated in a herb salt substitute, sauce or gravy; the stemless leaves, in a herb pillow; the young stems as a pleasantly tasting nibble and the later ones, dried and ground, as an extra seasoning aid; the bark, to season the aforementioned foods, and powdered as an insect powder. The coarsely cut bark has been employed for centuries to detoxify the system and blood stream, as a spring tonic, and in stomach, cold-cough and kidney remedies. A strained warm infusion of the pitch is mucilaginous and thus becomes a most efficacious eye lotion. A yellow dye is obtained by boiling the wood and bark of Sassafras.

25—Do dye with herbs. Samples of colors and the plants: yellow: flowers of Zinnia, Marigold and St.-Johns-wort, bark of Sassafras and Barberry, and Onion skins; violet; Elderberries and Wild Grapes, Iris petals; red: fruits of Black Currant and Poke, flowers of Hollyhock and Coreopsis; green: Nettle, Goldenrod and Mullein; gray: leaves of Horsetail, Blueberry, Butternut; brown: Sumac fruits and bark, Walnut hulls, Hickory bark. Dyeing is a fascinating and highly remunerative hobby.

26—Do remember that herbs offer thirty-two uses: *Candies, Clothing materials, Cosmetics, Deodorants, Disinfectants, Flower arrangements, Food supplements, Foods, for the Bath, Ground covers, Hair preparations, Health teas, Historical backgrounds, Insect repellents, Jams and Jellies, Pickles, Pillows, Potpourris, Preserves, Remedies, Remedies for animals, Sachets, Salt substitutes, Seasonings, Soil enrichers, Sprouts, Tea and Coffee substitutes, Tints and Dyes, Tobacco substitutes, Vinegars, Weather forecasters, and Wines and Beer.*

27—Do freeze these high potency foods in leak-proof material: the inner (root) shoots of Cattails, the upper leaf portions of Purslane (Pussley), Peppergrass, Wintercress, Lamb's-quarters and Japanese Knotweeds, Wild Onion, Wild Garlic; the early leaves of Dandelion, Chicory, Nettle, Yellow Dock, and Burdock; the early shoots of Milkweed; the ground peels of Orange, Lemon, and Tangerine.

28—Do gather Stinging Nettles by cutting them with a long knife or scissors so that the herb falls on newspapers spread beneath. (Be sure to wear gloves.) Then fold and tie the newspapers with string. Dry by suspension in a warm area (attic or cellar), then strip the leaves and fruits, and label. The fresh leaves are steamed a few minutes and eaten with other cooked vegetables; be sure to ingest every drop of the remaining liquor. Use the ground leaves in herb teas and as extra nutrient in omelets, soups, casseroles, and powdered, in a herbal salt substitute or food supplement in gelatin capsules obtainable from your pharmacist.

29—Do use your juicer and blender to obtain the optimum nutrients (minerals, vitamins and enzymes) from your native herbs: Dandelion, Burdock, Yellow Dock, Pennycress, Watercress, Sorrel, Purslane, Amaranth, Lamb's-quarters, Violets, Peppergrass, et al. (The beginner should mix the extraction with an equal amount of the juice of fresh Celery, Carrot, Kale, Parsley and Cabbage).

The juice contains 75 percent of the nutrients. It is diluted with three parts of water and if sipped *slowly,* on an empty stomach, is assimilated within an hour. Prepare only enough juice as needed—do not store.

The blendered herbs to be taken as foods are diluted with two (or more parts) of water and stirred well. Then the diluted concentrate is slowly *eaten* in teaspoonful amounts, i.e., mixed well with the saliva before swallowed.

30—Do plant aromatic herbs as companions to your cultivated vegetables. They serve either as soil enrichers or repellents of *harmful* insects and worms (e.g. nematodes). Several examples: Sage and Rosemary for Carrots and members of the Cabbage family, Summer Savory for Pole and Bush Beans, Peas, and members of the Onion family, Dill for the Cabbage family, Chamomile for Onions and Garlic, Nasturtium for Broccoli and Apple trees, Basil for Asparagus and Tomato, and Marigold for Tomato and Potato. (See #17)

31—Do tenderize your meat and fish with large grape leaves. Steam them as jackets for meat or with other vegetables, or cut them into small pieces for soup, stew, omelet, etc. And include a few of the washed tendrils in a vegetable salad, cole slaw, and other dishes. Love them as a passing nibble.

32—Do use American Ivy (American Woodbine, Virginia Creeper): the leaves in a tea (tisane), the stems for skin and blood disorders, the whole herb as an expectorant in bronchial complaints. It's a good alternative and substitute for American Sarsaparilla. The small, dark purplish-blue fruits have been syruped and given in feverish complaints.

Locate this proliferating ground cover and transplant a few feet of the stems (plus its tendrils) to a bare spot in your garden. And, too, let it ramble over your stone walls and fences and ascend nearby trees.

33—Do consider lichen, a fungus found on tree, rocks and walls, a herb. It has been used effectively in skin disorders (psoriasis and eczema) and recently was shown to yield an antibiotic which inhibited the activity of the *staphylococcus* bacteria.

34—Do save and use all Acorns. Remove the tannic acid content of the meats by gently simmering them (twenty minutes) in water to which bits of charcoal have been added. Rinse in tepid-cool water and include in bread, pastry, soup, stuffing, casseroles and in all cooked meat/fish dishes. An ideal replacement for Chestnuts. The tannic acid liquid is a fair tan tint or dye.

35—Do eat the fresh leaves of garden-cultivated residents: Pansy, Violet, Nasturtium, early Hollyhock, and flowers of the latter, Yucca and Rose. Chop the spring-gathered leaves of your Water Lily and use it either in a sandwich or salad or steam-cooked; the unopened flower buds are also steamed in soup, or pickled to become a satisfying relish.

36—Do enjoy the fruitfulness of Marigold flower heads. A weak infusion of the florets has been much used for reddened or inflamed eyes. Alone they're an acceptable substitute for the expensive Saffron to color and season baked foods, starches like Rice and Potatoes, and everyday recipes (e.g. soup, chowder).

Prepare your own antiseptic astringent lotion by covering the dried petals with rubbing alcohol (ethyl) or Witch Hazel extract for a week. Apply the strained solution to cuts and pimples;

use it as a cosmetic skin cleanser. Simmer the petals also in cold cream or unsalted lard and use in all external skin problems.

37—Do aromatize a room with herbs. Combine any three or four of these herbs: a tablespoonful each of Basil, Rosemary, Oregano, ground Cinnamon, Bayberry, Sweet Fern, Citrus rinds; a scant teaspoonful of Dill and Fennel seeds, and a half teaspoonful of Juniper berries. Stir well a cupful of the mixture in about a quart of hot water and let rest over a warm stove or next to a warm radiator. Very soon the undesirable malodors in the room have been overcome and are no more. Remember: in the summertime, place a few sprigs of the herbs in the direct sunlight of your windows.

38—Do prepare your own herbal aromatizer for the bath or shower. Use any mixture of the herbs mentioned under room aromatizer (#37), herb pillow (#21), plus Catnip, Lemon Balm, Spice Bush, Dill herb, Parsnip leaves, and a little Sage. Stuff the foot of a nylon stocking or a small cloth or linen bag and tie to the faucet or shower head. Sponge the body gently with the enveloped herbs.

39—Do include the fresh or dried, resinous exudations of Spruce, Larch and Pine trees in your skin healing lotions, creams or ointments. Use rubbing alcohol (ethyl), lanolin (cream or ointment) and unsalted lard. If either of these bases is warmed, you may also add Saint-John's-wort flowers, Oak or Sumac bark, late Sweet Fern, and Cinquefoil stems.

40—Do go to your library every week and find a book on herbs and their various benefits until you have exhausted the supply. Read Gerard, Coles, Parkinson, Culpeper, Withering et al., and cross index your findings on three-by-five file cards. Become an expert.

41—Do grow these useful herbs in your rock garden: Pennyroyal, Thyme and Marjoram. If you've not enough room in the garden or window areas, consider a roof garden. Use small barrels, wooden tubs, quart tins and other containers mentioned under fall-winter gardening (#3). The herbs? The same ones cultivated in the ordinary herb garden.

42—Do transplant or cultivate several well-known wildlings in your herb garden: Yarrow, Mints, Catnip, Iris, Meadowsweet and Spireas, Forget-me-nots, Violets, Wild Geranium, Blue Vervain, Purple Cone-flower, and Black-eyed Susan. All have specific therapeutics and especially are the Black-eyed Susan's roots (as a decoction) much used in blood and skin diseases. You may include all its parts in your herb teas and internal remedies.

43—Do purchase your (food seasoning, aromatic) herb seeds wherever they're sold—herb sellers and health food stores (they usually sell organically raised ones), drug and hardware stores, and garden centers. By planting them in poor, well-drained soil and adopting a non-fertilizing attitude toward soil and plant, you may obtain a better strain of seeds.

44—Do ascertain the many values of all uninvited guests found in your garden spaces before you discard them as worthless. Most of these weedy nondescripts have been in constant use for many centuries and their profitable applications are indicated under the uses of herbs in #26.

45—Do remember that thorny or prickly herbs—Barberry, Nettles, Rasp- and Blackberry, Hawthorn, Motherwort and others—foretell their therapeutic "signature" in *painful* conditions. Actually the herbs are not anodynes or pain-relievers per se but do try to reach the *cause* of the troubling pain. Therefore, one should eat much of their fruits and leaves and drink teas of their herb parts.

46—Do make use of the shrubs and small trees on your property. A few examples: Quince's fruits as food, seeds for hand lotions and cough syrup; Privet's leaves and stems as a remedy to heal mouth sores, stomach ulcers, and bowel complaints; Barberry's parts and the bark of the Flowering Ash in stomach/liver conditions; the leaves and bark of Birches to bathe skin eruptions; the leaves of Pine to stuff a pillow and its exuding pitch in skin remedies; fruits of Mountain Ash in sauce, jellies and preserves, etc.

47—Do sprout your fall collection of (dried) seeds. Use ordinary garden soil and a minimum of fertilizer. When the sprouting greens are 2 inches high, expose them to full sunlight. Soil-sprouted greens offer easily digested and assimilated minerals and vitamins and may be eaten as is, juiced or blended, added to salads, finished soups, stews, omelets, or steamed vegetables.

These seeds are ever available: Amaranth (Pigweed), Yellow Dock, Dandelion, Burdock, Lamb's-quarters, Peppergrass, Plantain, assorted Clovers, Sunflower, Parsley, Radish, Fenugreek, and Alfalfa. The latter two and unhulled Sesame and Buckwheat should also be water-sprouted. Buy these four from an organically-raised source to assure that they have not been chemically treated.

48—Do make a cough remedy out of your fever-and-cold tea by syruping with enough honey. Example: Stir well one-half teaspoonful each of Boneset, Thyme, Aniseeds, and Mallow in a cup of hot water. Cover until cool and strain. Add sufficient honey to provide a syrupy consistency. Sip a tablespoonful slowly every hour.

49—Do use every part of Milkweed. The early shoots, flowers and seedpods are nutritious foods; the dried, larger-sized pods can be painted for ornamental value; the early morning gathering of the flowers and the adhering dew are boiled to produce a thin syrup; the silk is used as extra stuffing for a herb pillow; the cut roots provide new plants and material for diaphoretic or expectorant remedies. Commercially, the seeds are a source of animal feed and vegetable oil comparable to Soybean oil and the stalks and silk have been processed into drugs, plastic, insulating materials and clothing.

50—Do use Blueberry's fruits *and* leaves. The former are best eaten uncooked and *without* sugar. They may be incorporated in native jellies, jams, or preserves, in baked goods and puddings. The fruits are often used alone or combined with Elderberries and other fruits to yield a satisfying wine. The leaves enter a simple herb tea and are often included in diuretic or blood detoxifying remedies with Burdock, Thyme, Watercress, Nettles, Sassafras, and Dandelion; in an anti-diabetic tea, with Stinging Nettles, Thistle, and other herbs. The leaves have anti-lithic properties and thus are helpful in kidney problems when stone-forming deposits need to be removed from the urinary tract.

Sun-dry the fruits for ten days (or use the attic or the space over the oil burner).

Better, i.e. more nutrient-packed, fruits are found in limestone areas, on low bushes and on a high hill.

(continued on page 296)

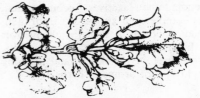

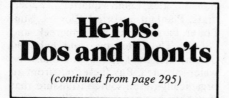

Herbs: Dos and Don'ts

(continued from page 295)

Don'ts

1—Don't ridicule the "quaint" or strange (to us) folklore, thoughts or conclusions of old-time herbalists and Indian medicine men. Their observations, trial-and-error practices, and acceptable miscalculations have led to modern medical discoveries: the Walnut tree's *juglone,* a powerful fungicide and parasiticide; Plantain, an adsorbent in painful, inflammatory conditions (boils, ulcers, et al.); a Fern extractive, a worm expellant; Stamonium, a narcotic and pain reliever, etc....

2—Don't neglect the herbs of your immediate neighborhood. Don't seek herbs from other areas, cities, or lands. Should you become ill or wish to stay well where you live—say New England—then use the herbs found there or in your immediate environs. Remember: "Farfetcht is dearly bought."

3—Don't be misled by "miracle herbs," or by "sure-cures" arising from the use of herbal remedies. Don't consider herbs as a cure-all or panacea. They do *not* do everything like DUZ does; they have their limitations, but "work" better if taken on an empty stomach and if other factors are also considered. Equally as important as herbs: eating organically raised foods, good dietary habits, exercise, sleep, taking no drugs or medications, fasting, etc.

4—Don't mix aromatic seeds (Anise, Caraway, Cumin) with other herbs, unless the latter are reduced to the size of the seeds or are finely ground. Otherwise the seeds may remain at the bottom of the container and not be included in the required teaspoonful dose for an herb tea. Or when you're making the tisane, add a few seeds to the herbs in the cup, pour the hot water over and stir *all* ingredients.

5—Don't use laxative-cathartic herbs as are frequently and rashly recommended. They are apt to weaken the intestines and cause the taker to be dependent upon laxatives. Recommended: As complete an abstinence from manmade foods as possible, a changeover to fresh uncooked vegetables and fruits, more exercise (walking), and drinking tepid teas of aromatic herbs.

Herbal no-nos:
Black Root (Culver's Root)
Boxwood
Bryony
Cascara
Jalap (also Wild Jalap)
Mandrake
Rhubarb leaves
Senna Leaves
Wahoo
Yellow Toadflax

6—Don't drink herb teas (decoctions, powders, or capsules) of *only* Horsetail, Bearberry (Uva Ursi), Horseradish root, or Juniper berries. Taken alone, either as tea or powder, these herbs may irritate the delicate linings of the urinary passages. Always balance with at least equal parts of demulcents (Mallow, Hibiscus, Hollyhock, Sassafras) and aromatics (Mints, Marjoram, Chamomile).

7—Don't call any plant a "weed." Almost every one so maligned—especially those that abound in your vegetable patch—has a purposeful use for us if only we'll take time to research its past and future applications.

Don't relegate these poor relations to the dump or waste areas until you have made sure of their identity and their English and Latin names; then consult various herb books and herbalists to discover their many uses.

8—Don't drink teas of *only* Red Clover, Sweet Clover or Alfalfa. Such solo herb teas may cause slight discomfort or headache. Use an equal part of Mint, Catnip or other aromatics to enhance the complete assimilation of their high-potency nutrients.

9—Don't neglect your reading about historical backgrounds and earliest uses of commonly known herbs (flowers, garden plants), as practiced by the ancient Chinese, Egyptians, people of biblical times and primitive societies, the Druids, the early Greek and Roman doctors, the American Indians and the colonial settlers.

10—Don't let salt and spices nullify the true aromatizing effect of your food-seasoning herbs. Either abstain completely from using them or use a bare minimum. Put a "For External Use Only" label on both. They're medically forbidden in most organic ailments and therefore should be rejected by healthy people.

Don't use even so-called Garlic, Celery or Onion salt. Their content is mostly the forbidden chemical.

11—Don't use the leaves and flowers of the fully grown Tansy for internal purposes. They're too irritating to the gastrointestinal and urinary passages. Consult a herbalist before using. But don't neglect them altogether. The finely powdered parts are mixed with powdered Fleabane and Pennyroyal to yield a good flea and insect chaser. For many years, we have used the freshly dried herb as a worthy moth repellent in our attic. And see Arbor Vitae (#14). However, the five to eight-inch leafy shoots of Tansy may be substituted for Sage and Cinnamon.

Don't be misled by non-herbalist authors who would consider Tansy *(Tanacetum vulgare)* another synonym for Yarrow *(Achillea millefolium).* Europeans may have used both herbs for similar purposes but recognized their differences in appearance, taste, odor, and therapeutics and perhaps suggested its Yarrow-like action.

12—Don't crowd your medicinal and savory herbs when you are drying them. Don't let them overlap, lest they mold. String-tie a small bundle and suspend them overhead, stems up, in a warm, air-circulating room, attic, cellar or over or near a warm stove, radiator or oil burner.

Don't leave drying or dried herbs in direct or even in indirect sunlight. This preserves their original appearance and nutrients.

Don't dry aromatic herbs near or with heat.

13—Don't use such possibly harmful or dangerous herbs as Poke, Bush Clover, Buttercup, Bittersweet, Dogbane, Stramonium and relatives, Mandrake, Buttonbush, Green and other Hellebores, Mountain Laurel.

Don't take chances. If a formula calls for any one of them, substitute an aromatic or demulcent, or consult a herbalist.

14—Don't discard the cuttings of your Arbor Vitae (Yellow Cedar) hedge. Dry and cover a cupful of the dried, ground leaves with rubbing alcohol (ethyl) and seal for a week, shaking it every day. Strain and use for scratches, cuts and simple skin affections. Place foot-long sprigs in the direct sunlight of attic windows and the diffusing oil will act as an insect-moth deterrent. And to disinfect or spread its antiseptic vapors throughout a given area, stir well a tablespoonful each of the herbs Rosemary, Tansy and a few Juniper berries in an open pan containing a pint of boiling water.

Don't use the Arbor Vitae leaves for internal purposes. They are far too strong and irritating to the innards.

15—Don't let a constantly damp spot in your garden go to waste. Plant these excellent dividend-payers: Mint, Spicebush, Daylily, Bee Balm, and Lady Slipper.

16—Don't cook or warm Chervil, Chives, Nasturtium, Sorrel or Watercress. While they do possess medicinal virtues, their true place is in the vegetable category and should always be eaten uncooked, to prevent losing their valuable nutrients. So ingested they are your health-protectors, your disease-preventors, your ounce of self-reliance.

17—Don't keep herbs over three years. That is time enough to have used them for dozens of purposes. At the end of that period, transfer all the remaining herbs to your jar of herbs intended for tea (tisane) and mix them with the contents. Aromatics belong there, too, but may be vinegared or wined.

Fleshy roots like Burdock and Dandelion should be kept only two years, and well protected from insect invasion by a small moth ball.

Label each container with name and date and location of collection. Store your herbs in a cool place.

18—Don't drink cold or iced tea—or hot either. Hot and cold drinks may destroy the gastric (food digesting) enzymes. Drink the infusion tepid or lukewarm. It will keep you warm in winter and cool in summer.

Don't gulp. Sip slowly, slowly, and it will help the processes of elimination, the glandular system and relax the nerves. A slow cup of herb tea is a welcome companion for an inner calm.

19—Don't chew *fresh* leaves of Wintergreen (Checkerberry) continually. I've had many reports that chewing them without a stop for two or three hours or more has caused painful headaches.

Don't drink a tea with Wintergreen the sole ingredient. Use an equal amount of Mint, Catnip, Chamomile, or food seasoner (Fennel, Lemon Balm, Marjoram). Why not stir a half teaspoonful of its ground leaves in a cup of plain everyday tea?

20—Don't use seeds of Cumin, Anise, Caraway and Fennel as is. Before using, pound them or break them up even slightly via a meat grinder, blender or coffee/spice grinder. Thus, the ground herb is dispersed throughout the food being prepared. Ingested whole, the seeds have been known to irritate the delicate linings of the gastro-intestinal canal.

Small rounded seeds like Poppy or Celery may be used whole.

21—Don't expect various herbs (Boneset, Yarrow) or food-seasoners (Marjoram, Sage, Thyme) to completely cure all your ailments.

Don't you sit back and do the "heavy-looking-on." To feel better *all over*, (1) don't season your foods with salt, spices, and assorted condiments. (2) Don't eat white flour and sugar and their products, or fried, greasy or over-boiled foods, or canned, packaged or boxed goods, or the stimulating tea, coffee or colas, or desserts (desert them!) or any more nutritionless man-made food "creations" than you can help. (3) Don't miss a day without some exercises—yoga or calisthenics or even walking—and if you're over 50, have an occasional afternoon nap and an earlier retiring hour.

22—Don't expect to learn *all* about herbs from books (many of which are written by non-herbalists) or from one or two lectures on the subject. Ask a nearby herbalist to teach you and other health-minded friends the basics, lore, various applications and therapeutics of weeds, cultivated herbs and everyday foods and the various ways of preparing herbal remedies and products.

Don't miss the field trips during the summer-fall season. Don't let a clear day go by without collecting and pressing some specimens; "weedy plants," flowers and pertinent parts of shrubs and trees. Learn which offer the greatest utility and then use them as supplemental foods, as ingredients of a multitude of remedies, as external preparations and in other ways, such as a fertilizing solution, herb pillow, flea chaser, aromatizer, and so on.

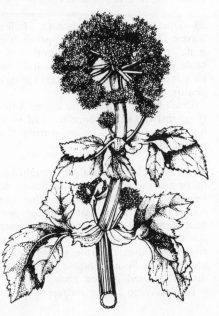

23—Don't grow flowers or shrubs just for aesthetic reasons. Make sure that the denizens of your garden pay rent for the space they occupy and earn their keep and care. Examples: Arbor Vitae's leaves may be used externally in various skin diseases and as a room disinfectant; the stately Hollyhocks as an excellent food source and demulcent in cough and kidney remedies. Hawthorn fruits go into sauces, jams, and jellies and in remedies for kidney, coronary, and high blood pressure. A garden should be as useful as it is beautiful.

24—Don't neglect the often discarded peels of Orange, Lemon, Lime, Tangerine, and Grapefruit. Consider them as herbs, too. Space each rind well apart from the others and let dry uncovered at room temperature. Store in a clean, *dry* jar and label with date. Then when you're ready to use, grind coarsely or finely, and only enough for present needs. Refrigerate the excess in a covered bottle. The peels may be used (whole, ground or powdered) to flavor baked goods, stuffings, soups, casseroles, meat or fish dishes, herb vinegars, and wines and marinating and basting liquids.

25—Don't let your hedges serve only to keep out the neighbor's kids and roaming dogs. Do not neglect the useful dollar-saving virtues of especially Barberry and Privet. The former's football-shaped fruits are ingredients of jellies, preserves, sauce and syrup; its twigs and roots, are remedies for stomach, liver and gallbladder problems, and as a yellow dye. An infusion of Privet's leaves and stems (bark) help to heal minor ulcerations of the mouth and stomach, bleeding and spongy gums, sore and irritated throat.

26—Don't consider your study of herbs a summertime thing, a passing fancy. Once your herb specimens have been properly identified—by herbalists, school or college teachers, grandparents et al., Latin and English names assigned and date and location of collection recorded, don't let a day go by without further researching their many uses.

27—Don't overcook edible herbs (except to prepare a decoction) or destroy their nutrients by drowning them in boiling water. The health-fortifying vitamins, minerals, and other nutrients will be lost, leaving the foods flat and tasteless. At least drink the remaining pot-liquor or save it for soup in other recipes.

(continued on page 298)

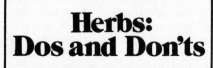

Herbs: Dos and Don'ts

(continued from page 297)

28—Don't transplant the early seedlings of Anise or Cumin. Their roots are a mesh of fine, almost delicate, threads that may not recover easily from the trauma of transplanting. Plant their seeds where they are to grow. That way you'll prevent damage.

29—Don't use spices in your herbal teas or remedies (except in sachets or potpourris). Used to season foods, and ingested consistently, they are liable to irritate the gastrointestinal mucous linings. An exception to the rule: A small stick of Cinnamon and *one* Clove, to gently flavor tea and used only for an occasion.

30—Don't waste the usually neglected space beneath a tree or shrub. Underplant with such useful herbs as Mints, Sedums, Violets, Lily-of-the-Valley.

Don't worry about garden bald spots or shady places. Use these ground covers: Periwinkle, Bugle, American Woodbine or Thyme. They need very little care and offer many values.

31—Don't forget that modern medical science has used the knowledge of how to heal diseases with herbal remedies and has produced drugs with the same properties as those herbs which were used for centuries to cure the ailments now succumbing to their new chemical forms. Cinchona, a source of quinine, is used for malaria; Digitalis for heart and dropsy problems; Rauwolfia for high blood pressure; Sarsaparilla for psoriasis; Soapwort as an antibiotic; Squill and Lobelia as expectorants; Cascara Sagrade for a tonic laxative; and Periwinkle and Mandrake as sources of anti-cancer medication. There are many more examples of old wives' tales leading to life savers. Herbs and herbalists deserve respect.

32—Don't take the juice of Aloe internally. Recent authors (not herbalists) have extolled its virtues and have recommended its dried juice as a purgative. (See #5). The freshly expressed juice may be used for chapped hands, insect bites, scratches and bites, scald and sunburn, "crow's feet" eye wrinkles, and in all skin problems; but *not* for internal purposes, unless a herbalist has been consulted.

33—Don't eat the large leaves (over six inches) of Comfrey. True, farm animals are fond of them, as they are of other *fresh* greens, grains, and grasses; but do Comfrey-eaters consume such herbage *uncooked*—as do our bestial friends?

There may arise a very possible danger from eating the fully-grown leaves as a steady diet, over an extended period of time. The mature plant contains two highly poisonous alkaloids, consolodine and symphytocynoglossine. The writings of Switzerland's Dr. Alfred Vogel gave American authors the opportunity to copy, almost word-for-word, the "sure-cure" wondrous phases of Comfrey *without paying too much attention to the possible harmful aftereffects.* But it is understood, according to Dr. Vogel, that on a long-range basis, these two alkaloids produce an "undesirable effect on the central nervous system." And Prof. Heber W. Youngken, this country's foremost authority on herbal medicine (pharmacognasy), noted their *nerve depressant* action. Beware: This is enough warning to warrant all health enthusiasts to forsake Comfrey's large-sized leaves as an edible herb.

34—Don't throw away the coarse stems of aromatic herbs: Oregano, Basil, Sage, Thyme, Rosemary, Oregano, et al. As such, they may be used to flavor cider, malt or wine vinegar. Or you may dry them thoroughly, reduce or grind them to a suitable size to incorporate in your herb-tea mixture; or powder them sufficiently for your herbal salt-substitute. Commercial herb importers and millers do not include only the leaves in a herb package but as much of the coarse stems as the law will permit. Another good argument for growing your own food-seasoning aromatics.

35—Don't neglect autumn's fallen leaves. They'll serve as a protective mulch to the last planting in your vegetable garden and blanket the soil and keep it comfortably soft for next spring's planting.

Don't forget to pack the leaves solidly against the stone foundation of your house as extra insulation during the winter months.

36—Don't plant Jerusalem Artichokes in, or even adjacent to, your flower or vegetable garden. When planting the tubers (roots) of this fast spreader, prevent them from taking over the growing spaces. Confine them within stone barriers in an unused fertile spot—preferably in an adjoining house lot or in a distant, unused garden area.

Don't say no to the nutrients of the tubers, a very good food: sliced raw in a vegetable salad, steamed or baked and mashed, used instead of Water Chestnuts in Chinese recipes, and diced, either as an ingredient in Bean, Pea or vegetable soup or added as a garnish to the soup when served.

37—Don't annoy your rock garden with mere do-nothing ornamentals. Begging to reside there and pay you good dividends are Sedums, Pinks, Marjoram, Pennyroyal, Mints, Thyme, Bloodroot, Sweet Alyssum.

Don't neglect that space.

38—Don't let the services of your garden's cast of floral characters go to waste: Bugle (astringent, for all internal and external bleedings), Geum species (tonic-aromatic, for stomach and bronchial disorders and feverish colds), Nasturtium (leaves, a good nutrient-packed edible), Yucca flowers (another good food), the ornamental Crabapple and Hawthorn trees (the tart fruits, a satisfying nibble, and costless ingredients of jellies, preserves, pickles, etc.), Marigold flowers (a dye/tint and food aromatizer), Gentian (an excellent stomachic, digestant and tonic), Hepatica (liver and bronchial affections) or Hollyhock (ingredient of salad, soup and healing remedies).

39—Don't linger too long under a Wild Cherry tree or Elder shrub on a hot sticky day. Beware the exuding hydrocyanic acid vapors that may cause a slight but lingering headache.

40—Don't gather aromatic herbs until the third consecutively dry day, and until between ten o'clock and twelve noon. No dew or dampness may be present lest mold be generated. Gathered in the afternoon, the herb's aromatic principles appear to wane. It is best to gather fragrant plants just before the flowers expand.

Don't gather perennial fragrant herbs but once. Cut their foliage two or three times during the growing season, a process that promotes new growth.

Don't cut all plants. Let a few go to seed.

Don't forget to remove a few plants to your window garden in anticipation of the approaching winter months.

41—Don't think of your flowering Rose bush as only decorative. Don't let go to waste the unopened and opening flower buds, the falling petals, the leaves, and later, the hips (fruits). The closed buds are much used with other aromatics (herbs and spices) in sachets, potpourris, and herb pillows; with citrus peels and Pine leaves, for a bath or shower; and with food seasoners like Thyme, Marjoram and Rosemary to aromatize a room.

Don't overlook the eatability of Rose petals and fruits. The latter's vitamin C content surpasses that of Tomatoes and Red Pepper; its vitamin P is remarkably high, and it offers a higher source of iron, calcium, and phosphorus than do Oranges. They are prepared as puree, jam, syrup, soup, wine, and vinegar.

Don't discard the loose or recently fallen petals: use them as a nibble, dipped in honey, to prepare an eye lotion, to apply wet to a recent scratch or skin irritation, or use the leaves, the dried and cut stems, and the coarsely ground hips, as a pleasantly near-tart tisane.

42—Don't worry about the truly poisonous weed-like herbs. Out of 300 that abound in New England, only a mere handful may be so labeled, if taken internally: Stramonium, Henbane, Water Hemlock, fresh Indian Turnip, Dogbane, Bush Clover, Saint-John's-wort, Poison Ivy, Dog's Mercury, Cowslip, Buttercup, Hellebore, Nightshade(s), Bloodroot, Baneberry. (See #13)

43—Don't use American Hellebore (nor the Black or Green varieties) despite "authoritative" remarks. Beware its properties: emetic, narcotic and cardiac (heart) depressant. It can cause severe skin reactions, poisoning and possible death.

Don't use the roots of Blue Flag (Iris) as an internal remedy. It is too strong in ordinarily recommended doses.

Don't use Bloodroot. It's a bit too dangerous for the neophyte herb-user.

Don't use Celandine *(Chelidonium majus)* until you've consulted a professional herbalist. Its rather laxating property should be considered. I call it a 5 percent herb, i.e., one part is thoroughly mixed with nineteen parts of mild, aromatic and demulcent herbs.

44—Don't neglect the late-summer and fall gathering of seeds of the worthy commoners: Dandelion, Lamb's quarters ters, Burdock, Yellow Dock, Amaranth and other prolific weedy growers. (Don't forget Parsley, Nasturtium and various Cresses.) They will do fine indoors in ordinary soil. Enjoy their greens and sprouts during the winter months.

45—Don't eat young Jewel Weed as some writers have suggested. It's far too laxating for the average constitution. And in any formula calling for the dried herb, use only one part mixed

well with fifteen or twenty parts of *non*-laxating herbs. (See #5.)

46—Don't overcook the leaves of Lamb's-quarters, Sorrel(s), Poke and Yellow Dock, (also, Spinach, Beet, Chard and Rhubarb stalks). Steam them two to three minutes, just long enough to soften. Long cooking may prevent the desired absorption of their calcium content.

47—Don't use "strong" herbs like Sage, Boneset, Wormwood, Rosemary, or Vervain alone. Before using either as tisane (herb tea) or in a remedy, modify it with equal parts of one or more parts of an aromatic (Mint or Marjoram) and of a demulcent (Mallow, Hollyhock, or Sassafras leaves).

48—Don't introduce these dangerously toxic herbs as flowering plants to your garden: Aconite, contains a potent narcotic; Daphne (Mezereon), whose root often blisters the skin, and the berries are purgative; fresh Lobelia, if chewed, may cause vomiting and giddiness; Castor, whose seeds contain a violently active poison.

Others to be avoided: Foxglove (Digitalis), Oleander, Autumn Crocus (Colchicum), Larkspur (Delphinium), Christmas Rose. They are really as dangerous as they are beautiful and though they enjoy the role of "medicinal herb," they should not be used except as a vegetal ornamental. If they're out of mind, out of sight and out of garden, then you are out of danger.

49—Don't gather Mushrooms, Puffballs, or Morels unless your guide has known and used them for many years. My experiences as an herb consultant over forty-four years have warned me against foraging for them. While, of 4000 different species, there are "only" forty to fifty that are truly lethal, poisonous or so suspected, *beware!*

Don't eat so-called edible, wild Mushrooms until you've studied their color photos, and can recognize them without hesitation. Consult the horticulturist at your local County Extension Service. Or learn to cultivate these fungi at home.

50—Don't eat recently gathered Butternuts and Black Walnuts until they've aged for two or more months.

Don't dry or store them in air-tight containers. Ventilation is necessary to prevent mold.

Don't collect the nuts unless you wear gloves. Their juice stains the hands dark brown. ☼

Herbs, Astrology Rhythm of Life

(continued from page 169)

credence to astrology, will damn it before he knows anything of its methods, its history or traditions, has no poetry in his soul, to say the least. My main purpose here is to record some of the ancient, beautiful beliefs about the herbs which grow around us, and their link with astrology. If, in doing so, I interest you and entertain you and make you begin to think about alternative ways to "be," other ways to think, different rhythms to adopt in your life, then I have satisfied myself that this little book has served a marvellous purpose.

For, as my ancestor, Jasper Petulengro, once said in Borrow's Lavengro: "Life is sweet, brother . . ." But the knowing of that sweetness, the learning of it, needs a special effort on the part of many a modern human being, trapped in the concrete landscape of city life. To walk on grass, breathe sweet air, has become something of a privilege, almost an impossible dream to millions of us. Many, of course, do not want or need such an existence, having been horribly conditioned by now to the diesel-poison of polluted air, the hard, springless arid waste of city sidewalks. If only they knew, if only they could know, what pleasure is to be had from regaining knowledge of old country lore, of cooking with herbs, eating them fresh in salads, using them for gentle medicaments against ill health, instead of rushing to the harsher, faster methods of modern science.

If only . . . then they would rediscover a most pleasant land — the land of tranquility, of the rhythm of life as my people once knew it.

The secret is everywhere . . . perhaps you will make a start now and learn about the riches that our ancient herbal lore has to offer in this computer age.

May I wish you *kooshti sante* — good health in mind and body, and a long and happy life. ☼

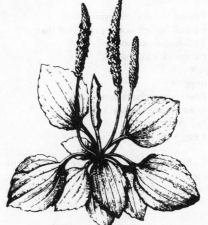

Herb Bouquets and Herb Soups

(continued from page 175)

Aromatic Seasoning
1 ounce nutmeg
1 ounce mace
2 ounces cloves
2 ounces peppercorns
1 ounce dried bay leaves
2 cloves of garlic
3 ounces basil
3 ounces marjoram
2 ounces winter savory
3 ounces thyme
1/2 ounce cayenne pepper
1/2 ounce grated lemon peel

All these ingredients must be well pulverized in a mortar and sifted through a fine wire sieve. Put in dry corked bottle for use.

Herb Soups

No. 1 *(stock)*

4 pounds rump beef
5 quarts cold water
2 teaspoons salt
3 medium onions
2 carrots, scraped
1 turnip, quartered
1 parsnip, cut in strips
1 small head of celery, sliced
Cloves
Herb bouquet

Wipe beef. Cover with cold water. Bring to boiling point and skim carefully. Simmer 2 hours. Add salt and vegetables. Stick an onion full of cloves; add herb bouquet and simmer gently 1 hour. Remove vegetables and meat. Season to taste. Serve in a separate dish.

Herb bouquet: thyme, winter savory, and fennel is a good soup combination.

No. 2 Herb Soup

1 head lettuce, shredded
1 small bunch watercress, cut fine
3 tablespoons butter
6 cups chicken stock
salt
pepper
1 teaspoon chervil, minced
1 teaspoon parsley, minced
1/2 cup cream
1 egg yolk

Cook lettuce and watercress in the butter for 5 minutes, being careful not to brown the herbs. Add stock and seasoning to taste. Cook half an hour, then add chervil and parsley and cream mixed with egg yolk. Stir until heated but do not boil.

No. 3 *(with sorrel and spinach)*

1/2 cup sorrel, finely shredded
1 cup spinach, finely shredded
1 head lettuce
1 leek
4 tablespoons butter
4 medium potatoes
3 teaspoons salt
2 quarts boiling water
1 tablespoon chervil, minced

Use fresh sorrel, spinach, and inside leaves of lettuce; wash and shred, discarding tough midribs. Cut leek into thin slices; cook in butter 15 minutes, being careful not to brown. Add potatoes, salt, and boiling water; boil quickly; reduce heat and boil gently for 1 hour. Crush the potatoes with a fork, add the chervil, and simmer 5 minutes longer. Turn into a soup tureen, add fried croutons, and serve.

If preferred the soup may be rubbed through a puree sieve, returned to the fire, and when boiling hot be poured onto the yolks of 2 eggs mixed with 2 tablespoons milk.

This soup may be varied indefinitely. Any number of green vegetables can be used, care being taken to use only a small quantity of those of pronounced flavor.

No. 4 *(with vegetables)*

3 heads lettuce
4 stalks celery
2 onions
1 handful sorrel
1 handful chervil
1 quart water
3 sprigs thyme
3 sprigs tarragon
1/2 cup cream
2 egg yolks
salt
pepper

Shred the lettuce, cut up celery, onions, sorrel, and chervil, and boil in water with thyme till well stewed. Strain off the herbs a half hour before dinner; add tarragon and let the soup cool, then add cream stirred in egg yolks. Season to taste. Stir well, and put it on the fire to heat but do not let boil.

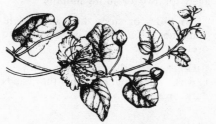

Herb Teas

(continued from page 177)

FENNEL TEA is also reputed to help the digestion, increase mother's milk, and be sedative. Steep 1 teaspoon seeds in 1 cup boiling water.

FENUGREEK TEA has been used since ancient times, and is supposed to be good for the digestion, colds, sinus troubles and fevers. Steep 1 teaspoon seeds in 2 cups boiling water.

GINGER TEA is made by steeping fresh or dried ginger root in boiling water for a pleasant spicy brew which is supposed to be useful for nausea and indigestion. It warms in cool or damp weather, too.

GOLDENROD TEA made from the dried flowers is recommended for ulcers, kidney problems, exhaustion, colds and fatigue. Boil 1 teaspoon dried flowers for 1 minute, steep for 15 and strain.

HOREHOUND TEA is a remedy for colds, coughs and asthma. When brewed very strong it can be laxative. 1 teaspoon leaves should be steeped in 2 cups boiling water for 20 minutes. One recipe for a bedtime tea calls for 1 cup horehound tea with a dash of cayenne and a teaspoon of vinegar, sweetened to taste with honey.

LEMON GRASS TEA is a delightful drink hot or iced. West Indian natives spice their brew with a clove or two.

LICORICE TEA is naturally sweet, but very thirst-quenching. Cold licorice tea replaces water for workers in some European iron mills. It also has a slight laxative effect.

LINDEN TEA (LIME FLOWER TEA) is said to be very soothing to the nerves, and to relieve coughs and nausea. Flowers and leaves are boiled together and strained.

NETTLE TEA is believed to have been used since Roman times as a blood tonic and preventive for kidney problems. Steep 1 teaspoon leaves in 2 cups boiling water for 15 minutes.

PARSLEY TEA is rich in vitamins and minerals and is reputed to be useful against fatigue, kidney stones, rheumatism and to be good for eyesight. Steep 1 teaspoon dried leaves in 2 cups boiling water 15 minutes.

PENNYROYAL TEA is supposed to be good for colds, constipation, insomnia, headaches, and "the evils induced by ladies' thin shoes." Steep 1 tablespoon leaves in 2 cups boiling water. Strain and serve. Leftover tea may be rubbed on the skin as an insect repellent.

PEPPERMINT TEA is probably the best known and most popular of herb teas. It is said to relieve colds, indigestion, headache, nervousness and nausea. It is also used to flavor blander herb teas. Brew 1 tablespoon leaves in 2 cups boiling water to desired strength. Peppermint tea is an ancient preparation, and is the preferred drink in many parts of the world.

RASPBERRY LEAF TEA is said to be efficacious for pregnant women, and has been used in Europe for centuries. One or two cups daily is recommended. One teaspoon dried leaves is steeped in 1 cup boiling water for 15 minutes.

RED CLOVER BLOSSOM TEA was very popular in the late 19th century. High in iron, red clover tea is considered a tonic to purify the blood and quiet the nerves. It is also reported helpful for ulcers, colds, weakness and fatigue. Boil 2 tablespoons dried blossoms in 3 cups boiling water for 1 minute and steep for 10 minutes. Strain and serve hot or cold.

ROSE HIP TEA is a delicious, ruby-colored beverage which is high in vitamin C. Steep 1 tablespoon dried rose hips in 2 cups boiling water for 20 minutes. It is said to be good against colds and kidney infections.

SAGE TEA is an aid to digestion. 1 tablespoon dried sage is steeped in 2 cups boiling water for 20 minutes. In Europe, sage is mixed with equal parts of balm (melissa).

SARSAPARILLA TEA is made from dried roots. It has a reputation as an aphrodisiac. The dried root requires long steeping and an early American recipe calls for equal parts of sarsaparilla and sassafras, and 1/2 part Virginia snakeroot.

SASSAFRAS TEA is made from the root bark of the American sassafras tree. An American Indian remedy for pain, colic, colds, fever, and the rash of measles, sassafras tea also has a reputation as a spring tonic. Boil chopped bark until a reddish-amber color appears.

SLIPPERY ELM TEA is a tea made from bark that was used by the American Indians to relieve sore throats and digestive ailments. It is also said to be good for nerves and rheumatism. Steep 1 ounce of dried inner bark in 1 pint of boiling water for 10 minutes.

SPEARMINT TEA is similar to peppermint, but rather milder in flavor.

THYME TEA is reputed useful against coughs, throat problems, nervousness and chills. Steep 1 teaspoon fresh or dried leaves in 1 cup boiling water for 15 minutes.

VIOLET LEAF TEA is rich in vitamins A and C and is said to ease colds and headaches. Steep 1 teaspoon chopped leaves in 2 cups boiling water for 10 minutes.

YARROW TEA has been used by Swiss mountaineers as a stimulant and tonic and is said to alleviate colitis. The chopped leaves are steeped in hot water for 10 minutes.

YERBA MATÉ TEA is a popular drink in South America. It is lower in tannin than Oriental tea, and is pleasantly bitter. Use 1 tablespoon yerba maté to 2 cups boiling water. Steep 5 minutes and strain.

YERBA SANTA grows in California and was used by Indians there against respiratory problems.

Mix or Match Teas

REDNESS
1/2 ounce peppermint leaves
1/2 ounce lemon grass
1/4 ounce hibiscus blossoms
1/4 ounce rose hips, seeded
1/4 ounce lemon verbena
1/8 ounce cloves

This is very good as an iced tea with the addition of slices of lemon, lime and orange.

DIXIE LAND
1 ounce spearmint leaves
1 ounce catnip
1/2 ounce rose buds
1 ounce lemon balm (melissa)
1/4 ounce cinnamon bark
a few cardamom pods

PANACEA
a tiny fishing village near Tallahassee
1 ounce chamomile
1 ounce passion flower
1/2 ounce dried orange peel
1/2 ounce dried lemon peel
1 ounce catnip

ROCKY TOP
1 ounce ginseng tops (Appalachian Mountain ginseng preferred)
1 ounce raspberry leaves (preferably from Virginia)
1 ounce sassafras root
1/2 ounce great burdock root
1 ounce dried elderberries
1 ounce wintergreen leaves
1/2 ounce sarsaparilla root

This is an Appalachian Mountain blend, using herbs that grow wild on the mountain slopes.

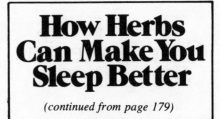

How Herbs Can Make You Sleep Better

(continued from page 179)

☐ The most effective herb sleep-producer in my view is *valerian*, from the Latin *valere*, "to be in health"; it was known to the Greeks as a nerve calmer. There are no bad aftereffects from the use of this herb. It was prescribed to relieve strain brought on by the air raids in the Second World War, and even single doses proved helpful, as it quiets the nervous system and the brain. Valerian grows in profusion in Derbyshire, and is also cultivated for world-wide sale. Unfortunately it has a bad smell. It comes in coated capsules from many herbal pharmacies, however, and can be used alone or with other sleep-producing herbs, either in capsule or tea form.

☐ *Peppermint tea* is a delicate and aromatic bedtime drink, and can also be used, as can chamomile, or lime flowers (linden) for babies' sleep and teething problems. Chamomile tea is a traditional tranquillizer and linden or lime (known by its Latin name as *Tilia*) is another effective soothing tea. Even today French mothers give *Tilia* to a crying child, especially at bedtime. Honey from lime flowers is highly regarded for its flavor, and is used in many medicines and liqueurs. Prolonged bathing in lime flower infusion is a folk remedy to calm hysteria. Make sure that you have a good supplier for lime-flower tea, as flowers that are too old can produce symptoms of narcotic intoxication. For an old, effective teething remedy combine a tablespoon of peppermint, skullcap and pennyroyal in a pint of boiling water. Steep for 30 minutes, strain and use warm, with honey for sweetening, 1 teaspoon at a time.

☐ *Aromatic woodruff* can greatly improve, and even prolong, one's sleep. To make the tea, use only hot, not boiling, water. According to the English herbalist Gerard, pouring woodruff into wine will "make men merry."

☐ A hot mull which will put you to sleep is warm cider plus a few cloves, a stick of cinnamon and a touch of woodruff. Another sleep-producing drink is a toddy with apple juice, and 6 cloves, 6 coriander seeds, 1 stick of cinnamon, a tablespoon of honey, the yolks of 2 eggs, juice of ½ lemon and a touch of woodruff.

☐ *Wild lettuce* is narcotic, and all lettuce possesses some of this narcotic juice—not enough to make you drugged, of course. But the ancients held lettuce in high esteem for its cooling and refreshing qualities. In

(continued on page 302)

fact the Emperor Augustus attributed his recovery from a dangerous illness to lettuce, and built an altar and erected a statue in its honor. Eau de laitre is water distilled from lettuce, and is used in France as a mild sedative in doses of 2 to 4 ounces. Certainly if you have an urge to eat something before you go to bed, try slowly chewing lettuce leaves, although the teas I have mentioned, plus honey, would be more effective.

□ *Sage* is yet another favorite sleep-producer, and a cup of sage tea plus honey will bring on a sense of calm. We always had several "sleep jars" in the house when I was a child, and one jar always contained a teaspoon of sage and rosemary to every 2 tablespoons of peppermint. Use only 1 teaspoon of the combined herbs for your steeped, strained tea before going to sleep.

□ The early American settlers used both *red bergamot tea* and *pennyroyal tea* for relaxed sleep. But a herb that does double duty in relaxing and picking up is *lemon balm*. It doesn't put you to sleep but rather removes any spasms and tensions which prevent sleep; and it can also be used as an early morning tea to overcome a feeling of tiredness.

□ Father Kunzle has two suggestions for harmless sleeping potions. He recommends 4 parts of golden rod to 1 part juniper, or a calming tea of lady's mantle and cowslips combined. Cowslips (*Primula veris*) have been used for centuries in England for nightly tea. Use flowers or root—preferably flowers.

□ The American herbalist Jethro Kloss advises a warm bath and hot tea for immediate sleep, and he suggests any of the following herbs steeped in a cup of boiling water for 20 minutes: lady's slipper, valerian, catnip, skullcap or hops, especially hops. He says that these herbs will not only induce sleep but will tone up the stomach and nerves, and never leave any bad aftereffect. If none of these herbs is available, hot lemonade, or hot grapefruit juice, either with or without honey, is an excellent substitute.

□ The Germans use ground anise with honey in warm milk as their bedtime drink, and the Dutch use another version, a tablet of aniseed in a glass of hot milk. Many Indians, I am told, use nutmeg oil on the forehead to induce sleep. The volatile *oil* does contain an intoxicant principle, but even grated nutmeg with lemon and boiling water can sometimes be used as a nightcap.

□ Many botanical sources and herb pharmacies have their own combinations for sleep. They are frequently made up in the form of capsules.

□ Dr. Jarvis, author of *Folk Medicine*, prefers apple, grape and cranberry juice to citrus juices. Since a great deal of nightly and other unease is due to an overalkaline reaction of the blood, these juices will undoubtedly help. Dr. Jarvis also suggests a daily drink of 2 teaspoons of cider vinegar in a glass of water before breakfast each morning. If you find this difficult to take, try a tablespoon of the cider vinegar and a tablespoon of honey (preferably uncooked honey) to a glass of water, which reconstitutes to a rather apple-juice taste. It is marvelous for getting the body started in the morning, and is an effective cure for constipation—another problem which can affect sleep.

Herb Pillows

□ Did your grandmother have a sleep pillow—a tiny, slender herb cushion covered with muslin and gay fabric? These are particularly good for invalids, babies and anyone in need of extra help in sleeping. They are a lovely present for anyone bedridden or old. The gentle aroma emanating from the pillows soothes the nerves, and often helps overcome the sickroom smell.

□ My favorite of all is lavender, or lavender with crushed rosebuds, or equal parts of sage, peppermint and lemon balm with or without lavender. Add some powdered orrisroot to "fix" the aroma, or a drop of simple or compound tincture of benzoin, when you crush the herbs in the mortar. You can also add a pinch of any of the following: rosemary, lemon verbena (a heavenly clean smell), angelica, tarragon, woodruff, marjoram, dill, thyme, hops.

□ You can make an entire pillow of hops, or of woodruff, or indeed of any of the herbs mentioned before as herb teas. Crush the dried leaves a bit, add a fixative, enclose in two men's handerchiefs, and add a washable "pillowcase" covering of a patterned fabric. These should be quite flat and slender to be comfortable. In order not to lose them every time you change your pillowcase, attach with a safety pin to the pillow ticking. ☼

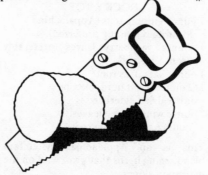

An Approved Receipt Against That Troublesome Complaint, Called the Teeth Set on Edge

Purslain, Sorrel, Sweet or Bitter Almonds, Walnuts, or burnt Bread, chewed, will certainly remove this disagreeable sensation.

—The Toilet of Flora, 1779

Toothbrushes Can Be Made

By cutting Licorice or Lucern or Marshmallow roots into pieces six inches long, and then boiling them in water for a long time; these are then drained, the ends carefully slit with a pen knife and the brushes dried. Dip your brush into some tooth powder and brush your teeth.

Throats can be considerably improved in their appearance if a pencil is rolled back and forth between the teeth several times a day. Sit up straight, head up and shoulders back when you perform this simple exercise.

The throat area can be exceedingly smoothed with frequent applications of vitamin E. Try massaging a fresh Avocado pit in circles on your throat. Make a cream of 1 tablespoon Avocado or ripe Banana mashed with a teeny bit of anhydrous lanolin and apply generously in the throat area. Massage the cream in with the pit.

Artichokes also contain nourishing materials for the skin. Cook your chokes in water, Celery tops, and Parsley plus 1 tablespoon Olive oil per choke. Eat the Artichokes and save one heart for your throat. Mash ¼ of the heart with 1 teaspoon organic whole egg mayonnaise. Use this beneficial cream to gently massage into the throat area with upward and outward movements. Leave it on for 10 minutes and give yourself a facial sauna so that the Artichoke cream can penetrate, or wipe off the excess and leave the residue on overnight. Then rinse your face and throat and spray with mineral water.

Behind-the-ear blackheads can be removed with a hot compress of Parsley juice placed over the area until the skin is soft and the pores are open.

Or make a solution of 1 tablespoon epsom salts, 1 drop white iodine, and ½ cup of boiling Violet water. Keep the solution hot, dip cotton balls into it and place them on the blackhead; press the blackhead out by spreading the fingers on either side. Don't ever press directly down on a blemish for you might spread the infection; instead press from the sides and up. Because it is so difficult to get to this area of the body ask help from your wife or husband (boy or girl friend will also do). After removing, astringe with Lemon juice or buttermilk.

Natural cosmetics The juice that issues from the Birch Tree, when wounded with an augur in spring, is detersive and excellent to clear the complexion: the same virtue is attributed to its distilled water. Some people recommend Strawberry-water; others the decoction of Orpiment,[1] and some Frogspawn water.

— *The Toilet of Flora, 1779*

Or, as *Delights for Ladies* puts it: "The sappe that issueth out of a Birch tree in great abundance, being opened, in March or April, with a receiver of glasse set under the boring thereof to receive the same, doth perform the same most excellently, & maketh the skin very cleer. This sap will dissolve pearle; a secret not known unto many."

Proper breathing is essential for health and handsomeness. It takes just 10 concentrated minutes a day. You could be giving yourself a facial at the same time: Lie down with your legs raised. Breathe in through the nostrils and let the air expand into your abdomen rather than into your lungs, breathe in 7 seconds, hold it for 3 and exhale slowly through the mouth.

For a quick face massage while showering, let a warm water spray flow over your face for 5 minutes. This is very stimulating. You can follow your Shower Facial Massage with an astringe of ice. First cover your skin with flannel or muslin and rub the ice over the fabric and *not* directly over your skin. If you rubbed your skin directly with ice it could cause enlarged blood vessels.

Face fresheners of sparkling mineral water are also nice. Try Evian, Vichy, or Perrier. Fill a plant mister with the water and spray the face after applying make-up to set it, after washing to freshen it and after swimming to remove salt.

Uncle Ed's Secret of Health and Beauty
I went to visit Uncle Ed when I was young and instructive but he was so old that before I could show him where it was at, he forgot what he was looking for. But he died only when he was very old, and his secret for youthful vigor was to walk outside in the snow naked every night and after shaving, wipe his face with icewater or snow, or take a cold shower daily. ☼

[1]*Orpiment is a mineral containing arsenic or the flowers of Sedum acre.*

Growing Herbs

(continued from page 183)

as plants from herb nurseries—as the seeds are not always easy to obtain.

Angelica	Mints
Chives	Pot Marjoram
Costmary	Sage
Fennel	Salad Burnet
Hyssop	Sweet Cicely
Lemon Balm	Tarragon
Lemon Verbena	Thyme
Lovage	Welsh Onion

Herb shrubs
And some herbs are shrubs or trees which are also obtainable from general nurseries.

Bay	Rose Geranium
Lavender	Rosemary

Having put into groups the best herbs for the purpose, it should be stressed that you do not need to have a garden in order to cultivate and sell your herbs. Many of the herbs listed can be grown in containers of one kind or another.

The whole idea of growing and selling your own herbs is open to apartment dwellers with space on their window sills both inside and out, and may be followed by those whose town garden consists of a small backyard, a patio, three bare walls or just a balcony. Here you can accommodate herbs in tubs, boxes and large pots as well as many other types of plant holders.

Lastly there are other advantages in growing herbs which are quite apart from any monetary profit you may make.

You will find you get much pleasure from your herbs with their beautiful leaves and flowers, and their heady scents. When you pass by a plant touching the leaves you will immediately be surrounded by its lovely perfume. One or two of the stronger herbs have an almost exotic scent. You will be able to try out the various herbs in your cooking, adding new tastes to old established dishes, and discovering how each plant has its own unique flavor.

You can enjoy making gifts for friends or family using your own fragrant herbs. A bunch of sweet smelling herbs is one of the nicest gifts to give to a blind person, who will get such pleasure from the many different scents. ☼

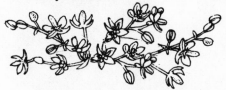

Herbal Baths

(continued from page 185)

Good for itching skin following a course of antibiotics.

Cammy Bath
This formula was especially created for a friend who was worried about her oily skin which seemed to be getting wrinkled and old-looking before its time. Mix together the following ingredients. Enough for 2-4 baths.

1/4 cup lavender
1/4 cup orange buds
1/4 cup rose buds
1/4 cup rosemary
1/4 cup eucalyptus leaves
1/4 cup linden
1/4 cup oil bark
1/4 cup camomile

Simple Bath Liquid
Mix together equal quantities of sage, rosemary, and lavender.

Bath Herbs for an Unhappy Little Girl
It is my feeling that simply the smelling of and the bathing in herbal ingredients can keep one in good health provided one eats a simple wholesome diet. When we were in Hawaii, my little girl got bitten about fifty times by mosquitoes the first night out. She scratched and scratched and is one of those children who can't seem to leave sores or bites alone. By the fourth day her bites seemed infected and pus was oozing from many of them. I had brought along one of my simple bath herb mixtures and made a deep warm bath for her, meanwhile simmering the herbs in water, and then had her soak in it for twenty minutes. The next day her sores stopped oozing, the pus was gone, and they were well on their way toward healing. The long soaky bath also stopped the itch and provided a night of restful sleep. If you don't have a bath or shower, simply simmer the herbs in a bit of water for ten minutes and then wet a washcloth with them and hold it to the bites or sores for as long as you can, once or twice a day. I used rose buds, orange peel, rosemary, alfalfa, mint, eucalyptus, camomile, and some of the licorice-smelling herbs. This mixture could be made up as you went along with whatever herbs or teas you had available at the moment. Probably even grass from a field would make an effective wash for sores and bites to stop incipient infection. ☼

Section Sixteen

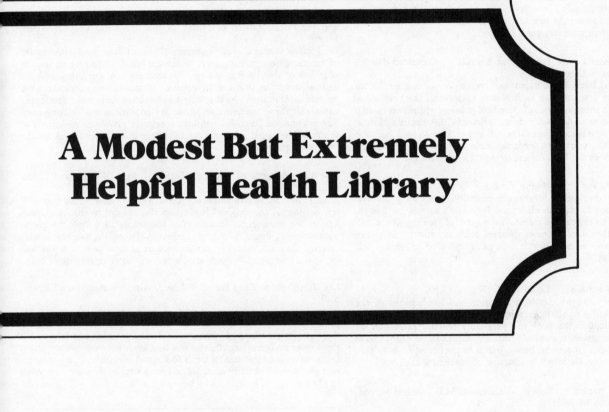

A Modest But Extremely
Helpful Health Library

Nutrition Manuals

Nutrition in a Nutshell Roger J. Williams, Ph.D. (Doubleday, $1.95)
Roger Williams is the man who discovered pantothenic acid, and was a pioneer in the research on folic acid, which he named. The clinic which he helped found is responsible for the discovery of more vitamins than any other laboratory. This authority is also a talented writer, whose basic guide to nutrition is easily understandable and applicable. He discusses the function of vitamins and minerals, as well as the need for supplementation. Indexed.

Gayelord Hauser's New Treasury of Secrets Gayelord Hauser (Farrar, Straus & Giroux, $8.95)
The author has been a consistent spokesman for natural health for more than fifty years, and an enthusiastic example of the benefits of pure foods and living habits. All based on good nutrition, he reveals the secrets of how to deal with various ailments, the hazards of dead foods, how to plan better menus (recipes given), how to look better—anything, in fact, you might want advice about. Anecdotes of personal experiences are both informative and entertaining.

Feel Like a Million Catharyn Elwood (Pocket Books, $1.75)
A complete one-volume education in nutrition, describing the elements in proper foods, the effects of their deficiencies on health, and programs to repair and maintain the state of "feeling like a million." The author also discusses diseases such as cancer and arthritis and conditions of poor health such as allergies, tooth decay, hair loss and tension.

Know Your Nutrition Linda Clark (Keats, $3.50)
This is a basic course describing the uses and interactions of the elements of nutrition: vitamins, minerals, power foods and proteins. Since its publication the book has become a popular reference for finding out, for instance, in what foods a vitamin can be found, what the vitamin does in the body, how much is required, and what other vitamins and minerals help it to function at maximum capacity.

Nutrition and Health Robert McCarrison, M.D., and H.M. Sinclair (Faber, out of print)
Sir Robert McCarrison, a physician who pioneered in human nutrition when he was Director of Research on Nutrition in India, discovered that "the greatest single factor in the acquisition and maintenance of good health is perfectly constituted food." He arrived at this conclusion from studying the lack of specific nutritional components and combinations that caused vulnerability to infection, and such deficiency diseases as beri-beri. A classic.

Health through Nutrition Lelord Kordel (Manor, $1.75)
A basic primer on how the body functions, and how foods can affect appearance, retard aging, and spur activity and productivity to new levels. The author describes the impact of food intake and nutritional choice on each condition—heart trouble, chronic fatigue, blood pressure, arthritis and even eyestrain. A sensible, direct and easy-to-use reference.

Nutrition and Your Body H.L. Newbold, M.D. (New Age Press, $3.95)
The addition of "Body" to the title indicates a special feature of this book: it orients the reader within the realm of anatomy and physiology, instead of leaving him stranded in intercellular space. What vitamins and minerals are doing is explained, not in a vacuum, but in the body. This is a basic general nutrition book, supplemented with food tables and technical references, photographs and line drawings, a bibliography and index.

Look Younger, Feel Healthier Carlton Fredericks, Ph.D. (Grosset & Dunlap, $2.95)
Based on the premise that Americans consume the most depleted, chemically altered, nutritionally empty food, this book helps the reader to discover his own particular needs not being met by the foods he eats. Diabetics, the obese, the old, hypoglycemics and many others learn how a more selective diet proves helpful. There are lists of supplements, additives, and even the insecticides legally allowed in the most commonly eaten fruits and vegetables. The transcript of a hearing on nutritional reform makes clear our government's attitude toward food and health.

Mental and Elemental Nutrients Carl C. Pfeiffer, M.D., Ph.D. and the Publications Committee of the Brain Bio Center (Keats, $9.95)
Dr. Pfeiffer was one of the pioneers of the orthomolecular treatment of mental illness, particularly the schizophrenias. He reveals the importance of vitamin B-6 and zinc for treating many health problems, and discusses the role and function of all the known nutrients, from protein and vitamins to the little-known trace minerals. The applications of these nutrients to particular conditions are documented. Suggestions are given for helping to remedy problems of aging and senility. The book goes into detail, but is not too technical for the interested reader.

The Encyclopedia of Natural Health Max Warmbrand (Pyramid, $4.95)
A basic natural health reference book for everyday home use written by one of the original leaders in the natural health field, well known for his success in restoring hopelessly ill people to health without using drugs or patent medicines. Digestion, the respiratory system, diabetes, arthritis, the heart and general nutrition (including special diets and recipes) are all part of this comprehensive book.

Let's Eat Right to Keep Fit Adelle Davis (New American Library, $1.95)
A great work on applied nutrition. Although the author presents complicated and difficult material, her clarity of explanation of the actions and interactions of vitamins, minerals, proteins and fats within the human body has kept this book a best seller for over twenty years. Davis advocated the use of fresh foods and nutritional supplements in a well-balanced daily diet. She outlines succinctly what is needed to maintain good health, and where to find it.

Environmental Considerations

Silent Spring Rachel Carson (Fawcett, $1.75)
As she was dying of cancer, Ms. Carson, a respected marine biologist, wrote the cornerstone of the ecology movement. In lyrical prose and with scientific accuracy she outlines the dangers of our increasingly polluted environment. Searing chapters on the destructiveness of pesticides and the dangers of eating a salad with "tolerance residues" of different pesticides on every ingredient are based on carefully researched work.

Food for Nought Ross Hall (Random, $3.95)
Ross Hall is shaking us from a nightmare of self-defeat, from the improvement of our food *industry* and the destruction of food's value. As a biochemist he warns that the abuse of hormones to fatten and tenderize livestock, the use of gasses to artificially ripen fruit, and the many more chemical aids employed to benefit size and appearance and to streamline harvesting and marketing, accomplish only deprivation of vital nutrients—disease and death. A well-documented technical survey, with notes, glossary and index.

Consumer Beware! Your Food and What's Been Done to It
Beatrice Trum Hunter (Bantam, $1.95)
A well researched indictment of the food industry and its manipulation of the consumer through advertising and promotion, while the quality of food continues to deteriorate. The author discusses such topics as the chemicals fed to beef, the freezing of "fresh" fish caught in contaminated waters, the physical conditions under which poultry is mass produced, the nutritional value of milk after pasteurization and separation. She calls for government agencies willing to work for better food, not engaged in disguise or substitution.

The Closing Circle   Barry Commoner (Bantam, $1.95)
"We have broken out of the circle of life." We are going broke getting wealth from the environment. The regular flow of life is being disrupted and perverted, and Barry Commoner tells us *what* has gone wrong, *why* it happened and *how* we can put it right. The urgency of our present condition is clearly communicated. Lucid information that is carefully annotated and indexed.

Unfit for Human Consumption   Ruth Mulvey Harmer (Prentice-Hall, $6.95)
"How the unrestricted use of pesticides menaces the health of us all" sums up the overwhelming case of the people vs. "wanton dissemination of pesticides in the environment." Ruth Harmer details the alternative, natural, nonpolluting enemies of insects. She gives advice on what to do about protecting your plants on an individual and commercial scale (giving case histories), and on what political measures an individual citizen can take.

The Chemical Feast   James Turner (Grossman, $.95)
Written by a member of the Ralph Nader study group assigned to report on the Food and Drug Administration, this sounds the cry for true and better food standards and safety laws, emphasizing the politics of nutrition as well as the actual condition of our food. It includes topics such as: Enforcement, Industry, Fraud, FDA Mythology, and Self-Defense in relation to the food made available to American citizens. Aimed at doers rather than watchers.

The Poisons in Your Food   William Longgood (Pyramid, $.95)
Here is clear documentation of the role we are forced to play as human guinea pigs for food additives that have not been adequately tested. Mr. Longgood also discusses the pesticides, excess sugar, and refining processes that contribute to the undermining of our nation's health. The conflicting results of laboratory tests often allow the food industry to choose the favorable test, while ignoring signs of danger. He offers suggestions for changing this deadly situation.

Hypoglycemia and Refined Carbohydrates

The Saccharine Disease   T.L. Cleave, M.D. (Keats, $4.95)
This name is given to a group of major diseases characteristic to western civilization, that are caused by the consumption of refined carbohydrates. Lack of fiber in the diet is responsible for diabetes, coronary disease, diverticulitis, peptic ulcer and obesity, among many others. Man has not been able to adapt to these refinements as quickly as they have been forced upon him. Dr. Cleave discusses specific diseases and his findings concerning their treatment, uncovering the common causative factor in all of them.

Sweet and Dangerous   John Yudkin, Ph.D. (Bantam, $1.95)
John Yudkin, professor of physiology, indicts sugar as the leading villain in many of the degenerative diseases that plague modern society. Through his own and others' well-documented research, he makes a powerful case for the exclusion of sugar from the diet. Dr. Yudkin also describes the efforts of the sugar industry and the food processors who strive constantly to deny his findings. Indexed.

Body, Mind and Sugar   E.M. Abrahamson, M.D. and A.W. Pezet, M.D. (Pyramid, $1.50)
E.M. Abrahamson was the first to bring to our attention the condition of hypoglycemia (called hyperinsulinism in his book). He explains it thoroughly, with descriptions of symptoms and effects, and relates this common disease to other problems such as chronic fatigue, allergies, alcoholism, and insanity. Many case histories are included, as well as dietary advice.

Low Blood Sugar and You   Carlton Fredericks, Ph.D. and Herman Goodman, M.D. (Grosset & Dunlap, $2.95)
One person in every ten, according to the authors, has hypoglycemia or low blood sugar. Their book was one of the first to identify the many hypoglycemic symptoms, frequently misdiagnosed as caused by mental illness. Charts of case histories include diagrams of glucose-tolerance tests; recommendations for diets and living programs include recipes and compensations for deficiencies. The book is valuable for anyone who has and is not aware of a hypoglycemic condition.

Sugar Blues   William Dufty (Warner, $1.95)
The author's personal suffering from being hooked on sugar led to an investigation of the "multiple physical and mental miseries caused by human consumption" of sugar, a chemical which he contends is both a drug and a poison. The sugar industry is powerful and to a large degree prevents accurate labelling, protective legislation, and straightforward information of medical facts from being made public. Meanwhile, mental illness and crime rates as well as diabetes are all gaining rapidly, fueled by sugar. Mr. Dufty's account is electrifying.

Nutrition and Healthier Children

Better Food for Better Babies and Their Families   Gena Larson (Keats, $1.25)
Believing that a child will inherit the kind of health that his parents have been maintaining during their lifetimes, the author offers a nutritional program for everyone, but most especially for the mother-to-be, beginning with her health before conception and continuing through her child's preschool years. Her goal is to "give every child born a body free of inborn illness and imperfection, with built-in resistance to disease and premature aging," and her book inspires the reader with the ambition to raise the quality of life for coming generations.

Let's Have Healthy Children   Adelle Davis (New American Library, $1.95)
This book's recommendations are confined to the nutrition of infants and children, properly starting with the health of the mother *before* conception. There are sections on diet during pregnancy, weight control, and diets for nursing mothers. The book follows through with "the requirements of a good formula" and the nutritional supplements needed by babies. The nutritional needs of the child through the preschool years are examined, and advice given on producing healthy youngsters.

Nature's Children: A Guide to Organic Herbal Remedies for Children   Juliette de Bairacli Levy (Schocken, $4.95)
The author and her children lived a wandering, gypsy life in Europe, using natural herbal remedies, a vegetarian (often raw) diet, and the country lore they picked up from the people they met. This method of raising children may seem strange at first, but much can be learned about the value of sun and air baths, a plain diet and joyous exercise, or the importance of communicating the loveliness of nature to young children. Anyone bound to jars of baby food or play pens might benefit from this exposure to a simpler life.

Cookbooks

Putting Food By   Ruth Hertzberg, Beatrice Vaughan and Janet Greene (Bantam, $2.50)
This is a classic guide to storing and preserving all kinds of food. Every conceivable method of food preservation is presented in detail. There are even directions for making several types of root-cellars, and how-tos for rendering lard, making soup, and making various types of sausage. Salted and smoked meats are all cured without sodium nitrate or sodium nitrite. A sprouting guide is included, as well as a section of recipes. Profusely illustrated with drawings and charts that make preserving fool-proof.

Good Food, Gluten Free   Hilda Cherry Hills (Keats, $3.50)
This is the only book we know of that is written for celiacs (those who are allergic to the protein in wheat, barley, rye, oats and sometimes buckwheat). It includes explanations, and about 300 recipes for gluten-free main dishes, soups, breads and biscuits, desserts and salads. Other diseases and conditions may benefit from the diet, such as multiple sclerosis, schizophrenia, rheumatoid arthritis, regional enteritis, autism and diabetes. Findings are thoroughly documented.

The Natural Foods Cookbook   Beatrice Trum Hunter (Pyramid, $1.25)
One of the first natural foods cookbooks to appear after the revolution and introduction of convenience, packaged and frozen foods, this now-famous book is a comprehensive collection of recipes and methods using wholesome ingredients, with an appeal to taste. Detailed descriptions of the making of cheese, yogurt, sauerkraut and yeast, along with methods of sprouting beans are unique, and a treasure to find in the same book as the usual recipes.

Cooking for Life   Michel Abehsera (Avon, $3.95)
A popular cookbook for those who have already adopted (or want to know more about) the macrobiotic way of life. Discusses the culinary meaning of Yin and Yang, the "Ten Commandments of Health," and includes hundreds of recipes, menus and cooking tips. Abehsera also wrote the book that started it all in this country—*Zen Macrobiotic Cooking.*

Great Meatless Meals   Frances Lappé & Ellen Ewald (Ballantine, $1.75)
This book follows *Diet for a Small Planet* and *Recipes for a Small Planet,* yet there is no redundancy. It contains recipes for thirty high-protein meals. The authors have also listed the grams of protein per serving with each recipe, and given clear and simple instructions. The recipes reflect wide research in their creative, international scope, and are cross-referenced for easy "mixing and matching" for your choice of complete-protein meals.

The New York Times Natural Foods Cookbook   Jean Hewitt (Avon, $1.95)
A chubby little book that contains more recipes than most, this offers a commendable variety. Jean Hewitt does not stick to one kind of health diet, such as *only* grains and vegetables, or *only* European peasant food, but includes some of everything that a natural foods orientation could offer. Not the most pure, the recipes do use sugar (though "raw" or "date sugar" is always indicated) and a particular brand of baking powder is recommended. So many recipes full of fine foods, that this inclusion does not detract.

Our Daily Bread   Stella Standard (Berkley, $2.95)
A recipe for every day of the year, using wholesome ingredients. There are recipes from many countries all over the world, using different kinds of grains and flours and including yeast breads, quick breads, pancakes, rolls, cakes and local specialties. Helpful extras are nutrient charts, a source list for flours and a high altitude guide to baking.

Whole-Grain Baking Sampler   Beatrice Trum Hunter (Keats, $2.25)
A complete baking book based on whole grain flours, natural unrefined sweeteners and yeast instead of baking powder or soda, this primer presents a large variety of breads, rolls, crackers, flat breads, cookies and confections, even including brioche and croissant. There is a helpful essay for the novice in breadmaking and another on the adaptation of cookie recipes to natural food standards.

Eat, Drink and Be Healthy   Agnes Toms (Pyramid, $.95)
A basic, but healthier, cookbook with over 2,000 recipes using ingredients unspoiled by additives or artificial coloring or flavoring. A chapter on nutrition gives good advice on planning balanced meals; on raw foods, delicious blender drinks and suggestions for raw vegetable main courses; on vegetables, the best cooking methods to preserve nutrients. There are also helpful timetables for cooking meats, fixing a smorgasbord and making party hors d'oeuvres.

Tassajara Cooking: A Vegetarian Cookbook   Edward Espe Brown (Shambhala, $3.95)
Cooking without meat—vegetables, fruits, pasta, grains. The first section of this cookbook deals with individual vegetables and the last part is recipes. There is much advice about how to cut and prepare the vegetables, and about the kitchen equipment needed. There are chapters on meal planning, dairy products (including the making of yogurt) and seasonal specialties. Illustrated with line drawings.

The Natural Foods Blender Cookbook   Frieda Nusz (Keats, $1.50)
Formerly two books, *Wheat and Sugar Free* and *Blenderbusz,* this is a collection of blender recipes and a great deal of general advice about the preparation of food from natural ingredients, as quickly and easily as possible. The author's nutritional knowledge is based on long experience in avoiding processed foods. Included are hard-to-find recipes such as how to make butter, ice cream using snow, or cabbage juice (for ulcers).

The Vegetarian Epicure   Anna Thomas (Vintage, $4.95)
Offering some of the *best-tasting* recipes around, this book is a standard with many people. The food lives up to standards of gourmet eating, without being extreme or aimed at anything but an ordinary person's palate (vegetarian or otherwise). It tends toward hearty, simple casserole-type dishes, with much emphasis on soups, beans and potatoes. The only serious lack is an absence of grain recipes other than vegetarian pasta dishes.

Recipes for a Small Planet   Ellen Ewald (Ballantine, $1.95)
Subtitled "The Art and Science of High Protein Vegetarian Cookery," this is a sequel to *Diet for a Small Planet.* Using the principles of protein complementarity, Ms. Ewald creates a wealth of recipes, each stating the number of grams of protein per serving, and the directions for preparation. There are appendices of useful kitchen tips, and a glossary of the foods used. The index is comprehensive.

Let's Cook It Right   Adelle Davis (New American Library, $1.95)
This goes beyond the ordinary health-oriented cookbook. There is information on the "whys" of cookery and on the "hows." The author also covers related topics, such as finding your nearest supplier of nutritional supplements. Nor are her recipes meant to be nutritionally good only; Chapter 3 is entitled "Make Delicious Gravies or None at All!" Each recipe includes several variations, leaving room for revision or creation.

The Tassajara Bread Book   Edward Espe Brown (Shambhala, $3.50)
Breads, with and without yeast, filled and unfilled, sourdough, rolls, pastry, muffins, desserts (including a foray into ice cream) and hiker's mix and granola. Instructions are simple enough to take the terrors out of baking. The line drawings are extremely helpful and prolific. More detailed step-by-step directions for beginners than in most other cookbooks. While emphasizing pure whole-grains, the novice can, using this book, become a pro.

The Deaf Smith County Cookbook   Marjorie Wynn Ford, Susan Hillyard, Mary Faulk Koock (Macmillan, $3.95)
A big, handsome, basic vegetarian cookbook using natural foods. Besides the usual hors d'oeuvres to desserts, there are helpful chapters on children's foods and camping and cooking out. The book is of Texan origin, so there are special southwestern recipes such as guacamole, enchiladas and deep-fried squash blossoms. It is lovely, being illustrated with nature photographs; and practical, with a comprehensive glossary of natural foods.

The Natural Foods No-Cook Book   John Tobe (Greywood, $1.25)
This is based on the principle that "no food is ever nutritionally improved by heating." That in fact much of its nutritional virtue is destroyed by cooking. There are menus and recipes for three meals a day for 365 days, as well as short discussions on the purpose, results and methods of eating raw foods. Most of the foods are easily obtainable and are suited to the seasons of the year. The menus are balanced to provide enough quality proteins, carbohydrates and fats each day.

Natural Beauty

My Secrets of Natural Beauty   Virginia Castleton (Keats, $2.95)
A handbook of natural beauty care written by a noted beauty expert who gives formulas for skin cleansers, creams, lotions, masks and wrinkle chasers made from simple home ingredients such as oatmeal, honey, cucumber, brewer's yeast, eggs and many more that are easy-to-find. She also gives recipes for complexion-improving and figure trimming salads and exercises for problem spots. This is a no-nonsense, practical collection of beauty aids that are within the realm of everyday use.

The Complete Herbal Guide to Natural Health and Beauty
Dian Dincin Buchman (Doubleday, $6.95)
A herbal expert discusses in detail the care of the skin and body using natural organic ingredients that, in many cases, have been used for hundreds of years. Specific chapters are devoted to various parts of the body and include exercises, advice from specialists and nutritional suggestions as well. An additional chapter describes the making of perfumes, potpourris and scent balls. Emphasis is on making your own medicinal and cosmetic preparations.

Face Improvement through Exercise and Nutrition   Linda Clark (Keats, $1.75)
A systematic approach to the care and exercise of every part of the face with illustrations demonstrating each exercise, and advice about diet and supplements. The material is gathered from experts, all of whom seem to agree that a pretty face needs pleasant thoughts, the right food and enough sleep, but that facial exercises are imperative for maintaining good looks.

Stay Young Longer   Linda Clark (Pyramid, $1.50)
The goal in this book is to show how people can continue to lead satisfying lives as they grow older. The interdependence of nutrition, exercise, emotions and attitudes, and their presence or lack affect the physical symptoms that frequently appear with aging. There is documented specific advice here for fatigue, the menopause, depression, falling hair, impotency, faulty memory and other indications of deficiency in some department of living.

A Guide to Natural Cosmetics   Connie Krochmal (Quadrangle, $8.95)
A formula-tested guide to the making of cosmetics from plants and other natural ingredients. Well illustrated, it recounts the history of cosmetics since Egyptian days and describes and illustrates procedures, tools, ingredients and their sources. In addition to the more conventional creams and lotions, there are less familiar nail preparations, shaving creams, toothpastes and mouthwashes. The author is a botanist and an expert on plant use.

Nutrition & Healing

You Are Extraordinary   Roger J. Williams, Ph.D. (Pyramid, $1.25)
Roger Williams has demonstrated that no two people are alike, any more than are two snowflakes. In ways of sleeping, nervous response, eating, working, or recuperating from illness no one resembles anyone else except in the broadest terms. Special treatment which considers the individual's particular biochemical make-up and needs is, therefore, necessary. The author does discuss common diseases in general terms, but also gives case histories of unique reactions to substances or treatments.

Mega-Nutrients   H.L. Newbold, M.D. (Wyden, $11.95)
Dr. Newbold is a psychiatrist who diagnosed his own case of hypoglycemia. The subsequent failure of his colleagues to even recognize it, motivated him to research and write a reference manual for home health care that tells you all you need to know about nutrition. He helps you to establish a personal vitamin and mineral regimen, suggesting a variety of tests that you can give yourself, or that you should ask your doctor to authorize. Tips on saving money on health care, beauty care, and other related subjects.

Health and Light   John Ott (Devin-Adair, $7.50)
John Ott reminds us that we take light for granted. We shield ourselves from natural light (with glasses and sunglasses, windshields and windows), and bathe ourselves in artificial light. Startling studies and case histories as well as current experiments show some resulting changes in, among other things, children's ability to be productive in school, a person's response to stress, our endocrine systems, our biological time clocks and even our personalities.

Better Eyesight without Glasses   W.H. Bates, M.D. (Pyramid, $1.75)
We do not usually imagine that we can volitionally improve the health and ability of our eyes. Yet, in his classic work (first published in 1920) Dr. Bates explains how eye exercises *can* help us. He also pioneered the development of methods of mental relaxation, focusing techniques and other aids. The book teaches us how the eye works and what errors in refraction are, and how they can be treated. Includes a large fold-out eye chart.

Food Facts and Fallacies   Carlton Fredericks, Ph.D. (Arco, $1.45)
Here are the essential facts about what we should eat under what circumstances and conditions. For example, take the usual prescription to eat pureed foods for diverticulitis: it has been discovered by nutritionists that refined foods *cause* diverticulitis, and the way to avoid it is to include bran, or other fiber in your diet. Mr. Fredericks balances the nutritionists' points of view against conventional methods concerning heart disease, diabetes, sterility, cancer prevention, and so on. He also includes recommendations on food preparation, and appropriate menus.

A New Breed of Doctor   Alan Nittler, M.D. (Pyramid, $1.50)
With much emphasis on prevention, this nutritional doctor discusses a dietary program for total body harmony and maintenance musts. Insight and development of the program have come from the realization that nature has its own built-in balance of safeguards and remedies. Drugs and other chemicals are now more wisely and sparingly administered by many members of the medical profession, in deference to the more effective use of natural biological solutions.

Food Is Your Best Medicine   Henry Bieler, M.D. (Random, $1.95)
Dr. Bieler holds the belief that disease is a toxic condition that results in actual cellular damage. Most medicines also attack some cells. Food does no attacking, and Dr. Bieler feels that herein lies the best possible medicine. This seems radical, but is concluded from extensive information on human physiology, and from the author's fifty years of successful nutritional therapy. Indexed.

The Stress of Life   Hans Selye, M.D. (McGraw-Hill, $2.95)
A thoroughly researched analysis of stress, bad (*dis*tress) and good (*eu*stress) as it affects body and mind, this book was a breakthrough to a new concept of health and disease. The body combats stress by using particular hormones. Overuse and imbalance of hormonal action can cause disease. The aim, therefore, is to learn to strengthen the body's individual defenses against stress through body chemistry. A well-annotated bibliography, glossary and index are included.

Your Body Is Your Best Doctor   Melvin E. Page, D.D.S. and H. Leon Abrams, Jr. (Keats, $1.25)
During his practice as a dentist, Dr. Page discovered that he could diagnose the metabolism of a patient using certain body measurements and tests for body chemistry, and that he could correct a glandular imbalance indicated by those measurements by administering small doses of glandular extract and banning sugar, artificial sweeteners, white flour, milk and stimulants from the diet. The degenerative diseases so prevalent today can be prevented, he believes.

New Hope for Incurable Diseases   E. Cheraskin, M.D., D.M.D. and W.M. Ringsdorf, Jr., D.M.D. (Arco, $1.65)
Modern medical research indicates that disease may be the result of a lack of resistance, often caused by poor or inadequate nutrition. The authors present scientific proof that nutrition can play a dramatic role in the prevention and cure of such diseases as multiple sclerosis, alcoholism, glaucoma, schizophrenia, atherosclerosis. Diet, sometimes in conjunction with traditional medication, is the chief "medicine" used by Dr. Cheraskin in the treatment of these diseases.

Nutrition and Your Mind   George Watson, Ph.D. (Bantam, $1.95)
During his treatment of mental illnesses, Dr. Watson's research led to the discovery that in some people symptoms are caused by a psychochemical reaction to the wrong type of food for the patient, or an allergic-type reaction to certain common substances. Among the mentally ill there are fast oxidizers and slow oxidizers according to the way the body burns sugar. When oxidation is normalized by the right nutrients, behavior also returns to normal. The book includes tests to help the reader identify his psychochemical type, appropriate diets and an appendix illustrating typical experiments.

Nutrition and Physical Degeneration   Weston Price, D.D.S. (Price-Pottenger, $15.50)
Through long and intense observation of primitive peoples, Dr. Price collected masses of evidence on diet and living habits—and photographs of subjects before and after exposure to processed foods and soft drinks. The evidence is clear: natural foods result in healthy people, while refined and convenience foods produce imperfect minds and bodies *in one generation*. Mental capacity degenerates and crime increases as well. Dr. Price suggests nutritional programs to mend the damage done.

Diet and Disease   E. Cheraskin, M.D., D.M.D.; W.M. Ringsdorf, Jr., D.M.D.; J.W. Clark, D.D.S. (Keats, $5.95)
A holistic overview of nutrition, weaving together seemingly unrelated observations and illnesses. The concept behind the work is that diseases do not exist separately, but come in clusters—such as heart disease ± diabetes ± gout ± obesity. The authors reveal interrelationships existing in many areas of the life sciences, one such area being food: defining the combined functions of carbohydrates and proteins, or carbohydrates and minerals. The book also is a systematic and thorough study of specific diseases.

Let's Get Well   Adelle Davis (New American Library, $1.95)
People tend to ignore their health until they lose it. *Let's Get Well* gives sound nutritional advice on coping with problems of ill health. From allergies to surgery, Davis outlines the nutritional aids which will help the body to cope with trauma and aid in preventing future problems—leaning heavily toward preventive nutrition as well. The chapters segment the book by specific ailments, making it simple to use. Comprehensively indexed.

Encyclopedia of Common Diseases   Staff of *Prevention* magazine (Rodale, $11.95)
From alcoholism to weight problems, here are 1,296 pages of well-arranged information about diseases or conditions bordering on disease. Each entry gives the diagnosis, symptoms, the effects of natural treatment (except for external accessories such as eyeglasses or hearing aids), and kinds of treatment. Excerpts from articles are included and often describe research, experiments and clinical analysis.

Toxemia Explained   J.H. Tilden, M.D. (Keats, $3.50)
Dr. Tilden believed in one theory about disease—that it is always caused by toxemic poisoning, by inadequate elimination and the build-up of poisonous waste products in the body. The one disease with the one cause can be cured by bed rest, relaxation, hot baths and only fruit or vegetable juices for food. He stresses a daily diet of fruits, vegetables and whole grains in the proper combinations; exercise; and emotional and mental control and balance.

Handbook of Natural Remedies for Common Ailments   Linda Clark (Devin-Adair, $9.95)
A reference for people suffering from the most common ailments who want to help themselves by natural means. Tried remedies, often in clinical experimentation, are listed in case histories of each ailment. Fatigue, cancer, hypertension and asthma are among those with documented evidence of relief: case histories of the ways people have tried or doctors have recommended.

Psychodietetics   E. Cheraskin, M.D., D.M.D.; W.M. Ringsdorf, Jr. D.M.D., M.S.; with Arline Brecher (Bantam, $1.95)
The premise states that nutrition can prevent and cure emotional disorders. In some case histories the absence of a single nutrient proved to be the factor controlling mental stability. An Optimal Diet is recommended to promote and maintain mental and physical health. Question and answer sections guide the reader through a wealth of nutritional information to an understanding of proper diet. A simple, understandable and flexible guide to health stability.

Nutrition against Disease   Roger J. Williams, Ph.D. (Bantam, $1.95)
Roger Williams theorizes that health results only when your particular nutritional needs are met, and that these needs can vary greatly among individuals. He explores diseases "from the standpoint of what various nutrients can do when tested under conditions that allow nutrients to function co-operatively." Some of the health problems that can be helped by nutrition include: birth defects, heart problems, dental caries, alcoholism and aging. Finally, he writes about the food industry and food faddism.

Supernutrition   Richard Passwater (Dial, $7.95)
The author believes that millions of Americans suffer from diseases that nutrition could prevent. He outlines a vitamin program based on a quiz whose answers can then be used to fit the needs of each individual. The program consists of taking vitamins, minerals and food supplements, gradually increasing the amount until the test shows the optimum results for health. The need for megavitamins, particularly in combating heart disease, cancer, hypoglycemia and mental and emotional problems, is demonstrated in separate chapters on these diseases.

Eating Your Way to Health   Ruth Kunz-Bircher, Ralph Bircher, Alfred Kunz-Bircher and Dagmar Liechti-Von Brasch (Penguin, $1.75)
The ideal Bircher-Benner diet does not include meat in its organically grown, vegetarian group of foods, but it does claim to provide facts and recipes for a basic complete diet. Special diets are given to alleviate problems of diabetes, allergies and obesity, including a salt-free diet, as well as the perfect diet for children. A generous assortment of menus and recipes beneficial for all needs, and all are based on the pure foods, Bircher-Benner approach which has been used with good results since the turn of the century.

Organic Gardening

Gardening Without Poisons   Beatrice Trum Hunter (Houghton Mifflin, $6.95)
Here is an alternative to the use of poison in your garden. Use age-old biological methods: control the water, light, soil and temperature, and then rely on a healthy plant's natural resistance; use insects that are natural enemies of the offenders, as well as plants that repel insects. (Here is weed control as well. Encourage animals and insects to do the dirty work.) Secondly, by applying current research in the use of sound waves, control insects, the study of population dynamics and so on.

The Organic Gardener   Catherine Osgood Foster (Vintage, $3.95)
A handsome book, with knowing discussions and advice on subjects ranging from soil composition, to composting, to growing high quality vegetables. Includes a comprehensive bibliography and directory listing almost every type of assistance a novice or experienced organic gardener would need. Line drawings on almost every page—of tools, garden plots, life and seasonal cycles, pests and much more.

Nutrition and the Soil   Lionel Picton (Devin-Adair, out of print)
This is a classic pioneer organic book. Starting with "Factors of Health Conveyed by the Soil," the relationship between dirt and our more complex human dust is explored, with discussions on the mycorrhizal association formed between fungi and roots, the difference of quality between seeds and the importance of the seed bed, and the role of minerals in plant and animal biology. One of the last chapters suggests, "Let Us Prevent Famine of Quality."

How to Have a Green Thumb without an Aching Back   Ruth Stout (Exposition, $4.00)
This manual revolutionized the gardening of countless people over the last quarter of a century. Miss Stout wanted to garden when she grew old, "and I don't mean from fifty to seventy, I mean from seventy to ninety." Now well into her nineties, she is still enjoying her non-digging, non-cultivating system of keeping soil fed, friable and weedless by covering it with kitchen and garden waste and hay. Furthermore, this is a guide for growing specific fruits, flowers and vegetables; and provides delightful reading.

Encyclopedia of Organic Gardening   J.I. Rodale and Staff (Rodale, $14.95)
A reference book by long-time organic gardening specialists, the jacket boasts over 300 illustrations and more than 1,490 topics. Seventy-six popular fruit and nut trees, 60 popular and unusual vegetables, and more than 850 popular flowers. The book emphasizes the organic point of view, with discussions on composting and mulching, and a section on soil that is a book in itself. It offers much how-to advice.

Good Food Naturally   John B. Harrison (Keats, $3.95)
Organic gardening firsthand, by a successful commercial organic farmer of thirty years standing. His farm in Canada is a showplace and a classroom for students wanting to learn how to grow nourishing food and keep soil productive. The author explains how soil and plants interact, how to plant and grow, deal with pests, harvest, store and cook. Helpful to the novice are the plans for garden plots, the work calendar and the details for compost making and mulching.

Companion Plants   Helen Philbrick and Richard Gregg (Devin-Adair, $3.95)
An alphabetized list of plants with emphasis in the descriptions on which other plants thrive or do poorly in their presence. This symbiosis or antagonism among plants has been neglected as an ecological force until recently and is important in affecting crop yield. Also important is the effect certain plants have in discouraging pests. If the advice in this book is carefully used, organic gardens should improve appreciably as a result.

Plowman's Folly   Edward H. Faulkner (University of Oklahoma, $2.95)
"The most important challenge to agricultural orthodoxy that has been advanced in this century." This was true in 1943 when the book was first published, and is still true printings later. Very simply, Faulkner stated that there was no scientific reason to plow at all. In imitation of minimal, almost primitive methods, Faulkner simply cut through the sod with a disk harrow, which creates no deep furrows, nor does it turn the soil inside out on itself. He went on to prove how destructive plowing could be, leading to erosion and soil depletion, and upsetting some of the important and beneficial natural cycles and processes taking place in the soil.

Vegetarianism

Super Soy!   Barbara Farr (Keats, $3.50)
This lowly bean is unveiled, and its nature revealed as a super source of protein (twice as much per weight as steak), vitamins A, B-complex, and when sprouted, vitamin C, and minerals (soybean curd is equivalent in calcium to cow's milk). The soybean supplies essential fatty acids while being low in cholesterol, provides dietary fiber, and one acre can produce almost thirty times as much soy-protein as beef-protein. The author explains *why,* then gives a whole book of *how.* Recipes from appetizer, through main course, to dessert.

Diet for a Small Planet   Frances Lappé (Ballantine, $1.95)
This seminal work explains what is meant by "protein complementarity." Ms. Lappé shows the ease and benefit of reducing one's dependency on meat as a source of protein, and demonstrates how incomplete protein from vegetables, grains, nuts and seeds may be augmented by serving these foods in combinations, to arrive at a complete-protein meal. The book contains recipes, arranged by complementarity. Each recipe lists the grams of protein in common foods, and relative costs.

The Vegetable Passion   Janet Barkas (Scribners, $8.95)
About vegetarians, this is a richly documented and readable history of individuals and groups who have raised philosophical objections to a diet that includes any slaughtered creatures. Their practice is based on conviction rather than tradition or economy. The author is especially intrigued with the variety of groups—from Pythagoreans to Seventh-day Adventists—and the dissimilarity of individuals—Leonardo da Vinci, Shelley, Hitler, Ghandi.

Minerals

The 12 Tissue Salts   Esther Chapman (Pyramid, $.95)
Tissue salts are inorganic minerals which already exist in the body, and which, in deficiency, can cause an abnormal or diseased condition, according to the famous findings of Dr. W.H. Schuessler in 1873. The author adds her own list of discoveries. She catalogues the properties of the tissue salts, the conditions which they help, and in what amounts, and appropriate nutritional advice. Mrs. Chapman contends that the curative power of tissue salts is miraculous, particularly in the treatment of radiation sickness.

The Trace Elements and Man   Henry Schroeder (Devin-Adair, $7.95)
This unfolds some of the mysteries of life, going back to the time when an organism first crawled out of the sea to roam the earth. Sea water had been supplying his system with a rich mixture of minerals and trace elements—now the less-rich sources of fresh water, plants and other creatures would have to meet the demand. This is scholarly and fascinating writing about our past, present, and future, and the bleak prospect of industry exposing man to deadly minerals. Indexed.

Minerals: Kill or Cure?   Ruth Adams and Frank Murray (Larchmont, $1.65)
We usually think of minerals and trace elements as something we do not get enough of. The authors point out that this is only partly true, as they teach about mineral pollutants that are being poured into our environment, and which they believe are seriously undermining our health. The book includes many different studies, on both sides of the mineral question, including the fluoridation controversy.

Biological Transmutations   Louis Kervran (Swan House, $2.75)
This is a detailed account of Kervran's research and discoveries on a controversial subject: the ability of a living organism to take one substance and transform it into another, quite different. For instance, the change of organic manganese to iron in the body. This somewhat mysterious-sounding ability has been appreciated and utilized by physicians and agronomists in France primarily, but interest in the process has been spreading throughout the world.

Herbals & Wild Food

Herbs, Health and Cookery   Claire Loewenfeld and Philippa Back (Universal, $1.95)
This is an extensive survey of the many uses of herbs, covering cookery to healing. There are descriptions of 24 herbs generally utilized in cooking, with recipes for each. In addition, much attention is paid to the requirements of special diets, and the methods of brewing herb teas. Many health properties that are attributed to herbs are listed, as well as methods for using them to maintain health and to effect cures.

Eat the Weeds   Ben Charles Harris (Keats, $1.50)
Descriptions of, and recipes for 150 wild edible plants frequently ignored or considered pests. Listed are synonyms for their names, where they can be found, the parts of the plant to be used, when to collect them and how to prepare them. Some uses are new, such as maple seedlings used in salad or steamed with other vegetables. Others are part of traditional country lore. Many plants grow uninvited outside the kitchen door, and offer great nutritional benefit— for the learning of it.

Back to Eden   Jethro Kloss (Woodbridge, $2.25)
Almost 800 pages of information about herbal medicine, natural remedies for illnesses, general health rules, vegetarian recipes and essays on such cures as compresses, baths, massage, and so on. Brought up on herbal lore, and accustomed to a natural way of living on their farm in Wisconsin, Jethro Kloss went on to become a renowned natural healer whose use of herbs, in particular, is hardly paralleled. Millions of copies of the book have been sold in the years since it was first published.

Ginseng and Other Medicinal Plants   A.R. Harding (Emporium, $4.00)
Complete information about ginseng, considered by the Chinese to be a panacea—its properties, cultivation, diseases, medicinal qualities, marketing, etc. The author (the book was originally written in 1908) grew ginseng and successfully treated the sick with it. He describes many other medicinal plants from swamp, forest, dry soil, moist soil, thickets and so on, always giving other common names, habitats, descriptions of plant and root and information on harvesting and use. Each plant is illustrated.

Common Herbs for Natural Health   Juliette de Bairacli Levy (Schocken, $2.45)
This is a herbal arranged in traditional style, with plants listed alphabetically by common name. Each is followed by its Latin name, where it is found, its usage and dosage, and some tantalizing folklore. One index deals with the confusing issue of the quicksilvery names of herbs, and another with herbal cures of disorders and ailments. Actually a handbook, going into detail on related subjects such as cosmetic recipes, companion planting and planting by the moon, and herb preservation.

The Complete Herbal for the Dog   Juliette de Bairacli Levy (Arco, $9.75)
The natural rearing of dogs, according to the author, includes a diet of raw meat, whole grains, dandelions or other herbs, homemade whole wheat bread and one day of fasting a week, also fasting when ailing. Cooked meat, canned dog food with preservatives and made into mush, cut off half the possible life of a dog and half his vitality while he *is* alive. She lists most canine ailments and herbal remedies.

Stalking the Healthful Herbs   Euell Gibbons (McKay, $3.95)
Once Euell Gibbons made a meal from wild foods collected in New York's Central Park, proving that they can be foraged almost anywhere. In this book he examines the nutritional and medicinal attributes of wild plants. From horseradish and stinging nettle to basswood trees and skunk cabbage, he tells us what plants have to offer. Also, fascinating lore, and information on the conservation of our wild heritage.

Foods and Juices

Live Food Juices   H.E. Kirschner (Kirschner Pub. $3.00)
Oriented toward healing, the author discusses the values of individual juices and how they are useful in ameliorating various health conditions. He tells about new and almost miraculous cures, and cites many case histories. A table of nutritional values of juices stresses their everyday dietary value. Also included is a brief chapter on low-protein dieting.

Soybeans for Health and a Longer Life   Philip Chen, Ph.D., with Helen Chung, M.S. (Keats, $1.50)
Dr. Chen has been a prominent force in making the soybean one of the top products in the United States today. His book aims to prove that a more liberal dietary use of this almost nutritionally perfect food is an economical way to promote health and longevity. To help the soybean expand from its present limited use in industry and in animal feed, he analyzes its nutritive value, describes its different uses as a food product, and its culture and preservation—in addition to presenting about 150 recipes.

The Beansprout Book   Gay Courter (Simon & Schuster, $2.95)
This is a small goldmine of information of the what, how and why of sprouting, containing virtually everything a novice sprouter needs to know. It goes from a discussion of the nutritional, economical and ecological benefits of sprouting, to a collection of sprout recipes. A dictionary of various sprouting materials and a list of suppliers complete the information.

Add a Few Sprouts   Martha Oliver (Keats, $1.50)
Sprouts can provide the protein content of meat, without waste of energy or resources, and are exceptionally high in vitamins C and B. Unlike most other foods, sprouts suffer practically no nutritional loss from marketing, storing, preparing or cooking. Mrs. Oliver describes the many medical functions that the nutrients in sprouts can aid, the biochemistry of sprouting and methods of sprouting, with illustrations of various types of sprouters. The recipe section covers main dishes, soups and salads, breads and stuffings. An extensive annotated bibliography.

Yogurt, Kefir and Other Milk Cultures   Beatrice Trum Hunter (Keats, $1.50)
A convenient manual for identifying, making and using most cultured milk products, particularly yogurt, kefir, cheese and whey. These dairy foods establish healthy bacteria in the colon and intes-

tine which fight off infection; they are powerful bactericides (eight ounces of yogurt have the effect of fourteen units of penicillin); and they restore the digestive system to normal after antibiotics have been used. Mrs. Hunter explains how to make the cultures and includes recipes for their use.

Raw Vegetable Juices   N.W. Walker (Pyramid, $1.25)
First published in 1939 the principles herein advocated have more than stood the test of time, and this is still one of the standard popular works on the subject. A foundation is laid with solid information on the value of juices, their content and effect, and builds with discussions on specific juices. The author also considers the use of juices in healing many ailments, from acidosis to varicose veins, and provides 87 different juice-mixture formulas.

Specific Vitamins

The Healing Factor: "Vitamin C" against Disease   Irwin Stone (Grosset & Dunlap, $1.95)
It is proven in thorough documentation of experiments and case histories that man, unlike other animals, cannot manufacture his own ascorbic acid; and that ascorbic acid, or vitamin C, is vital to good health. Without planned supplementation we receive only one to two percent of the amount we need. Study has been done on the relation of vitamin C to specific illnesses including poliomyelitis and cancer, as well as to aging, cigarette smoking and environmental pollution.

Vitamin C and the Common Cold   Linus Pauling, Ph.D. (Bantam, $1.95)
Linus Pauling is responsible for publicly introducing vitamin C into average household conversation. His book starts with the "discovery of vitamins" and the biochemical properties of ascorbic acid, and then considers vitamin C and its relation to our everyday health. Also included are: chapters on buying vitamin C; further studies in ascorbic acid and its relation to the common cold; the government and vitamin C; and a reference section.

The Heart and Vitamin E   Evan Shute, M.D.   (Keats, $4.95)

A classic work on vitamin E, which was first published in 1956, has gone through several editions since. The "Outline of the Clinical History of Vitamin E" at the back of the latest edition furnishes a fascinating overview of the systematic and determined approach of Evan Shute and others to discovering all that vitamin E means to health. Experiment after experiment was undertaken—until the broad picture of the uses of vitamin E emerged. The book explains their findings; comprehensive and comprehensible.

The Doctor Who Looked at Hands   John Ellis, M.D. (Arco, $1.65)
Dr. Ellis discovered the uses of vitamin B-6 after a tedious search of many years. This is an autobiographical account of the initial phases of his work with the vitamin, often called "the musician's vitamin" because of its effect on the functioning of hands. Among its many virtues, he found that B-6 relieves edema in pregnancy, and forestalls eclampsia. He believes that quantitative accuracy is the secret of good nutrition, and that we constantly have to force useless calories out of the diet.

Body, Mind and the B Vitamins   Ruth Adams & Frank Murray (Larchmont, $1.95)
Exploration of the B vitamins has not yet reached its peak. The last few years have seen ever widening fields of use, especially in the treatment of mental disorders. This book has sold hundreds of thousands of copies, and the 1976 edition is expanded, in an attempt to keep up with research. Each of the B components is discussed at length and in such a way as to give laymen a firm understanding and background knowledge. A most useful reference, and enjoyable education.

Vitamin E: Your Key to a Healthy Heart   Herbert Bailey (Arco, $1.65)
Bailey, a veteran medical writer, makes a well researched case for the use of vitamin E in the prevention and treatment of heart ailments. The author clearly documents and offers insight into the work of the pioneers in vitamin E therapy. Bailey also points out the methods by which the medical establishment has kept vitamin E a controversial commodity.

Dr. Wilfrid E. Shute's Complete Updated Vitamin E Book   Wilfrid E. Shute, M.D. (Keats, $8.95)
Research and information have increased, and clarified confusing issues. Some interesting new topics include vitamin E and: hypertension, diabetes mellitus, dermatology, and the controversy over cholesterol. There is a discussion on the commercialization of vitamin E, its "fad" aspects and government control. Dr. Shute also talks about vitamin E as a *vitamin,* not just a cure.

Quality Survival

Farming for Self-Sufficiency   John and Sally Seymour (Schocken, $4.95)
An encouragingly clear book, the Table of Contents lists, chapter by chapter: Land, Horse, Cow, Pig, Grass, Fruit and Nuts, and so on. The straightforward approach is carried through into the text, offering the beginning back-to-the-lander a handle on a confusing topic. For the more experienced, this serves as a useful outline, but will require some fleshing-in with additional research. The authors provide a complete bibliography.

Recipe for Survival   Doris Grant (Keats, $3.95)
An English nutritional expert presents facts about the destruction of food values in modern processing which has led to specific diseases such as cancer, diabetes and the mental illnesses which have increased the crime rate and suicide. Doris Grant's "recipe" includes every aspect of nutrition, from meal planning to shopping to storage and preparation. In the section on food recipes is her famous "Grant Loaf." References come from scientific sources.

A Sand County Almanac   Aldo Leopold (Ballantine, $1.95)
Aldo Leopold, of the Conservation Hall of Fame, questions the quality of the American standard of living and answers that "the opportunity to see geese is more important than television," and that "diminishing returns," not just diminishing beauty, is the result of man's conflict with the natural universe. The book presents an alternative vision, relates that vision to the current issues of conservation, and finally argues their priority on the basis of rational philosophical principles.

Go Ahead and Live!   Mildred Loomis (Keats, $.95)
A blueprint for independent living, written by experts and centered on an undisclosed couple whose main concern is to find and practice good answers to the question: *How* should people live so as to be involved in growth and peace instead of destruction? They are given specific advice toward this end by doctor, lawyer, sociologist, psychologist, economist, architect and so on, and carry it out to demonstrate the workability of positive living. Helpful books are listed for additional reading in various areas.

The Wheel of Health   G.T. Wrench, M.D. (Schocken, $1.75)
Convinced that the way to cure disease is to study health, Dr. Wrench found that the healthiest people in the world are the Hunzas in the northwest corner of India. Long-lived, energetic and free of disease, their way of life demonstrates the connection between healthy soil, healthy food and healthy people. In Hunzaland, all waste is returned to the soil, mineral silt washes down on the crops from the mountains; the crops are as free from blight and disease as the people. Simple, active and nutritionally pure lives insure the health of generations ahead.

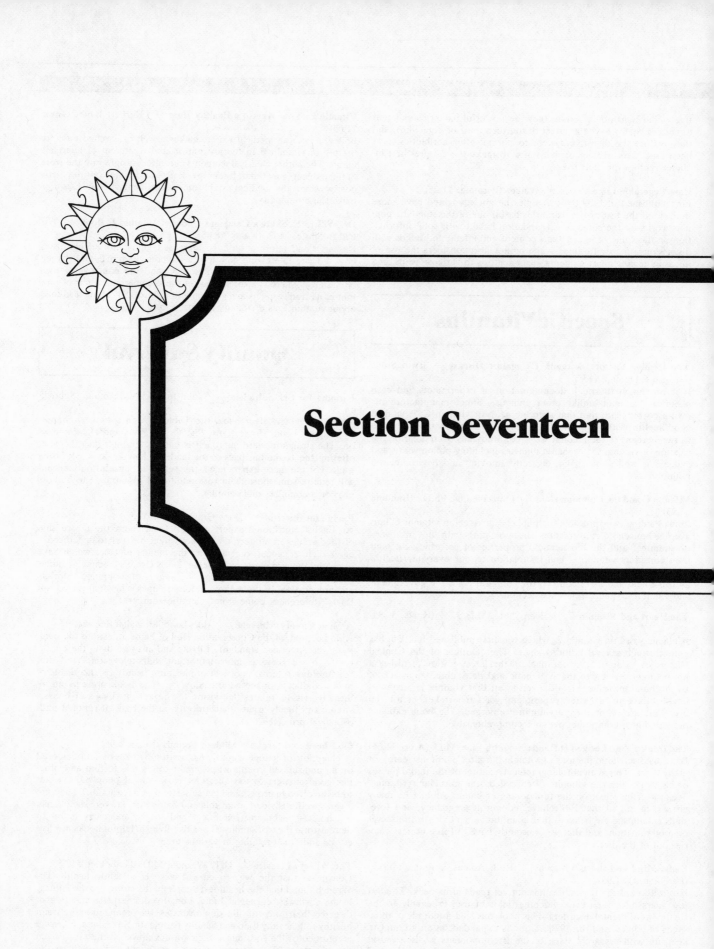

Section Seventeen

Health Sources
of Interest,
With Help If You Need It

a. Publishers of health books
b. Magazines and publications in the field
c. Associations, periodicals and meetings

Publishers' Addresses

Arco Publishing Co., Inc., 219 Park Ave. So., New York, NY 10003

Avon Books, 959 Eighth Ave., New York, NY 10019

Ballantine Books, Inc., 201 E. 50th St., New York, NY 10022

Bantam Books, Inc., 666 Fifth Ave., New York, NY 10019

Berkley Publishing Corp., 200 Madison Ave., New York, NY 10016

Devin-Adair Co., Inc., Sound Beach Ave., Old Greenwich, CT 06870

Dial Press, 1 Dag Hammarskjold Plaza, New York, NY 10017

Doubleday & Co., Inc., 245 Park Ave., New York, NY 10017

Emporium Publications, Inc., 28 Sackville St., Charlestown, MA 02129

Exposition Press, Inc., 900 So. Oyster Bay Rd., Hicksville, NY 11801

Faber & Faber Ltd., 3 Queen Sq., London, England (WC1N 3AU)

Farrar, Straus & Giroux, Inc., 19 Union Sq. W., New York, NY 10003

Fawcett World Library, 1515 Broadway, New York, NY 10036

W.H. Freeman and Company, 660 Market St., San Francisco, CA 94104

Greywood Publishing Ltd., 101 Duncan Mill Rd., Don Mills, Ont., Canada (M3B 1Z3)

Grosset & Dunlap, Inc., 51 Madison Ave., New York, NY 10010

Grossman Publishers, 625 Madison Ave., New York, NY 10022

Harper & Row, Publishers, 10 E. 53rd St., New York, NY 10022

Houghton Mifflin Co., 1 Beacon St., Boston, MA 02107

Keats Publishing, Inc., PO Box 876, New Canaan, CT 06840

Larchmont Books, 25 W. 45th St., New York, NY 10036

Macmillan Inc., 866 Third Ave., New York, NY 10022

McGraw-Hill, Inc., 1221 Ave. of the Americas, New York, NY 10020

David McKay Co., Inc., 750 Third Ave., New York, NY 10017

Manor Books, Inc., 432 Park Ave. So., New York, NY 10016

New Age Press, 4636 Vineta Ave., La Canada, CA 91011

New American Library, Inc., 1301 Ave. of the Americas, New York, NY 10019

Penguin Books, 74 Fifth Ave., New York, NY 10011

Pocket Books, 630 Fifth Ave., New York, NY 10020

Prentice-Hall, Inc., Englewood Cliffs, NJ 07632

Price-Pottenger Foundation, 2901 Wilshire Blvd., Suite 345, Santa Monica, CA 90403

Pyramid/Harcourt Brace Jovanovich, Inc., 757 Third Ave., New York, NY 10017

Quadrangle/The New York Times Book Co., 10 E. 53rd St., New York, NY 10022

Random House, Inc., 201 E. 50th St., New York, NY 10022

Rodale Press, 33 E. Minor St., Emmaus, PA 18049

Schocken Books, Inc., 200 Madison Ave., New York, NY 10016

Charles Scribner's Sons, 597 Fifth Ave., New York, NY 10017

Shambhala Publications, Inc., 2045 Francisco St., Berkeley, CA 94709

Shute Foundation For Medical Research, 10 Grand Ave., London, Ont., Canada (N6C 1K9)

Simon & Schuster, Inc., 630 Fifth Ave., New York, NY 10020

Swan House Publishing Co., 1852 E. 7th St., Brooklyn NY 11223

Universal Publishing & Distributing Corp., 235 E. 45th St., New York, NY 10017

University of Oklahoma Press, 1005 Asp Ave., Norman, OK 73069

Vintage/Random House, 201 E. 50th St., New York, NY 10022

Warner Books, Inc., 75 Rockefeller Plaza, New York, NY 10019

Woodbridge Press, PO Box 6189, Santa Barbara, CA 93111

Peter H. Wyden, Inc., 750 Third Ave., New York, NY 10017

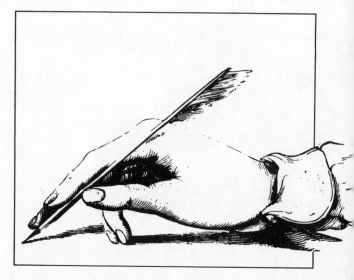

Magazines and Publications in the Field

Acres U.S.A., PO Box 9547, Raytown, MO 64133

Alive and Well, Box 8092, Waco, TX 76710

Alternatives: (Perspectives on Society and Environment), Trent University, 705, Peterburgh, Ontario, Canada

Annals of Allergy, 2117 River Road, N, Minneapolis, MN 55411

Bestways, 466 Foothill Blvd., La Canada, CA 91011

Better Nutrition, 25 W. 45th St., New York, NY 10036

Better Times, 225 Park Ave. S, New York, NY 10003

Carlton Fredericks Newsletter of Nutrition, Box 100, New York, NY 10956

East West Journal, 29-41 Farnsworth St., Boston, MA 02210

Energy and Character: journal of bio-energetic research, Abbotsbury, Weymouth, Dorset, England

Executive Health, Pickfair Bldg., Rancho Santa Fe, CA 92067

Frontiers, 19th St. & Parkway, Philadelphia, PA 19103

Good Earth, Box 2605 W, Melbourne, 300 Victoria, Australia

Health Magazine, 76 Avenue Rd., Toronto, Ontario, Canada M5R 241

The Health Quarterly, 36 Grove St. (Box 876), New Canaan, CT 06840

The Healthline Newsletter, PO Box 548, Belmar, NJ 07719

Herb Grower Magazine, Falls Village, CT 06031

Human Ecology Forum, Cornell University, Ithaca, NY 14850

Journal of Agriculture and Food Chemistry, American Chemical Society, 1155 16th St. NW, Washington, DC 20036

Journal of American Institute of Homeopathy, 1541 State St., Schenectady, NY 12304

Journal of Community Health, Human Science Press Periodicals, 72 Fifth Ave., New York, NY 10011

Journal of Physical Education and Research, 1201 16th St. NW, Washington, DC 20036

Let's Live, 444 N. Larchmont Blvd. (Oxford Industries), Los Angeles, CA 90004

Life and Health, 6856 Eastern Ave., Washington, DC 20012

The Maine Organic Farmer and Gardener, PO Box 373, Kennebunk, ME 04046

Medical World News, 1221 Ave. of the Americas, New York, NY 10020

Mother Earth News, PO Box 70, Hendersonville, NC 28739

Natural Living, 1560 Broadway (EVR Productions), New York, NY 10036

Naturopath and the Natural World, 1920 Kilpatrick, Portland, OR 97217

New England Journal of Medicine, 10 Shattuck St., Boston, MA 02115

Newspaper of Consumer Action Now, Inc., 78 E. 56th St., New York, NY 10022

Nutrition Actions, Center for Science in the Public Interest, 1779 Church St. NW, Washington, DC 20036

Nutrition Reports International, PO Box 1608, Los Altos, CA 94022

Organic Directory, Rodale Press, Emmaus, PA 18049

Organic Gardening and Farming, Rodale Press, Emmaus, PA 18049

Prevention, Rodale Press, Emmaus, PA 18049

Radionic Quarterly: an approach to health and harmony, Field House, Peaslake, N. Guildford, Surrey, England GU5 9SS

Research Recovery and Energy Review, Box 1144, Darien, CT 06820

Seed: journal of organic living, 8A All Saints Rd., London, W.11 England

Strength and Health Magazine, Box 1707, York, PA 17405

Today's Nutrition, 25 W. 45th St., New York, NY 10036

Vegetarian Nutritional Guide, Box 5, Pacific Palisades, CA 90272

Vegetarian Times, Box a3104, Chicago, IL 60690

Vegetarian Voice, 501 Old Harding Highway, Malaga, NJ 08328

Well-Being: a healing magazine, Box 7455, San Diego, CA 92107

Yoga and Nutrition, Box 35340, Vancouver, British Columbia, Canada

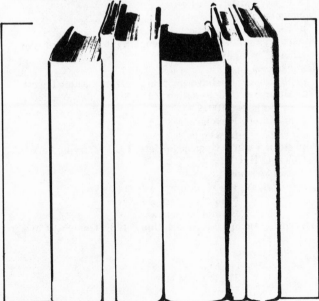

Associations, Periodicals and Meetings

Academy of Orthomolecular Psychiatry, 1691 Northern Blvd., Manhasset, NY 11030

Adrenal Metabolic Research Society of the Hypoglycemia Foundation 1 Park La., Box 98, Mount Vernon, NY 10552
annual symposium
publications: Homeostasis Quarterly

Air Pollution Control Association, 4400 Fifth Ave., Pittsburgh, PA 15213
annual meeting: June
publications: Journal of the APCA
Directory of Government Air Pollution Agencies
Directory and Resource Book
Proceedings Digest

American Association for Comprehensive Health Planning, 801 N. Fairfax St., Alexandria, VA 22314
annual meeting
publications: Health Planning in Transition
American Journal of Health Planning

American Board of Nutrition, Dept. of Medicine, University of California, Davis, CA 95616
annual meeting

American Board of Preventive Medicine, 615 N. Wolf St., Baltimore, MD 21205
semiannual meeting: December and June, Washington, DC

American Chiropractic Association, 2200 Grand Ave., Des Moines, IA 50312
annual meeting: June
publications: Healthways
Journal of Chiropractic

American College of Preventive Medicine, 801 Old Lancaster Rd., Bryn Mawr, PA 19010
annual meeting
publications: Newsletter

American Foundation for Homeopathy, 4701 Willard Ave., Chevy Chase, MD 20015
annual meeting
publications: The Layman Speaks, a Homeopathic Digest

American Health Foundation, 1370 Ave. of the Americas, New York, NY 10019
publications: Preventive Medicine
Newsletter

American Natural Hygiene Society, 1920 W. Irving Park Rd., Chicago, IL 60613
annual meeting
publications: The Healthways Advisor
Natural Hygiene Educator
Natural Hygienews

American Osteopathic Association, 212 E. Ohio St., Chicago, IL 60611
annual meeting
publications: Newsbriefs
The D.O. Monthly
Journal

American Physical Fitness Research Institute, Inc., Box 49024, Bel Air, CA 90049
publications: Bulletin

American Podiatry Association, 20 Chevy Chase Circle NW, Washington, DC 20015
annual meeting
publications: Journal of the American Podiatry Association
educational material

American Society of Chinese Medicine, PO Box 555, Garden City, NY 11530
publications: American Journal of Chinese Medicine

American Society for Preventive Dentistry, 435 N. Michigan Ave., Chicago, IL 60611
annual meeting
publications: Journal

American Vegan Society, PO Box H, Malaga, NJ 08328
annual meeting
publications: Ahimsa

American Vegetarian Union, PO Box 68, Duncannon, PA 17020
World Congress: July 1978
publications: American Better Health
American Vegetarian Hygienist

Association & Directory of Acupuncture, 2 Harrowby Court, Seymour Pl., London SW1V 4EU England
annual meeting
publications: Newsletter

Bio-Dynamic Farming and Gardening Association, 308 E. Adams St., Springfield, IL 62704

Brain Bio Center (biochemical research), 1225 State Rd., Princeton, NJ 08540

Brother's Brother Foundation (preventive medicine), 824 Grandview Ave., Pittsburgh, PA 15211
annual meeting: December
publications: Newsletter

Center for Light Research, 666 Elm St., Buffalo, NY 14263
publications: Newsletter

Center for the Study of Responsive Law (Ralph Nader), PO Box 19367, Washington, DC 20036
associated groups: Connecticut Citizens Action Group
Corporate Accountability Research Group
Health Research Group

Citizens for Clean Waters, 301 Lloyd Bldg., Seattle, WA 98101

Clayton Foundation Biochemical Institute (nutrition), Experimental Science Bldg., University of Texas, Austin, TX 78712

Community Systems Foundation (nutrition), 2200 Fuller Rd., Ann Arbor, MI 48105

Consumer Federation of America, 1012 14th St. NW, Suite 901, Washington, DC 20005
annual meeting
publications: News
Directory of State and Local Government and Non-Government Consumer Organizations
Annual Voting Record of U.S. Congress

Consumer Union of the United States, Inc., 256 Washington St., Mount Vernon, NY 60550
annual meeting
publications: Consumer Reports
Teaching Tools for Consumer Reports

Federation of Homemakers, 4338 N. Fairfax Dr., Alexandria, VA 22203
publications: Newsletter

Henry Doubleday Research Association, 20 Convent La., Bocking, Braintree, Essex, England
publications: Newsletter

Herb Society of America, Horticultural Hall, 300 Massachusetts Ave., Boston, MA 02115
annual meeting
publications: Newsletter
Herbarist

Hippocrates Health Institute, 25 Exeter St., Boston, MA 02116

Homeopathic Council for Research and Education, 66 E. 83rd St., New York, NY 10028
annual meeting

Homeopathic Foundation, 3 E 85th St., New York, NY 10028

Human Dimensions Institute, 4380 Main St., Buffalo, NY 14226
publications: Human Dimensions Publication

Hunza Health Research Society, 410 W. 45th St., New York, NY 10036
annual meeting: autumn, New York City

Huxley Institute for Biosocial Research, 144 First Ave., New York, NY 10021
affiliated division: American Schizophrenia Association
publications: Newsletter
Journal of Orthomolecular Psychiatry
(lending library)

Institute for Environmental Awareness, 113 Beacon St., Greenfield, MA 01301
annual meeting
publications: Environmental Awareness Newsletter

Institute of Nutritional Research, Box 3414, Los Angeles, CA 90028

International Academy of Preventive Medicine, 871 Frostwood Dr., Houston, TX 77024
semiannual conference
publications: Newsletter
Journal
Conference Proceedings

International College of Applied Nutrition, PO Box 386, La Habra, CA 90631
annual meeting
publications: Newsletter
Journal of Applied Nutrition

International Institute for Biological and Botanical Research, Box 912, Brooklyn, NY 11202

The International Naturopathic Association, 3519 Thom Blvd., Las Vegas, NV 89106

Life Extension Foundation, 11 E. 45th St., New York, NY 10017

National Association of Naturopathic Physicians, 609 Sherman Ave., Coeur d' Alene, ID

National Council on Wholistic Therapeutics & Medicine, G.P.O. Box H, Brooklyn, NY 11202
conferences and symposia

National Environmental Health Association, 1600 Pennsylvania Ave., Denver, CO 80203
annual meeting
publications: Journal of Environmental Health

National Institute of Medical Herbalists, 19 Cavendish Gardens, Bocking, Essex, England
annual meeting
publications: Health from Herbs
Herbal Practitioner

National Interagency Council on Smoking and Health, 419 Park Ave. S, New York, NY 10016
publications: Bulletin
Smoking and Health Newsletter

National Nutritional Foods Association, 7727 S. Painter Ave., Whittier, CA 90602
annual meeting
publications: Health Food Age
Health Foods Business
Health Foods Retailing
Newsletter

Natural Health Federation, Box 688, Monrovia, CA 91016

Natural Food Association, PO Box 210, Atlanta, TX 75551
annual convention and *regional meetings*
publications: Natural Food and Farming
Natural Food News

Nutrition Foundation, 489 Fifth Ave., New York, NY 10017
annual meeting
publications: Nutrition Reviews

Nutrition Today Society, 101 Ridgely Ave., Annapolis, MD 21404
publications: Nutrition Today

On Noise as a Public Health Hazard, 6570 AMRL (BBA), Wright-Patterson AFB, Dayton, OH 45433

Price-Pottenger Nutrition Foundation, 5622 Dartford Way, San Diego, CA 92120
publications: Newsletter

Society for the Protection of the Unborn through Nutrition, 17 N. Wabash St., Suite 603, Chicago, IL 60602
publications: SPUN Reports

Soil Association, Walnut Tree Manor, Haughley, Stowmarket, Suffolk, England
annual conference
publications: Mother Earth
Span

Soil Conservation Society of America, 7515 NE Ankeny Rd., Ankeny, IA 50021
annual meeting
publications: Journal of Soil and Water Conservation

Vegetarian Society of New York, 277 Broadway, New York, NY 10007
monthly meetings
publications: Vegetarian Courier

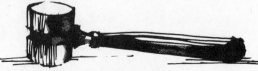

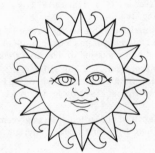 # Acknowledgments

Acknowledgments

Credits are arranged in the same order in which the articles appear in the Table of Contents

"A Handy Guide to the Familiar Supplements" by Barbara Farr from *Super Soy!*. Copyright © 1976 by Barbara Farr. Published by Keats Publishing, Inc.

"Before Vitamin Was a Household Word" by Melvin E. Page, D.D.S. and H. Leon Abrams, Jr., from *Your Body Is Your Best Doctor*. Copyright © 1972 by Melvin E. Page, D.D.S. Published by Keats Publishing, Inc.

"Vitamins: Should You Take Them and How Much?" by Linda Clark from *Be Slim and Healthy*. Copyright © 1972 by Linda Clark. Published by Keats Publishing, Inc.

"Can Mineral Supplements Improve Your Health?" by Carlson Wade from *Healthful Living Today*, May-June 1973. Copyright © 1973 by Keats Publishing, Inc.

"The Almost Miraculous Qualities of Vitamin E" by Wilfrid E. Shute, M.D., from *The Complete Updated Vitamin E Book*. Copyright © 1975 by Wilfrid E. Shute, M.D. Published by Keats Publishing, Inc.

"Hypoascorbemia — A New Slant on Vitamin C" by Irwin Stone from the *Bulletin* of The National Health Federation.

"Powerful Twosome: Calcium and Magnesium" by John Hildebrand from *Healthful Living Today*, Summer 1974. Copyright © 1974 by Keats Publishing, Inc.

"Does Your Diet Include Enough Vitamin E?" by Beatrice Trum Hunter from *Healthful Living Today*, Summer 1974. Copyright © 1974 by Keats Publishing, Inc.

"Vitamin F, New Hope for Cholesterol Control" by Carlson Wade from *Nutritional Update*, June 1973. Copyright © 1973 by Keats Publishing, Inc.

"High-Power Foods for High-Powered Health" by Linda Clark from *Know Your Nutrition*. Copyright © 1973 by Linda Clark. Published by Keats Publishing, Inc.

"Grandma Ate Flowers!" by Lelord Kordel from *Natural Folk Remedies*. Copyright © 1974 by Lelord Kordel. Reprinted by permission of G.P. Putnam's Sons.

"Soybeans: Nature's Ally against Disease" by Philip S. Chen, Ph.D. with Helen D. Chung, M.S., from *Soybeans for Health and a Longer Life*. Copyright © 1973 by Philip S. Chen, Ph.D. Published by Keats Publishing, Inc.

"Piima, Remarkable Culture from Nomad's Land" by Gena Larson from *The Health Quarterly*, Third Issue. Copyright © 1976 by Keats Publishing, Inc.

"Garlic . . . Don't Put It Down!" by Lloyd J. Harris from *The Book of Garlic*. Copyright © 1974, 1975 by Lloyd J. Harris. Reprinted by permission of Holt, Rinehart and Winston, Publishers.

"Remarkable Miso" by William Shurtleff and Akiko Aoyagi from *The Book of Miso*. Copyright © 1975 by the authors. Published by Autumn Press, Inc. Reprinted with their permission and by arrangement with Westbrae, Natural Foods, Inc.

"Advice Is Easy to Give" by Roger J. Williams from *Nutrition in a Nutshell*. Copyright © 1962 by Roger J. Williams. Published by Doubleday & Company, Inc.

"What Makes People Sick?" by E. Cheraskin, M.D., D.M.D. and W.M. Ringsdorf Jr., D.M.D., from *New Hope for Incurable Disease*. Copyright © 1971 by E. Cheraskin, M.D., D.M.D., and W.M. Ringsdorf Jr., D.M.D., M.S. Published by Exposition Press.

"Toxemia, the One Disease Everyone Has" by J.H. Tilden, M.D., from *Toxemia Explained*. Copyright © 1976 by Keats Publishing, Inc.

"Nutrition and Your Baby's First Years" by Gena Larson from *Better Food for Better Babies*. Copyright © 1972 by Gena Larson. Published by Keats Publishing, Inc.

"Cholesterol and the Frequently Maligned Egg" by Carl C. Pfeiffer, Ph.D., M.D., from *Mental and Elemental Nutrients*. Copyright © 1975 by Carl C. Pfeiffer, Ph.D., M.D. Published by Keats Publishing, Inc.

"Optimum Foods for Optimum Health" by Henry G. Bieler, M.D., from *Dr. Bieler's Natural Way to Sexual Health*. Copyright © 1972 by Henry G. Bieler, M.D. Published by Charles Publishing Company, Inc.

"Grandma's Natural Remedies: Time-Tested and Still Trusted" by Kurt W. Donsbach, D.C., N.D., from *Preventive Organic Medicine*. Copyright © 1976 by Kurt W. Donsbach, D.C., N.D. Published by Keats Publishing, Inc.

"Meet My Wonder Foods" by Gaylord Hauser from *Gaylord Hauser's New Treasury of Secrets*. Copyright © 1951, 1952, 1955, 1961, 1974 by Gaylord Hauser. Reprinted with the permission of Farrar, Straus & Giroux, Inc.

"Iodine in Our Diet — Too Little or Too Much?" by Beatrice Trum Hunter from *The Health Quarterly*, Second Issue. Copyright © 1976 by Keats Publishing, Inc.

"The Real Reason Why You Are Overweight" by Linda Clark from *Be Slim & Healthy*. Copyright © 1972 by Linda Clark. Published by Keats Publishing, Inc.

"Supernutrition and Staying Young Longer" by Richard A. Passwater from *Supernutrition*. Copyright © 1975 by Richard A. Passwater. Reprinted by permission of The Dial Press.

"When You Fast . . ." by Allan Cott, M.D. with Jerome Agel and Eugene Boe from Chapter 4, "When You Fast" in *Fasting: The Ultimate Diet*. Copyright © 1975 by Jerome Agel. Published by Bantam Books, Inc.

"The Stepchild of Medicine: Hypoglycemia" by Paul Talbert from *The Health Quarterly*, First Issue. Copyright © 1975 by Keats Publishing, Inc.

"Danger: The Water You Drink" by Allen E. Banik, O.D., with Carlson Wade from *Your Water and Your Health*. Copyright © 1974 by Allen E. Banik, O.D. Published by Keats Publishing, Inc.

"Diet, Eyesight and Common Sense Care" by Nancy Morrison from *The Health Quarterly*, First Issue. Copyright © 1975 by Keats Publishing, Inc.

"New and Natural Hope for the Arthritic" by Max Warmbrand, N.D. from *Overcoming Arthritis & Other Rheumatic Diseases* by Max Warmbrand. Copyright © 1976 by Max Warmbrand, N.D. Reprinted by permission of The Devin-Adair Company, Old Greenwich, CT.

"Acupuncture, Science or Superstition?" by Charles Ewart from *The Healing Needles*. Copyright © 1973 by Charles Ewart. Published by Keats Publishing, Inc.

"The Healing Benefits of Acupressure" by F.M. Houston, D.C., from *The Healing Benefits of Acupressure*. Copyright © 1958, 1972, 1974 by F.M. Houston, D.C. Published by Keats Publishing, Inc.

"Shiatzu: An Introduction to the Japanese Version" by Yukiko Irwin with James Wagenvoord from *Shiatzu*. Copyright © 1976 by Yukiko Irwin. Reprinted by permission of J.B. Lippincott Company.

"A Polluter's Garden of Verses — And More Pollution" by Barbara Jurgensen and Murray Goodwin from *A Polluter's Garden of Verses*. Copyright © 1975 by Barbara Jurgensen and Murray Goodwin. Published by Keats Publishing, Inc.

"Oh, How You'll Love to Get Up in the Morning" by Nikki and David Goldbeck from *The Good Breakfast Book*. Copyright © 1976 by Nikki and David Goldbeck. Published by Quick Fox.

"The Magic of Sprouting" by Martha H. Oliver from *Add a Few*

Sprouts. Copyright © 1975 by Martha H. Oliver. Published by Keats Publishing, Inc.

"**Some Treats from Aunt Tilda**" by Karen Kelly and Joan Hopkins from *Tilda's Treat, A New Way to Eat.* Copyright © 1975 by Karen Kelly and Joan Hopkins. Published by Keats Publishing, Inc.

"**How to Sweet Talk That Sweet Tooth**" by Eunice Farmilant from *The Natural Foods Sweet-Tooth Cookbook.* Copyright © 1973 by Eunice Farmilant. Used by permission of Doubleday & Company, Inc.

"**Honey: Sweetheart of the Kitchen**" by Agnes Toms from *Meals & Menus for All Seasons.* Copyright © 1973 by Agnes Toms. Published by Keats Publishing, Inc.

"**Liquid Lunches for Better Health**" by Ed Flynn from *The Health Quarterly,* Second Issue. Copyright © 1976 by Keats Publishing, Inc.

"**Me Eat Weeds? You've Got to Be Kidding!**" by Ben Charles Harris from *Eat the Weeds.* Copyright © 1961, 1969, by Ben Charles Harris. Published by Keats Publishing, Inc.

"**Soybeans and Nutrition**" by Barbara Farr from *Super Soy!* Copyright © 1976 by Barbara Farr. Published by Keats Publishing, Inc.

"**Those Sugar Blues and How We Get Them**" by William Dufty from *Sugar Blues.* Copyright © 1975 by William Dufty. Reprinted with the permission of the publisher, Chilton Book Company, Radnor, PA.

"**If You Don't Want It, Don't Eat It**" by T.L. Cleave, M.R.C.P., from *The Saccharine Disease.* Copyright © 1974 by John Wright & Sons, Ltd. Published by Keats Publishing, Inc.

"**Hunza Food: Recipes for the Beautiful Life**" by Renée Taylor from *Yoga, the Art of Living.* Copyright © 1975 by Renée Taylor. Published by Keats Publishing, Inc.

"**Vegetarianism: From Ben Franklin to Dick Gregory**" by Janet Barkas from *The Vegetable Passion.* Copyright © 1975 by Janet Barkas. Reprinted by permission of Charles Scribner's Sons.

"**Macrobiotics: The Cerealean's Dictionary**" by Michel Abehsera from *Cooking for Life.* Copyright © 1970, 1972 by Michel Abehsera. Reprinted by permission from Swan House, PO Box 170, Brooklyn, NY. A completely revised edition will be coming out in June, 1977.

"**Some Low-Sodium Recipes**" by Gena Larson from *Better Foods for Better Babies.* Copyright © 1972 by Gena Larson. Published by Keats Publishing, Inc.

"**Why Organic Gardening?**" by John B. Harrison from *Good Food Naturally.* Copyright © 1972 by John B. Harrison. Published by Keats Publishing, Inc.

"**A Talk about Organic Gardening**" by John B. Harrison from *Healthful Living Today,* Summer 1974. Copyright © 1974 by Keats Publishing, Inc.

"**Starting an Organic Garden**" by Ken and Pat Kraft from *Good Food the Natural Way.* Copyright © 1974 by Ken and Pat Kraft. Published by Doubleday & Company, Inc.

"**The Pleasures of Container Gardening**" by Sharon Cadwallader, selection from *In Celebration of Small Things.* Copyright © 1974 by Sharon Cadwallader. Reprinted by permission of Houghton Mifflin Company, Inc.

"**How Does Your Garden Grow?**" by Ruth Stout from *I've Always Done It the Easy Way.* Copyright © 1975 by Ruth Stout. Published with permission of Exposition Press.

"**Companion Plants and Bio-Dynamic Gardening**" by Helen Philbrick and Richard Gregg from *Companion Plants* by Helen Philbrick and Richard Gregg. Copyright © 1966 by The Devin-Adair Company. Reprinted with permission from The Devin-Adair Company, Old Greenwich, CT.

"**Composting in Your Living Room**" by Walter Harter from *Organic Gardening for City Dwellers.* Copyright © 1973 by Warner Books, Inc.

Published by Warner Paperback Library.

"**Taking the Mystery Out of Mulching**" by Malcolm Margolin, selection from *The Earth Manual.* Copyright © 1976 by Malcolm Margolin. Reprinted by permission of Houghton Mifflin Company.

"**Pests Are Pests — Man Made Them So**" by John B. Harrison from *Good Food Naturally.* Copyright © 1972 by John B. Harrison. Published by Keats Publishing, Inc.

"**How to Resist the Resisters**" by Catharine Osgood Foster from *The Organic Gardener.* Copyright © 1972 by Catharine Osgood Foster. Reprinted by permission of Alfred A. Knopf, Inc.

"**What's an Herb to Do With?**" by Euell Gibbons from *Stalking the Healthful Herbs.* Copyright © 1966 by Euell Gibbons. Reprinted by permission of David McKay Company, Inc.

"**Herbs, Astrology and the Rhythm of Life**" by Leon Petulengro from *Herbs and Astrology.* Copyright © 1977 by Leon Petulengro. American edition published by Keats Publishing, Inc.

"**Harvesting, Drying and Storing Herbs**" by Claire Loewenfeld and Philippa Back from *The Complete Book of Herbs and Spices.* Copyright © 1974 by Claire Loewenfeld and Philippa Back. Reprinted with permission of G.P. Putnam's Sons.

"**The Medicinal Qualities of Ginseng**" by A.R. Harding from *Ginseng and Other Medicinal Plants.* Unabridged and unaltered 1972 edition published by Emporium Publications.

"**Herbs, Fines Herbs, Soup Bags and Herb Soups**" by Irene Botsford Hoffman selection from pp. 11-15 of *The Book of Herb Cookery.* Copyright © renewed 1968 by Irene Botsford Hoffman. Reprinted by permission of Houghton Mifflin Company, Inc.

"**How Herbs Can Make You Sleep Better**" by Dian Dincin Buchman from *The Complete Herbal Guide to Natural Health and Beauty.* Copyright © 1973 by Dian Dincin Buchman. Reprinted by permission of Doubleday & Company, Inc.

"**Everything above the Collarbone**" by Jeanne Rose from *Jeanne Rose's Herbal Body Book.* Copyright © 1976 by Jeanne Rose. Used by permission of Grosset & Dunlap.

"**Herbs for Pleasure and Profit**" by Philippa Back from *Choosing, Planting and Cultivating Herbs.* Copyright © 1977 by Philippa Back. American edition published by Keats Publishing, Inc.

"**Herbal Baths**" by Jeanne Rose from *Herbs & Things.* Copyright © 1972 by Jeanne Rose. Used by permission of Grosset & Dunlap. **Sections Eleven and Twelve** contain excerpts from articles that have appeared in *The Health Quarterly.*

Section Thirteen: Where not credited here, recipes come from articles that have appeared in various issues of *The Health Quarterly.*

"**Soups, Beautiful Soups**" are taken from the following books: *Better Food for Better Babies* by Gena Larson; *Recipe for Survival* by Doris Grant; *Three Worlds Cookbook* by Gayle and Robert Fletcher Allen; *Meals & Menus for All Seasons* by Agnes Toms; *Add a Few Sprouts* by Martha H. Oliver; *Super Soy!* by Barbara Farr.

"**Salads, Salads, Raw, Raw, Raw!**" by Gena Larson from *Better Food for Better Babies.* Copyright © 1972 by Gena Larson. Published by Keats Publishing, Inc.

"**Sandwiches to Love**" by Agnes Toms from *Meals & Menus for All Seasons.* Copyright © 1973 by Agnes Toms. Published by Keats Publishing, Inc.

"**What to Do With Yogurt and Kefir**" by Beatrice Trum Hunter from *Yogurt, Kefir & Other Milk Cultures.* Copyright © 1973 by Beatrice Trum Hunter. Published by Keats Publishing, Inc.

"**Yesterday's Cranks Are Today's Prophets**" by Doris Grant from *Nutritional Update,* Spring 1975. Copyright © 1975 by Keats Publishing, Inc.

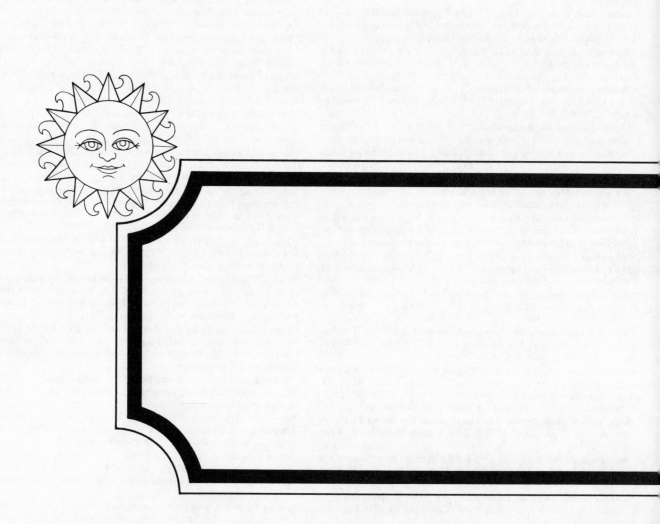

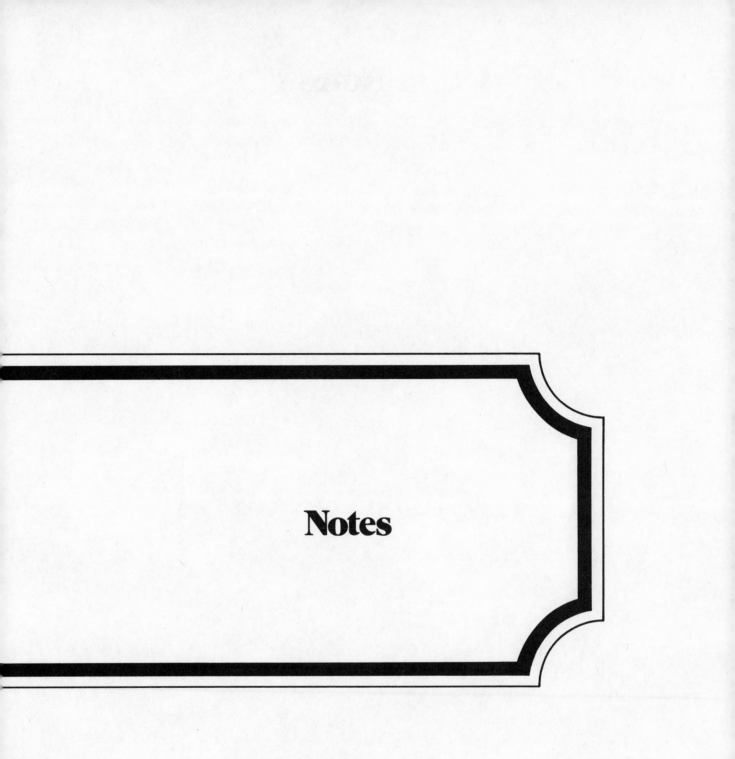

Notes

Notes

Notes

Notes

Notes

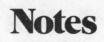

Notes

Notes

Notes

Notes

Notes

Notes

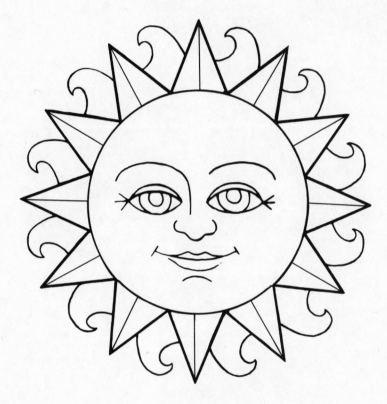